PHEOCHROMOCYTOMA

William Muir Manger
Ray W. Gifford, Jr.

PHEOCHROMOCYTOMA

with 132 figures and 28 color plates

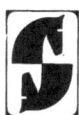

Springer Science+Business Media, LLC

William Muir Manger, M.D., Ph.D., F.A.C.P.,
  F.A.C.C.
Associate Professor of Clinical Medicine
Department of Medicine and Institute of
  Rehabilitation Medicine (Research
  Assignment)
New York University Medical Center, and
Assistant Attending Physician, Nephritis
  Hypertension Clinic
Columbia Presbyterian Medical Center
  New York, New York

Ray W. Gifford, Jr., M.D., F.A.C.P., F.A.C.C.
Head of the Department of Hypertension
  and Nephrology
Cleveland Clinic
Cleveland, Ohio
With technical assistance of Mr. Sydney
  Dufton, Mrs. Mildred Hulse, Mr. Craig J.
  Hart, Miss Irene von Estorff, and Mr.
  Thomas W. Rock

Designer: Howard Liederman

Library of Congress Cataloging in Publication Data
Manger, William Muir.
  Pheochromocytoma.
  Bibliography: p.
  Includes index.
  1. Pheochromocytoma.   I. Gifford, Ray W., Jr.,
joint author.   II. Title.
RC280.A3M36   616.1'32   77-8628

9 8 7 6 5 4 3 2 1

© 1977 by Springer Science+Business Media New York
  Originally published by Springer-Verlag New York Inc. in 1977
Softcover reprint of the hardcover 1st edition 1977

ISBN 978-1-4612-9902-8   ISBN 978-1-4612-9900-4 (eBook)
DOI 10.1007/978-1-4612-9900-4

This monograph is dedicated to four doctors whose lives have been so largely given to teaching, encouraging, and inspiring their fellow men. Their compassionate concern for others and their remarkable sensitivity to the needs of both students and associates bring to mind a quotation from Ecclesiasticus (38:2): "For Of The Most High Cometh Healing."

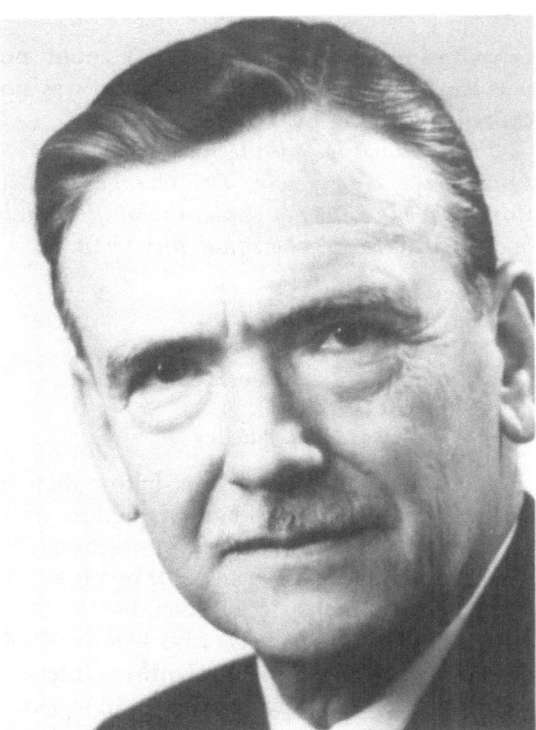

Ulf Svante von Euler
(Physiologist and Teacher)
1905—

Unquestionably, one of the most accomplished and illustrious scientists of our time is Professor Ulf Svante von Euler. His scientific genius has produced an incredible array of elegant pioneering investigations of extreme importance to the concepts of sympathetic nerve function. (It is particularly fitting that Professor von Euler be included in the dedication of this monograph, since he has also contributed significantly to the chemical detection and localization of pheochromocytoma and to an understanding of its biochemistry and pathophysiology.) Furthermore, he was the first to identify prostaglandin in human semen.

For his contributions in the field of catecholamines, including his discovery in 1946 that the neurotransmitter of the sympathetic nervous system was norepinephrine, he shared the Nobel Prize for Physiology in 1970.* Professor von Euler has also served with distinction as chairman of the Nobel Prize Committee for Medicine and as President of the Nobel Foundation. He has been honored by

---

* It is noteworthy that his father, Hans von Euler, had previously received a Nobel Prize in Chemistry in 1929.

outstanding awards and honorary degrees throughout the world.

The quality, precision, reliability, and rigid objectivity of his studies have established a mark of excellence revered by all those involved in catecholamine research. Equally impressive is the quality of his character. Despite his fame, he remains unimpressed by his achievements. His calm dignity, sincerity, deep sense of integrity, graciousness, warm hospitality, and deep concern for his fellow men impart a nobility of character rarely observed. His remarkable career and character have set an inspiring example to all those privileged to know him.

Albert Schweitzer has said that example is not the most important thing in influencing others; it is the *only* thing.

William Muir Manger

Dr. Irvine H. Page has enjoyed a warm friendship with Ulf von Euler *for many years. The esteem of one great scientist for another (expressed below by Dr. Page) is particularly appropriate and inspiring.*

From about 1920 to 1945, a cluster of highly gifted investigators fashioned a body of knowledge concerned with the neural transmitter of the sympathetic nervous system. It was my good fortune to have known almost all of them personally although their work often lay outside my field. There were Cannon, Dale, Holtz, and von Euler, to mention only the most important. It is von Euler to whom this book is dedicated.

I first met Dr. von Euler's father in Munich, Germany, in the late 1920s when I was working at the Kaiser Wilhelm Institute. A year or two later it was my good fortune to meet Ulf when we both were working at the University College in London.

Over the years I have learned that Dr. von Euler epitomizes two essential qualities of greatness: humility and the sharp cutting edge of thought. Always, his work has been thorough and creative—little wonder that the scientific and medical communities have recognized his greatness. In my long journey up and down the peaks and canyons of this highly emotive as well as intellectual world, I have known only a few the equal of Ulf von Euler. His work has spoken for itself and so clearly that it needs no advocacy from me. His humanity has withstood the test of time—no small achievement for anyone.

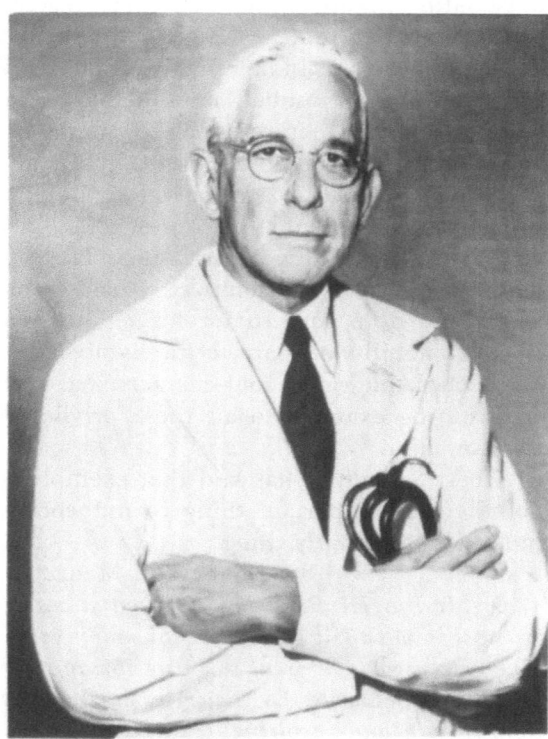

Robert Frederick Loeb
(Internist and Teacher)
1895–1973

Anyone fortunate enough to have come into intimate contact with Dr. Loeb recognized his extraordinary brilliance and inflexible integrity. Rarely in a lifetime does one meet a human being with such boundless talent. His magnetism, charm, and style were pure delight to his house staff and professional associates. His inspiration as a teacher created a matchless aura of excitement and dedication. In 1969 he was cited by Harvard University as "A man whose career epitomizes both the compassion and brilliance of medical science."

As a deeply grateful former student and house staff officer of Dr. Loeb, I would simply say:

> He gave us knowledge-
> He gave us wisdom-
> He gave us direction-
> He gave us flight.

William Muir Manger

(Dr. Loeb, despite illness, had kindly agreed to critically review this monograph before it reached the publisher. His comments would have been exceedingly helpful, to say the very least. Unfortunately, because of further incapacitation from his illness, he could not perform this service since he felt he was not capable of giving his best effort.)

The following tribute to Dr. Robert F. Loeb was expressed by Dr. George H. Mc-Cormack, Jr., a former student who ultimately became Dr. Loeb's personal physician.

> Robert F. Loeb
> 1895–1973
> ". . . whose transmitted effluence cannot
>   die so long as fire outlives the
>   parent spark"
>   *Adonais*, Shelley

Each of us differs from his fellow man in a multitude of ways and our common traits are few; fewer still, traits approaching the universal—and their ranks thin fast. As a people, we increasingly resemble William Irwin Thompson's insects, who live out their lives in weeks but pass on acquired information to succeeding generations in written records. The winter's generation writes of cold and laughs at the summer's concern with heat. The transmitted word thus becomes absurd and finally perishes, the fire of learning threatens never to exceed its parent spark, and we search for someone like Robert F. Loeb, who for nearly forty years created common bonds between students year after year at Columbia's College of Physicians and Surgeons and who now, 15 years after the end of his academic career at the university, remains for all those students and colleagues who knew him, an ideal and an unfailing inspiration.

One cannot do his memory justice. A listing of his achievements and honors comes no closer to describing his impact on those around him than measurement of rainfall tells the story of a storm.

He was Bard Professor of Medicine at Columbia University from 1947 to 1960 and then held the same title Emeritus until his death; but surely he counted titles as of smallest importance. He devoted his life not to the acquisition of honors, although they certainly came, but rather to the understanding of disease, to the relief of suffering, and to teaching others to carry on the work when he had gone; and he achieved each of these goals in a manner and to a degree better than did anyone else in his own time and for time yet unknown to come; and he did all this without losing personal contact with and a feeling of responsibility for every member of his department—Nobel laureates who worked with him and the people who cleaned glassware in his laboratories.

He inspired the fiercest of loyalties, and that, too, lives on, with a thousand memories of things that he did and thought more ably than anyone else. He carried out studies that led to a successful treatment of Addison's disease and a rational therapy for the ketoacidosis of diabetes mellitus, and in these and other similar areas unfailingly minimized the importance of his work—and would have been astonished to realize that he had cultivated followers who will not let those accomplishments be forgotten.

I was privileged to be his student, later the resident in his department, and, still later, his physician. In the last years of his life he asked me to take on that latter role and it is most memorable to me that he seemed surprised that I was willing. I know he never imagined, not for a moment, that I valued that role and service as none other, guarded it jealously, and thereby having the chance to spend time with him to the end, as few outside his family did, got more than I gave—as was usual with the Professor. The memory of that time remains as clear as yesterday and is, as everything about him was to me and his colleagues, unforgettable and rewarding, a different and more ideal level of experience, a measure of our later decline, for which there is only thanks.

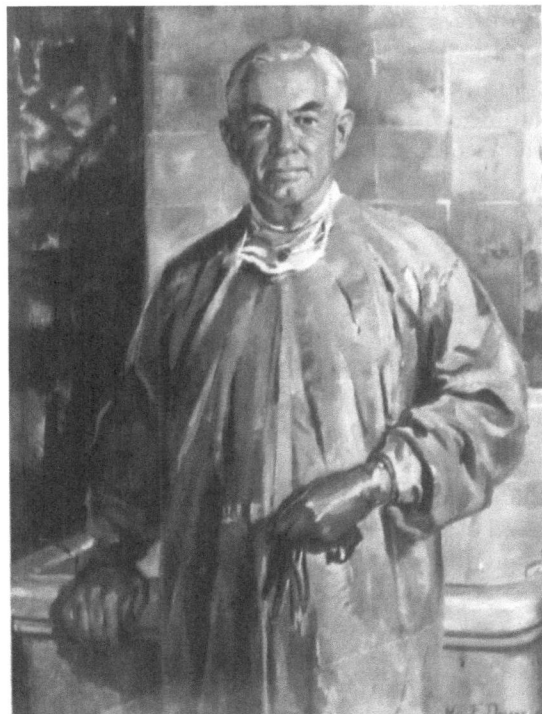

Charles William Mayo
(Surgeon and Teacher)
1898–1968

Dr. Charles W. Mayo was a highly competent surgeon who contributed importantly to the advancement of his profession. This was evidenced by his publications, service to country, and numerous accolades. He was loved by his patients because of his extraordinary kindness and because he so naturally practiced his creed: "To imagine the kind of doctor I'd like if I were sick, and then to be that kind of doctor."

"Though I speak with the tongues of men and of angels, and have not charity, I am become a sounding brass or a tinkling cymbal"
Saint Paul

For those who had the pleasure of knowing him personally, he will always be remembered for his warmth, his delightful sense of humor, and his disarming simplicity—reminiscent of Will Rogers. However, above all, he will be remembered for possessing that rarest of all qualities, a genuine and deep concern for the welfare of others. He was "A Man for All Seasons."

William Muir Manger

The above is a photograph of a painting that was given to me following an illness of Dr. Mayo in New York City in June 1959 when he and his wife, Alice, asked me to care for him. The original painting by William F. Draper hangs in the library of the Mayo

Clinic. (It is an interesting coincidence that this monograph is dedicated to Dr. Charles W. Mayo, since in 1927 his father, Dr. Charles Horace Mayo, was credited with first successfully removing a pheochromocytoma from a patient at the Mayo Clinic.)

Shortly after Dr. Mayo's death in 1968, the following remarks by one of his closest friends, Dr. Howard A. Rusk, appeared in Medical World News (August 30, 1968):

Along the road of life, you are sometimes fortunate to meet a person who enriches the lives of others with a special aura of warmth and friendliness. One of those rare individuals was Dr. Charles W. Mayo. His recent death leaves an emptiness in the hearts of his colleagues, friends, and patients all over the world.

It was my good fortune to room next to Chuck Mayo in medical school at the University of Pennsylvania. He was always great company. He had a permanent twinkle in his eyes and a touch of whimsical mischief that endeared him to young and old.

A young man carrying the mantle of a great name never has an easy time. And the Mayos of Minnesota have always stood for the great and good things in medicine—scientific pioneering, honesty, dedicated patient service mixed with compassion. His mother had been Rochester's first trained nurse and anesthetist. Chuck's father, Dr. Charles Horace Mayo, his uncle, Dr. Will Mayo, and his grandfather, Dr. William W. Mayo, founded the Mayo Clinic in 1889. Professionally and philosophically, they were all greats in medicine. And Chuck was born to accept this responsibility.

But he always had an eye for mischief. Once he dyed chicken eggs blue and put them in the nest of his father's imported pheasants, who had failed to lay any eggs. His understanding mother saved him from punishment by pointing out to his irate father the imaginative side of the prank.

I remember his description of a Christmas vacation during the years together in medical school. "This has been the worst holiday ever," he said. "I couldn't wait to get back to school. My father had an important doctor from Europe visiting us. On the first morning of vacation, when father was up early, he saw that the doctor had put his shoes outside the door to be polished.

"That morning my father did it. The rest of the vacation, I had to do it very early in order to get them back before our guest arose. When you get in from a dance at 2 a.m. and have to polish shoes at 6 a.m., it's no fun."

His father—"Dr. Charlie"—occasionally visited the medical school during our student years. When he did, he lived in the fraternity house, ate with us, and counseled us. Sitting at the feet of this great human being was a highlight of our medical education.

During his active days at the clinic Chuck developed into a distinguished abdominal surgeon and carried a tremendous clinical load. When World War II started, he headed a unit from the clinic. After spending months in a staging area in the South, he complained bitterly to the Surgeon General that this highly qualified professional team was being wasted.

Within days, the Mayo unit was on its way to the jungles of New Guinea, headed for facilities that were only in the planning stage. For the first few months in the Pacific, Chuck and the other chiefs of service ran tractors and bulldozers to help build the hospital in which they would eventually work.

In 1953, President Eisenhower appointed him alternate delegate to the Eighth General Assembly of the United Nations. It was a wise choice. His career at the UN hit its dramatic high point when he confronted the Communists with a report on the brain-washing methods they were using to extract "confessions" from American prisoners.

"The total picture presented," he said, "is one of human beings reduced to a status lower than that of animals: filthy, full of lice, festered wounds full of maggots: their sickness regulated to a point just short of death; unshaven, without haircuts or baths for as much as a year; men in rags, exposed to the elements, fed with carefully measured minimum quantities and lowest qualities of food and unsanitary water, served often in rusty cans; isolated, faced with squads of trained interrogators, bullied incessantly, deprived of sleep, and browbeaten into mental anguish."

"We must remember that all this was not done as mere senseless brutality; it was done for one single purpose: to make free men serve Communist ambitions."

Three years later, President Eisenhower

designated Chuck and his wife as personal representatives to the coronation of the King of Nepal. "You should have seen me riding that brocaded elephant," he said. "I was scared to death, but never had so much fun in my life."

As a member of the board of governors of the Mayo Clinic and the board of regents of the University of Minnesota, he made significant contributions to medical education and to the delivery of medical services. He also served on the advisory committees to the Veterans Administration and the American Legion. There he helped mold the policy that created the splendid medical services in the VA today. He was editor of *Post-graduate Medicine* and wrote hundreds of scientific papers that were published in the major journals.

During his long career, Chuck Mayo saved the lives of many people. He added joy, color, and fun to the lives of many more.

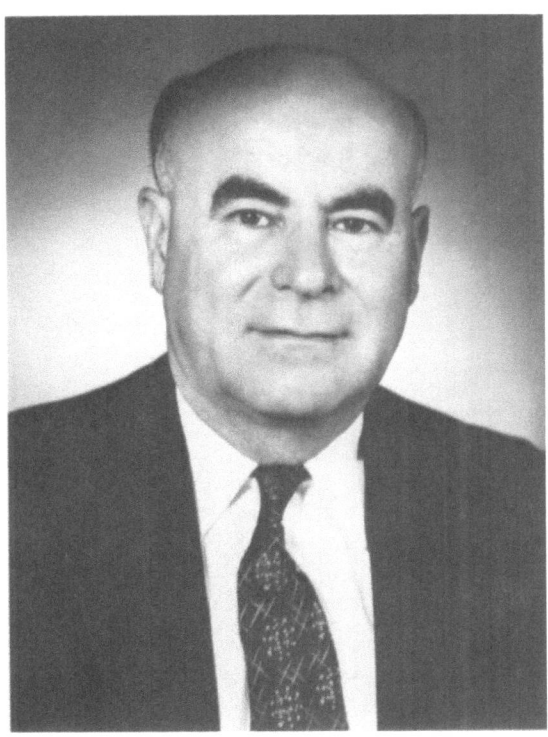

Khalil George Wakim
(Physiologist and Teacher)
1907–

My close friendship with Dr. Wakim makes it all but impossible to avoid using superlatives in dedicating this book to this very noble human being. Dr. Wakim is a remarkably able teacher and an investigator with unlimited energy and inspiring integrity. Yet, even more impressive is the fact that his greatest happiness comes from service to his fellowmen. The very purpose of his life has been largely concerned with the development and guidance of his students and research associates. While Dr. Wakim was a professor of Physiology at the University of Indiana, he placed a sign above his door which read "Never too busy to see a student." He cares little for his own advancement; his main satisfaction rests on the achievement and success of the young men he has trained. Those of us who were privileged to work with Dr. Wakim are eternally grateful for his influence and guidance. He continues to enrich the lives of all his associates not only by his counseling, patience, understanding, and warm affection, but also by adherence to a level of ethical and moral standards of the very highest order.

It is noteworthy that Dr. Wakim and his associates were among the first in the United States to study the effect of various physiologic procedures on the concentrations of plasma catecholamines as determined by fluorometric chemical assay.

William Muir Manger

Dr. Wakim is held in the very highest esteem by his colleagues at the Mayo Clinic. Their expression of admiration is indicated in the statement made by the staff of the Mayo Clinic when Dr. Wakim attained emeritus status after serving 25 years as a full Professor of Physiology. The citation reads:

"A Tribute of Esteem and Appreciation to Khalil George Wakim, Doctor of Medicine and Doctor of Philosophy—presented to him by the Staff of the Mayo Clinic in the course of its Annual Meeting, Rochester, Minnesota, November 11, 1971. His colleagues present this token of their esteem and of their gratitude for his undeviating allegiance to the pursuit of truth, whether in the carefully designed experiment of the laboratory or in the endless complexity of human affairs, for his delight in and his mastery of the art of teaching whereby he imparted to others the demands of excellence and the excitement of discovery, for his varied and revealing studies of renal and hepatic physiology, for his distinguished service to those distant lands where he was born for which they honored him with knighthood and medallion, and for his ardent support of that living body of high principles which were initiated by the Founders William James Mayo and Charles Horace Mayo and which now clearly are recognized as the ideals of the Mayo Clinic and the Mayo Foundation."

Perhaps the most fitting of all is a statement made by one of Dr. Wakim's teachers which was quoted by the noted physiologist, the late Dr. Frank C. Mann:

I have never known so exceptional a man. He is totally absorbed in his work. He is highly qualified by virtue of his dedication and his phenomenal intellectual ability. He is motivated by a compelling scientific curiosity and Christian compassion for his fellowman. As author and co-author of more than 300 published articles on his medical research, his influence is national and international; and he is on call for lectures, teaching, and daily consultation by telephone from all parts of the country. His wide acquaintance with the humble and the great is astounding, and his modesty and humility are simply devastating to anyone with pretensions. It is providential that a youth with such potential should come from the obscurity of a Lebanese village and by a fragile chain of circumstances make such an exceptional contribution to humanity.

Preface

This monograph, which was more than five years in preparation, represents a very detailed account of pheochromocytoma, a tumor that is almost invariably lethal if untreated. In addition to its definitive presentation of the subject, this volume contains the most current information regarding the diagnosis and management of pheochromocytoma. It is important to reemphasize the seriousness of diagnosing and treating pheochromocytoma with the aphorism of Esperson and Dahl-Iversen that although a pheochromocytoma may be morphologically benign it is physiologically malignant (280) and with Aranow's characterization of this tumor as a "veritable pharmacological bomb" (20). If managed appropriately by a highly skilled and professional "bomb squad," this tumor can be removed and the patient cured in at least 90 percent of cases. The secret lies in first suspecting and recognizing the patient who has pheochromocytoma and then offering the expert management such a patient requires. These facts more than justify this publication, since the internist, pediatrician, obstetrician, ophthalmologist, otolaryngologist, urologist, neurologist, surgeon, anesthesiologist, dermatologist, psychiatrist, radiologist, and also the dentist must be made acutely aware of the varied manifestations of this condition and of the pathologic entities which sometimes coexist with pheochromocytoma. Furthermore, they should have a thorough knowledge of the sophisticated methods of diagnosis and treatment of patients with pheochromocytoma in order to minimize the potential dangers. In addition, the pathologist, oncologist, geneticist, pharmacologist, physiologist, biochemist, and those involved in neuroscience will also benefit from some of the information contained in this book.

The extreme variety of the manifestations of pheochromocytoma has rightfully given this disease the title of "the great mimic" (215) and may leave the diagnostician in a state of utter bewilderment. Yet, if he is aware of the pathophysiologic alterations which this tumor may cause and if he understands the embryonic and genetic implications of this condition, he will make order out of confusion and arrive at the correct diagnosis.

> Not chaos-like, together crushed and
>   bruised,
> But, as the world harmoniously confused;
> Where order in variety we see,
> And where, though all things differ, all
>   agree.
>   Alexander Pope

Special attention has been given to the current status of diagnosis and treatment of these tumors. In addition to the traditional approach of presenting medical information, we have included a large number of instructive figures and have emphasized teaching tables. These tables should aid the physician and student in comprehending and retaining valuable information in diagnosing and treating patients with pheochromocytoma. It is our hope that this concept of communicating medical information will prove effective and time saving. The data presented in the tables are displayed clearly and concisely and represent the findings of many investigators, in addition to our experience with approximately 150 patients seen at the Mayo and Cleveland clinics, and at Columbia Presbyterian and other medical centers in the New York City area, where the pathologic diagnoses of pheochromocytoma were confirmed. The bibliography contains most of the information reported and supports the views expressed.

Because of the vast and almost endless ramifications of pheochromocytoma, and because of the extreme seriousness of this condition, which is curable in a high percentage of cases, we have found it necessary for this volume to be of considerable size and definitive scope. It is our hope that with the guidelines set forth in this book, plus a measure of God's grace, the physician will gain much expertise in detecting and managing the patient with pheochromocytoma.

William Muir Manger
Ray W. Gifford, Jr.

Acknowledgments

The superb technical assistance of Mr. Sydney Dufton in performing determinations of plasma and tumor catecholamines cannot be overstated. His diligence and rigidly accurate technique in fluorometric analysis have been outstanding.

I wish also to express my deep appreciation to my secretary, Miss Rose Hurwitz, for countless hours of remarkably skillful assistance in typing this monograph. My deep gratitude also goes to my research associates, Mrs. Mildred Hulse, Mr. Craig Hart, Miss Irene von Estorff, and Mr. Thomas W. Rock, for assistance in studying some of our patients and in preparing some of the figures and tables. Without the extraordinary aid of Mrs. Hulse and Mr. Hart in preparing, proofreading, and editing this manuscript, the task would have have been far less enjoyable and the publication considerably delayed. Their constructive criticisms and efficiency have been inestimable.

Special thanks are given to Dr. Meyer M. Melicow for extremely helpful consultation and for allowing us to reproduce pathologic data compiled by him from the records of patients with pheochromocytoma seen at Columbia Medical Center. Dr. Melicow has contributed greatly to the pathologic characterization of this tumor. Special thanks also goes to my close friend and colleague, Dr. Gabriel G. Nahas. His collaboration in studies on adrenergic mechanisms has been invaluable.

Grateful acknowledgment is expressed to all those physicians who have permitted us to include photographs, photomicrographs, tables, and charts of studies relating to pheochromocytoma.

In addition to others who helped, the following contributed significantly to this monograph:

For consultation and advice:

Dr. E. A. Banner, Dr. M. Bessis, Dr. H. Blaschko, Dr. R. J. Crout, Dr. R. Esser, Dr. M. Gertler, Dr. G. Grotte, Dr. D. A. Holub, Dr. R. F. Loeb, Dr. M. Madayag, Dr. N. E. Naftchi, Dr. M. Nickerson, Dr. E. F. Osserman, Dr. I. H. Page, Dr. D. Pertsemlides, Dr. J. T. Priestley, Dr. P. J. Puchner, Dr. S. G. Sheps, Dr. M. Tannenbaum, Dr. L. Triner, Dr. R. Weinshilboum, and Dr. C. E. Wolf.

For reading portions of the manuscript and making helpful comments we are especially grateful to:

Dr. J. Axelrod, Dr. M. Bosniak, Dr. H. B. Burchell, Dr. S. E. Gitlow, Dr. B. Hoffman, Dr. R. Hollenhorst, Dr. R. Lennon, Dr. F. L'Esperance, Dr. G. G. Nahas, Dr. S. W. Peart, Dr. R. Pruitt, Dr. M. Sandler, Dr. A. D. Smith, Dr. U. S. von Euler, Dr. K. G. Wakim, and Dr. H. Weil-Malherbe.

For providing the opportunity of studying their patients:

Dr. L. Baer, Dr. J. Baldwin (deceased), Dr. S. E. Gitlow, Dr. M. Grumbach, Dr. D. Holub, Dr. T. Killip, Dr. J. H. Laragh, Dr. J. Lowenstein, Dr. H. W. Neuberg, Dr. D. Pertsemlides, Dr. P. J. Puchner, Dr. S. S. Scheidt, and Dr., S. S. Yormak.

For assistance in editing and publication:

I particularly wish to deeply thank my former English teacher, Mr. Ferdinand E. Ruge (Head English Master at Saint Albans School in Washington, D. C.) for his extraordinary expertise, diligence, and kindness in editing the manuscript of this monograph. Had it not been for his patience and understanding, and for the training and guidance he gave me at Saint Albans School many years ago, it is very likely it would never have been written. Mr. Ruge died a few months before this book was published. In a memorial tribute Canon Charles Martin (Headmaster, Saint Albans School) read the following, which Mr. Ruge had composed: "His joy in life was teaching. His reward in life was to have his former students or their parents come up to him, remembering. And if he was impatient or dictatorial in life it was because he believed everyone had a certain divinity within himself to be and do the best he possibly could under any circumstances."

Working with the staff of Springer-Verlag and their free-lance consultant, Dr. Lester Hoffman, has been a thoroughly delightful association. Their direction and perception were invaluable and their able assistance was greatly appreciated.

For aid in statistical analysis:

The Department of Biostatistics, Mayo Clinic, Rochester, Minnesota (Dr. J. Berkson, Mrs. V. Golenzer, Dr. W. F. Taylor); The Statistics and Epidemiologic Unit of the New York University Cancer Center (Dr. N. Dubin); Miss I. von Estorff, and Mr. C. J. Hart.

For aid in preparation of figures and book cover, and for photographic assistance:

Miss Nina Barbaresi, Mr. V. Oberwiler, Mr. C. Poole, Mr. S. D. Simmons, Mr. W. E. Slue, Jr., Mr. S. A. Willard, and Mr. R. G. Wilson.

For assistance in catecholamine determinations:

Mrs. M. Hulse, Dr. C. C. Manger, III, Dr. J. Manger, Mr. T. W. Rock, and Dr. K. Steel.

For assistance with securing patients' records:

Mrs. M. T. Smith.

For assistance in assembling references, typing, proofreading, or translating foreign journals:

Mr. J. Birkner, Reverend Don A. Bundy, Mr. R. B. Elson, Mr. J. T. Epstein, Mr. C. J. Hart, Dr. G. G. Nahas, Miss E. E. Pasmik, Dr. H. Sell, Miss G. Soss, Mr. R. A. Weiss, Mr. R. J. Weiss, Mr. S. Wilson, and Mr. J. P. Campbell.

For financial support:

Support for the research and studies reported in this monograph came largely from the Mayo Clinic and Foundation, The William Muir Manger Research Foundation, and the Hypertension Fund of the Institute of Rehabilitation Medicine. Without the encouragement and interest of Dr. Howard A. Rusk and the laboratory facilities he made available to me at the Institute of Rehabilitation Medicine, many of the studies would not have been possible.

Finally, I wish to thank my wife, Lynn, and my children, William, Lala, Shep, and Charles, for their understanding and patience while I spent innumerable evenings and weekends preparing this book.

William Muir Manger

Foreword

It is wise to look back the better to understand the present and the future. To prevent intellectual chaos from the multiplicity of facts accumulated by scientists, general principles—universals if you will—ultimately must be drawn.

Oddly, the science of hypertension and even its clinical manifestations, including vascular disease, were largely neglected until the 1920s. Essential and malignant hypertension had been described but the terms were ill defined. In 1922 L'Abbé noted paroxysmal attacks due to pheochromocytoma and proved them to be caused by adrenal medullary tumors. Then an image of hypertension began to develop. Roux's demonstration that extirpation cured the attacks was convincing enough to stimulate gently the slow process of unravelling, and then refashioning, this enormously important problem.

But in one way those important observations got us off on a partially wrong tangent. Renal parenchymal disease and juxtaglomerular tumors produced an angiotensin-dependent hypertension; adrenal cortical tumors, a steroid-dependent hypertension; salt, a volume-dependent hypertension; coarctation, a hemodynamic-dependent hypertension. Therefore, it was often assumed that there must be a single cause for all hypertensions, but time and hard work have shown all of these to be secondary hypertensions and to be relatively uncommon.

Some 25 years after the initial work it became apparent that essential hypertension had many causes and usually there were several to be found in the same individual. While "essential" in this case is expected to mean "having no obvious exciting cause," it might have better meant, "Your guess is as good as mine." The deeply entrenched idea of a single cause for a single disease began to lose its sanctity. Now it is being accepted that essential hypertension belongs in a new category of disease, a "disease of regulation." Since the body has many ways to regulate tissue perfusion and consequently arterial pressure, multiple highly disparate mechanisms—humoral, neural, structural, and hemodynamic—have been identified and their malfunction often corrected with gratifying return of blood pressure to normal. That these varied mechanisms work in unison and are equilibrated has been graphically portrayed as a mosaic—hence, the "mosaic theory of hypertension."

If this is all so—and there is much evidence that it is—then a catecholamine-producing tumor fits well into the overall scheme of things. Such a tumor is one of many identifiable causes of hypertension, and research on it has provided an invaluable contribution to the great body of knowledge concerning these important diseases—reason enough for a good book on pheochromocytoma.

My friends William Manger and Ray Gifford have written just such a book. It happily combines basic science and clinical discussion as all good books should. I happen to know, or have known, all of the men to whom the book is felicitously dedicated. This is a heart-warming innovation begun several years ago by Dr. Manger in another of his books. Medicine and science reflect people.

Praise makes good men seem better and mediocre ones worse. On this basis, I feel free to offer my sincere congratulations to the two authors who wrote the book by themselves, a custom and feat rare these days. This is no ordinary book and I believe time will prove it. I predict that it will be read by your successors, but in the meantime don't wait to read it yourself.

Irvine H. Page, M. D.

Contents

PHEOCHROMOCYTOMA

Background and Importance

CHAPTER ONE

INTRODUCTION

Pheochromocytoma is perhaps the most fascinating of all tumors. Its clinical expressions, often dramatic and explosive, are so variable that it has rightly earned the title of the "Great Mimic" (215). The manifestations of this neoplastic endocrinopathy and its associated disorders are almost endless. It is equally perplexing that the pathologist is unable to differentiate histologically whether a pheochromocytoma is benign or malignant.

Uniquely, although 10 percent of these neoplasms are pathologically malignant (as evidenced by metastasis), lethal complications from the effects of excessive circulating catecholamines (epinephrine and norepinephrine) almost invariably result if the disease is not appropriately treated. This latter fact boldly underscores the importance for extreme vigilance by the physician in an attempt to recognize those harboring pheochromocytoma since potentially 90 percent of patients can be cured. The secret for the clinician lies in sharpening his index of suspicion. With the diagnostic modalities now available, there can be no excuse for missing the diagnosis. Despite the magnitude of the hypertensive problem currently faced throughout the world, and despite the relatively low incidence of pheochromocytoma, all patients who have manifestations which even remotely suggest pheochromocytoma must be properly screened for this disease.

MAGNITUDE OF THE HYPERTENSIVE PROBLEM

A study performed by the Health Examination Survey revealed that hypertension was the most common chronic disease in the United States (1961–1962). It was reported that 15.3 percent of persons 18 to 79 years of age had systolic blood pressures of 160 mmHg or more, diastolic pressures of 95 mmHg or more, or both. Ten percent of persons in this age range had diastolic hypertension. Today it is estimated that roughly 23 million adults (one in every six!) in the United States have hypertension. About 15 million of these have diastolic hypertension; the remainder have only systolic hypertension caused mainly by atherosclerosis or occasionally by an elevated cardiac output or an increased stroke volume. An insidious and ubiquitous disease, which is particularly virulent in the black population, hypertension may contribute to the death of 750,000 and the disability of another 750,000 Americans each year. Only about 80 percent of the hypertensive population of this nation know they have this disease and, tragically, probably 30 percent or less of these afflicted persons are receiving adequate treatment, which has proved so effective in reducing morbidity and mortality. In one sense it is extremely unfortunate that the vast majority of hypertensives are "symptomless," since irreversible cardiovascular damage and death may occur before the condition is recognized.

The magnitude of this health program is especially evident when one appreciates that approximately 95 percent of persons with diastolic hypertension are incurable (except very rarely by renal transplantation). It is estimated that 15 percent of all cases of incurable diastolic hypertension result from bilateral renal parenchymal disease, whereas 80 percent are due to primary (essential) hypertension (Table 1.1A). Only 5 percent of patients have other causes of diastolic hypertension which are sometimes curable (Table 1.1C).

INCIDENCE OF PHEOCHROMOCYTOMA

Although the precise incidence of pheochromocytoma is unknown, it is reasonable to assume that the incidence of pheochromocytoma may be at least as great as 0.1 percent in the population with diastolic hypertension. Minno and coworkers (668) found that in 15,984 consecutive (i.e., deaths from all causes) autopsies performed at the Mayo Clinic between 1928 and 1951, there were 15 subjects (i.e., about 0.09 percent) who had adrenal pheochromocytoma (extraadrenal chromaffin tumors were not included in their series). Similarly, Schlegel found 23 cases of pheochromocytoma in 25,274 autopsies performed between 1945 and 1958 at the Pathological Institute of the University of Zurich, Switzerland; this 0.09 percent incidence included both intra- and extraadrenal tumors (866). Berkheiser and Rappoport (61) reported a 0.25 percent incidence of these tumors in 2012 autopsies, whereas Blacklock and coworkers (79) discovered no pheochromocytomas in 2994 autopsies.

Adrenal pheochromocytomas were discovered eight times in 1700 patients with hypertension subjected to bilateral lumbodorsal sympathectomy, an incidence of 0.47 percent (392). A similar incidence (0.5 percent) had been reported in 1950 by Smithwick in 1200 of these patients (918). With additional experience an incidence of 0.4 percent was reported in 1964 by Greer, Robertson, and Smithwick (400). These were patients with severe sustained hypertension and would not be representative of the overall hypertensive population in this country. Furthermore, this incidence would not take into account approximately 50 percent of the patients with these tumors who have only paroxysmal hypertension; nor would it include any patients who may have had extraadrenal pheochromocytomas. On the other hand, this was not the experience at the Lahey Clinic, where, in approximately 1200 splanchnicectomies for hypertension, no pheochromocytomas were found during careful adrenal gland exploration (469).

In 1956 one of us (W.M.M.) with our associates at the Mayo Clinic reported discovering

Table 1.1 *Causes of Diastolic Hypertension*[a]

A. Primary (essential, idiopathic) hypertension, (80 to 90% of all patients)
B. Bilateral renal parenchymal disease, (5 to 15% of all patients)

Incurable

Chronic glomerulonephritis
Chronic pyelonephritis
Polycystic disease
Diabetic nephropathy
Systemic lupus erythematosus
Amyloidosis

Multiple myeloma
Scleroderma
Wegener's granulomatosis
Goodpasture's disease
Periarteritis nodosa
Balkan nephritis

Sometimes incurable

Acute glomerulonephritis
Hypercalcemic nephropathy
Renal cortical necrosis

Renal involvement in gout
Toxic nephropathy

C. Other causes

Incurable

Cerebral ischemia (vertebrobasilar)[b]
Hyperdynamic β-adrenergic circulatory state[b]
Autonomic (diencephalic) seizure
Pseudohermaphroditism (↑ androgenic steroids)
Turner's syndrome (with or without coarctation)

Myxedema
Tabetic crisis[b]
Dysautonomia[b]
Abdominal angina
Inappropriate vasoconstriction
Spinal cord lesion (noxious stimulus)[b]
Acute intermittent porphyria[b]

Sometimes curable

Unilateral renal parenchymal disease (including renal transplant rejection)
Occlusive renovascular disease
Thyrotoxicosis
Cushing's syndrome (hydrocortisone and corticosterone)
Primary aldosteronism (Conn's syndrome)
Acute coronary insufficiency[b]
Coarctation of aorta (above renal arteries)
Hypersensitivity reactions[b]
Encephalitis[b]
Acromegaly
Renal tumors or renin-secreting tumors (e.g., Wilms tumor; juxtaglomerular cell tumor; renal carcinoma)
Excess deoxycorticosterone (or ? another mineralocorticoid); [enzyme defect (e.g., adrenogenital syndrome with 11β- and/or 17α-hydroxylase deficiency)]
Ovarian tumors (sometimes ↑ steroids)
Hypercalcemia
Obesity
Excess ingestion of
    Licorice
    Carbenoxolone
    Sodium bicarbonate

Expansion of blood volume
Hypothalamic tumor[b] or dysregulation[b]
Poisoning with
    Thallium
    Carbon monoxide
Fibrosarcoma pulmonary artery[b]
Pork sensitivity[b]
Iatrogenic [birth control pills; corticosteroids; methylphenidate; deoxycorticosterone; vasopressor drugs (including *catecholamines*); monoamine oxidase inhibitors + tyramine or some *sympathomimetics*[b]]
Pheochromocytoma[b]
Increased intracranial pressure[b]
Hypoglycemia[b]
Intracranial lesions[b]
Neuroblastoma,[b] *ganglioneuroblastoma,*[b] *ganglioneuroma*
Lead poisoning[b]
Acrodynia
Carcinoid[b]
Clonidine withdrawal[b]
Tetanus[b]
Factitious[b]
Toxemia of pregnancy[b]
Guillain-Barré syndrome[b]

[a] Conditions in italics may have increased excretion of catecholamines and/or metabolites.
[b] May have paroxysmal hypertension.

51 patients with pheochromocytoma in 7993 patients screened (primarily with pharmacologic tests and occasionally with plasma catecholamine determinations) for hypertension (534). It is interesting that Helmer reported a parallel experience: in about 7000 hypertensive patients whose urine was screened using an aortic strip bioassay, he identified 47 cases of pheochromocytoma—an incidence of 0.67 percent (360). The incidence of 0.64 percent which we reported is admittedly greater than would be expected in the entire hypertensive population, since our patients were usually screened because there was some suspicion that a pheochromocytoma might be responsible for symptomatology and/or sustained or paroxysmal hypertension. Similarly, Gitlow and associates felt that the 0.7 percent incidence of pheochromocytoma which they detected in 1500 consecutive hypertensives was somewhat high, since many of the patients had been referred to their laboratory to confirm or exclude the diagnosis of pheochromocytoma (358). Such a preselection probably explains the 2.2 percent incidence of this tumor reported in hypertensive patients studied by Goodall and Stone (385). Hume found one patient with pheochromocytoma in 317 hypertensive patients (an incidence of 0.32 percent) screened for this tumor by quantitating urinary catecholamines (466).

It seems likely from the foregoing data that a rough estimate of the incidence of pheochromocytoma in the population in the United States with any degree of sustained diastolic hypertension might be somewhere between 0.1 and 0.2 percent. (This incidence would undoubtedly be greater if only patients with moderate and severe diastolic hypertension were included.) However, this would account for only about half the number of persons harboring pheochromocytoma in the United States, assuming 50 percent of patients with pheochromocytoma have only paroxysmal hypertension. In addition, some pheochromocytomas, found at autopsy, have been considered nonfunctioning, since they apparently caused no symptoms (668, 988). It would appear that pheochromocytoma may occur more frequently than thought by most physicians. Van Way and associates estimated that there are 75,000 patients with pheochromocytoma in the hypertensive population of the United States (990); our guess is that there may be 36,000 persons harboring this treacherous tumor (assuming an incidence of 0.1 percent in 18 million persons with sustained diastolic hypertension and assuming that 50 percent of patients with pheochromocytoma have paroxysmal hypertension). The relatively high incidence (0.09 percent) of pheochromocytomas found in the large series of consecutive autopsies cited above suggests that a significant number of these tumors may cause very minor manifestations and/or they may secrete little if any catecholamines into the circulation.

In 1964 deGraeff and Horak reported results of an extensive 10-year survey in the Netherlands which indicated that pheochromocytoma could be the cause of hypertension in roughly six per 1000 hypertensives (218). From a survey of the literature, McNeill and associates estimated that one new case harboring this tumor may occur each year in a population of one to two million (645).

The annual death rate from pheochromocytoma is difficult to assess since the precise incidence of the tumor is unknown. Furthermore, it is likely that a significant number of patients die from a pheochromocytoma which is never recognized. In 1944 MacKeith pointed out that in a series of 165 patients with pheochromocytoma, 78 percent were diagnosed at autopsy (598), and in 1951 Graham estimated that approximately 600 to 800 patients in the United States die annually of hypertension due to pheochromocytoma (392)! This estimate was based on a pheochromocytoma incidence of 0.47 percent in the hypertensive population and a death rate from hypertension in this country of 175,000 individuals per year. The DeCourcys, in 1952, and also Barbeau, in 1967, estimated that each year there are probably about 1000 deaths from pheochromocytoma in the United States (39, 215).

Schäfer reported in 1959 that in Germany approximately 100 patients die annually of pheochromocytoma (860). In 1972 Ross estimated that in England and Wales about 50 persons die unnecessarily each year from undetected pheochromocytomas (812).

The exact prevalence of pheochromocytoma remains uncertain. In addition to the reports of its incidence cited above, it is reasonable to assume that a significant number of persons may die annually from complications of pheochromocytoma without recognition of the tumor. Once again, it should be reiterated that *the extreme importance of this condition is that it is curable in about 90 percent of patients but will eventually be lethal in almost all cases if untreated.* As has been aptly said of pheochromocytomas: "Histologically, they are usually benign; physiologically they are malignant" (18, 48).

For those who may encounter patients with pheochromocytoma the following dictum is particularly appropriate: "Think of it, confirm it, find it, and remove it" (812).

HISTORICAL

A chronological review of the historical highlights which have so elegantly led to an understanding of the pathophysiology and biochemistry of pheochromocytoma is herewith presented.

In 1886 Frankel first described pheochromocytomas which were found at autopsy in both adrenal glands of an 18-year-old girl who had died suddenly in collapse. This girl gave a 1-year history of recurrent episodes of palpitations, headache, vomiting, and pallor, accompanied by a hard, noncompressible pulse and retinitis. Her kidneys revealed arterial changes characteristic of hypertensive vascular disease, and myocardial hypertrophy was also present (325). In 1893 Manasse (610) reported a patient with pheochromocytoma and in 1896 he demonstrated that a similar tumor from another patient could be stained a brownish color when exposed to chromium salts (611). Previously this histochemical "chromaffin" reaction [which is a reduction phenomenon (715) due probably to the presence of catecholamines] had been known to occur only in the adrenal medulla; however, in 1902 Kohn (519) found this reaction could be demonstrated in cells in other parts of the body. This latter finding suggested a common embryologic origin of these cells.

Marchetti in 1904 (629) first described bilateral adrenal pheochromocytomas which may possibly have been familial; however, the first case documented as familial pheochromo-

cytoma was reported by Hyman and Mencher in 1943 (470). In 1908 Alezais and Peyron introduced the term "paraganglioma" to designate extraadrenal chromaffin tumors arising in paraganglia (6). In 1910 Pick coined the term "pheochromocytoma" to indicate tumors whose cells had an affinity for chromium salts (751). In the same year Suzuki first reported the occurrence of pheochromocytoma and neurofibromatosis in the same patient (957). The frequent combination of these tumors, which has been validated by many reports, appears related to a common neuroectodermal origin of the tumor cells. Subsequently, Glushien in 1953 reported the association of pheochromocytoma and angiomatosis retinae (von Hippel's disease) (371), and it had been previously noted that approximately 20 percent of patients with von Hippel's disease developed hemangioblastoma of the cerebellum (Lindau's disease). DeCourcy and DeCourcy in 1952 (215) and Sipple in 1961 (897) pointed out the increased incidence of thyroid carcinoma associated with pheochromocytoma. In 1962 parathyroid adenomas were reported by Cushman (199) and by Manning and associates (627) to occur as a third tumor in some patients harboring both pheochromocytoma and thyroid carcinoma.

Only about 55 years ago, in 1922, L'Abbé and his colleagues first made the fascinating observation that paroxysmal crises of hypertension occurred in a 28-year-old woman who was found at autopsy to have a pheochromocytoma (536). Volhard in 1907 (996) and Helly in 1913 (432) had apparently described the clinical syndrome earlier. A few years later, in 1926, this syndrome was firmly established by Vaquez and Donzelot (991), and shortly thereafter a pheochromocytoma was removed successfully by Roux (826) in Switzerland, and by C. H. Mayo at the Mayo Clinic (636). Both of the patients harboring these tumors had paroxysmal episodes of hypertension, which ceased following removal. Pincoffs is credited with first recognizing a pheochromocytoma preoperatively in 1929 (755); subsequently that year Shipley operated on the patient and successfully removed the tumor, which was located in the adrenal gland and had become adherent to the vena cava (892). Rabin in 1929 found that a pheochromocytoma contained a pressor agent in excess of that occurring in the normal adrenal medulla and suggested that this might account for the clinical manifestations (777). A few years later, in 1936, crystalline epinephrine was isolated from a pheochromocytoma by Kendall (506). A pressor substance occurring in the plasma during a hypertensive crisis in a patient with pheochromocytoma was first demonstrated in 1937 by Beer et al. (53). They employed a bioassay technique to detect this substance, which they believed was epinephrine. Two years later Strombeck and Hedberg, using a chemical assay, reported a marked increase in the concentration of blood epinephrine in a patient with this tumor (944). In 1938 the occurrence of sustained hypertension was reported in one patient at the Mayo Clinic with an adrenal pheochromocytoma (72), and in another patient with a paraganglioma (731).

In 1945 Roth and Kvale discovered that histamine would precipitate an attack of marked hypertension and symptomatology in patients with pheochromocytoma (822). The use of the histamine test proved a valuable aid in detecting patients with pheochromocytoma (who had paroxysmal hypertension) when the blood pressure was normal or only slightly elevated. Other than the histamine test, only the glucagon test for pheochromocytoma, introduced in 1967 by Lawrence (555), has proved relatively reliable as a provocative test.

In 1947 Goldenberg, Snyder, and Aranow found that the intravenous administration of the adrenergic blocking agent benzodioxan would dramatically lower the blood pressure of patients with pheochromocytoma, whereas no decrease in blood pressure was observed when this drug was administered to patients with essential hypertension or to normotensive individuals (381). With the aid of this new pharmacologic test and radiologic studies, a preoperative diagnosis of pheochromocytoma was made and subsequently two separate tumors were removed in 1948 by Cahill from a 12-year-old girl who had persistent hypertension (341). This appears to have been the first surgical cure of multiple pheochromocytomas.

Although other pharmacologic tests have been used to detect the presence of pheo-

chromocytoma, the most reliable and commonly used drug which characteristically and dramatically lowers an elevated blood pressure due to the presence of increased circulating catecholamines is phentolamine (Regitine)—first used by Iseri and coworkers in 1951 (473).

Norepinephrine, although synthesized as long ago as 1904 (940), attracted remarkably little attention until 1946, when von Euler (287, 288), and Holtz and coworkers (458), independently reported its occurrence in the body. Von Euler discovered that norepinephrine is in fact the neurotransmitter of the sympathetic nervous system. In 1947 Holtz and coworkers (458) found that the adrenal medulla contained both epinephrine and norepinephrine, and Holton first demonstrated in 1949 the presence of norepinephrine in pheochromocytomas (456).

In 1950 and 1951, von Euler and coworkers showed that patients with pheochromocytoma excreted increased quantities of epinephrine and/or norepinephrine, and sometimes hydroxytyramine (dopamine, the precursor of norepinephrine), in the urine (263, 285, 295). Evidence for the presence of dopamine in normal urine had been obtained by Holtz and coworkers in 1942 (457). The diagnostic value of an increased urinary output of epinephrine and norepinephrine was emphasized. Shortly thereafter, Lund, in 1952, reported elevations of epinephrine and norepinephrine in the blood as well as in the urine of patients with pheochromocytoma (590).

Subsequently, in 1954, Goldenberg and coworkers reported the results of chemically screening the urine for epinephrine and norepinephrine in a series of 16 patients with pheochromocytoma (380). The same year, Manger and coworkers reported the results of fluorometric quantitation of plasma epinephrine and norepinephrine in a group of 13 patients with pheochromocytoma (616). These latter investigators also pointed out the diagnostic value of quantitating epinephrine and norepinephrine during a hypertensive episode provoked by the administration of histamine to some patients with pheochromocytoma and paroxysmal hypertension. Manger, Flock, and coworkers also first demonstrated the rare occurrence of dopamine in an extract of a pheochromocytoma (616). This latter finding has also been noted by others (586, 644, 1014). In 1956 Weil-Malherbe identified the presence not only of dopamine but also of dihydroxyphenylalanine (dopa) in a pheochromocytoma. More recently, dopa has been demonstrated in one malignant (16) and two benign pheochromocytomas (586).

Studies by Armstrong and coworkers in 1957 (23) and 1959 (22) demonstrated that 3-methoxy-4-hydroxymandelic acid (VMA) was present in increased concentrations in the urine of patients with pheochromocytoma and was a major metabolite of epinephrine and norepinephrine. In 1958 Axelrod and coworkers (33, 537) established that O-methylation was the principal pathway for the metabolism for these catecholamines in the blood and some tissues. Also in 1958, LaBrosse and coworkers reported increased urinary concentrations of both VMA and normetanephrine (O-methylated norepinephrine) in patients with pheochromocytoma (538). The other major pathway for catecholamine metabolism had been demonstrated by Blaschko and coworkers in 1937 to be oxidative deamination caused in a number of tissues by amine oxidase (83). With these discoveries, and with the development of methods for measuring catecholamines, their metabolites, and the enzymes involved in their metabolism, Sjoerdsma (905, 910), as well as Crout and Gitlow and their coworkers, significantly clarified aspects of metabolism, function, and chemical diagnosis of pheochromocytomas (191, 195, 360, 910).

Subsequently Smith and Winkler have contributed importantly to a better understanding of the mechanism whereby catecholamines are released from pheochromocytomas (916).

It is an impossible task to acknowledge adequately all those who have played a role in advances in the diagnosis and management of patients with pheochromocytoma and those who have contributed to a better understanding of the pathophysiology and biochemistry of this tumor; however, in addition to those already cited, the following doctors should be mentioned:

Clinicians: E.V. Allen, A. Barbeau, K. Engelman, A.D. Goodman, H. Hermann, C.E. Jackson, M.R.A. Khairi, R. Mornex, L.B. Page, W.S. Peart, S.G. Sheps, G.W. Sizemore, R.H. Stackpole, and A.N. Steiner.
Ophthalmologists: G.M. Bruce, R.W. Hollenhorst, D.M. Robertson, and F. Rodin.
Surgeons: J.B. Graham, D.H. Hume, J.T. Priestley, W.H. Remine, H.W. Scott, Jr., and R.H. Smithwick.
Anesthesiologists: V. Agpar, A. Faulconer, Jr., E.P.W. Helps, R. Katz, E.M. Papper, A.I. Robertson, N. Schnelle, and C. Wolf.
Pharmacologists and physiologists: A. Pekkarinen and L. Stjärne.

Those who have made significant contributions to the pathology of pheochromocytoma and some of its complications and associated conditions are J.A. Carney, R.E. Coupland, R.J. Gorlin, J.E. Leestma, M.M. Melicow, A.M. Minno, M. Tannenbaum, and P.D. Van Vliet.

William James has said that "the purpose of life is to spend it for something that outlives you." The contributions to an understanding of pheochromocytoma by those mentioned above have established an eternal foundation on which subsequent generations of investigators can securely and skillfully build.

Catecholamine Metabolism: Biosynthesis, Storage, Release, and Inactivation

CHAPTER TWO

GENERAL REMARKS

NOMENCLATURE, OCCURRENCE, AND METABOLISM

Basic to an understanding of the pathophysiology of pheochromocytoma is a knowledge of the biosynthesis and inactivation of the catecholamines. The term "catecholamine" refers to any compound composed of a catechol nucleus (a benzene ring with two adjacent hydroxyl groups) and an amine-containing side chain; these substances are of low molecular weight. The catecholamines known to occur in man are dopamine, norepinephrine, and epinephrine. They are importantly involved in neural and endocrine function.

Dopamine appears to serve as a neurotransmitter in the central nervous system and, to a minor extent, in some sympathetic ganglia. There is accumulating evidence that dopaminergic nerves and receptors exert unique functions in the brain and elsewhere (374, 683, 684); however, this amine functions as a precursor for norepinephrine. Epinephrine and norepinephrine are of major importance in affecting metabolism and cardiovascular physiology. Biosynthesis of these amines occurs in the sympathetic neurons (mainly the nerve endings), brain, and chromaffin tissue. Both norepinephrine and epinephrine are synthesized in some chromaffin cells and parts of the brain, whereas only norepinephrine is synthesized in the postganglionic sympathetic nerves, where it serves the important function of the neurotransmitter (mediator of nerve activity) at most postganglionic sympathetic endings in the autonomic nervous system. It has been proposed that some norepinephrine synthesized in the region of the cell nucleus may be transported via axoplasmic flow to sympathetic nerve endings (201). However, all the enzymes necessary for conversion of the amino acid L-tyrosine to norepinephrine are present in the nerve ending, where the bulk of norepinephrine is synthesized and stored. Tyrosine is derived from dietary or tissue tyrosine or from dietary phenylalanine which is metabolically converted to tyrosine in the body (683, 684). Neurons which liberate catecholamines are called "sympathetic" or "adrenergic neurons.' In the fetus the adrenal (452, 1029) and organ of Zuckerkandl (collections of chromaffin cells located anterior to the abdominal aorta just above its bifurcation and extending to the origin of the inferior mesenteric artery) (1029, 1030) contain only norepinephrine; however, epinephrine also appears in these organs within 1 year following birth (1030). The sites of norepinephrine storage in tissue is indicated in Table 2.1.

Although norepinephrine and epinephrine are secreted into the blood, where they can be demonstrated in minute concentrations, the presence of dopamine in the blood of normal subjects was not quantitatively reported until 1973 (153). More recently, with the use of a very sensitive assay, dopamine has been detected, although only sporadically, in a few normotensive and hypertensive subjects, and it has been suggested that the plasma concentration of this amine is independent of sympathetic activity (214). All three catecholamines are, however, present in urine. Since none of the catecholamines are capable of crossing the blood-brain barrier, it is likely that catecholamine metabolism and turnover in the brain are not reflected by the level of these amines in the urine.

Table 2.1 *Sites of Norepinephrine Storage in Tissue*[a,b]

Organ	Cell	Relative amount	Present in granulated vesicle
Brain and spinal cord	Adrenergic neuron:		
	Cell body	Moderate	No
	Nerve ending	Very large	Partly
Sympathetic ganglia	Adrenergic neuron:		
	Cell body	Small	No
Organs with sympathetic innervation (i.e., heart, spleen, liver, kidney, muscle, salivary gland)	Adrenergic neuron: Sympathetic nerve ending	Very large (most of the norepinephrine in the body)	Yes (adrenergic vesicle)
	Extraneural pool (in parenchymal cells)	Small	No
Adrenal medulla (and extramedullary chromaffin cells)	Chromaffin cell	Very large	Yes (chromaffin granule)
Uterus	Parenchyma (?)	Moderate	No

[a] From Wurtman, R. F. *Catecholamines.* Courtesy of Little, Brown and Co. 1966. p. 17.
[b] Note: The concentrations of norepinephrine in the adrenergic cell body and nerve ending have been estimated to be 10–100 μg/g and 10,000 μg/g, respectively.

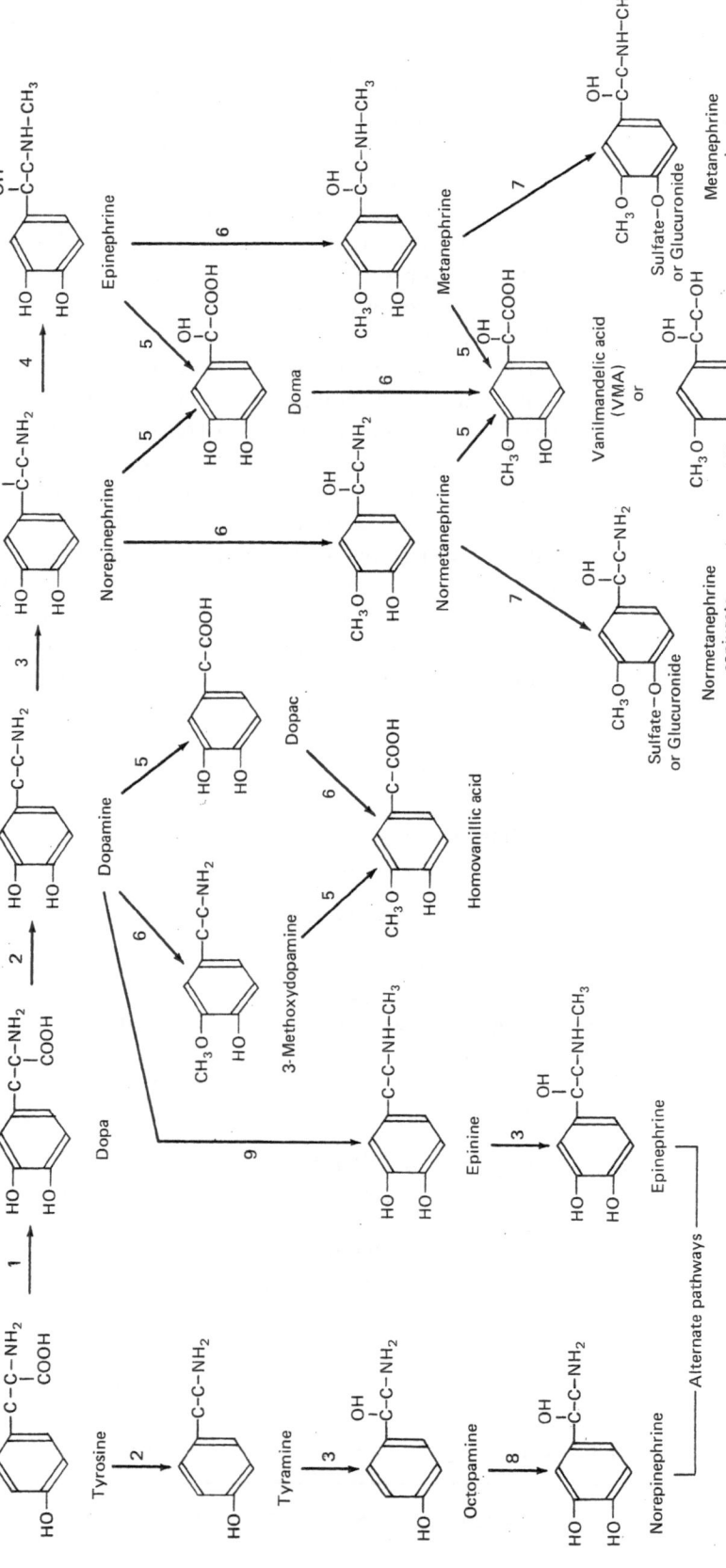

Fig. 2.1 Pathways of synthesis and metabolism of catecholamines with enzymes catalyzing various reactions. 1-Tyrosine hydroxylase; 2-aromatic amino acid decarboxlyase; 3-phenylamine-β-hydroxylase; 4-phenylethanolamine-N-methyltransferase; 5-monoamine oxidase plus aldehyde dehydrogenase; 6-catechol-O-methyltransferase; 7-conjugating enzymes; 8-rabbit-liver enzyme; 9-rabbit-lung enzyme.

Figure 2.1 reveals the pathways of biosynthesis and metabolism of catecholamines and indicates the enzymes catalyzing the various reactions. The biosynthesis, storage, release, and inactivation of the catecholamines in sympathetic nerves, chromaffin cells, and pheochromocytomas will now be considered in detail.

SYMPATHETIC NERVES

BIOSYNTHESIS, STORAGE, AND RELEASE OF NOREPINEPHRINE

Figure 2.2 reveals a schematic representation of the biosynthesis, storage, and secretion of norepinephrine in a sympatheic nerve ending. Each sympathetic nerve may contain as many as 25,000 varicosities (or "buttons"), which simply represent thickenings or bulges, at the nerve endings and along the course of the fibers, where norepinephrine is synthesized and stored in granulated vesicles. In addition to the norepinephrine contained in these latter organelles (i.e., synaptic vesicles) an intracellular pool of "free" norepinephrine is also assumed to exist (683, 684). Most of the varicosities, which contain high concentrations of norepinephrine, lie in close proximity to effector (target) cells and represent synaptic regions of the sympathetic nerve terminals (463).

L-Tyrosine from the blood is thought to be transported across the membrane of the sympathetic nerves by a special concentrating mechanism. It is then converted by the enzyme tyrosine hydroxylase, which is found only within catecholamine-producing cells, to L-dihydroxyphenylalanine (dopa). This reaction, which requires tetrahydropteridine as a cofactor, proceeds slowly in vivo and is considered the rate-limiting step in the biosynthesis of the catecholamines (500, 572). Tyrosine hydroxylase is inhibited by catecholamines and this inhibition appears important in controlling the rate of biosynthesis of norepinephrine in the sympathetic nerves (694). Dopa, in turn, is rapidly decarboxylated to L-dihydroxyphenylethylamine (dopamine) by aromatic l-amino acid decarboxylase in the cytoplasm of the neurons. This second step proceeds rapidly and requires pyridoxal phosphate as a cofactor. Dopa decarboxylase is widely distributed even in tissues that do not normally synthesize catecholamines, and its high activity in kidney may explain the large amounts of dopamine found in urine.

Dopamine then enters minute granulated vesicles (400–600 Å) in the sympathetic nerve terminals, where it is then finally hydroxylated by dopamine-β-hydroxylase (DBH) to l-norepinephrine. DBH is found only in cells that produce norepinephrine. This third

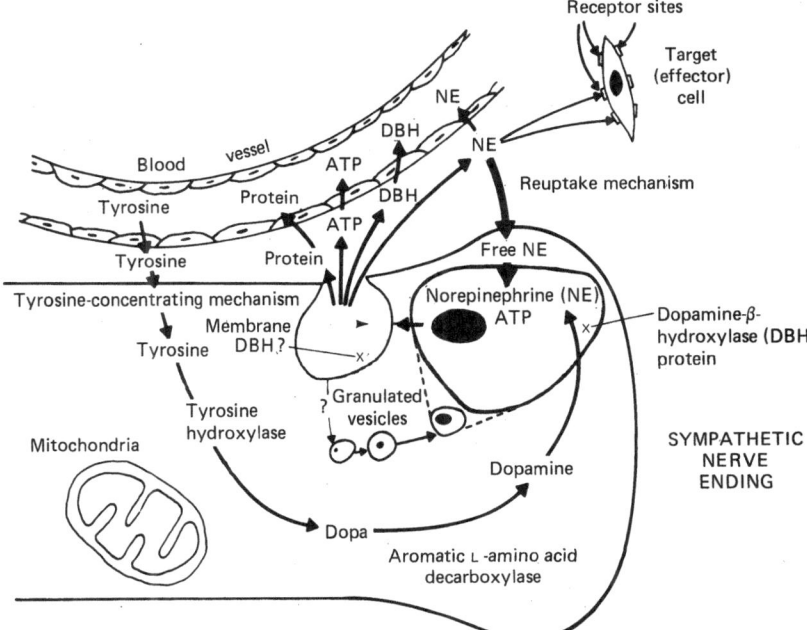

Fig. 2.2 Intracellular movements of substrates in the biosynthesis of norepinephrine; secretion via exocytosis of storage granules, and theoretical "recycling" of granule.

enzymatic reaction requires O_2 and ascorbic and fumaric acids as cofactors. Norepinephrine, the neurotransmitter, remains inactive and protected in these storage vesicles until released by activation of the sympathetic nerves. A small amount of norepinephrine leaks from these granules into the surrounding cytoplasm, but these vesicles also have the capacity to take up and bind norepinephrine from the cytoplasm. It is believed that excitation of the sympathetic nerves results in a process of exocytosis (emiocytosis, or "cell vomiting") whereby storage granules move, perhaps via microtubules, to the surface of the sympathetic nerve membrane, where they expel their contents into the extracellular fluid and circulation (1020). Berl and co-workers have suggested that actomyosin-like protein may function in the release of transmitter material at synaptic endings; exocytosis could occur by a "mechanochemical interaction between the vesicle and synaptic membrane with resultant conformational changes in the interacting membranes leading to extrusion of vesicle contents" (62). The contents of these vesicles consist of norepinephrine and adenosine triphosphate (ATP) in perhaps a 4:1 molar ratio, plus soluble DBH, and a small amount of protein (other than DBH) which is called chromogranin. It is possible that the empty vesicles are then re-utilized (recycled) for the synthesis and storage of norepinephrine. This latter possibility seems likely since 90 percent of DBH is in bound form, remaining in the vesicle's membrane, and the estimated half-life of the sympathetic nerve vesicle is 3 weeks (200).

Primarily because of an efficient reuptake mechanism, a relatively small fraction of physiologically active neurotransmitter reaches receptors on the target (effector) cells and thereby activates these cells (e.g., vascular smooth muscle, myocardium, adipocyte, myometrium, or hepatocyte; there is some evidence that receptors exist at presynaptic neural sites). Even intense activation of the sympathetic nervous system may cause no appreciable increase in the plasma concentration of norepinephrine (621). This finding is probably explained by the efficient reuptake mechanism and enzymatic degradation which prevent norephinephrine from overflowing into the circulation in significant amounts. It

is assumed that the relatively small amount of norepinephrine which reaches the circulation does so by a process of diffusion; however, we are unaware of any experimental studies which either validate or refute this concept.

The physiologic response of target cells to injected or secreted catecholamines depends on (1) the fraction of catecholamine delivered to the target cell (this can vary with the state of the circulation); (2) ability of the cell to inactivate the delivered catecholamines; and (3) sensitivity of the target cell (1059, p. 33).

Release of norepinephrine and DBH is enhanced by calcium ions, and also by some α-adrenergic blocking agents (e.g., phenoxybenzamine and phentolamine). This enhanced release can be inhibited by prostaglandin E_2, perhaps due to prostaglandin's interference with availability of Ca^{2+} (30).

During the past few years evidence has accumulated for the existence of a presynaptic regulation of norepinephrine release from adrenergic nerves (545a). It has been postulated that norepinephrine released by nerve stimulation (once it reaches a threshold concentration in the synaptic gap) activates presynaptic α-receptors, triggering a negative feedback mechanism which inhibits further release of the neurotransmitter. Compatible with this hypothesis is the fact that α-receptor agonists inhibit, whereas α-receptor antagonists enhance, norepinephrine release by nerve stimulation. It now appears that, in addition to α-receptors in adrenergic nerve endings, there are dopaminergic and muscarinic receptors which are inhibitory to neurotransmitter release, and also nicotinic receptors which elicit norepinephrine release (545a). The existence of a presynaptic β-adrenergic receptor seems to be an equally plausible concept: stimulation of a presynaptic β-receptor would enhance the norepinephrine release during adrenergic stimulation and thus constitute a positive feedback control of neurotransmitter secretion. Recently, Stjärne and Brundin have demonstrated a dual adrenoceptor-mediated control of norepinephrine secretion from human vasoconstrictor nerves, i.e., a facilitation by β-receptors and an inhibition by α-receptors in the presynaptic region. From their elegant experimental observations it was suggested that the low sensitivity for α-adrenoceptors can only be triggered by high concentrations of norepinephrine occurring in the synaptic cleft. On the other hand, the extremely high sensitivity of β-adrenoceptors should enable them to detect physiologic concentrations of circulating catecholamines. These latter receptors may thus subserve the function of enhancing secretion of norepinephrine from synaptic nerves during conditions of increased secretion of epinephrine from the adrenal medulla (938a). However, high epinephrine concentrations may depress norepineprine secretion from synaptic nerves by stimulating the less sensitive α-adrenergic-mediated control mechanism (938a).

INACTIVATION OF NOREPINEPHRINE

Catabolism Inactivation of norepinephrine occurs in several ways. The norepinephrine which is free in the cytoplasm of sympathetic nerves may be deaminated by monoamine oxidase (MAO) plus aldehyde dehydrogenase in mitochondria to form an unstable aldehyde, which can then be oxidized to an acid, 3,4-dihydroxymandelic acid (DHMA or DOMA); or, norepinephrine may be reduced to an alcohol, dihydroxyphenylglycol (DHPG). The reduction product predominates in the rat, whereas the oxidation product predominates in man (34).

MAO, which is widely distributed and is particularly abundant in the brain, liver, and kidney, was once considered to play a key role in terminating the physiologic action of the catecholamines. This enzyme is now thought to be primarily concerned with disposing of excess stores of catecholamines (522). On the other hand, the norepinephrine which is released into the circulation is largely converted by meta-O-methylation to normetanephrine by the action of catechol-O-methyltransferase (COMT) (33, 537). COMT, first identified by Axelrod (28), is present in almost all tissues and particularly concentrated in liver and kidney. Studies on the subcellular distribution of this enzyme indicate its occurrence not only as a soluble fraction but as a membrane-bound fraction in red blood cells and a microsomal fraction in the liver. Although COMT has been considered to be located in extra-neuronal sites, there is recent evidence of an intraneuronal location in some tissues (373); it does not, however, appear to be present in very significant amounts in sympathetic nerves. COMT requires S-adenosylmethionine as the methyl donor. The biosynthesis, storage, secretion, and catabolism of norepinephrine in the sympathetic nerve is diagrammatically illustrated in Figure 2.3.

Further degradation of normetanephrine and metanephrine by MAO and of 3,4-dihydroxymandelic acid by COMT in cells elsewhere in the body results in the formation of 3-methoxy-4-hydroxymandelic acid (VMA). A small amount of methoxyhydroxyphenyl

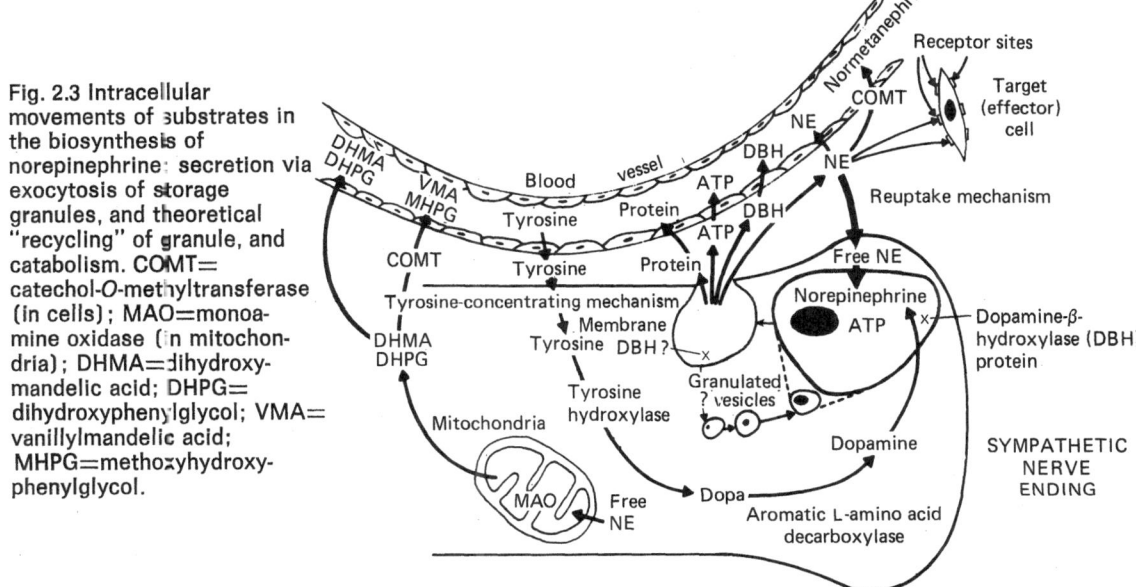

Fig. 2.3 Intracellular movements of substrates in the biosynthesis of norepinephrine; secretion via exocytosis of storage granules, and theoretical "recycling" of granule, and catabolism. COMT= catechol-O-methyltransferase (in cells); MAO=monoamine oxidase (in mitochondria); DHMA=dihydroxymandelic acid; DHPG= dihydroxyphenylglycol; VMA= vanillylmandelic acid; MHPG=methoxyhydroxyphenylglycol.

glycol (MHPG) is generated by the enzymatic reaction of MAO with metanephrine and normetanephrine, and by the reaction of COMT with dihydroxyphenylglycol. Some free norepinephrine and normetanephrine are converted to glucuronide and/or sulfate conjugates, which are biologically inert, as are the metabolites formed by the action of MAO and COMT (305, 537). Generally, the total catecholamine concentration (i.e., free and conjugated) in urine is 1.5 to 3 times as high as that for the free amine; this appears to hold true for norepinephrine as well as for epinephrine (286, p. 286).

Uptake and binding The inactivation of catecholamines entering the blood is extremely rapid. For example, radioactive norepinephrine and epinephrine, when injected into animals in physiologic concentrations, have an initial half-life of 10 to 30 sec (1017, 1033, 1059). Vendsalu reported the half-life in plasma of norepinephrine infused into humans to be 2.3 min (992). In man the disappearance of intravenously infused 7-^{3}H-epinephrine occurs in at least two phases—a rapid decay with a half-life of 1.2 min, and a slower one with a half-life of 75.3 min, consistent with binding and slow release of epinephrine from various tissues (540).

The fate of intravenously administered ^{3}H-epinephrine in the rat is indicated in Table 2.2. In the untreated rat, 69 percent of the administered dose appeared in the urine as the O-methylated derivative, and 8 percent was deaminated. Iproniazid (a MAO

blocker) treatment resulted in an increased O-methylation and a decreased deamination, whereas the reverse was found when pyrogallol (a COMT blocker) was used. Deamination occurs both intra- and extraneuronally, but O-methylation occurs mainly extraneuronally (521).

The fate of the catecholamines in the circulation depends largely on the organs to which they are delivered (1059, p. 27). Organs richly innervated with sympathetic nerves (e.g., heart and spleen) take up circulating catecholamines and bind most of them in a physiologically inactive form in the storage vesicles of sympathetic nerve endings. On the other hand, organs containing relatively high concentrations of COMT and MAO (e.g., liver and kidney) convert the catecholamines to their metabolites (i.e., normetanephrine, metanephrine, VMA, or MHPG). Because of the blood–brain barrier, only the hypothalamus takes up detectable amounts of catecholamines (1017).

Manger and coworkers (624, pp. 292–300) and LaBrosse and Hertting (539) demonstrated the remarkable ability of the liver to clear 85 percent or more of the catecholamines from the circulation. Effective clearance by the liver continues until relatively high rates of catecholamine infusion are reached (624, pp. 292–300). The heart extracts 70 to 80 percent of these amines from the circulation during a single passage (1062).

Rapid removal and physiologic disposition of catecholamines from the circulation cannot be entirely accounted for by sympathetic

Table 2.2   *Fate of Intravenously Administered ^{3}H-Epinephrine in the Rat*

Treatment	Free	Conjugated	O-Methylated	Deaminated
	Percent administered dose excreted in urine			
Untreated	9	5	69	8
Iproniazid (MAO Inhibitor)	10	4	82	1
Pyrogallol (COMT Inhibitor)	27	5	17	29

^{a} Data taken from Kopin, I. J., Axelrod, J., and Gordon, E. *J. Biol. Chem.* **236:** 2112, 1961. With permission of the copyright owner: The American Society of Biological Chemists, Inc.

nerve uptake (986). Avakian and Gillespie (26, 27) found that norepinephrine is taken up in vitro, not only by adrenergic nerves but also by smooth muscle, collagen, and elastic tissue, and they suggested that smooth muscle cells have a transport mechanism for intracellular norepinephrine uptake (27). Kaumann (501) obtained results consistent with a saturable extraneuronal mechanism with high affinity for norepinephrine. Even catecholamine entry into blood cells has been demonstrated (613, 620, 624, pp. 172–174). This can be dramatically shown by incubating blood cells in the presence of high concentrations of catecholamines and then examining them with a fluorescence technique (613) (Figs. 2.4 and 2.5). When blood cells are incubated in high concentrations of catecholamines, simple diffusion undoubtedly accounts for a large percentage of the catecholamine which enters the cells. This is suggested by the fact that incubation at 0°C (which should block active uptake by cells) does not appreciably alter the intensity of the fluorescence in the cells. In vivo, blood cell uptake of circulating catecholamines can occur by an energy-requiring mechanism as well as by diffusion.

Thus, there are "specific" (neuronal) and "nonspecific" (extraneuronal) catecholamine storage sites. The uptake of catecholamines by sympathetic nerves (uptake$_1$) and extraneuronal uptake of catecholamines (uptake$_2$) have been reviewed and studied by Iversen (477); however, the mechanisms and import-

Fig. 2.4 Photomicrograph of peripheral blood cells and platelets (1,000×) of 3-year-old female with congenital hemolytic anemia and postsplenectomy thrombocytosis (RBC 3,800,000, platelets 600,000, and 20,000 WBC/ml^3 with 85 percent polymorphonuclear leukocytes, 9 percent monocytes, and 6 percent lymphocytes). Cells had been incubated in plasma containing dopamine (500 μg/ml), and then exposed to paraformaldehyde vapor. Note intense fluorescence in polymorphonuclear leukocyte—especially in the nucleus. Nuclei in mononuclear cells were moderately fluorescent but cytoplasmic intensity was mild. Platelets were mild to moderately fluorescent but RBC did not fluoresce, since fluorescence is obscured by hemoglobin. From Manger, W. M. and Bessis, M., unpublished.

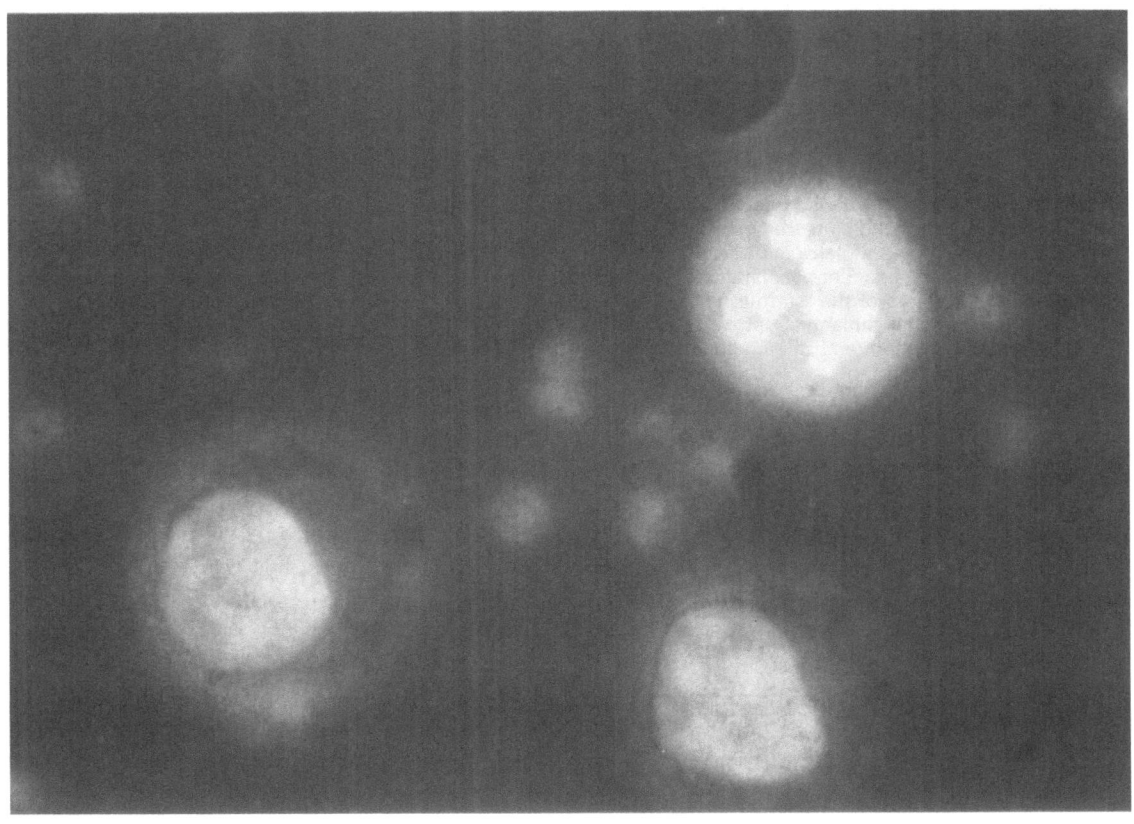

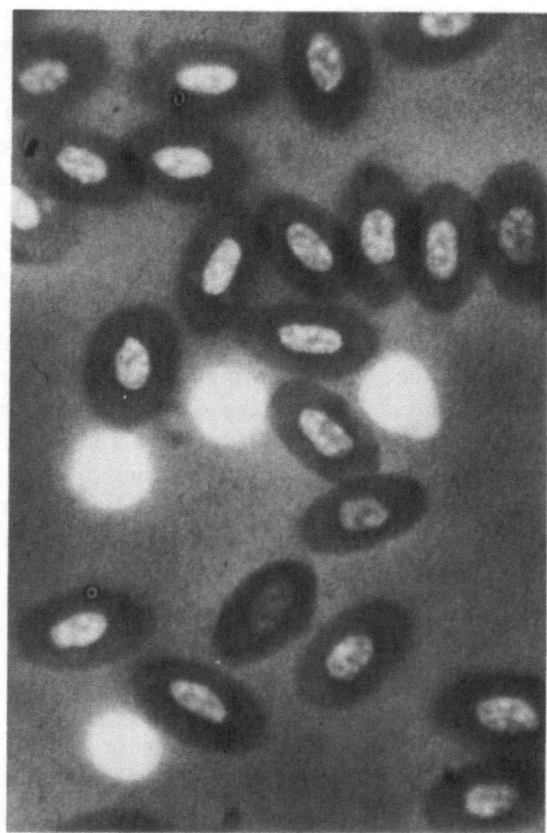

Fig. 2.5 Photomicrograph revealing fluorescence in WBC and in nuclei of RBC of frog's blood (250×). Blood (0.2 ml) was mixed with 0.2 ml of normal saline containing 200 μg dopamine and incubated for 30 min at 37°C. Cells were removed after centrifugation and a smear of the cells was exposed to vaporized paraformaldehyde. Entry of catecholamines into frog RBC can be demonstrated, since hemoglobin did not obscure fluorescence in RBC nuclei. From Manger, W. M. and Bessis, M., unpublished. (These studies were performed at the Institut de Pathologie Cellulaire in Paris. We are most grateful for the excellent assistance we received from the staff of the Institut in performing in vitro studies on catecholamine uptake by blood cells. William Manger, Jr. and Lala Manger helped with the frogs.)

ance of extraneuronal catecholamine uptake are complex and have not been adequately investigated. The most important mechanisms for removing and inactivating circulating catecholamines are uptake into sympathetic nerves and metabolic degradation by the enzyme COMT (31).

Only about 2 to 4 percent of infused norepinephrine or epinephrine appears in the urine as free catecholamines, and several investigators have reported that roughly 30 to 35 percent is excreted as VMA and 50 to 55 percent as metanephrine or normetanephrine (22, 32, 514, 540). However, as pointed out by Crout, various approaches used to assess the relative proportion of each catecholamine metabolite in the urine do not yield identical results (185). This is readily apparent in Table 2.3, where the pattern of metabolites appearing in the urine after infusing the D,L-isomer of $2\text{-}^{14}\text{C}$-epinephrine is compared with the pattern following infusion of $l\text{-}7\text{-}^{3}\text{H}$-epinephrine. Apparently, optical isomers of the catecholamines may not be metabolized in a quantitatively identical fashion (185). The excretion patterns in normal subjects and patients with pheochromocytoma are also shown in the table.

Reuptake mechanism Of major importance in terminating the physiologic action of norepinephrine released at the sympathetic nerve terminals is the neuronal reuptake process. This high-affinity neuronal uptake is stereoselective and requires sodium; it can be utilized by other amines structurally similar to norepinephrine (e.g., epinephrine, dopamine, tyramine, α-methylnorepinephrine, metaraminol, and amphetamine) (30). These structurally related amines can also be taken up by the storage vesicles and displace norepinephrine. Potter and Axelrod demonstrated that organs having extensive sympathetic nerve innervation take up and store circulating catecholamines in a chemically unchanged form in granulated vesicles of sympathetic nerve terminals (768). Moskowitz and Wurtman have imaginatively likened the release and reuptake of the neurotransmitter to the behavior of a sponge: "the wave of depolarization squeezes the metaphoric sponge, causing catecholamine molecules to drip out into synapses; with repolarization the sponge snaps back into shape, sopping up the catecholamines in the synaptic cleft" (683).

Perhaps as much as 80 percent of norepinephrine liberated from synaptic nerves into the extracellular fluid is taken up into adjacent synaptic nerve terminals by an active transport mechanism (321). Such a reuptake mechanism is of great value to the economy and efficient function of the sympathetic nervous system. To emphasize the importance of the reuptake process in terminating the action of norepinephrine, it should be appreciated

Table 2.3 *Relative Excretion of Catecholamines and Metabolites: Comparison of Values Found under Differing Experimental Conditions[a]*

Situation	\multicolumn{4}{c}{Percent of total excreted as[b]}	$\dfrac{VMA}{NE(E)}$	$\dfrac{VMA}{NMN(MN)}$
	NE(E)	NMN(MN)	VMA	Other		
Normal Subjects:						
Endogenous excretion	1.1	7.6	91	—	83	12
d,l-NE-2-C^{14} infusion	4	22	32	40	8	1.5
d,l-E-2-C^{14} infusion	4	47	27	22	6.7	0.57
l-E-7-H^3 infusion	4	34	55	7	14	1.6
Pheochromocytoma Patients:						
"Low" group	5	25	70	—	14	2.8
"High" group	1.7	27	71	—	42	2.6

[a] Abbreviations: NE = norepinephrine; E = epinephrine; NMN = normetanephrine; MN = metanephrine; VMA = vanilmandelic acid. "Low" = tumors with low total catecholamine content but rapid turnover. "High" = tumors with high total catecholamine content but slow turnover. From Crout, J. R. Chap. I. Catecholamine metabolism in pheochromocytoma and essential hypertension. *In: Hormones and Hypertension.* Courtesy of C. C. Thomas, 1966, p. 15.

[b] In studies of radioactive NE and E, total excretion represents total radioactivity in the urine. In all other studies, total excretion was taken to be the sum of NE + E + NMN + MN + VMA.

that the biologic activity of the catecholamines is promptly terminated even if catabolic degradation is pharmacologically blocked. Hypersensitivity of sympathetically denervated structures to catecholamines may partly be explained by degeneration of sympathetic nerves and disappearance of storage vesicles following nerve section. As a consequence, vesicles are not available to take up the catecholamines, and therefore an excess of these amines is available to stimulate the adrenergic receptors of the denervated structure.

CHROMAFFIN CELLS

BIOSYNTHESIS, STORAGE, RELEASE, AND INACTIVATION

The biosynthesis, release, and metabolism of norepinephrine in chromaffin cells is essentially the same as that in the sympathetic nerves; however, some chromaffin cells (e.g., certain cells in the adrenal medulla) have the capacity to convert l-norepinephrine to l-epinephrine This reaction is brought about by the enzyme phenylethanolamine-N-methyltransferase (PNMT), which transfers a methyl group from S-adenosylmethionine to the nitrogen position of norepinephrine. In mammalian tissues, only the heart, adrenal medulla, brain (29), and brainstem (831) have

measurable amounts of this epinephrine-synthesizing enzyme (PNMT) (29). Since PNMT, when present, is located in the cytoplasm of chromaffin cells, norepinephrine must migrate from the chromaffin granule to the cytoplasm for methylation, and then return to the granule for storage. The irreversibility of the conversion of norepinephrine to epinephrine has been confirmed in a patient with pheochromocytoma in whom no significant amount of norepinephrine-^{14}C was detected in the urine after infusion of d,l-epinephrine-2-^{14}C (910).

It is noteworthy that enzymes (tyrosine hydroxylase, DBH, and PNMT) controlling catecholamine biosynthesis in the adrenal medulla are under hormonal control. Hypophysectomy causes a decrease in the amount of these enzymes and epinephrine and also a diminished secretion of adrenal catecholamines resulting from insulin hypoglycemia. Restoration of the enzyme activity, at least in part, may be achieved by administration of ACTH or glucocorticoids (30). Some recent evidence suggests that glucocorticoids modulate transsynaptic induction of tyrosine hydroxylase in sympathetic ganglia as well as in the adrenal medulla (725).

It has been claimed that insulin hypoglycemia selectively releases epinephrine from the adrenal medulla, and it has been conjectured that two chromaffin cell populations exist (277). Our own studies in dogs indicated that hypoglycemia releases both epinephrine and norepinephrine from the adrenal medulla (132). Hillarp and Hökfelt presented cytological findings suggesting that epinephrine and norepinephrine are formed in different cells in the adrenal medulla (444, 445). There is also experimental evidence, involving a variety of adrenal medullary stimuli, that these two populations of cells can release their respective hormones independently. This latter observation supports the concept that cells containing norepinephrine have a separate innervation from those containing epinephrine (286). However, indisputable evidence is not available to demonstrate that some cells contain only norepinephrine, and that others contain epinephrine and PNMT and little, if any, norepinephrine.

Eighty to 85 percent of the catecholamine content of the adult human adrenal medulla is epinephrine and 15 to 20 percent norepinephrine. Plasma and urinary levels of norepinephrine correlate reasonably well with sympathetic nerve activity, since norepinephrine enters the circulation mainly as an "overflow" from the adrenergic nerves. Catecholamines released from the adrenal glands are inactivated mainly by COMT and MAO in the liver.

Bilateral adrenalectomy markedly reduces the concentration of epinephrine in the urine of man, whereas the norepinephrine concentration is not significantly altered (293, 379). Any remaining epinephrine (perhaps one-fifth of that normally excreted in the urine) is presumed to come from chromaffin cells present elsewhere in the body (286, p. 287). It should be pointed out that the adrenal medulla can be viewed as a sympathetic ganglion which is innervated by preganglionic cholinergic fibers. These latter fibers release acetylcholine, which causes secretion of catecholamines by a process of exocytosis from the chromaffin cells of the adrenal medulla. The control of secretion from other chromaffin cells has not been adequately elucidated.

Secretion of catecholamines by a process of exocytosis was first studied in the adrenal medulla, where it appears to be responsible for the release of catecholamines from these chromaffin cells (234, 994).

The imaginative approach and elegant studies of Douglas and his associates have uncovered several factors in the chain of events linking stimulus to secretory response (stimulus-secretion coupling) in the chromaffin cell of the adrenal medulla (234). He coined the term "stimulus-secretion coupling" after the phrase "excitation-contraction coupling," which had previously been introduced to describe related events in the field of muscle physiology (234). From results of electrophysiologic experiments, Douglas summarized the consequences of exposing chromaffin cells to acetylcholine as follows:

Interaction between acetylcholine and the plasma membrane of the chromaffin cell

↓

Altered membrane chemistry (conformation?)

↓

Increased membrane permeability

↓

Entry of sodium and calcium ions

↓

Depolarization (without impulse formation)

Action potentials were never observed in adrenal medullary cells in response to acetylcholine; thus, it appears that spike generation is not involved in stimulus-secretion coupling in the chromaffin cell (234). It was further demonstrated that the presence of calcium was not only essential but was itself sufficient for the secretion of catecholamines in response to acetylcholine; other ions (potassium, sodium, chloride, and magnesium) were not necessary (234). Secretion of adrenal catecholamines caused by other substances (e.g., histamine, serotonin, angiotensin, and bradykinin) appears to depend on depolarization of the chromaffin cells and the entry of calcium, the latter being a critical event in stimulus-secretion coupling of chromaffin cells (234).

Douglas and associates showed that the molar ratio of catecholamines to ATP and metabolites in the venous effluent of the adrenal gland following stimulation was similar to that found within chromaffin granules. Moreover, when cellular ATPase was inhibited, stimulation of the adrenal medulla was accompanied by release of unhydrolyzed

ATP. This sophisticated detective work, plus the knowledge that ATP and other adenine nucleotides traverse cell membranes poorly, led Douglas (234) to conclude that the content of the chromaffin granule must be extruded directly to the cell exterior, without traversing the cytoplasm, by a process known as reverse micropinocytosis, exocytosis (216), or emiocytosis (541).

Exocytosis consists of the migration of the chromaffin storage granule, perhaps via a system of microtubules, to the cell surface, where the membrane of the granule fuses with the plasmalemma and escape of secretory product occurs through an aperture in the fused membranes (234). The possibility that the entire chromaffin granule is extruded intact seems excluded by the finding that the phospholipids and cholesterol of the granule membrane are not released during adrenal medullary secretion (234). In addition, electron micrographs of adrenal medullary cells frequently reveal cystoplasmic structures resembling empty secretory granules (176, 178, 226, 230). The fate of the emptied granule is uncertain; it may be recycled and refilled with catecholamines, or, possibly, the membranes may be destroyed by lysosomal enzymes.

A similarly important role for calcium in stimulus-secretion coupling which involves exocytosis has been demonstrated in cholinergic and adrenergic nerves, where the respective neurotransmitters, acetylcholine and norepinephrine, are contained in membrane-limited structures (synaptic vesicles). Finally, a variety of other secretory cells appear to have similar secretory mechanisms (234). It has been speculated that calcium may induce exocytosis by permitting an interaction between ATPase in the chromaffin granule membrane and ATP in the cell membrane (234); however, the precise role of calcium in effecting exocytosis is not yet clear.

In Figure 2.1 it can be seen that metabolic degradation of epinephrine results in metanephrine and VMA; some of the epinephrine and metanephrine is conjugated to form glucuronides and sulfates. The turnover rate for all the catecholamines in the adrenal medulla is quite slow, the half-life being about 7 to 10 days. In the sympathetic nerves, the half-life for one pool of norepinephrine appears to be about 4 to 6 hr, whereas the half-life for another pool is approximately 1 day (111). Storage granules in the adrenal medulla are usually several times larger than the storage vesicles in the sympathetic nerves.

PHEOCHROMOCYTOMAS
BIOSYNTHESIS

There is evidence that pheochromocytomas have the various enzymes necessary for the conversion of tyrosine to catecholamines, and the level of activity of some of these enzymes (tyrosine hydroxylase, dopa decarboxylase, and DBH) is high (383, 545). Furthermore, compared with the amount of catecholamine synthesized in bovine adrenal medulla, the amount synthesized in pheochromocytomas may be considerably greater [e.g., in one tumor, the concentration of catecholamines synthesized in 1 hr was approximately 27 times that in a normal bovine adrenal (81)]. The biologic half-life of tumor norepinephrine has been found to be on the order of 8 to 12 hr (905). Most tumors contain a smaller concentration of epinephrine than does the normal adrenal medulla, or even no epinephrine. Of interest, and of some chemical importance, is the fact that, with rare exceptions, pheochromocytomas which secrete at least some epinephrine are located in the adrenal gland (193, 299). Crout and Sjoerdsma studied 75 patients and reported that 42 percent had elevated concentrations of epinephrine in the urine and that 95 percent of tumors in patients with increased epinephrine excretion occurred in the adrenal; of those having elevations only of urinary norepinephrine, 67 percent of tumors were in the adrenal area (193).

Some investigators have stated that two out of three pheochromocytomas store and secrete both epinephrine and norepinephrine, whereas the remaining tumors contain and secrete only norepinephrine; only very rarely has a tumor proved to contain and secrete only epinephrine (299, 385).

In our experience, 84.6 percent of tumors in patients with sustained hypertension contained both epinephrine and norepinephrine, whereas both amines were present in 100 percent of the tumors from patients with paroxysmal hypertension. On the other hand, only 44.4 percent of patients with sustained hypertension (all with actively secreting tumors) had elevations of both catecholamines in their plasma. With regard to patients with paroxysmal hypertension, when blood pressures were close to the normal range, 35.7 percent had plasma elevations of both catecholamines; however, when tumors in this paroxysmal group were actively secreting catecholamines (spontaneously or induced by tumor manipulation or drug administration), 64.3 percent of these patients had elevations of both catecholamines in their plasma.

Since occasionally some extraadrenal pheochromocytomas (located, for example, in the hilus of the liver, thorax, urinary bladder, the organ of Zuckerkandl and other intra-abdominal sites) have been found to contain epinephrine (268, 332, 624, 662, 872), one must not rely too securely on the fact that an epinephrine-secreting tumor is almost invariably adrenal in origin. The catecholamine content of pheochromocytomas varies considerably (even in the same tumor), usually being between 1 and 8 mg per g of tumor. These values are significantly greater than the catecholamine concentration of the normal human adrenal medulla, which is said to contain from 0.9 to 1.5 mg per g of tissue (115, 872, 882); the total content in the normal human adrenal medulla is about 6 mg (292). It is important to appreciate that there is no good correlation between the size of a tumor or its catecholamine concentrations and clinical or laboratory manifestations. The severity of symptomatology depends mainly on the amount of catecholamine liberated into the circulation.

CONCENTRATION OF BIOGENIC AMINES, METABOLITES, AND DOPA

Most pheochromocytomas secrete a combination of norepinephrine and epinephrine; however, usually norepinephrine is liberated in considerably larger concentrations than is epinephrine. Some tumors secrete only norepinephrine; a few tumors secrete only epinephrine. Very rarely, dopamine, dopa, and serotonin (5-HT) may be elaborated by pheochromocytomas (Table 2.4). It has been suggested that the elaboration of dopa can occur only in a malignant pheochromocytoma (16); however, two benign pheochromocytomas

have been reported which secreted catecholamines and dopa (586). It is noteworthy that although increased urinary excretion of dopamine and its metabolite 4-hydroxy-3-methoxyphenyl acetic acid (HVA, i.e., homovanillic acid) rarely occurs in patients with pheochromocytoma (see Chapter 6, Biochemical Tests), increased excretion of these substances occurs frequently in patients with other neural crest tumors (see Chapter 5).

About 80 to 85 percent of the total catecholamines in the normal adrenal medulla is epinephrine (882). The activity of the enzyme PNMT, which is required for the methylation of norepinephrine to form epinephrine, depends on the presence of high concentrations of corticosteroids, such as occurs in adrenal blood (630, 1061). Therefore, it is understandable why many pheochromocytomas, particularly those in extraadrenal locations, where the blood concentrations of corticosteroids are relatively low, contain little if any epinephrine. Wurtman has suggested that the occasional occurrence of high concentrations of epinephrine in pheochromocytomas, in extraadrenal tumors, might be explained by a noninducible PNMT enzyme (i.e., a PNMT enzyme whose activity does not require the presence of corticosteroids) (1064).

Winkler and Smith have estimated that 2 to 14 percent of the epinephrine content of the human adrenal gland is secreted per 24 hr (1053), a figure similar to that of the rat adrenal medulla (558). However, estimates of the 24-hr catecholamine turnover in pheochromocytomas have ranged from 0.4 to 768 percent (195, 283a, 437, 809, 858, 1052). Hence, in some of these tumors catecholamine synthesis is markedly increased above the rate in the normal adrenal.

Table 2.4 reveals the content of various substances reported in pheochromocytomas by a number of investigators. The concentrations of epinephrine and norepinephrine in pheochromocytomas in several large series of patients reported by other investigators are included at the bottom of the table for comparison. Manger and coworkers analyzed the catecholamine content in their tumors fluorometrically and, in nearly all instances, the catecholamines were identified chromatographically. In one tumor discovered at post mortem, dopamine was detected for the first time by paper chromatography (616). However, the occurrence of dopamine in pheochromocytomas has been discovered in only a few of these tumors, and the concentration of this amine has usually been relatively low, as noted in Table 2.4. Only in one pheochromocytoma reported in the world literature was dopamine the major amine (644). Dopa, the metanephrines, VMA, and serotonin (5-HT) have been detected in some of these tumors (Table 2.4) (195, 586); however, except for serotonin these substances are biologically relatively inert.

In 1964, Hermann and Mornex reviewed the literature and reported that the catecholamine concentration in 88 pheochromocytomas ranged from 0.076 to 73.5 mg/g of tissue, but that most of them contained 0.5 to 5 mg/g; 72 percent of the tumors contained higher concentrations of catecholamines than the normal adrenal medulla (437). Crout and Sjoerdsma reported a concentration of catecholamines which ranged from 0.7 to 19.6 mg/g in 24 tumors, with epinephrine composing 0 to 56 percent of the total content (195).

To explain the enormous capacity of some pheochromocytomas to synthesize catecholamines in the presence of huge amine concentrations in many of these tumors, it has been postulated that feedback inhibition of tyrosine hydroxylase may be lacking or in-

Table 2.4 *Contents of Various Substances In Pheochromocytoma Tissue ($\mu g/g$)[a,b]*

Authors	No. of cases	NE	E	Dopa	Dopa-mine	Meta-nephrines	VMA	5-HT
McMillan (644)	1	150	0	0	1970	—	—	0
Weil-Malherbe (1014)	2	722;764	106;115	8;147	41;494	—	—	—
Sato et al. (851)	3	624–4250	68–5100	—	—	6.7–19.7	0.3–0.73	—
Page and Jacoby (729)	2	1185;1326	590;5180	—	—	1.54;2.3	0.57(1)	—
Donath et al. (232)	2	2245–5140	25;76	—	3.4;9.4	—	—	—
Rosenthal et al. (809)	1	354	19	—	—	246	—	—
Ziegler et al. (1071)	18	100–10,000	0(4)–9514	—	0(4)–37	—	—	0(13)–1.8
Anton et al. (16)	2	1125;1470	37;150	<25	<25	15.5	<50	—
Voorhess (998)	4	367–6486	0(1)–7221	—	0	—	<0.5	—
Falck et al. (307)	2	3500;5600	1330;1350	—	5;12.7	—	—	0.3;0.9
Bohuon (86)	1	49	0	0.05	0.15	—	—	—
Hintersberger et al. (449)	4	41–7700[c]		—	0(2)–0.1	—	0	—

(Above data from Winkler, H. and Smith, A. D. Chap. 20. *In: Catecholamines.* Courtesy of Springer-Verlag, 1972, p. 905.)

Manger et al. (616)	10	500–5400	0–4490					
Bollman et al. (91)	54	300–17,500[c] (NE concentration varied from 7 to 100%)						
Crout and Sjoerdsma (195)	24	340–11,400	0–8200					
Louis et al. (586)	6	1100–8300	1000–3100	90–160	200–230			
Manger and Gifford (present report)	22	0–5060	0–5040					

Content of Normal Suprarenal Tissue ($\mu g/g$)

von Euler (284)		44–160	220–840					
Flock		0–75[d]	100–500[d]					
Anton and Sayer (17)		87	1173					

[a] Abbreviations: Dopa = 3,4-dihydroxyphenylalanine; VMA = vanilmandelic acid; 5-HT = 5-hydroxytryptamine; E = epinephrine; NE = norepinephrine.

[b] Numbers in parentheses next to data indicate number of observations.

[c] Total of NE and E.

[d] Results of chromatographic analysis of suprarenal glands removed from four patients with metastatic carcinoma. Courtesy of Dr. Eunice V. Flock, Emeritus Professor of Biochemistry, Mayo Clinic, unpublished data.

efficient (446, 695, 825, 1052). Relatively low concentrations of MAO (10, 115, 345) and COMT (910) have been detected in tumor tissue.

Since the O-methylation reaction could be demonstrated only when tumor tissue was presented with S-adenosylmethionine, it is uncertain whether pheochromocytomas are capable of synthesizing this methyl donor (905). The presence of COMT and MAO accounts for the occurrence of the metanephrines and VMA in some pheochromocytomas (Table 2.4). Other metabolites, i.e., 3-methoxy-4-hydroxyphenylglycol (523, 910), N-methyl-metanephrine (475), and homocystine (75), have been detected in low concentrations in some tumors. Further studies on quantitating the enzymes responsible for metabolizing catecholamines in pheochromocytomas are indicated, since they may shed additional light on tumor metabolism and the mechanism of catecholamine release from these tumors.

DIFFERENCES BETWEEN ADRENAL MEDULLA AND PHEOCHROMOCYTOMA IN STORAGE, RELEASE, AND INACTIVATION OF CATECHOLAMINES

Since the adrenal medulla and pheochromocytoma are both composed of chromaffin cells, it is appropriate to discuss differences in storage, release, and inactivation of catecholamines in these structures under the same heading. Apparent differences can thus be better emphasized and clarified.

The normal adrenal medulla is innervated by the splanchnic nerve, which is a preganglionic (cholinergic) portion of the sympathetic nervous system. Therefore, activation of the splanchnic nerve induces a release of acetylcholine at its nerve terminals which, in the presence of calcium, causes secretion of catecholamines (mainly epinephrine) from the adrenal medullary cells via the process of exocytosis.

Electrical stimulation, many forms of physiologic stress, and a variety of drugs are known to cause a release of catecholamines from the sympathetic nervous system and adrenal medulla. One of us (W.M.M.) and coworkers have demonstrated that a number of drugs cause a release of catecholamines (mainly epinephrine) even from the isolated

perfused adrenal medulla of the dog (Table 2.5) (697). Whether release of epinephrine and norepinephrine in this perfused adrenal was caused by the direct effect of drugs on the adrenal medullary cells, or resulted from activation of remnants of the severed splanchnic nerve, was not clear. With regard to release of catecholamines from the adrenal medulla, it is noteworthy that a significant decrease in the number of catecholamine granules in the medullary cells is evident after a procedure known to cause secretion of these amines. For example, we have noted such a decrease after perfusing the isolated adrenal gland with an acid solution (Figs. 2.6 and 2.7). It is also possible that acidosis may cause a release of catecholamines from the sympathetic nerve terminals and extraadrenal chromaffin cells. There is evidence that hypoxia is accompanied by catecholamine release from extraadrenal chromaffin tissue (255) as well as from the adrenal medulla (133).

The mechanism whereby catecholamine release from pheochromocytomas is triggered remains obscure. In one tumor, electron microscopy demonstrated a nerve with small synaptic vesicles in contact with cells containing catecholamine vesicles (597). However, there is no convincing evidence that pheochromocytomas have any nervous innervation (56, 178, 782), and it is unlikely that activation of the sympathetic nervous system could explain the release of catecholamines directly from pheochromocytomas. It is therefore difficult to explain the sudden secretion of catecholamines into the circulation that is sometimes precipitated by an emotional upset, hypotension, or hyperventilation.

The granules in the normal adrenal medulla, in addition to containing high concentrations of catecholamines and small amounts

Fig. 2.6 A. Electron micrograph of a section of normal canine adrenal medulla. The adrenal was fixed in vivo with buffered glutaraldehyde. Cells are seen between a venule (V) and a sinusoid (S).
B. Electron micrograph prepared from an adrenal gland which was perfused in vitro with diluted homologous blood at normal pH for 2 hr. Portions o two chromaffin cells are seen around a sinusoid (S). From Nahas, G. G., Zagury, D., Milhaud, A., Manger, W. M., and Pappas, G. D., *Am. J. Physiol.* 213: 1188, 1967.

Table 2.5 *Effect of Acetylcholine, Angiotensin, Tyramine, and Histamine on the Catecholamine Output of the Perfused Isolated Canine Adrenal Gland*[a,b]

Drug	Dose (mg)	Adrenal catecholamine output (ng/gland/min)			
		Control	3' $\overline{p}$ Injection	5' $\overline{p}$ Injection	8' $\overline{p}$ Injection
Acetylcholine	1.0 (3)	75 (24–150)		2004 (687–3575)	
Angiotensin	0.006 (1)	150	740	215	
	0.0125 (1)	15	141	108	55
	0.025 (1)	54	738	271	130
Tyramine	0.25 (3)	30 (18–48)	402 (47–1066)	112 (41–240)	54 (35–90)
	0.50 (2)	48 (39–56)	86 (64–109)	66 (47–84)	52 (40–63)
Histamine	0.01 (2)	85 (74–96)	125 (96–154)	108 (80–136)	69 (62–76)
	0.05 (2)	72 (65–79)	82 (50–115)	80 (77–82)	78 (64–91)

[a] From Nahas, G. G., Zagury, D., Milhaud, A., Manger, W. M. and Pappas, G. D. *Am. J. Physiol. 213:* 1190, 1967.

[b] Values are averages and ranges. Numerals in parentheses following dose represent number of glands. Acetylcholine, angiotensin, and tyramine, but not histamine, produced significant increases in adrenal catecholamine output.

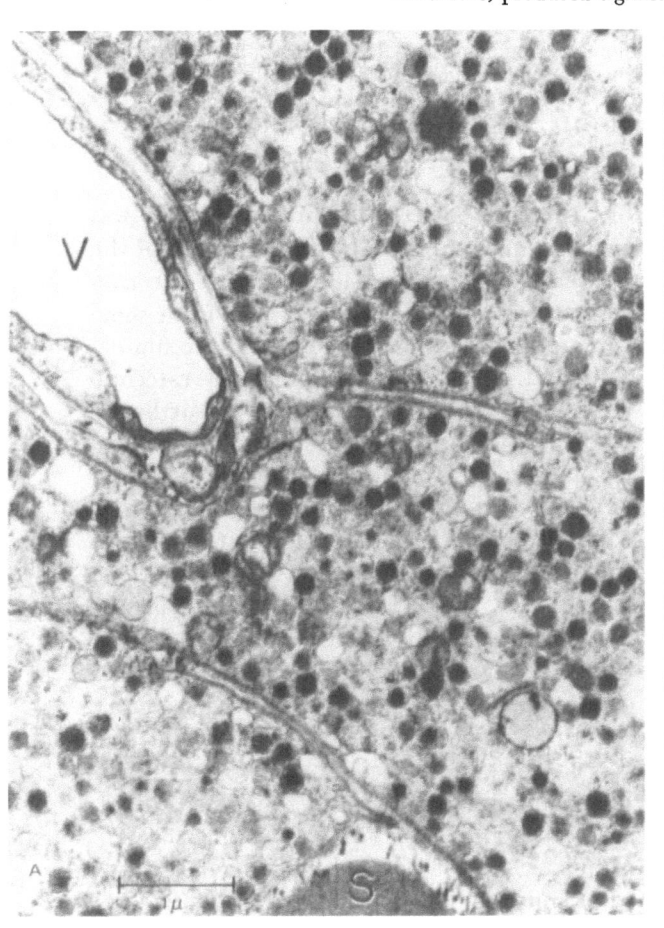
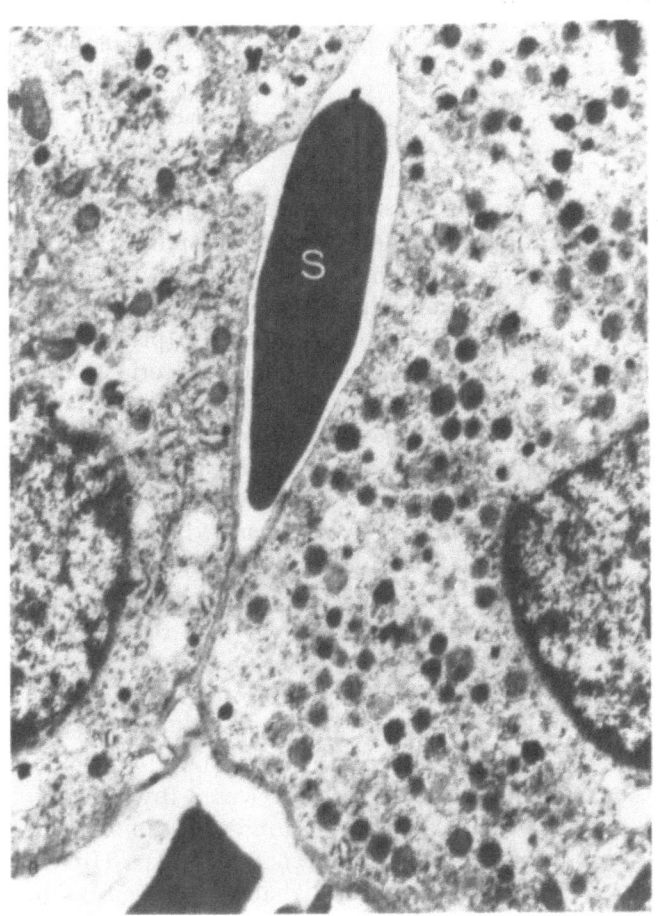

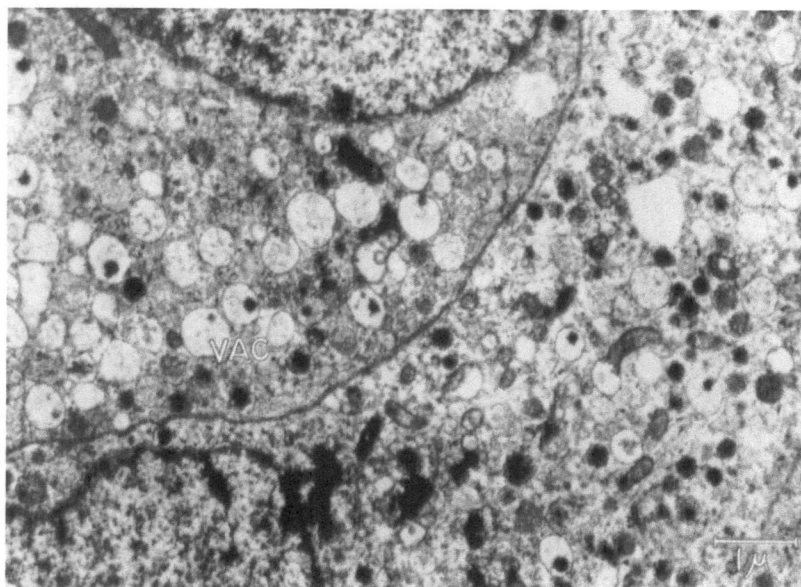

Fig. 2.7 Chromaffin cells of a canine adrenal gland perfused for 90 min with acid blood (pH 7.0, pCO₂ 98 mmHg). Wide areas of degranulation are present with vacuolar appearance (VAC=vacuole).

When perfused at a normal pH adrenal catecholamine output averaged 70 ng/gland/min. Catecholamine output increased by 100 percent following perfusion with hypercapnic mixtures at a pH of 6.96–7.10 (pCO₂ 70 to 118 mmHg) and by 660 percent with a mixture at a pH of 6.79 to 6.92 (pCO₂ 125 to 210 mmHg). The increase in adrenal catecholamine output was primarily due to a rise in epinephrine concentration. Similar results were obtained following perfusion with media made acid by addition of lactic acid. The results indicate that increase in hydrogen ion [H⁺] directly stimulates adrenal medullary secretion. From Nahas, G. G., Zagury, D., Milhaud, A., Manger, W. M., and Pappas, G. D., *Am. J. Physiol. 213*: 1191, 1967.

of protein, also contain the highest concentration of adenosine triphosphate (ATP) known in biology.

Adenosine triphosphate appears to play a role in binding catecholamines (probably to the negative charges of the nucleotides) in a storage complex in the granules of the normal adrenal medulla. This binding appears to occur in a ratio of approximately 4 moles of epinephrine or norepinephrine to 1 mole of nucleotide (82). Gélinas (345) and Schümann (872) found that the molar ratio of catecholamines to ATP in chromaffin tumors varied from about 10 to 1 to 35 to 1, considerably greater than the ratio of 4 to 1 in the normal adrenal medulla. A deficiency of ATP in pheochromocytoma cells (442) suggested that the catecholamines may be less securely bound and more easily released (by a variety of stimuli) from these chromaffin tumors than from the normal adrenal medulla. Hillarp and coworkers found that the concentration

of ATP in some pheochromocytomas was sufficient to bind only 13 to 23 percent of the total catecholamines (446), and that the constant liberation of catecholamines from some tumors may result from excessive accumulation and an overflow of unbound catecholamines into the circulation (446). Further, a study of the storage granules of a pheochromocytoma revealed that only a minor amount of the catecholamines in the tumor could be stored by a mechanism requiring a stoichiometric relationship between these amines and ATP (939). Schümann has suggested the possibility that the parallel loss of ATP and catecholamines from the granules of the adrenal might be related to a secretory as well as a storage function of this nucleotide (872). However, Stjärne and coworkers noted that the rates of loss of ATP and catecholamines from the granules of a pheochromocytoma were not parallel, and may be somewhat independent of each other (939).

Table 2.6 *Properties of Chromaffin Granules from Pheochromocytoma[a,b]*

	Pheochromocytoma (human)	Adrenal medulla (ox, horse, and pig)
Catecholamine/ATP (molar ratio)	8–35 (6)[c,d] 4.7–6.5 (5)	5.3 (human)[c]
μmoles catecholamine/mg protein nitrogen	4.3–27.7 (5)	6.8–15.7
Cholesterol/lipid phosphorus (molar ratio)	0.5 (1)	0.48–0.53
Lysolecithin: % of total lipid phosphorus	11.7–23.8 (3)	7.1–16.8
% of soluble protein	63 (1)	57–74
% catecholamine released per hr at 37°C	27–33 (2)	25–30

[a] Adapted from Winkler, H. and Smith, A. D. Phaeochromocytoma and other catecholamine-producing tumours. Chap. 20. *In: Catecholamines.* Courtesy of Springer-Verlag, 1972, p. 908.

[b] The number of tumors investigated is indicated in parentheses. Except where indicated, values included in this table are taken from Blaschko, H., Jerrome, D. W., Robb-Smith, A. H. T., Smith, A. D., and Winkler, H., *Clin. Sci. 34:* 453–465, 1968; and from Winkler, H., Zeigler, E., and Strieder, N., *Klin. Wschr. 45:* 1238–1241, 1967.

[c] Values taken from Schümann, H. J., *Klin. Wschr. 38:* 11–13, 1960.

[d] Values taken from the following: Gélinas, R., Pellerin, J., and D'Iorio, A., *Rev. Canad. Biol. 16:* 445–450, 1957; Leduc, J. and D'Iorio, A., *Rev. Canad. Biol. 19:* 34–52, 1960; and Stjärne, L., Euler, U. S. von, and Lishajko, F., *Biochem. Pharmacol. 13:* 809–818, 1964.

Table 2.6 is adapted from a study by Winkler and Smith (1053); it compares the properties of chromaffin granules from pheochromocytoma with those from the adrenal medulla of the ox, horse, and pig. The fact that most of the catecholamines from the adrenal medulla or from pheochromocytomas are sedimentable indicates that these amines occur in particles; however, as pointed out by Smith and Winkler, it is uncertain whether the unbound catecholamines represent soluble cytoplasmic amines or whether they are due to a leakage from catecholamine-containing particles during homogenization and centrifugation (916). It has been shown that chromaffin granules of the normal adrenal medulla are very similar to those from pheochromocytomas with respect to fragility, weight, density, and electron microscopic appearance (82, 1053). Also, it has been shown that in several species norepinephrine-containing granules have a greater density than epinephrine-containing granules of the adrenal medulla (247, 873, 1051). Winkler

and Smith have emphasized that although some tumors have a deficiency of ATP in their chromaffin granules, others do not (1052). Furthermore, the catecholamine content (per mg of protein-N) varied over a wide range but was similar to that in normal granules which, they felt, indicated a normal capacity of tumor granules to store catecholamines (1052). In addition, water-soluble proteins and their amino acid content in adrenal chromaffin granules of animals and pheochromocytoma granules were identical (943).

Winkler and Smith indicated that some investigators have shown the catecholamine release from tumor and from normal adrenal medullary granules in vitro to be similar (Table 2.6); yet since these studies were performed on granules relatively rich in ATP, they suggest that comparative studies should also be performed on tumor granules deficient in ATP to ascertain whether catecholamine release can be affected by the level of ATP (1053).

Clinical evidence that catecholamine secretion from pheochromocytomas does not result from activation of the sympathetic nervous system was presented by Hermann and Mornex (437). They detected no increase in urinary excretion of catecholamines in two patients with pheochromocytoma in whom hypoglycemia was induced by injecting insulin. Hypoglycemia in the dog has been shown to activate sympathetic pathways in the central nervous system, which results in secretion of adrenal medullary catecholamines into the circulation (132).

Not infrequently, release of catecholamines from a pheochromocytoma with precipitation of a hypertensive crisis may be induced by some circumstance or maneuver which manipulates and compresses this richly vascularized tumor, and thereby expels catecholamine-rich blood into the circulation. It should be recalled that some tumors contain sinusoidal spaces (178) with blood rich in catecholamines which can easily gain access to the circulation.

The mechanism whereby certain drugs (e.g., histamine, glucagon, and tyramine) release catecholamines in patients with pheochromocytoma remains uncertain. Drugs may possibly cause a direct stimulation of chromaffin cells of these tumors and cause a liberation of catecholamines; or, possibly, some drugs may cause a significant vasodilatation with an increased blood flow to the tumor, which "flushes" catecholamine-rich blood into the circulation. The fact that histamine does not cause a significant increase in the catecholamine output from the perfused isolated adrenal gland (697) indicates that this drug, at least, does not directly stimulate normal adrenal medullary cells to secrete catecholamines (Table 2.5); furthermore, it seems unlikely that histamine would cause direct stimulation of pheochromocytoma cells. Histamine may, however, evoke adrenal medullary secretion by an indirect effect mediated through splanchnic stimulation (936); furthermore, it has been shown by a technique of intracellular recordings, that histamine may have a direct action on normal chromaffin cells in tissue culture (235).

It is reasonable to assume that the sympathetic nerve terminals in some patients with pheochromocytoma have accumulated excessive stores of catecholamines, such as occur in patients receiving norepinephrine infusion (691, 945), and that, therefore, any drug stimulating the sympathetic nervous system directly or reflexly (e.g., from hypotension caused by drug-induced vasodilatation) could release excessive quantities of catecholamines into the circulation and produce a hypertensive crisis.

Conceivably, of course, any combination of these mechanisms of catecholamine release may be operative.

It is possible that in some patients with pheochromocytoma hypertensive crises induced by emotional upset, pain, hyperventilation, or anesthesia may result from stimulation of the adrenergic nervous system and release of excessive stores of catecholamines from sympathetic nerve vesicles. Tilting a patient with pheochromocytoma from a horizontal to an upright position has been shown to cause an exaggerated increase in urinary norepinephrine not seen in subjects without this tumor (421). This latter finding might conceivably result purely from a mechanical effect (compression of the tumor with expulsion of blood); however, reflex activation of the adrenergic system might also account for the results.

Winkler and Smith have presented an interesting explanation of why most pheochromocytomas continually release catecholamines without any apparent stimulus (1053). They acknowledge the possibility that exocytosis may occur in some tumors as it does in cells of the normal adrenal medulla; however, somewhat contradicting this concept is (1) the lack in these tumors of any nervous innervation (which initiates events culminating in exocytosis in the normal medullary cells), and (2) the much faster catecholamine turnover in tumors (sometimes 100 times greater) than in the normal adrenal medulla. Further, it has been reasoned that the striking increase in synthesis of catecholamines and proteins in some tumors would require a pronounced increase in the amount of endoplasmic reticulum, yet there is no morphologic evidence for this (1053).

Winkler and Smith have proposed that release of catecholamines from cells of pheochromocytomas may occur by diffusion through the cytoplasm and cell wall (1053). They postulated that the chromaffin storage granules (vesicles) may be filled to capacity and be unable to accommodate the rapidly synthesized catecholamines. In support of this contention they cite reports by Roth and coworkers and Nagatsu and coworkers which indicate that the enzyme tyrosine hydroxylase in pheochromocytomas lacks the sensitivity to feed-back inhibition found in the normal adrenal medulla (1053). They also cited the finding of Sjoerdsma and coworkers that α-methyltyrosine, an inhibitor of tyrosine hydroxylase, reduces the blood pressure and urinary catecholamines of patients with pheochromocytoma, whereas it does not have this effect with similar doses in other hypertensives (908). This finding was felt to suggest that the rate of release of catecholamines from pheochromocytomas depends on the rate of biosynthesis of these amines rather than on the size of the store.

Crout and Sjoerdsma (185, 195) reported studies on 22 patients with single pheochromocytomas and classified the tumors into two types (Table 2.7): (a) small tumors with "low" contents of catecholamines and rapid turnover rates (i.e., they released 68 percent of their catecholamine content per day) which released mainly unmetabolized catecholamines into the circulation (deduced by a relatively low ratio of concentrations of metabolites to catecholamines in the urine), and (b) relatively large tumors with "high" contents of catecholamines and slow turnover rates (i.e., they released 8.1 percent of their catecholamine content per day) which released mainly metabolized catecholamines into the circulation (deduced by a relatively high ratio of metabolites to catecholamines in the urine). Tumors classified in the low group had a mean rate of catecholamine turnover which was eight times greater than that of the tumors in the high group (195). The classification of pheochromocytomas into relatively small tumors with rapid catecholamine turnover and relatively large tumors with slow catecholamine turnover is graphically depicted in Figure 2.8. It is therefore no surprise that there is little if any correlation between the hormonal content of these tumors and the severity of symptoms.

The precise nature of the biochemical differences in these tumors is not clear, although they must be in part related to differences in storage and binding of the catecholamines. The paradox that small pheochromocytomas frequently produce the most pronounced

Table 2.7 *Tumor and Urinary Data in Two Groups of Patients with Pheochromocytoma*[a]

	Type of tumor[b,c]	
	"Low"	*"High"*
Tumor		
Number studied	13	9
Total NE + E Content (mg)	53 ± 6.9	2355 ± 1150
Weight of tumor (g)	29 ± 8.6	218 ± 89
% of NE + E in tumor released/day	68 ± 16	8.1 ± 2.4
Urine		
Total metabolites (mg/day)	28 ± 4.7	142 ± 75
NE + E (mg/day)	1.6 ± 0.32	1.2 ± 0.63
NE + E (as % of total)	5.1 ± 0.59	1.7 ± 0.63

[a] Modified from Crout, J. R. Chap. I. Catecholamine Metabolism in Pheochromocytoma and Essential Hypertension. *In: Hormones and Hypertension.* Courtesy of C. C. Thomas, 1966, p. 25. Data from Crout, J. R. and Sjoerdsma, A. *J. Clin. Invest. 43:* 94–102, 1964.

[b] Tumors were arbitrarily grouped on the basis of their total content of NE + E; tumors in the "low" group contained less than 100 mg total (range = 19 to 87 mg), and tumors in the high group contained more than 100 mg total (range = 329 to 10,600 mg).

[c] Numbers following ± are standard errors of the mean.

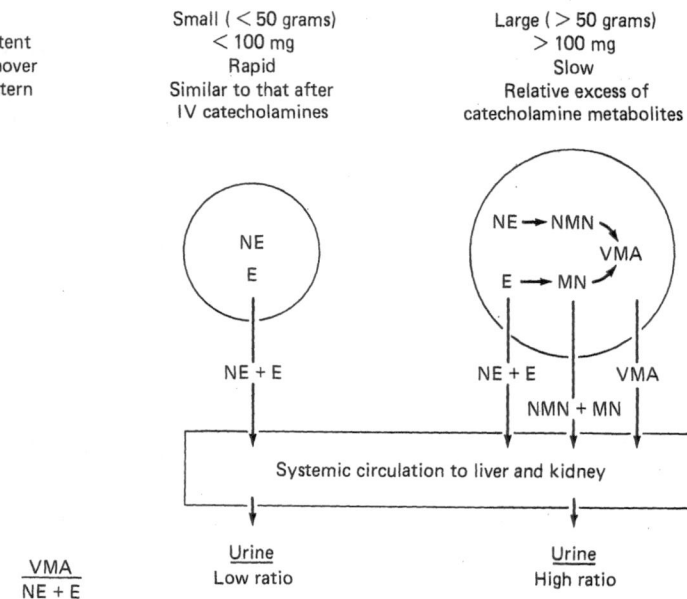

Tumor	Small (< 50 grams)	Large (> 50 grams)
Catecholamine content	< 100 mg	> 100 mg
Catecholamine turnover	Rapid	Slow
Urine excretion pattern	Similar to that after IV catecholamines	Relative excess of catecholamine metabolites

$$\frac{VMA}{NE + E}$$

Urine
Low ratio

Urine
High ratio

Fig. 2.8 Schematic illustration of the mechanism by which degradation of catecholamines within tumor produces a greater relative increase in urinary VMA than in free catecholamines. Tumor typical of "low" group in Table 2.7 is on left, and tumor representative of "high" group is on right. NE=norepinephrine; E=epinephrine; NMN=normetanephrine; MN=metanephrine; VMA=vanilmandelic acid. Adapted from Crout, J. R. Chap. I. Catecholamine metabolism in pheochromocytoma and essential hypertension. In: *Hormones and Hypertension.* Courtesy of C. C. Thomas, 1966, p. 24.

symptoms and may be discovered earlier than large tumors can be explained on a biochemical basis. If a pheochromocytoma metabolizes much of its catecholamines (perhaps up to 90 percent in tumors with slow turnover, according to Crout), the patient is protected to some degree from the pharmacologic and physiologic effects these amines exert when released into the circulation; however, as mentioned by Crout, the patient is placed in greater jeopardy from the standpoint of neoplasia and the compression effects of an expanding tumor mass (185). It is indeed fortunate that the larger tumors retain the enzymatic machinery for inactivating catecholamines in situ, since, if this protective mechanism were lost, the patient would most certainly succumb to massive liberations of catecholamines into the circulation. This latter point is worth recalling before administering blockers of the enzymes which catabolize catecholamines (e.g., MAO inhibitors) to hypertensive patients, even if the existence of pheochromocytoma is extremely remote. Whether these catabolic enzymes appear de novo or increase in concentration relatively more than do the catecholamines as pheo-

chromocytomas increase in size is unknown. However, in the great majority of patients, symptomatic attacks become more frequent and sometimes more severe. Only on extremely rare occasions do symptomatic attacks appear to lessen or cease to occur. These observations suggest that as these tumors grow the catabolic enzymes do not appear de novo and do not increase relatively more than do catecholamines.

Crout has stated that the pheochromocytomas harbored by children are almost always small in size and have a rapid turnover rate of catecholamines. In addition, he has pointed out that tumors producing excessive amounts of epinephrine as well as norepinephrine are more apt to be large and have a slow rate of turnover. With these exceptions, he observed little correlation between the type of tumor and the patient's age, sex, or clinical manifestations (185).

Winkler and Smith have cited the observations of Crout and Sjoerdsma as further evidence supporting the hypothesis that the bulk of the catecholamines released by pheochromocytomas bypass the storage granule (1053). They reasoned that tumors metabolizing much of their catecholamines in situ must contain considerable quantities of catecholamines which are not protected by the granule membrane. They suggested that the catecholamines in these pheochromocytomas are not secreted by exocytosis but bypass the storage site and diffuse out of the cell (1053). Furthermore they felt that even in small tumors with a rapid catecholamine turnover, secretion by exocytosis was unlikely. The observation that the chromaffin reaction is only rarely sharply localized in catecholamine-secreting tumors (in contradistinction to the relatively sharp localization seen in cells of the normal adrenal medulla) (370) is consistent with the hypothesis of secretion via diffusion proposed by Winkler and Smith.

The finding that serum DBH was not elevated in patients with pheochromocytoma is additional evidence that these tumors are not innervated and that exocytosis is not significantly involved in secretion of their catecholamines (342). It is noteworthy that in three of 11 patients with pheochromocytoma studied by Geffen and associates there was a relatively small decrease in plasma DBH concentrations postoperatively (342); therefore, according to the finding of these investigators, only a small degree of exocytosis may occur in some of these tumors. However, Lovenberg and coworkers have found serum DBH levels in six patients with pheochromocytoma to vary from the upper range of normal to about two times this upper limit (587). In two of these patients, removal of the tumor was accompanied by a decrease in serum DBH activity from 500 units/ml to 50 units/ml in one patient, and from 600 units/ml to 250 units/ml in the other. In the latter patient the half-life of DBH activity in plasma was found to be about 8 hr (587). Bohuon and associates (88) have found results similar to those reported by Lovenberg and coworkers. More recently, Stone and associates reported studies on eight patients with pheochromocytoma. They found that despite very elevated urinary catecholamine concentrations preoperatively the mean concentration of serum DBH was not significantly different from that of apparently healthy subjects. No remarkable change in DBH concentration was observed in three of four patients studied 1 week after tumors were removed; in the

fourth patient, however, there was a 60 percent decrease in serum DBH activity. They concluded that although diffusion across plasma membranes is the predominant mechanism of catecholamine release from pheochromocytomas, tumor heterogeneity may exist and that exocytosis may contribute to catecholamine release in some patients (940a). The question of exocytosis and DBH activity in patients with pheochromocytoma has apparently not been completely answered. It appears probable that certain pheochromocytomas exhibit some degree of exocytosis, whereas others do not. However, it is reasonable to imagine that exocytosis occurs to a small degree continuously in all these tumors due to spontaneous fusion of the chromaffin granule membrane with the plasma membrane.

Finally, the possibility of a relative lack of metabolizing enzymes within the tumor, which would permit diffusion of amines out of the cell without much degradation, has been proposed as an alternative mechanism causing continuous excessive catecholamine secretion (1053). This latter possibility has not been adequately explored.

In summary, the hypothesis has been presented that (1) catecholamine synthesis in pheochromocytomas is disassociated from their storage in chromaffin granules and that the released catecholamines bypass the storage granules, and (2) that the rate of release is dependent upon the rate of synthesis (1052). This has been contrasted to the normal adrenal, where catecholamine secretion rate is controlled by the activity of the nerves stimulating the chromaffin cells. Winkler and Smith have also suggested another minor route for release of catecholamines based on the finding that lysosomes of tumor cells often contain partly digested chromaffin granules (1052). Lysosomal destruction of granule membrane would permit the catecholamine content to escape from the granule and to diffuse out of the cell. The mechanism of catecholamine secretion from the normal adrenal medulla and the mechanism of release from pheochromocytomas suggested by Winkler and Smith are depicted in Figure 2.9.

The mechanism of catecholamine release proposed by Winkler and Smith would explain the continuous secretion of catechol-

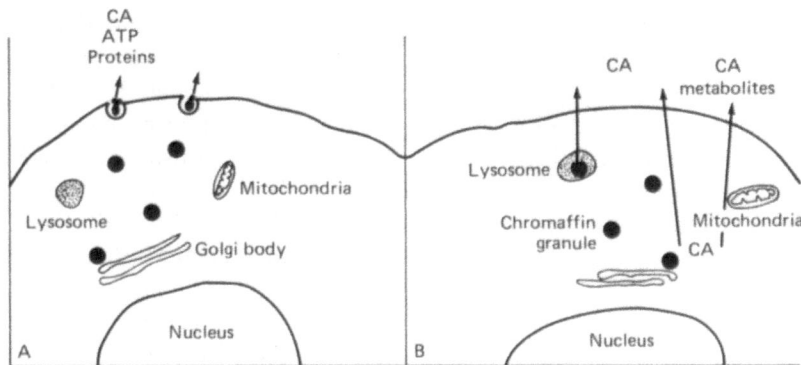

Fig. 2.9 Release of catecholamines (CA) from chromaffin cells of (A) normal adrenal medulla and (B) pheochromocytoma. A. Catecholamines are stored and transported in chromaffin granules and are secreted directly from the granules. B. Catecholamines are released after diffusion across the cell, bypassing the chromaffin granules (center arrow); some are metabolized by mitochondrial monamine oxidase (right arrow); some might also be released (left arrow) after digestion of chromaffin granules in lysosomes. From Winkler, E. and Smith, A. D., *Lancet 1:* 794, 1968.

amines which occurs with some pheochromocytomas; however, the sudden release of catecholamines into the circulation must be precipitated by other mechanisms. Sudden release of catecholamines may result from mechanical compression of a pheochromocytoma by a physical maneuver or palpation of the tumor. Winkler and Smith suggested an additional explanation for hypertensive crises that was mentioned previously. They postulated that increased amounts of catecholamines may accumulate in sympathetic nerves in patients with pheochromocytoma [as occurs during infusions of catecholamines (691)]. Any stimulus which activates the sympathetic nervous system might then release a greater-than-normal amount of catecholamines into the circulation, thereby causing a hypertensive crisis (1052).

In support of this latter hypothesis, Winkler and Smith cited the work of Engelman and Sjoerdsma, which revealed that tyramine injected into patients with pheochromocytoma caused an increased excretion of urinary catecholamines and their metabolites, an effect which persisted for several days after the tumors had been removed (274). In keeping with these findings, we found elevated venous plasma catecholamines in one patient on the sixth and the 10th days following removal of a pheochromocytoma, whereas the values were normal when the patient was seen 25 months postoperatively (624, p. 90).

On the other hand, we have noted that the cold pressor test (447), which activates the sympathetic nervous system, has been performed innumerable times in patients with pheochromocytoma without inducing a severe symptomatic hypertensive crisis. This observation agrees with the finding of Greer and associates that 76 percent of their patients with this tumor had a normal cold pressor response (i.e., the systolic and diastolic pressure elevations were less than 20 and 15 mmHg, respectively, as occurs in about 82 percent of normal subjects (400). It should be mentioned parenthetically that one patient with pheochromocytoma has been reported in whom the cold pressor test caused no blood pressure rise on one occasion, and a rise of 40/36 mmHg on another occasion (338).

It is only with the intravenous administration of a provocative agent (e.g., histamine or glucagon) that a typical hypertensive "attack" is induced. These findings suggest that patients with pheochromocytoma on whom the cold pressor test was performed either did not have excessive amounts of catecholamines in their sympathetic nerves or that this type of cold stress did not cause a release of the accumulated amines. Since nearly all patients on whom the cold pressor test was performed had paroxysmal rather than sustained hypertension, it is probable that the paroxysmal group, with only periodic secretion of their tumors, may have little or no accumulation of catecholamines in their sympathetic nerves.

Origin, Pathopharmacology, and Pathology

CHAPTER THREE

NOMENCLATURE

The term "pheochromocytoma," suggested in 1912 by Pick (751), derives from the chemical and pathologic characteristics of the cell ["pheochromocyte" = a cell which takes on a "dusky" color (from the Greek: *phaios*, meaning dusky + *chroma*, meaning color) when exposed to chromium salts, and "cytoma" = tumor]. It is a tumor of neuroectodermal origin which arises from the chromaffin cells (pheochromocytes) of the sympathoadrenal system. For this reason the tumors are sometimes referred to as chromaffinomas, or adrenergic tumors. The term "chromaffinoma" indicates a tumor with cells having an affinity for chromium salts (i.e., contact with buffered dichromate or dichromate in formalin causes the cells to be stained brown). The term "paraganglioma" has also been used to characterize pheochromocytomas originating in chromaffin cells adjacent to sympathetic ganglia or in other extraadrenal sites. Because of the confusing nomenclature, it has been proposed that these tumors having the same histologic pattern, regardless of location, be designated "paragangliomas," chromaffin or nonchromaffin type, and functional or nonfunctional (561). However, we believe that it is less confusing if all chromaffinomas which secrete catecholamines and cause manifestations of excess circulating catecholamines be regarded as pheochromocytomas and that subclassification be avoided.

EXTRAADRENAL PARAGANGLIOMAS OF UNCERTAIN CLASSIFICATION

Because of the continuing uncertainty in the classification of some extraadrenal paragangliomas, a detailed discussion of their origin, location, cytologic features, and clinical manifestations is presented herein.

Recently, an excellent review of the tumors of the extraadrenal paraganglion system (including chemoreceptors) was presented by Glenner and Grimley (370). They pointed out that this system can be grouped on the basis of anatomic distribution, innervation, and microscopic structure into four interrelated "families," as follows: (1) *branchiomeric;* (2) *intravagal;* (3) *aorticosympathetic;* and (4) *visceral-autonomic paraganglia.*

The *branchiomeric* group includes jugulotympanic, intercarotid (carotid body), subclavian, laryngeal, coronary, aorticopulmonary (which includes the aortic body), pulmonary, and perhaps orbital paraganglia; all of these paraganglia appear intimately associated with blood vessels. On the other hand, *intravagal paraganglia,* occurring along the distribution of the vagus nerve (interior to the perineurium), are not intimately associated with blood vessels; they have been described within the jugular ganglion, ganglion nodosum, and just inferior to the ganglion nodosum. (The branchiomeric and intravagal paraganglia are located in the head, neck, and superior mediastinum; their sites are indicated in Figure 3.1. Histologically branchiomeric and intravagal paraganglia are identical, but they can be distinguished from the adrenal medulla by the presence and "the arrangement of the chief cells (type 1 cells, epithelioid cells, or glomus cells) in compact microscopic nests (Zellballen). This organization reflects the presence of a second cell type known as sustentacular or type 2 cells, and they are homologous to the satellite cells of autonomic ganglia" (370) (Fig. 3.2).

Physiologic experiments have indicated that the carotid and aortic bodies are sensitive to fluctuations in pH and arterial oxygen tension (167), and that these paraganglia may

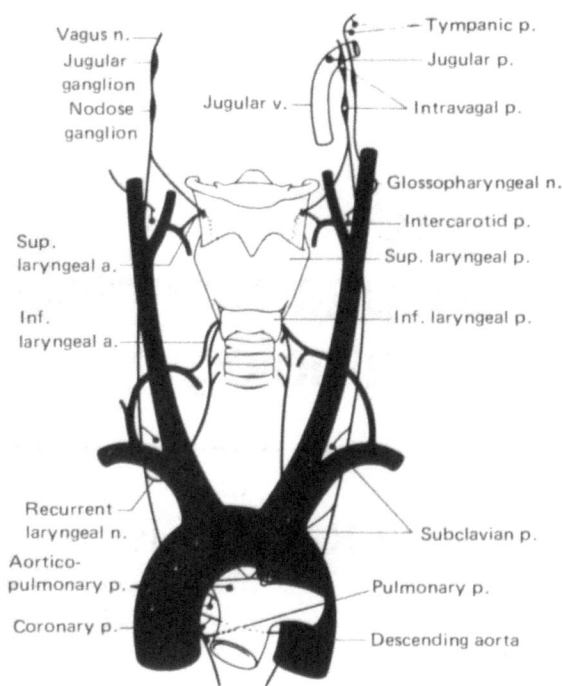

Fig. 3.1 Sites of branchiomeric and intravagal paraganglia. This diagram represents the branchiomeric and intravagal paraganglia and their anatomic relationships. a, artery; v, vein; p, paraganglia. (Based upon drawing for Fig. 6 from Kleinsasser, O. Das glomus laryngicum inferior. *Arch. Klin. Exp. Ohren Nasen, Kehlkopfheilkd. 184:* 214–225, 1964. Munich: J. F. Bergmann Verlagsbuch.) From Glenner, G. G. and Grimley, P. M. Tumors of the extraadrenal paraganglion system (including chemoreceptors). In: *Atlas of Tumor Pathology,* second series, fascicle 9. Courtesy of Armed Forces Institute of Pathology, 1974, p. 18.

be important in regulating the cardiorespiratory system in conditions associated with hypoxia [e.g., cardiovascular or pulmonary insufficiency, high altitudes, or sleep (74, 167, 405, 439)]. It is particularly fascinating that conditions causing hypoxemia have been shown to be associated with remarkable hyperplasia and enlargement of the carotid body (21, 250–252, 429).

The *aorticosympathetic paraganglia,* which are associated with the ganglia of the sympathetic chain and collateral ganglia, have cytologic features which resemble either the pheochromocytes of the adrenal medulla (e.g., the paraganglia associated with the superior cervical ganglia), or, if they contain chief and sustentacular cells, resemble the branchiomeric and intravagal paraganglia (e.g., the abdominal preaortic paraganglia). It is therefore understandable that paragangliomas in

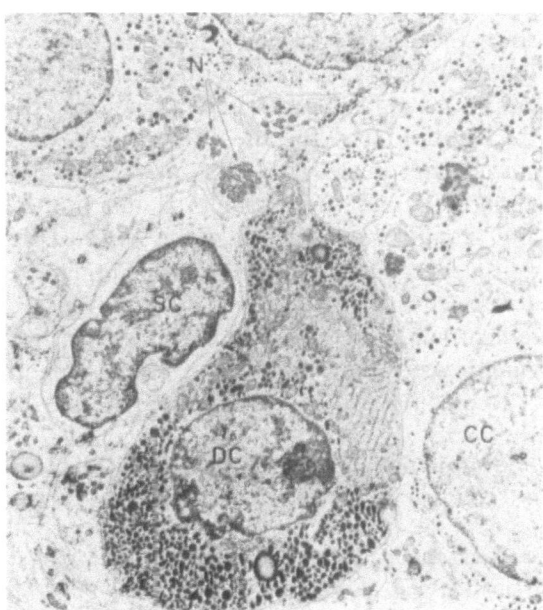

Fig. 3.2 Carotid body chief cell types. A dark variety of chief cell is situated adjacent to several typical chief cells. Note the relatively larger and more angular granules in the dark cell. CC=typical chief cell; SC=sustentacular cell; DC=dark variety of chief cell; N=nerve fibers in cross section (11,500×). From Glenner, G. G. and Grimley, P.M. Tumors of the extraadrenal paraganglion system (including chemoreceptors). In: *Atlas of Tumor Pathology*, second series, fascicle 9. Courtesy of Armed Forces Institute of Pathology, 1974, p. 22.

the retroperitoneum may have features of either pheochromocytomas or paragangliomas of the carotid-jugulare type (370).

The *visceral-autonomic paraganglia* have not been adequately characterized, but seem to occur in association with visceral organs and blood vessels (e.g., in the interatrial septum of the heart, in the liver hilus, in the bladder wall, in association with the mesenteric vessels, and perhaps in relation to the duodenal wall and peripheral vessels). Some of these structures have cells which appear to contain dense-cored vesicles and catecholamines (370).

It has been stated that "all paraganglia, including those which act as chemoreceptors, store catecholamines which are facultatively sequestered in dense-cored granules of the chief cells," and that "functional catecholamine-secreting neoplasms may arise in any paraganglion" (370). Controversy on these assertions continues to exist. It has been

claimed that catecholamines are present in human carotid bodies (413) and carotid body tumors (60, 368, 412, 772), and in glomus jugulare tumors (37, 239). In a study of the cytoplasmic granules in human specimens from seven carotid bodies, nine carotid body tumors, and six glomus jugulare tumors, Campella and Solcia demonstrated the presence of serotonin in a small proportion of carotid body cells, but failed to unequivocally detect catecholamines (134).

With regard to the chromaffin reaction, Glenner and Grimley and others have observed that even in the catecholamine-secreting pheochromocytoma the chromaffin reaction may not be demonstrable. They have suggested that the explanation for this observation "may relate to (1) differences in the nature and integrity of the protein granule retaining the reactive compound in cells from different tissues and tumors; (2) the concentration of the compound within the cells; or (3) the susceptibility of depletion of the store of catecholamines prior to histologic fixation." They have accordingly emphasized, as have others, that the absence of a positive chromaffin reaction cannot be considered solid evidence of the absence of a catecholamine or an indoleamine (370).

In a personal conversation, Dr. Raffaele Lattes (Chairman of the Department of Surgical Pathology, Columbia Medical Center, New York) cautioned that it may often be difficult, if not impossible, to verify the origin of paragangliomas in some locations. For example, a neoplasm near the region of the bifurcation of the common carotid artery may be considered a carotid body tumor when in fact it has its origin from other paraganglion cells. Dr. Lattes has had a wide and pioneering experience in the classification of nonchromaffin paragangliomas, including carotid body-like tumors (chemodectomas) (549, 550). The following is a personal communication regarding his concept of these tumors:

These are tumors originating, in different anatomic regions, from normal but poorly known structures. They morphologically resemble the carotid body situated at the bifurcation of the common carotid artery. It is probable that their main function is analogous to that of the carotid body, namely, that of chemoreceptor. Recently however, there has accumulated some evidence that these structures can contain catecholamines. Electron microscopically they show neuroendocrine granules in the chief cells. Likewise tumors originating from these structures occasionally can be shown by fluorescence microscopy and ultrastructural study to contain neuroendocrine granules of the norepinephrine type.

These structures, and their tumors, are associated with cranial nerves and with vessels of embryonic branchial arch origin. They have been found not only at the carotid bifurcation, but also in the ganglion nodosum of the vagus nerve, in the middle ear (tympanic nerve), the bulb of the jugular vein, the adventitia of the aortic arch and of the major pulmonary vessels, the paralaryngeal region, and the orbit. These tumors can be multicentric; this feature should not be interpreted as a proof that they can metastasize. A true malignant behavior for these tumors is extremely rare. The majority—if not all—of these tumors are nonfunctional, as contrasted with the chromaffin paragangliomas or pheochromocytomas.

Table 3.1 reveals the locations of nonchromaffin paragangliomas in a series of 253 cases studied at Columbia Medical Center. The largest number of these tumors occurred in the middle ear (43 percent) and the carotid body (34 percent); the third most common site was the aortic body (10 percent).

It is generally agreed that a positive chromaffin reaction in a cell is highly suggestive, although not absolute proof, that a catechol-

amine or an indoleamine is present; however, since the absence of the chromaffin reaction does not totally exclude the presence of these amines, Glenner and Grimley have expressed the opinion that the use of the term "nonchromaffin" to describe some of the paraganglion cells and their tumors is too limiting and should be discarded. They stressed the defect in a nosology based on dichromate reaction by citing the occasional occurrence of nonchromaffin catecholamine-secreting paragangliomas and adrenal medullary tumors.

According to Glenner and Grimley (370):

One of the outstanding light microscopic features of paragangliomas is their tendency to reproduce the architecture of the normal gland with sufficient fidelity that the overall organoid pattern is maintained. This usually gives the impression that the tumor represents a glandular hyperplasia or a proliferative caricature of the tissue of origin. A further feature is the frequently poor preservation or fixation of the cellular component of the tumor, which increases the difficulty in diagnosis. These tumors are characterized also by the absence of mucin and such cellular configurations as ribbons, festoons, and rosettes. Although in most cases the tumors are well defined by a condensation of connective tissue, they, like their organ of origin, do not have a prominent capsule. The surrounding connective tissue contains myelinated and nonmyelinated nerves, arteries, veins, lymphoreticular and mast cells, and occasional nerve bundles and ganglion cells. Nerve fibers have not been observed by electron microscopy within the tumor mass.

Most paragangliomas are quite vascular (with large or small blood spaces), and they may contain hemorrhagic foci and hemosiderin deposits. Nests of ovoid to polyhedral cells may appear in an alveolar pattern circumscribed by a reticulum network or occasionally bounded by hyaline or connective tissue bands; the organoid arrangement of these nests may "reproduce the classic 'Zellballen,' or basket pattern of the normal gland" (370). The cells have an eosinophilic cytoplasm (of variable staining intensity), and are mainly derived from chief cells; however, they exhibit greater pleomorphism than the normal cells. The nuclei of the tumor cells are ovoid or round and vary from vesicular to hyperchromatic; mitoses and cells resembling the normal sustacular cells are rarely

Table 3.1 *Nonchromaffin Paraganglioma*[a]

Location	No.
Carotid body (1 malignant)	85
Ganglion nodosum	9
Middle ear: glomus jugulare, glomus tympanicum (17 locally invasive, 1 with distant metastasis)	110
Larynx	3
Hypopharynx	3
Orbit	1
Bronchus and lung	3
Aortic body	25
Retroperitoneum	11
Multicentric	3
Total	253

[a] Courtesy of Dr. Raffaele Lattes, Columbia Presbyterian Medical Center, New York City, unpublished data on 253 cases recorded in the files of Surgical Pathology, College of Physicians and Surgeons (1974).

seen in paragangliomas, and the normal relationship of nerve fibers to chief cell nests is lacking. "Cellular vacuolization, shrinkage and pyknotic nuclei are a usual fixation artifact" (370).

Representative microscopic sections of paraganglions from four different sites are shown in Figure 3.3 (see p. 71).

Ultrastructural studies reveal cytoplasmic granules (varying from 100 to 300 μm in diameter—usually 150 μm) similar to those seen in the normal chief cells. These granules are characteristic of paragangliomas and, according to Grimley and Glenner, and Capella and Solcia, some of the larger granules may represent abnormal lysosomal fusion or concentrations of the primary secretory material (134, 403). A characteristic formalin-induced yellow-green fluorescence, consistent with the presence of catecholamines, may be demonstrated in some paragangliomas (Fig. 3.4, p. 72).

It may be helpful to the clinician to mention some of the clinical features encountered in patients with paragangliomas located in the neck or head. Tumors in these locations usually present with unique signs and symptoms resulting from compression of adjacent structures, although, rarely, they may cause manifestations of excessive circulating catecholamines. Since their classification still remains unsettled, a brief discussion of the clinical features of branchiomeric and intravagal paragangliomas is, therefore, included in this section rather than under manifestations of pheochromocytoma. The following remarks are based on the report by Glenner and Grimley in their monograph on extraadrenal paragangliomas:

Carotid Body Paraganglioma It is noteworthy that carotid body paragangliomas occur 10 times more frequently in Peruvians living at very high altitudes than in those living at sea level; these tumors also are reported more frequently at high altitudes in Colorado and Mexico. It has been postulated that hypoxia-induced hyperplasia of the carotid body may predispose to neoplastic transformation. Tumors are usually 3 to 6 cm in diameter but may be 15 cm or greater; their location at the bifurcation of the common carotid artery may be of value in the differential diagnosis.

Glenner and associates first described a norepinephrine-secreting carotid body tumor in 1961 (368, 369). This tumor contained 1.5 mg of norepinephrine per g of tissue and caused clinical manifestations typical of pheochromocytoma. Subsequently, two tumors secreting both norepinephrine and epinephrine (60, 332), and one tumor which secreted only norepinephrine (412) have been reported. Carotid body tumors containing norepinephrine may be capable of mimicking a pheochromocytoma.

Tumors have been reported in patients from 7 to 75 years of age, with an average age of 45 years. There is no sex predilection. Extension to the hypopharynx can cause hoarseness; pressure on cranial or cervical sympathetic nerves can produce vocal cord and/or facial paralysis and Horner's syndrome. A bruit is often heard over the mass, which is firm and does not move on swallowing. Carotid angiography can be a most valuable diagnostic aid. (See Preoperative Localization of Tumor—Radiographic Techniques, in Chapter 6).

Although malignancy in carotid body tumors has been reported as occurring in only 6.4 percent of all cases (932), yet in one series of 30 cases, followed for an average of 11 years, the incidence of malignancy was 23 percent. Metastases occur in regional lymph nodes and visceral organs, particularly in the lungs, and in the skeleton. The protracted interval between diagnosis of the primary tumor and the appearance of metastases (up to 35 years) has been emphasized (104). Only one malignant tumor which appeared to be functioning (secreting norepinephrine) has been reported. As is the case with pheochromocytoma, there are no reliable cytologic criteria to differentiate a malignant from a benign paraganglioma of the carotid body. Although extremely rare, the concurrence of carotid body tumor and pheochromocytoma has been reported (854).

Jugular Paraganglioma Paraganglia located along the course of the tympanic branch of the glossopharyngeal nerve or the auricular branch of the vagus nerve give rise to the jugular paraganglioma (glomus jugulare tumor), which is the most common tumor of the middle ear. Microscopically, it is identical to the carotid body tumors. This tumor may erode the floor of the hypotympanum and present as a mass in the middle ear or external canal, and it may cause enlargement of the jugular foramen and extend to the base of the skull. It has also been reported extending into the jugular vein and even as far as the heart (151). About 40 percent of these tumors extend intracranially.

Three functioning jugular paragangliomas have been reported and each of these secreted norepinephrine and caused clinical manifestations typical of pheochromocytomas. One of these tumors contained 14.1 mg norepinephrine and 0.55 mg epinephrine per g of tumor, whereas the others were found to contain only norepinephrine.

These tumors occur at any age, but most frequently between 25 and 65 years (average, about 50 years). Three-fourths of tumors occur in women.

Otologic signs and symptoms are common and consist of an aural polyp with a tendency to bleed following slight trauma, progressive loss of hearing, a sensation of fullness or pounding in the ear, chronic ear discharge, and facial paralysis and pain. With invasion of the posterior fossa, neurologic symptoms such as dysphagia and hoarseness may become manifest; invasion of the temporal bone may cause paralysis of the ninth through the 12th cranial nerves, whereas invasion of the mastoid may cause a facial nerve palsy. A high cervical mass may be palpated and a bruit may be detectable. Metastases to cervical lymph nodes and even to the liver have been reported (550).

Laryngeal Paraganglioma Laryngeal paraganglioma arise above the anterior end of the vocal cords, or between the thyroid and cricoid cartilage, or from paraganglia within the recurrent branch of the vagus nerve (intravagal paraganglioma). These soft and often encapsulated tumors vary in size from 6 mm to 6 cm and are located in the supraglottic or subglottic (tracheal) region. In addition to the usual alveolar pattern, there may be an eosinophilic fibrous connective tissue stroma surrounding nests, cords, and trabeculae of chief cells. Of the 12 patients reported to have laryngeal paraganglioma, only one had a metastasis (to a lymph node). The age of the

patients ranged from 14 to 67 years and no sex predisposition was apparent.

Patients may develop hoarseness and experience throat pain which occasionally is spasmodic and induced by swallowing. Because of the tendency of these lesions to bleed, biopsy must be performed with great caution. These tumors have not been reported to cause clinical manifestations associated with excess circulating catecholamines.

Supraaortic and Aorticopulmonary Paragangliomas Paragangliomas occurring in the anterior mediastinum above the bifurcation of the pulmonary artery or below the aortic arch may arise from paraganglia having a chemoreceptor function. Most frequently these tumors are attached to or located within the pericardium but they may lie anterior to the aorta. Occasionally they extend into the supraclavicular region. One tumor was found between the esophagus and the lower end of the trachea, and another encircled the subclavian artery. Usually, aortic body tumors are lobulated and measure 2 to 12 cm in length. Thirty cases had been reported up to 1974. Microscopically, aortic body tumors often have chief cells that appear larger than those of carotid body tumors (549); otherwise aortic and pulmonary paragangliomas are indistinguishable from carotid body tumors. Metastases may occur to regional lymph nodes. Because of their location and impingement on adjacent structures, respiratory distress is the most common symptom. A chest x-ray reveals that the mass is in the anterior mediastinum, and venography usually demonstrates that the mass is distinct from the aorta. Duke and associates described a norepinephrine-secreting glomic tissue tumor (chemodectoma) in a patient with hypertension. Their patient had both an aortic body tumor and a retroperitoneal paraganglioma (240).

Pulmonary Paraganglioma Pulmonary paragangliomas occur in the lung parenchyma and near the lung hilus. Some occur just beneath the visceral pleura and may reach 4 cm in size. Microscopically some of these tumors may resemble carotid body tumors; however, a variety of cellular patterns are seen and sometimes the nodules are composed mainly of spindle cells. Multiple minute pulmonary nodules were found most commonly in women (ranging in age from 39 to 84 years). Clinical symptomatology of excessive circulating catecholamines related to these paragangliomas has not been observed and no malignancies have been reported.

Orbital Paraganglioma Up to 1974 only five orbital paragangliomas (ranging in size from 2.4 to 4 cm) had been reported; these appeared in the retrobulbar area or involved the rectus muscles. Microscopically, they appear similar to carotid body tumors. No sex predilection was evident in these tumors, which were reported in patients ranging from 4 to 55 years (average, 38 years). Throbbing orbital pain and visual loss are the most common symptoms. Glaucoma can occur and macular degeneration may be observed if the optic nerve is involved. Malignant transformation does not seem to occur. Clinical manifestations of excess circulating catecholamines have not been reported.

Intravagal Paraganglioma Paragangliomas of the vagus nerve usually arise within the perineurium, just below or at the ganglion nodosum and near the jugular foramen. One tumor was described near the carotid bifurcation. They vary from 2 to 6.5 cm in size. Microscopically, they are similar to carotid body paragangliomas except for the frequent presence of prominent collagenous septa, which often are hyalinized. Dense core granules were identified in one of these tumors. Levit and associates have reported a functional tumor of the vagus nerve (571).

Twenty-six of 37 patients reported in the literature up to 1974 were women. Ages of patients ranged from 18 to 65 years (average, 37 years). Hoarseness and dysphagia (744) were often experienced and the most frequent finding was a mass in the anterolateral aspect of the neck, just beneath the ear. Medial displacement of peritonsillar structures may occur, and occasionally the tumor may bulge in the nasopharynx and extend to the base of the skull. Angiography is a valuable diagnostic aid. Extension of these paragangliomas into the cranium is a frequent cause of death. They have been reported to metastasize to the skull, vertebrae, and pelvis.

COMMENT
The exact classification of extraadrenal paragangliomas remains unsettled. Most of these are benign and nonfunctional. However, the important point to remember is that some of these tumors are capable of synthesizing and secreting catecholamines into the circulation. Consequently, these functional tumors may cause sustained and/or paroxysmal hypertension and other manifestations related to excessive concentrations of catecholamines in the circulation. One should, therefore, constantly keep in mind that functioning paragangliomas in a variety of locations may produce manifestations identical to those encountered with a functioning pheochromocytoma of the adrenal gland.

EMBRYOLOGY

The embryonic development of adrenergic cells and tumors is indicated in Figure 3.5. The sympathetic ganglia are formed in the fetus by cells of the neural crest which migrate from the thoracic region of the crest about the fifth week and locate dorsolaterally to the aorta to form the sympathetic chains (547). Some sympathetic neuroblasts migrate anterior to the aorta to form other ganglia. A second migration of neural crest cells occurs during the seventh week; they develop an affinity for chromium salts and have therefore been designated pheochromoblasts (597). Groups of these cells invade the developing adrenal cortex, which is of mesodermal origin, and form the adrenal medulla (438). Some pheochromoblasts form clusters of cells which become mature pheochromocytes at various levels of the paravertebral region, in the para-aortic area, and near the aortic bifurcation. Neuroblasts also migrate into the developing adrenal medulla and become mature sympathetic ganglion cells (438).

Certain cells of the neural crest form the primitive cell, the sympathogonia, which has a dense nucleus, rich in chromatin (Fig. 3.5). Whether this cell can differentiate into a sympathogonioma (a primitive cell neoplasm) is not entirely clear. The sympathogonia cell does, however, give rise to the sympathoblast (i.e., neuroblast, which is larger and contains

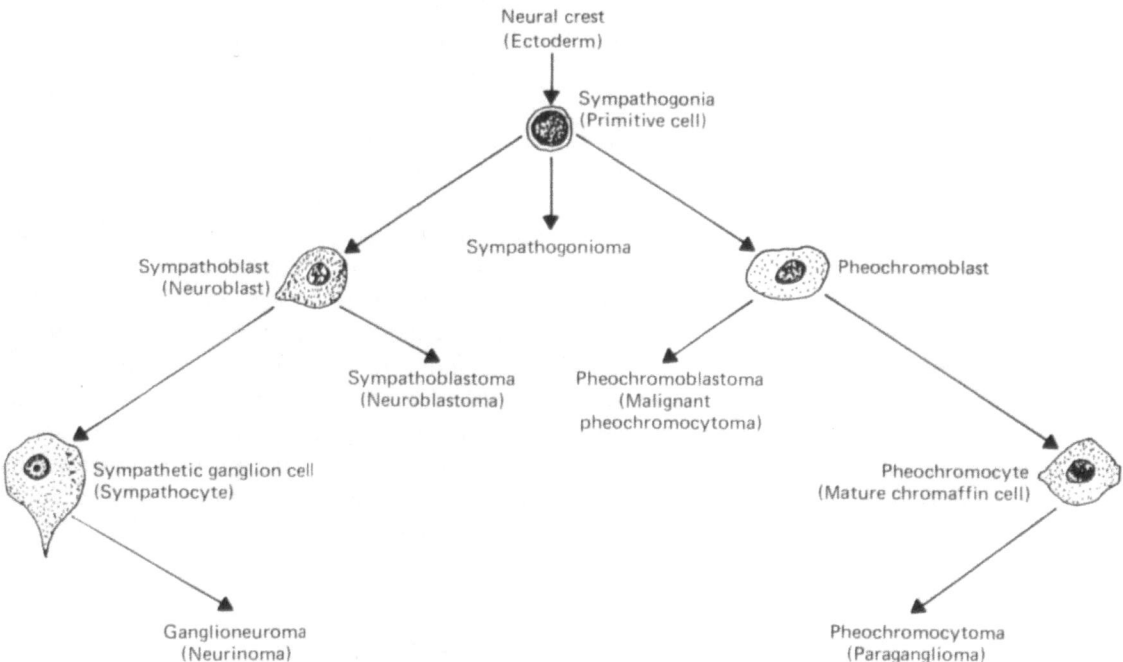

Fig. 3.5 Embryonic development of adrenergic cells and their tumors. Adapted from Karsner, H. T. Tumors of the adrenal. In: *Atlas of Tumor Pathology*, section VIII, fascicle 29, 1950, p. 33. Courtesy of Armed Forces Institute of Pathology and from *Käser, H., Pharmacol. Rev. 18*: 660, 1966. By permission of Williams & Wilkins Co.

less dense chromatin and more cytoplasm with a short cytoplasmic process) and also to the pheochromoblast. In turn, the sympathoblast differentiates into sympathetic ganglion cells, whereas the pheochromoblast becomes the pheochromocyte (the mature chromaffin cell, which contains a vesicular nucleus and granular cytoplasm and can be specifically identified by its affinity for chrome salts). The pheochromoblastoma (malignant pheochromocytoma, which is also chromaffinic) is said to arise from the pheochromoblast, and the benign pheochromocytoma from the pheochromocyte; but since the histology of the cells of malignant as well as benign tumors appears identical, it is impossible to be certain of the cellular origin of the malignant and benign pheochromocytoma. It seems likely that mature chromaffin cells as well as cells of a pheochromocytoma can differentiate and give rise to a malignant pheochromocytoma. According to the scheme in Figure 3.5, the neuroblastoma and ganglioneuroma are thought to arise, respectively, from the neuroblast and sympathetic ganglion cell; however, it appears that the sympathetic gan-

glion cell may differentiate into a neuroblastoma. A fascinating transformation of this latter malignancy into ganglioneuroblastoma or into benign cells (e.g., ganglioneuroma) can occur (246, 1039). We are not aware of any evidence that a pheochromocytoma may revert to mature chromaffin tissue.

From the foregoing it should be appreciated that, in addition to the simplified scheme of embryonic development of adrenergic cells and their tumors proposed in Figure 3.5, other pathways of cell differentiation and dedifferentiation may occur. The designation "pheochromocytoma" should probably include chromaffin cell tumors in any site (i.e., not only those arising from the adrenal medullary cells, where about 90 percent of these tumors occur, but also those arising from all extraadrenal sites in the abdomen, chest, and neck).

It should be emphasized that chromaffinity or "positive chromoreaction" [a brown or yellow-brown coloration of cells due to the oxidation of intra or extracellular catecholamines by dichromate, iodate (961), or other oxidants] is not specific for pheochromocytoma. The reaction occurs in all cells of the chromaffin system and other tissues which contain catecholamines, serotonin, or certain aromatic phenols and amines (890, pp. 258, 275). Pure norepinephrine-containing pheochromocytomas may yield a much lighter reaction with dichromate oxidation than tumors containing epinephrine or both catecholamines (890, p. 261). Appropriately, it has been suggested that the term "chromoreaction" be viewed as a color rather than a chromium specific reaction (890, p. 260). In the past, a commonly used substitute chromoreaction was produced with the Schmorl stain, a dilute Giemsa solution which colors the chromaffin cell green (890, p. 263).

The anatomic distribution of extraadrenal chromaffin tissue in the newborn, and the location of extraadrenal pheochromocytomas reported in the literature up to 1965, have been represented in composite figures by Coupland (178) (Fig. 3.6). The largest number of chromaffin cells occurs in the adrenal medulla. Another large collection of these cells composes the organ of Zuckerkandl, a bilateral structure frequently fused by an isthmus, which lies just anterior to the aorta in the region where the inferior mesenteric artery arises; it appears at the end of the second month and accounts for about one-half of the total mass of extraadrenal chromaffin tissue in the fetus (90). In the neonate the organ of

Fig. 3.6 A. The anatomic distribution of extraadrenal chromaffin tissue in the newborn. B. The location of extraadrenal pheochromocytomas reported in the literature up to 1965. From Coupland, R. *The Natural History of the Chromaffin Cell. Essex.* Courtesy of Longsman Green and Co., Ltd., 1965.

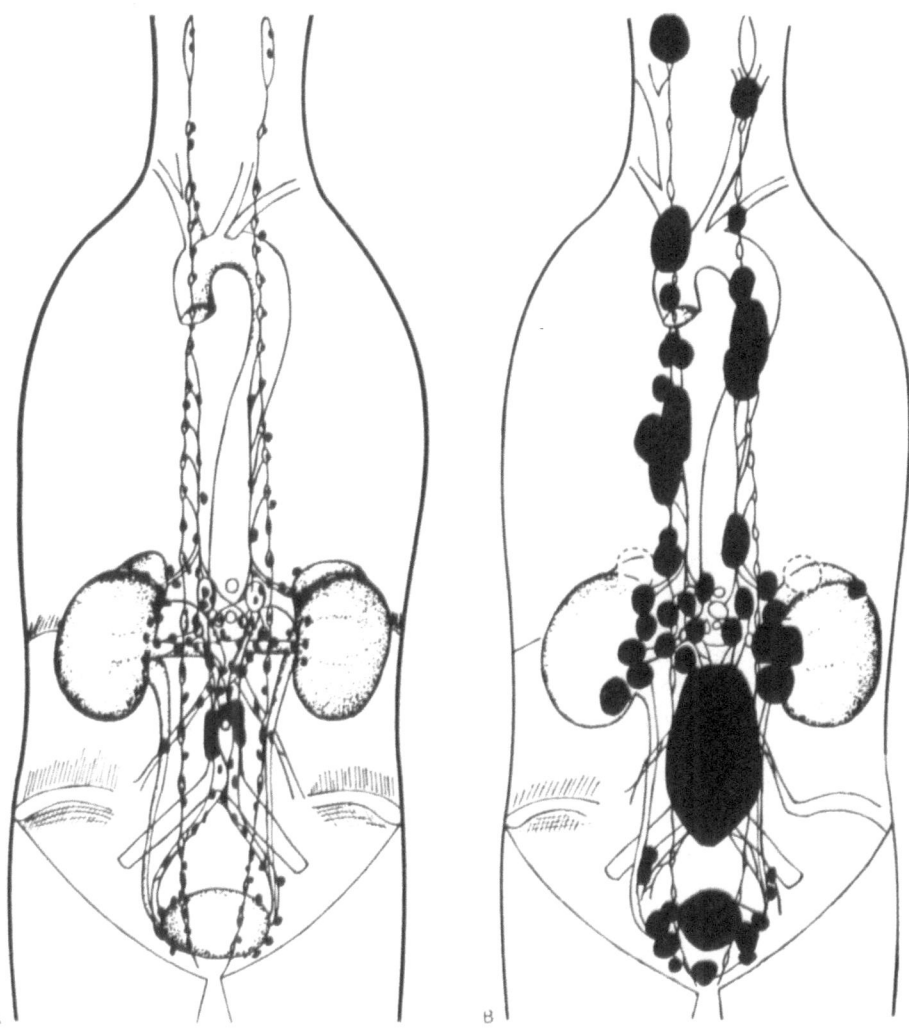

Zuckerkandl is consistently present in small nodular collections of chromaffin cells within peri-aortic fat; the organ is progressively replaced by fibrous tissue with aging into adulthood (890, p. 259); however, it appears that this collection of chromaffin tissue may contain the enzyme PNMT and may be able to secrete epinephrine, since the presence of epinephrine in blood and urine after bilateral adrenalectomy results from the secretion of extraadrenal chromaffin tissue including the organ of Zuckerkandl (296, 857, 1030). It usually disappears during early childhood, possibly by a dispersion of its cells along pre-aortic sympathetic nerve fibers (176, 177).

Catecholamine synthesis first appears in extraadrenal chromaffin cells about the eighth week of gestation, whereas a comparable degree of synthesis is not evident in the adrenal medulla until the 10th to 12th week (90). It is noteworthy that in the human during gestation and at birth the catecholamine content of the adrenal medulla and of the organ of Zuckerkandl is almost entirely norepinephrine; however, by 2 years of age the percentage of norepinephrine in both of these organs is only about 20 percent, whereas epinephrine accounts for about 80 percent of the total catecholamines (1030).

Chromaffin cells occur in association with the coeliac, mesenteric, renal, adrenal, hypogastric, testicular, and prevertebral sympathetic nerve plexuses. Chromaffin cells are also found adjacent to sympathetic nerves elsewhere in the body (e.g., those innervating the bladder, prostate, and other organs), and occasionally the cells occur ectopically. The major sites where pheochromocytomas occur are in the adrenal medulla, paraganglia cells of the sympathetic nervous system (sometimes referred to as "paragangliomas"), and the organ of Zuckerkandl. Less commonly, pheochromocytomas arise in chromaffin tissue found elsewhere, such as in the wall of the urinary bladder, para-aortic regions, behind the liver, in the hilus of the liver or kidney, in the region of the rectum, testicles, ovaries, and in the chest and neck. Additional exotic locations of origin have included the isthmus of a horseshoe kidney (709) and the spermatic cord (300). Pheochromocytomas have even been reported intracranially (122) but, to the best of our knowledge, these have always been

metastatic lesions. As can be seen in Figure 3.6, these pheochromocytomas can occur wherever chromaffin tissue exists. A tumor behaving clinically like a catecholamine-secreting pheochromocytoma (when manipulated) has also been described in the popliteal region; however, no pathologic study was performed on this tumor (personal communication, Dr. Robert F. Loeb, former Chairman of the Department of Medicine, Columbia Medical Center, New York).

As mentioned above, some tumors of the chemoreceptors (chemodectomas of the carotid and aortic body) or glomus jugulare complex (also called glomic tumors) have been reported to secrete epinephrine and/or norepinephrine and produce hypertension (60, 240, 368, 370, 571, 960, 1012). The precise classification of these tumors (discussed in detail at the beginning of this chapter) remains uncertain since some are chromaffin-positive and secrete catecholamines and resemble pheochromocytomas histologically, whereas others have none of these features (370, 403, 571). Sherwin emphasized that the presence of chromaffin cells within chemoreceptors has long been controversial and that so-called chromaffin cells in these tumors may in fact be mast cells (890, p. 259). It has been stated that carotid body tumors are sometimes familial and, if so, they are bilateral in 25 percent of cases (761).

It has been pointed out that a tissue which contains catecholamines may give a negative chromaffin reaction due to anoxic depletion of catecholamine granules or improper tissue fixation (368). However, the cells of some pheochromocytomas and one glomus jugulare tumor, which gave an equivocal or negative chromaffin reaction, became fluorescent when exposed to formaldehyde (221). This latter reaction is considered specific for the presence of biogenic amines and some of their precursors. The term "catecholamine-secreting paraganglioma" has been suggested for tumors of the chemoreceptors or tumors of other neurosecretory origin when they mimic pheochromocytoma (571). Table 3.2, which was prepared by Cobin and coworkers, reveals pertinent findings on patients reported in the literature who had carotid body or glomus jugulare chromaffinomas (160a). The patient of Cobin and associates who is included in

Table 3.2 Manifestations of Tumors of the Carotid Body or Glomus Jugulare Reported by Various Investigators[a,b]

Reported by	Age (years)	Sex	Tumor region	Neck mass	Horner's syndrome	Cranial nerve dysfunction	BP (mmHg)	Press on tumor BP change	Paroxysms of BP	Catecholamines		Chromaffin reaction
										Plasma and/or urine	Tumor	
Cragg (178b)	39	F	Carotid (and Zuckerkandl)	Yes	No	No	↑					−
Cone (168)	8	M	Carotid	Yes	Yes	No	↑		No	↑	+	
Berdal et al. (60)	66	M	Glomus	Yes	No	No	Normal	Preoperatively ↑	No	↑	+	−
Glenner et al. (368)	12	M	Carotid	Yes	Yes		↑	Preoperatively ↑	No		+	Weak +
Duke et al. (239)	33	F	Glomus	No	No	Yes	Normal	−	Yes	↑	+	−
Hamberger et al. (412)	65	M	Carotid	Yes			↑	During bronchoscopy and operatively ↑		↑	+	
Fries et al. (332)	21	M	Carotid	Yes	Yes	No	Normal	Operatively ↑	No		+	+
Levit et al. (571)	24	M	Glomus	Yes, eventually	No	Yes	Normal	Operatively ↑	Yes	↑	+	+
Manhart et al. (626)	16	F	Carotid	Yes, eventually	No	No	↑	No increase	Yes	↑		
Cobin et al. (160a)	19	F	Carotid	Yes, eventually	Yes	No	↑	No increase	Yes	↑	+	+

[a] Adapted from Cobin, R., Pertsemlidis, D., Gitlow, S., and Krieger, D. *Am. J. Med.* in press.
[b] + = Present; − = absent; ↑ = increased; BP = blood pressure; M = male; F = female.
[c] The tumors in region of the organ of Zuckerkandl gave a positive chromaffin reaction although no catecholamines were detected.

the table was also studied by us (patient No. 19 in Chapter 7). The common occurrence of a neck mass and the not infrequent presence of Horner's syndrome and/or cranial nerve dysfunction are noteworthy.

Adrenal medullary hyperplasia has been detected in two severely hypertensive children (71). Furthermore, on rare occasions it appears that the clinical picture of pheochromocytoma may be due to adrenal medullary hyperplasia (238, 674). In 1975 Carney and associates reported bilateral adrenal medullary hyperplasia in a 12-year-old girl who was normotensive; they hypothesized that adrenal medullary hyperplasia may be a precursor to familial pheochromocytoma (136). More recently, Carney and associates (135b) and Gagel and coworkers (340) have presented pathologic evidence to support this hypothesis; some of this evidence will be presented subsequently in this chapter.

ETIOLOGY (SPORADIC AND FAMILIAL)

Pheochromocytomas have been found to arise spontaneously in dogs, rats (particularly with aging) (1006), and a variety of domestic animals (e.g., horse, ox, sheep, and bulls, but very rarely in cows) (1031, 1040).

Dr. D. C. Twedt (D.V.M.) stated that during the past several years at the Animal Medical Center (N.Y.C.) the diagnosis of pheochromocytoma has been established at necropsy in approximately 50 dogs (personal conversation). These tumors have occurred in many different breeds of dogs, particularly when they become older (usually greater than 7 years). Some investigators have claimed that the boxer is particularly prone to pheochromocytoma; however, it should be recognized that this breed of dog is especially prone to a variety of tumors and ulcerative colitis, which may be related to a deficiency of the immune system. Characteristically, the dogs may be noted to have paroxysmal periods of panting, dyspnea, restlessness, hypertension, tachycardia, weakness, tremor, epistaxis, signs of congestive heart failure, seizure, and collapse (980) (Dr. D. C. Twedt, personal conversation). Dr. Twedt further stated that to his knowledge pheochromocytomas have been

found only in the adrenal gland of the dog and that the great majority of these tumors are benign (personal conversation). Occasionally the tumor may be large, calcified, and invade the inferior vena cava (980).

In the Wistar strain of rat with the propensity to develop pheochromocytoma, the tumor occurs in 80 percent of the animals over 25 months old (356). The tumor occurs more frequently in male rats, and is associated with a high incidence of adenomas of the pituitary, the islets of Langerhans, and interstitial cell tumors of the testis. In addition, pheochromocytoma, with or without other endocrine tumors, has been induced in rats by x-irradiation (1006).

The etiology of chromaffinomas remains unknown; they are relatively rare in both man and animal (178). Of particular interest and importance is the familial incidence of pheochromocytoma, which we believe may be as frequent as 10 percent. This estimate is based on reports that 10 percent of pheochromocytomas are bilateral, one-half of these are familial, and 50 percent of familial tumors are bilateral; there is no preponderance of right adrenal involvement, as occurs in nonfamilial (sporadic) cases of pheochromocytoma. The age at the time of diagnosis is usually younger in familial cases. Reports of familial pheochromocytoma first appeared in 1943 (470) and 1947 (126). A particularly remarkable example of this condition was seen at the Mayo Clinic where bilateral pheochromocytomas were removed from each of three siblings (821).

Studies of kindred with this tumor that have been reported suggest a dominant autosomal mode of inheritance with high penetrance (144, 865, 921a, 938). Smits suggested that familial pheochromocytoma is a monomeric, dominant, and autosomal inherited disease with variable expression in the phenotype (921). Strong support that familial pheochromocytoma is inherited in a dominant manner is indicated by the following: (a) the occurrence of this neoplasia in successive generations in the absence of consanguineous marriage; (b) the fact that approximately half the offspring from afflicted parents married to normals are proved or probable cases; (c) the fact that a parent of almost every patient with the neoplasm also has the tumor; and (d) the fact that there is a relatively high frequency of the neoplasm in the kindred (938). The male-to-male transmission excludes an X-linked mode of inheritance (938).

It is, of course, impossible to be certain of the exact incidence of familial occurrence since a careful survey and study of all relatives is rarely performed, and many familial cases have been mistakenly considered sporadic. A review of the world literature in 1960 revealed that there were only 22 patients having a familial history of pheochromocytoma (466). The tumors were bilateral in 11, multiple (i.e., other than bilateral adrenal) in two, and single in nine. There were three extraadrenal pheochromocytomas—two occurring in the thorax and one in the neck (466). Since that time, reports of familial pheochromocytoma have increased significantly (135a,b, 144, 232, 340, 437, 711, 799a, 865, 938).

In 1968 Steiner and coworkers stated that familial pheochromocytoma had been described previously in at least 25 families, involving 75 individuals. Furthermore, they reported a study of a kindred in which there were 10 proved and 15 probable cases of pheochromocytoma, five with medullary thyroid carcinoma, two with parathyroid hyperplasia, and one with Cushing's syndrome. Of the 10 proved cases, the tumor was bilateral in nine. The family was traced through seven generations and included 186 members (938). It is interesting that familial pheochromocytoma and medullary thyroid carcinoma have been reported in 17-year-old identical twins (84). In a report of familial pheochromocytoma and/or medullary thyroid carcinoma from the Mayo Clinic an examination of the adrenal glands of 19 patients with this familial endocrinopathy revealed the following: synchronously occurring bilateral pheochromocytomas in nine patients; asynchronous bilateral pheochromocytoma in one patient; unilateral pheochromocytoma with contralateral diffuse and nodular hyperplasia in two patients; unilateral pheochromocytoma with contralateral diffuse hyperplasia in two patients; unilateral pheochromocytoma in one patient; bilateral nodular hyperplasia in one patient; bilateral diffuse hyperplasia in one patient; and no abnormality in two patients (135b).

Evidence is accumulating which supports the concept that familial pheochromocytoma and medullary thyroid carcinoma (Sipple's syndrome) may originate respectively on a background of adrenal medullary hyperplasia and C-cell hyperplasia in the thyroid (135a,b, 136, 340, 1058). It has also been reported that pheochromocytomas from patients with Sipple's syndrome have higher concentrations of epinephrine than norepinephrine and may be different from pheochromocytomas in patients without this syndrome (852).

Recently, Baylin and coworkers reported findings that suggest a single clone origin for both medullary thyroid carcinoma and pheochromocytoma (51).

Hume has made the intriguing statement that "the high incidence of bilateral, multiple and ectopic pheochromocytomas in children, plus the rapid and intense course often seen, tend to suggest that the pathogenesis of the disease in childhood may involve factors which are not operative in the adult" (466). He has raised the possibility that endocrine changes associated with the advent of puberty may be a pathogenetic factor since the maximal incidence of the onset of the disease at ages nine to 11 is consistent with this view.

Nodular hyperplasia and an increase of norepinephrine in the adrenal medulla have been produced in rats by chronic injections of nicotine; however, no evidence for the induction of pheochromocytoma was cited and blood pressures were not recorded (278). Chronic thiouracil poisoning can produce hypertrophy of the adrenal medulla (631). Even more intriguing is the experimental production of pheochromocytoma by hormones. The finding of Moon and coworkers suggests that growth hormone may play a role in the pathogenesis of pheochromocytomas. They found that chronic injections of growth hormone over a 15-month period in male rats resulted in the development of adrenal medullary pheochromocytomas in nine of 16 animals, whereas no tumors occurred in the controls (675). Four of the rats had bilateral pheochromocytomas; however, none of the rats developed hypertension (675). Furthermore, Lupulescou has produced adrenal medullary changes in the rat varying from hyperplasia to pheochromocytoma by administering massive doses of growth hormone or estrogen for 5 months (595). The tumors contained increased catecholamine concentrations and hypertension developed.

Although the mechanism whereby growth hormone administration causes pheochromocytoma and other tumors in the experimental animal is unknown, some imbalance of hormonal secretions may be postulated, since these tumors cannot be produced in hypophysectomized animals (678).

Fifty years ago Lindau suggested that the rare occurrence of von Hippel-Lindau syndrome (i.e., retinal angiomatosis plus cerebellar hemangioblastoma) in association with pheochromocytoma and renal tumors and, sometimes, with cysts of the pancreas and the kidneys, may represent a generalized mesoblastic abnormality originating during early fetal development (575). This thesis, however, is untenable since it is recognized that chromaffin cells and the neurocutaneous abnormalities which sometimes occur in conjunction with pheochromocytoma are of ectodermal and not mesodermal origin.

AGE OF OCCURRENCE AND SEX PREDILECTION

Pheochromocytomas may occur at any age, the greatest frequency being in the fourth and fifth decades. The rare occurrence of congenital pheochromocytoma was reported in a premature girl who was found to have bilateral adrenal pheochromocytomas (352). Symptoms from a pheochromocytoma have been noted to have started in a 1-month-old child (577). The tumor has also been reported in two 81-year-old patients (61, 723) and one 82-year-old patient (256). However, only on extremely rare occasions will the tumor develop in the very young and the very old. Cone and coworkers could find only 11 patients under 10 years of age reported in the literature up to 1957 (169). In a series of 100 children (15 years of age or younger) with pheochromocytoma reported by Stackpole and Melicow, 68 were boys and 32 were girls, and 35 were younger than 10 years of age (933). The age distribution of these children is indicated in Figure 3.7.

Although there appeared to be no sex predilection in the adult patients we studied, or in the 92 patients with pheochromocytoma reported by Gitlow and associates (358), yet in 138 patients with this tumor seen at the Mayo clinic, 45.6 percent were males and 54.4 percent were females (784). These percentages are precisely the same as were observed at Columbia Medical Center: in 100 consecutive patients with pheochromocytoma, 47 were males and 53 were females (personal communication, Dr. Meyer M. Melicow, Given Professor Emeritus Uropathology Research, Columbia Medical Center, New York) (Fig.

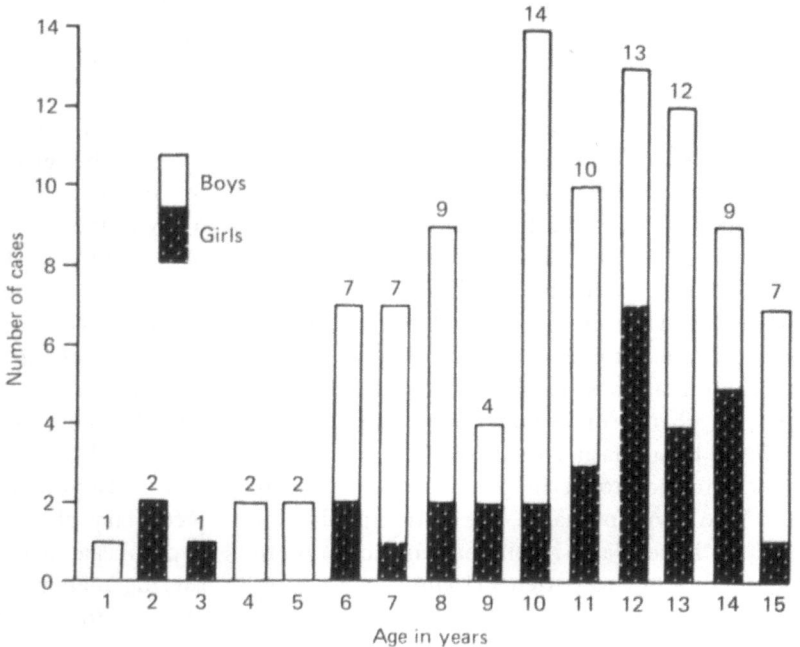

Fig. 3.7 Pheochromocytoma in children. Number of cases in boys and girls according to age. From Stackpole, R. H., Melicow, M. M., and Uson, A. C., *J. Pediatr. 63:* 321, 1963.

3.8). In a series of patients with pheochromocytoma reported by Scott and associates an even greater percentage were female (29 of 44 patients, i.e., 60 percent) (875a).

LOCATION

Approximately 99 percent of these tumors occur in the abdomen, and 85 to 90 percent of all chromaffinomas are located in the adrenal glands. Reports in the literature and our own experience indicate that pheochromocytomas occur more often in the right than in the left adrenal gland (122, 392, 784, 959).

In 76 patients (ranging in age from 12 to 77 years) studied at the Mayo Clinic, roughly two out of three tumors occurred in the right and one out of three in the left adrenal. In this series, when the tumor was in the right adrenal, paroxysmal hypertension occurred about twice as frequently as persistent hypertension, whereas the opposite was true when tumors occurred in the left adrenal. As pointed out by Gifford and coworkers (352), the significance of the latter finding (i.e., any correlation between the location of an adrenal pheochromocytoma and the pattern of hypertension) is doubtful. Of these 76 patients, two had solitary extraadrenal tumors, four had bilateral adrenal pheochromocytomas, one

Fig. 3.8 Distribution of 107 pheochromocytomas in 100 patients (47 male, 53 female) seen at Columbia Medical Center. Location: 98% in abdomen and 1 in thorax, 1 in bladder, 83 intraadrenal, and 17 extraadrenal. Eighty-six percent were functioning, 14 percent possibly nonfunctioning, 7 percent malignant, and 4 percent associated with neurofibromatosis. c.b.=carotid body; i.m.a.=inferior mesenteric artery. Courtesy of Dr. M. M. Melicow, Columbia Medical Center, New York City, unpublished.

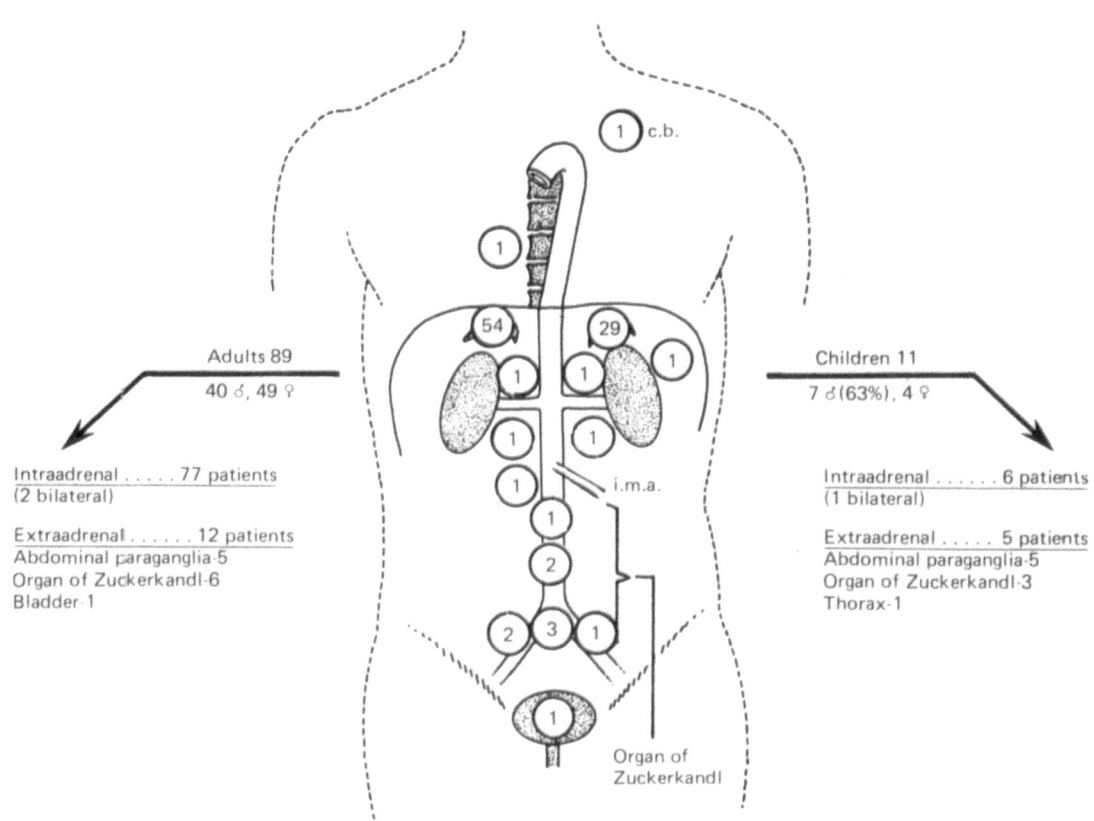

had tumors in both adrenals and at an extra-adrenal site, and two had one adrenal pheochromocytoma with multiple extraadrenal tumors (352). It is noteworthy that the average age of diagnosis in this series (almost all adults) was 45.1 and 39.4 years for those with paroxysmal and sustained hypertension, respectively (352).

In a more recent report of 138 patients (about 93 percent adults) with pheochromocytoma studied at the Mayo Clinic up to 1970, 90 percent of tumors were situated in the adrenal glands and 10 percent in extraadrenal locations in the abdomen. The commonest site of origin for extraadrenal tumors was the organ of Zuckerkandl. Since 1970 two patients with pheochromocytomas in the mediastinum and one patient with a tumor in the bladder have been encountered. Ninety-three percent of all tumors were single and 7 percent were multiple. Of the 128 patients with intra-adrenal tumors, 70 (56.5 percent) had the tumor in the right gland, 48 (38.7 percent) had the tumor in the left gland, and six patients had bilateral tumors (784). We know of one woman who developed hypertension due to a pheochromocytoma of the right adrenal, then became normotensive and remained asymptomatic for 2 years following tumor removal; at that time she became severely hypertensive and was discovered to have a pheochromocytoma of her left adrenal gland. It is conceivable that this patient had familial rather than sporadic pheochromocytoma, but this was not determined.

Localization of tumors in 204 patients (almost all adults) with chromaffinomas, reported by Graham (392), is indicated in Table 3.3. The distribution of 107 pheochromocytomas in 100 patients seen at Columbia Medical Center in New York City is shown in Figure 3.8. Eighty-nine patients were adults and 11 were children; 17 percent were black, which indicates no racial preference for pheochromocytoma, since the percentage of blacks in the New York City area is about 16 percent. Tumors were almost twice as common in the right as in the left adrenal gland. Tumors occurred slightly more frequently in females. Eighty-six percent of the tumors were clinically functioning, whereas no characteristic manifestations were recorded in 14 percent. It is evident that in patients with fa-

Table 3.3 *Localization of Tumors in 204 Patients with a Chromaffinoma[a]*

Tumor	No.
Pheochromocytoma	
Unilateral	162
Bilateral	19
Paraganglioma	
Lumbar-paravertebral	12
In front of the greater abdominal vessels	4
In the organ of Zuckerkandl	4
Thoracic-paravertebral	2
In the coeliac ganglion	1

[a] Adapted from data reviewed in Graham, J. B., *Int. Abstr. Surg. 92:* 106, 1951. By permission of *Surgery, Gynecology, and Obstetrics.*

milial pheochromocytoma and in children, there is an increased tendency to have bilateral adrenal tumors as well as synchronous and metachronous multiple extraadrenal tumors (135b, 875a).

A review of the literature up to 1967 revealed 205 cases of pheochromocytoma located in the following regions: 88 in the upper abdomen and 58 in the lower abdomen; 20 in the urinary bladder; four in the lower pelvis; 24 in the thorax; five in the neck; and six unspecified (332). Up to 1969, 26 patients with pheochromocytoma of the organ of Zuckerkandl had been reported (589).

Hume reported the location of pheochromocytomas in 76 children (Table 3.4), and Stackpole, Melicow, and Uson (933) indicated the location of chromaffinomas in a series of 100 children (Fig. 3.9). The significantly greater number of bilateral and multiple tumors in children as compared to adults is apparent. From our observations and the experience of others it appears that pheochromocytoma is multiple in about 8 percent of adults and 35 percent of children. Gitlow has placed these percentages at even higher levels, 15 and 40 percent, respectively (358). Hermann and Mornex reported that about 33 percent of these tumors in children are multiple (437, p. 76).

A number of intrathoracic pheochromocytomas have been reported (70, 76, 268, 604, 605, 643, 666, 726, 733, 749). However, less than 2 percent of pheochromocytomas orig-

Table 3.4 *Location of Pheochromocytoma in 76 Children*[a]

Location	No. of cases	
Right adrenal	25	
Left adrenal	11	
Bilateral adrenal	15	
Bilateral plus extraadrenal	3	
Right side, extraadrenal	1	
Left side, extraadrenal	6	
Multiple, right side	2	
Multiple, left side	1	
Right adrenal plus extraadrenal	4	
Left adrenal plus extraadrenaly	3	
Multiple extraadrenal	1	
Intrathoracic	1	
Aorta	3	
Total	76	
Multiple tumors	29	39%
Bilateral adrenal	18	24%
Extraadrenal, or extraadrenal plus a single adrenal tumor	11	15%
Single Tumors	47	61%
Adrenal	36	47%
Extraadrenal	11	14%

[a] Modified from Hume, D. M. *Am. J. Surg. 99:* 466, 1960.

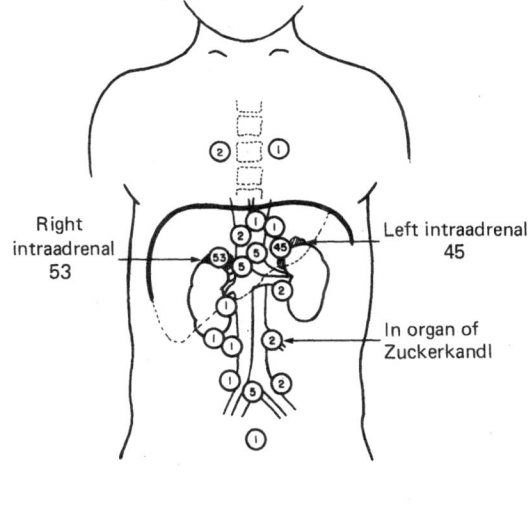

Tumor incidence

Single tumors - - - - - - - - - - - - - - - - - in 68 children
Multiple tumors - - - - - - - - - - - - - - - - in 32 children
Intraadrenal tumors only - - - - - - - - - in 70 children
Extraadrenal tumors only - - - - - - - - - in 22 children
Intra-and extraadrenal tumors - - - - - in 8 children

Fig. 3.9 Distribution of 140 pheochromocytomas in 100 children (69 boys, 31 girls). Note: The exact location of six extraadrenal tumors and the side of three intraadrenal tumors were not stated, and not included in the diagram. Courtesy of Dr. M. M. Melicow (with modification), Dept. of Pathology, Columbia Medical Center, New York, New York.

inate in the chest, where they occur in the posterior mediastinum and are paravertebral in location, since they arise from chromaffin cells along the sympathetic chain. A particularly unusual location was that of an intrapericardial tumor; its retrocardiac location resulted in physical and radiographic signs of mitral valve disease (70). One patient was described who had multiple pheochromocytomas in the thorax (76), and another patient had extraadrenal abdominal and thoracic tumors (178). Coupland stated that the intrathoracic tumors almost certainly arose from chromaffin cells associated with the sympathetic chain or splanchnic nerve and that branches of these nerves could usually be traced into these tumors; however, he further stated that there is no evidence that nerve terminals actually innervate the chromaffin cells of pheochromocytomas (178).

In 1970 McNeill and associates reviewed 22 cases of intrathoracic pheochromocytoma

reported in the literature and described an additional patient who had a pheochromocytoma in the chest and also in an ectopic adrenal gland situated in the hilum of the left kidney (645). Only one of the chest tumors in these patients was malignant. It was found that intrathoracic pheochromocytoma occurred mainly between the ages of 20 and 40 years in both sexes, but was more common in men (about 60 percent occurring in males) (645).

Seven of these 23 patients with intrathoracic pheochromocytomas were normotensive and four were asymptomatic. Tumors occurred with equal frequency in either hemithorax, and 65 percent were situated between the levels of the fifth and eighth thoracic vertebrae in the costovertebral angle. The majority weighed over 20 g. Additional benign pheochromocytomas were detected in four patients: one boy and one girl each had bilateral adrenal tumors, whereas the other two patients, a teen-age boy and a middle-age man, each had a single pheochromocytoma located in relation to a renal hilum (645). Pertinent information regarding the cases of intrathoracic pheochromocytoma reviewed by McNeill appears in Table 3.5. One patient with malignant pheochromocytoma reported by Olsen and coworkers was uniquely interesting in that the primary tumor occurred in the right atrium (721).

Less than 0.1 percent of pheochromocytomas arise from chromaffin tissue in the neck (168) and, as mentioned previously, some of these probably represent chemodectomas (240, 571). The occurrence of a pheochromocytoma in an intraspinal site has, very rarely, been reported (184, 745, 788), and even an intracerebral location in one patient has been mentioned (122). However, in the latter location, the tumor is probably always metastatic. Some pheochromocytomas may metastasize to the skull (649) and also to the meninges (320).

It is noteworthy that if an adrenergic tumor is epinephrine-producing it is almost always located in the adrenal gland. Occasionally, a tumor of the organ of Zuckerkandl may secrete epinephrine; very rarely other extraadrenal pheochromocytomas [e.g., in the hilus of the liver (624), in the urinary bladder (964), in the thorax, and behind the inferior vena cava (268)] have been reported to secrete predominantly epinephrine. As pointed out by Engelman and Hammond, secretion of epinephrine by some extraadrenal pheochromocytomas is inconsistent with the hypothesis (1060) that production of epinephrine in the adrenal medulla is a consequence of high local concentrations of glucocorticoids elaborated by the adrenal cortex (268).

WEIGHT AND SIZE

Pheochromocytomas vary considerably in weight and size but about 70 percent weigh less than 70 g and about 85 percent less than 200 g. Tumors may weigh as much as 3167 (668), 3500 (218), and 3600 g (165, 320). Two tumors weighing 1000 and 850 g contained, respectively, 20 and 10.6 g of catecholamines (concentrations of epinephrine and norepinephrine in the latter tumor were about equal) (55, 195). The tumor of one of our patients weighed 1330 g; however, about 90 percent of its weight was due to the fluid in a huge cyst. The weight of 68 pheochromocytomas seen at the Mayo Clinic is recorded in Table 3.6. The average weight was roughly 100 g—similar to that in a series of 37 pheochromocytomas reported by Zelch and associates at the Cleveland Clinic (1070).

Very rarely, microscopic pheochromocytomas have been demonstrated. Desai described a patient with paroxysmal hypertension and headaches resulting from a microscopic pheochromocytoma in the left adrenal gland which appeared entirely normal at laparotomy. In this case he demonstrated the crucial importance of sudden blood pressure elevations which occurred during palpation of the left but not the right adrenal gland. He indicated the value of manipulation of the adrenals in "betraying the invisible pheochromocytoma." Furthermore, he emphasized that, in the presence of a definite clinical diagnosis of pheochromocytoma, a pronounced elevation of blood pressure on adrenal palpation is an indication for removal of that adrenal despite a normal and innocuous appearance (227). Some microscopic lesions may possibly represent nodular hyperplasia (890, p. 274). Also, tumors the size of a football may be encountered. The average tumor size in 46 patients seen at the Cleveland Clinic was 4.5 cm (223).

PHYSIOLOGIC AND PHARMACOLOGIC EFFECTS

A knowledge of the physiologic and pharmacologic effects of norepinephrine and epinephrine on various effector systems, as outlined in Table 3.7, is of value in understanding some of the hemodynamic and clinical manifestations observed in patients with pheochromocytoma.

In addition to α- and β-adrenergic receptors, which respond to epinephrine and norepinephrine (see Table 3.7), a third type of adrenergic response, caused by dopamine, has been defined (476). Dopaminergic receptors have been identified in the brain and also in the renal vasculature, where dopamine causes vasodilatation.

A high degree of binding specificity and a strong affinity for catecholamines characterize the receptor-catecholamine interaction.

Table 3.5 *Intrathoracic Pheochromocytoma*[a]

Case no.	Authors[b]	Age and sex	Site[c]	Weight (g)	Catecholamine content (mg/g tumor) Nor-adrenaline	Adre-naline	Other pheochromocytomas	Other lesions	Remarks
1	Miller (1924)	39 F	Right, D.6	32	—	—	—	—	Pheochromocytoma detected at autopsy
2	Philips (1940)	39 M	Left, D.2	—	—	—	Both adrenal glands weighed 20 g	—	Pheochromocytoma detected at autopsy
3	Maier (1949)	25 M	Left, D.4–5	28	—	—	—	—	—
4	Nissen (1949)	22 F	Left	—	—	—	—	—	—
5	Overholt, Ramsay, and Meissner (1950)	16 M	Left, D.4–7	50	—	—	—	—	—
6	McLeish and Adler (1955)	19 M	Left, D.7	26	—	—	—	Café-au-lait pigmentation	—
7	Cone, Allen, and Pearson (1957) and Sjoerdsma, Leeper, Terry, and Udenfriend (1959)	8 F	Left, D.7–8	20	1.8	0	Both adrenal glands	Gangrene of ileum	Pheochromocytoma detected at autopsy. Familial: mother had bilateral adrenal tumors and sister multiple pheochromocytomas
8	von Euler and Ström (1957), and Björk, Linderholm, Lublin, Pernow, and Thornberg (1959)	31 M	Multiple	0.1–66	0.1–0.3	0	Metastases in bone, lungs, pleura, liver, lymph nodes, and retroperitoneum	—	Malignant pheochromocytoma
9	Silvestrini, Genesi, Sachsel, and Costa (1957)	39 F	Right, D.10–11	38	0.07	0.003	—	—	—
10	Maier and Humphreys (1958)	48 M	Right, D.7–8	—	—	—	—	Non-chromaffin paraganglioma of carotid body	—
11	Maier and Humphreys (1958)	13 M	Right, D.5–6	27	—	—	Attached to right renal vessels	—	Recurred 9 years later with extension into extradural space

continued on p. 50

Table 3.5 *Continued*

Case no.	Authors[b]	Age and sex	Site[c]	Weight (g)	Catecholamine content (mg/g tumor)		Other pheochromocytomas	Other lesions	Remarks
					Nor-adrenaline	Adre-naline			
12	Pampari and Lacerenza (1958)	64 M	Right, D.7–8	—	—	—	—	Vertebral erosion	—
13	de Graeff, Muller, and Moolenaar (1959)	17 M	Left, D.4–7	55	1.2	0	—	—	—
14	de Graeff, Muller, and Moolenaar (1959)	56 F	Left, D.9–10	22	5.1	0	—	—	—
15	Green and Bassett (1961)	63 M	Right, D.5	6	—	—	—	Lymphosarcoma and hemangioma of liver	Pheochromocytoma detected at autopsy
16	Wilson (1962)	28 M	Right, D.5	22	0.4	0	—	—	—
17	Luna, Katz, and Ernst (1963)	26 F	Right, D.10	80	2.34	0.3	—	—	—
18	Peiper and Golestan (1963)	36 F	Left, D.4–5	—	—	—	—	—	—
19	de Graeff and Horak (1964)	60 F	—	—	—	—	—	—	Pheochromocytoma detected at autopsy
20	Cueto, McFee, and Bernstein (1965)	47 M	Right, D.4–5	106	—	—	—	—	—
21	Downs and Schoemperlen (1966)	35 F	Right, D.7	—	5.6	0.6	—	—	—
22	Edmunds (1966) and Weber, Janower, and Griscom (1967)	9 M	Left, D.5–7	—	—	—	Both adrenals	—	Familial: mother had pheochromocytoma of right adrenal gland
23	Present report	47 M	Left, D.8	17	0.43	0.001	Hilum of left kidney in accessory adrenal gland	—	Tumor also contained VMA 0.035 mg/g

[a] From McNeill, A. D., Groden, B. M., and Neville, A. M. *Brit. J. Surg. 57*: 460, 1970.

[b] See original publication for complete references.

[c] Right and left refer to hemithorax; D refers to thoracic vertebra.

Table 3.6 Weight of 68 Pheochromocytomas Seen at the Mayo Clinic[a]

Weight (g)	Paroxysmal function		Persistent function	
	Tumors	Percent	Tumors	Percent
<5	1	3.0	0	—
5– 50	15	44.1	16	47.1
51–100	6	17.6	6	17.6
101–200	8	23.5	5	14.7
201–500	3	8.8	6	17.6
501–700	1	3.0	1	3.0
	34	100.0	34	100.0
Range	1.2–575		5–700	
Average	93		117	

[a] From Gifford, R. W. Jr., Kvale, W. F., Maher, F. T., Roth, G. M., and Priestley, J. T. *Mayo Clinic Proc. 39:* 300, 1964.

Table 3.7 Effects of Circulating Norepinephrine (NE) and Epinephrine (E) and Receptors Stimulated[a]

Effector system	Response and type of receptor stimulated[b,c]	
	NE	E
Isolated heart	Positive inotropic β and chronotropic β	Positive inotropic β and chronotropic β
Heart frequency in vivo	Bradycardia (vagal reflex)	Tachycardia β
Mean arterial blood pressure	Increase	Slight increase or decrease
Skeletal muscle	Vasoconstriction α	Vasodilatation β
Liver	Vasoconstriction α	Vasodilatation β
Skin	Vasoconstriction α	Vasoconstriction α
Kidneys	Vasoconstriction α	Vasoconstriction α
Sweat glands (localized[d] secretion)	Activation α	Activation α
Intestinal smooth muscle (decrease of motility and tone)	Relaxation α, β	Relaxation α, β
Pupils	Weak dilatation α	Dilatation α
Central nervous system	Slight or no effect ?	Apprehension, excitation ?
Blood sugar (glycogenolysis)	Slight increase β	Increase β
Free fatty acids (lipolysis)	Increase β	Increase β
Basal metabolic rate (with increased heat production)	Slight increase (mainly due to increased FFA)	Increase (mainly due to increased FFA?)
Blood eosinophils	Slight fall ?	Fall ?

[a] Taken partially from Euler, U. S. von, and Ström, G. Present status of diagnosis and treatment of pheochromocytoma. *Circulation 15:* 6, 1957. By permission of the American Heart Association.

[b] The receptors on which NE and E act can be classified as α and β receptors depending on the reaction of the effector organs to contact with these amines. β receptors have been subdivided into β_1, and β_2 (337). For example, cardiac inotropy and lipolytic effects of the catecholamines are β_1 responses whereas bronchodilatation and vasodilatation appear to be β_2 responses. Evidence suggests that in distal coronary resistance vessels there are α- and β-adrenergic receptors which on stimulation may, under some circumstances, cause vasoconstriction and vasodilatation, respectively (685a).

[c] Stimulation accounts for activation of sweat glands on palms and a few other regions but generalized sweating in patients with pheochromocytoma remains unexplained.

[d] ? = Mechanism uncertain.

This interaction is rapid and reversible. Only several thousand β-adrenergic receptors have been demonstrated in a single cell. These receptors are macromolecules which are located in the plasma membranes (563). Stimulation of adrenergic receptors results in a sequence of biochemical events that produce a biologic response. In many instances the sequence appears to be the following: The catecholamine (a so-called "first messenger") stimulates the enzyme adenylate cyclase, which is located on the internal surface of the plasma membrane of the target cell. This enzyme then accelerates the intracellular generation of a cyclic nucleotide (the so-called "second messenger"), which in turn activates enzymes known as protein kinases; the kinases then phosphorylate a wide variety of important substrates which appear to mediate the characteristic responses attributed to the catecholamines.

Epinephrine and norepinephrine have similar biologic activity except that epinephrine is metabolically 20 to 100 times more active (385). Norepinephrine is a potent generalized vasoconstrictor, whereas epinephrine causes vasoconstriction in some regions but vasodilation in others. As pointed out by Dustan and coworkers, the hemodynamic characteristics of hypertension associated with pheochromocytoma would be expected to represent a balance of effects of the catecholamines liberated into the circulation, since only rarely do the tumors secrete only one of these hormones (244). Studies by Dustan and coworkers on eight patients with pheochromocytoma revealed an increase in the mean heart rate, cardiac index, and rate of left ventricular ejection associated with a moderate rise in total peripheral resistance; however, since there was a wide range of values, results for patients with sustained and paroxysmal hypertension were averaged together (Table 3.8). Björk and coworkers reported that in a patient with pheochromocytoma and sustained hypertension the pressure in the pulmonary artery, and the pressure in the "wedge position" were higher than normal, and were markedly reduced by the intravenous administration of phentolamine (76). In contrast to the normal pulmonary artery pressure in patients with uncomplicated essential hypertension, pulmonary pressure in patients with sustained hypertension due to pheochromocytoma is increased, as it is in subjects receiving catecholamine infusions (378).

Kreul and associates performed hemodynamic, electrocardiographic, and catecholamine studies before and during removal of a pheochromocytoma in a 38-year-old woman with sustained hypertension. Plasma norepinephrine was seven times the normal value, and elevations of plasma dopamine and dopa were also detected. The patient had received phenoxybenzamine (30–60 mg/day orally) for 12 days up to the day of the operation, which was performed under enflurane anesthesia. Following removal of the tumor, the concentrations of plasma catecholamines and dopa returned to normal. Myocardial performance improved immediately after tumor removal; as blood pressure and peripheral resistance decreased the cardiac index increased, the pre-ejection period (PEP) shortened, the left ventricular ejection time (LVET) lengthened, and PEP/LVET decreased (528a). These in-

Table 3.8 *Hemodynamics in Eight Patients with Pheochromocytoma*[a]

Index	Average	Range	Normal for lab $\pm$ SE
Heart rate (beats/min)	81	72–112	68 $\pm$ 2
Blood pressure (mmHg)	167/98	133/83–190/132	
Cardiac index (liters/min/m²)	3.36	2.7–4.6	3.05 $\pm$ 0.09
Total peripheral resistance (units/m²)	37.6	26–51	30 $\pm$ 0.83
Mean rate left ventricular ejection (ml/sec/m²)	174	119–242	151 $\pm$ 4.2

[a] From Dustan, H. P., Tarazi, R. C., and Bravo, E. L. Physiologic characteristics of hypertension. *In: Hypertension Manual.* Courtesy of Laragh, J. H. ed., New York, Dun-Donnelley, 1974, p. 233.

vestigators cited a report in the literature of a patient with a pheochromocytoma which apparently secreted both epinephrine and norepinephrine. In this patient a shortened pre-ejection period was thought to indicate that the positive inotropic effect of catecholamines on the heart, due to β-adrenergic stimulation, was greater than the peripheral vasoconstriction from α-adrenergic receptor stimulation.

Despite the fact that epinephrine infusions in humans produce greater metabolic effects and more pronounced symptomatology than do similar infusions of norepinephrine, it is generally impossible to predict the secretion pattern of a pheochromocytoma on the basis of clinical manifestations. Yet, in some patients with tumors secreting only norepinephrine, paroxysmal symptoms and evidence of hypermetabolism and abnormal glucose tolerance may be conspicuously absent. Goldenberg noted that tumors containing 90 percent or more of norepinephrine and not more than a total of 80 mg of this catecholamine caused a syndrome with unimpressive metabolic features which mimicked essential hypertension; as the total amount of norepinephrine in the tumors increased hypermetabolism and hyperglycemia became more evident. Tumors containing predominantly epinephrine usually caused not only hypertension but also tachycardia and hypermetabolism. A surprising observation was that some tumors containing large amounts of epinephrine produced a clinical picture of essential hypertension without any metabolic disturbances (375). We (624) and other investigators (377, 466) found no precise correlation between the concentration of epinephrine and norepinephrine in pheochromocytomas and the presence of sustained and paroxysmal hypertension. Furthermore, it has been claimed that sweating and postural hypotension may be the only signs suggesting pheochromocytoma, and that sometimes these patients are clinically indistinguishable from those with essential hypertension (728).

In the few patients with pheochromocytomas secreting predominantly epinephrine, it has been reported that paroxysmal symptoms may be accompanied by an elevated hematocrit, white blood cell count, blood urea nitrogen, and bilirubin. However, of particular note is the fact that hypotension and shock sometimes occur (417, 728). On extremely rare occasions, during the course of bacteremia, abscess formation has been reported in some pheochromocytomas (437, p. 130).

GROSS AND MICROSCOPIC APPEARANCE

Usually the tumor is encapsulated, often by a thin, transparent, fibrocollagenous capsule. The cut surface appears pinkish or yellowish-brown (Fig. 3.10, p. 72), is highly vascular, and frequently contains hemorrhagic, friable, necrotic, and sometimes cystic areas which may contain dark brown fluid. Large tumors tend to develop cystic necrosis and to hemorrhage into the central portions of the neoplasm (784). Pheochromocytomas originating in the adrenal frequently compress and displace the normal gland to the periphery. Sometimes calcium may be deposited in these tumors (Fig. 3.11, p. 73), or they may become almost completely replaced by a large cyst (Fig. 3.12, p. 73). Histologic changes resembling "brown" adipose tissue have been described in the retroperitoneal fat in the region surrounding these tumors (648, 889), and it has been suggested that these changes represent the lipolytic effects of catecholamines (648). The cells of pheochromocytomas tend to be larger than those of the normal adrenal medulla and are usually pleomorphic, with extreme anisocytosis and poikilocytosis in some areas. Individual cells may be about 20 μm in diameter. They are generally polygonal (polyhedral) or spheroidal, with eosinophilic and/or basophilic cytoplasm containing multiple minute granules. Normal adrenal medullary cells usually show less pleomorphism than do cells of the tumor, and the latter sometimes contain multinucleated giant cells (890, p. 266). An example of a multinucleated giant cell is evident in Figure 3.13 (on p. 74, a photomicrograph of a section from the cystic pheochromocytoma shown in Figure 3.12). Colloid droplets, located in the cytoplasm and varying in size from fine granules to huge droplets, are especially common in pheochromocytoma (889). Although their function is not clear, these droplets may play a role in binding nonparticulate catecholamines (890, p. 266).

Symington and Goodall noted that some of the 12 pheochromocytomas they examined had a large alveolar character; mature chromaffin cells, containing basophilic granules, were arranged in trabeculae or alveoli, and there were large thin-walled sinusoids bounded only by tumor cells. These investigators also described a small alveolar type pheochomocytoma, devoid of sinusoids and with chromaffin cells arranged in compact alveoli. In addition, they observed a combination of these cellular patterns and sometimes noted trabeculae of compactly arranged cells which had more eosinophilic and less granular cytoplasm than did the alveolar cells. They suggested that eosinophilic staining may be associated with the more primitive cell type (pheochromoblast); however, they pointed out that eosinophilic and basophilic staining may depend not only on tumor cell maturity but also on the technical details of preparing the histologic section (959). The nuclei are of moderate size and occasionally multiple. Typically spherical and centrally located, they contain a remarkably large nucle-

olus. Considerable anisonucleosis is sometimes evident, and occasionally the nuclei may be eccentric. The variability in cellular patterns observed in pheochromocytomas is illustrated in Figure 3.14, which shows the histopathology of four pheochromocytomas. In the pheochromocytomas studied at the Mayo Clinic, three cellular patterns were observed: epithelial in 55 percent, pleomorphic in 43 percent, and spindle cell in 2 percent. The epithelial type consisted of cords and clusters of cells with abundant granular eosinophilic cytoplasm, moderate-sized ovoid nuclei, and occasional hyperchromatic degenerating forms. In the pleomorphic variety, cells were somewhat similar to the epithelial cells but more varied in shape and size, and their nuclei were more irregular and hyperchromatic; giant cells were frequent. It was remarked that "irregular hyperchromatic, degenerating nuclei were so common that on first observation a poorly differentiated neoplasm was suggested." The spindle cell variety was composed of plump spindle cells. Mitotic figures were rarely evident (784).

Fig. 3.14 Photomicrographs of different fields in pheochromocytomas to show different cellular types. (Contributed by Dr. E. M. Humphrey to *Atlas of Genitourinary Pathology*, American Registry of Pathology, p. 213, 1946.) A.F.I.P. Neg. Acc. No. 114159. From Karsner, H. T. Tumors of the adrenal. In: *Atlas of Tumor Pathology*, section VIII, fascicle 29. Courtesy of Armed Forces Institute of Pathology, 1950, p. 53. By permission of Williams & Wilkins Co.

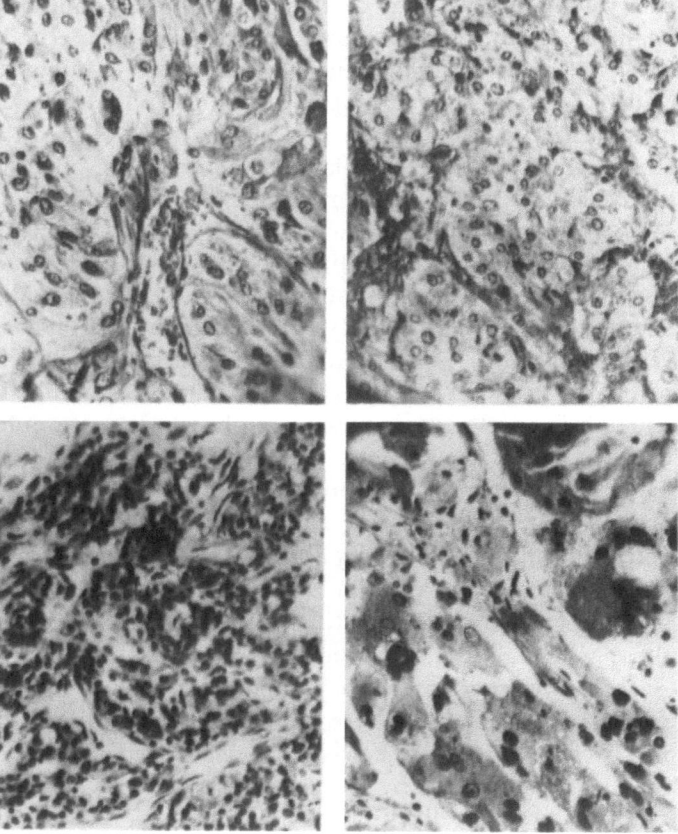

Both cytoplasm and intracytoplasmic secretory granules, which contain catecholamines, can be stained characteristically brown with chromium salts (Fig. 3.15, p. 75). Figure 3.15 is a photomicrograph of a pheochromocytoma which has been treated with chromate. The finding that some of the cells are not chromated may indicate that these cells are relatively immature; Coupland has pointed out that chromaffin granules are not normally found until pheochromocytes have reached a considerable degree of morphologic maturity (177). The greater diffuse chromaffin reaction in the cytoplasm of these tumor cells, as compared to the cells of the normal adrenal medulla, may possibly be explained by a deficient ATP binding capacity in the pheochromocytoma cells (178). As mentioned previously, the chromaffin staining reaction cannot be considered highly specific for the catecholamines, since serotonin and other phenolic amines will give a similar chemical reaction (279). A positive chromaffin reaction has been observed when medullary thyroid carcinoma tissue is treated with chromate, suggesting that this type of carcinoma and pheochromocytoma may derive from the same cellular system (581).

In the past 2 years pathologic evidence has accumulated which supports the concept that adrenal medullary hyperplasia is the precursor of familial pheochromocytoma (135b, 136, 340). Recently, Carney and associates at the Mayo Clinic reported a fascinating study on the adrenal glands of 19 patients or their primary relatives who had Sipple's syndrome, i.e., an endocrinopathy consisting of a combination of adrenal pheochromocytoma, medullary thyroid carcinoma, and occasionally hyperparathyroidism. This syndrome, which has also been designated multiple endocrine neoplasia (MEN–type 2), is usually familial and will be discussed in detail in Chapter 4. Grossly visible nodular or diffuse medullary enlargement of the adrenal glands was present in the majority of their cases. Seventy-three percent of affected adrenal medullas had multilobular pheochromocytomas, in contrast to the unilobular lesion of sporadic pheochromocytoma. Fifteen of their 19 patients had pheochromocytomas (defined as nodules measuring 1 cm or more in diameter), and 10 of these abutted directly on adrenal

cortical cells, which showed mild to severe pressure atrophy. In five patients the tumors penetrated through the tumor capsule or adrenal capsule and invaded periadrenal fat. In one patient there were multiple nonencapsulated nodules with hypertrophy and diffuse proliferation of the pheochromocytes. Five patients had metastatic spread of their pheochromocytoma.

Microscopically, the tumor cells in familial and sporadic pheochromocytomas appear to be similar in size, shape, nuclear pattern, staining characteristics, and arrangement. In the familial tumors studied by Carney and coworkers, the cytoplasm was generally granular and characteristically basophilic; however, the staining was highly variable, ranging from basophilic through amphophilic (i.e., stainable with either acidic or basic dyes), clear, or brown, to distinctly acidophilic, or mixed acidophilic and basophilic (135b). Rare vacuolization and eccentric nuclei simulated "signet ring" cells, and all tumors contained large or small intra- or extracytoplasmic hyaline globules scattered throughout the tumor. Vesicular nuclei were polymorphic (round, oval, or fusiform), and positioned centrally or eccentrically. Binucleated and multinucleated cells were evident in most tumors, and nuclear pyknosis was frequent. Giant and bizarre nuclei were occasionally seen in most tumors, but mitotic figures were absent in 40 percent of the tumors and infrequent in the remainder. Atypical mitoses were not found.

The vasculature was usually composed of small capillaries; large sinusoids occasionally gave an angiomatous appearance. Stroma was usually minimal, but in some tumors it constituted a major component; stromal calcification occurred in two tumors. Extensive necrosis was present in five tumors.

Carney and associates have pointed out that diffuse medullary hyperplasia may not be an absolute prerequisite to the development of medullary nodules in this syndrome, since diffuse medullary hyperplasia was not identified in one of their patients who had bilateral adrenal medullary nodules. They concluded that nodular medullary hyperplasia as well as diffuse medullary hyperplasia may precede the development of pheochromocytoma in the MEN–type 2 syndrome.

Of clinical importance with regard to the MEN–type 2 syndrome were the following findings:

1. Familial pheochromocytoma was responsible for a significant mortality [e.g., in five of the 17 patients (29 percent) studied by Carney and associates, and in 33 of 149 cases (32 percent) reported in the literature, the patient's death was attributed to the pheochromocytoma].
2. Unlike sporadic pheochromocytoma, moderately advanced pathology may exist in patients with the MEN–type 2 syndrome without producing any clinical or laboratory manifestations suggesting hyperfunctioning adrenal medullary tissue or a pheochromocytoma [e.g., seven of the 19 patients with MEN–type 2 studied by Carney and associates were asymptomatic and eight were normotensive; these patients were more apt to have variable or negative laboratory tests for pheochromocytoma than patients with the sporadic variety of the disease (898)].

Carney and coworkers have emphasized that, once the diagnosis of adrenal medullary disease is made in patients with the MEN–type 2 syndrome, total bilateral adrenalectomy should be performed with excision of any extraadrenal pheochromocytomas. [Extraadrenal pheochromocytomas have, on rare occasions, occurred in patients with the MEN–type 2 syndrome (218a, 631a).]

Their recommendation was based on the (1) likelihood of synchronously occurring bilateral adrenal medullary involvement, (2) risk of local recurrence if the entire gland is not removed, and (3) high mortality from pheochromocytoma in this syndrome (135b).

ULTRASTRUCTURE

Electron microscopy of the normal human adrenal medulla reveals that many of the cells have organelles (i.e., mitochondria, dense bodies, endoplasmic reticulum, lipid and osmiophilic or chromaffin granules scattered throughout the cytoplasm, and also a Golgi apparatus, which is juxtanuclear in position). These granules border on the limit of resolution with the light microscope, and contain lipids, protein, and catecholamines. (Lipids and catecholamines have an affinity for osmium and chromium salts, respectively.) They are spherical, rectangular, or oval sac-like structures 150 to 250 nm in diameter and are surrounded by a membrane. (These granules are 4 to 5 times larger than those found in the sympathetic axon terminals.) Some of the granules which have very dark electron-dense contents entirely or partially bounded by an electron-lucent zone store norepinephrine, whereas the other granules, which are completely composed of lighter electron-dense material, store epinephrine (176, 965). Fine particles, with diameters of 50 to 100 Å and with varying degrees of "packing," can usually be seen in the granules having no lucent area, but were not observed in the electron-dense material of granules having halos (Fig. 3.16) (965).

The first ultrastructure study of pheochromocytoma, with a demonstration of chromaffin granules, was reported by Kleinschmidt and Schümann in 1961 (516). A number of investigators have noted the presence of chromaffin granules varying from 100 to 300 nm (5, 45, 56, 82, 178, 397, 463, 551, 669, 729, 782, 809, 965, 1067).

Tannenbaum reported an elegant ultrastructural study of the normal adrenal medulla and of 14 pheochromocytomas in which he demonstrated a close correlation between the morphology of the catecholamine storage granules and the tissue concentration of epinephrine and norepinephrine (965). The ultrastructure of two pheochromocytomas containing almost entirely epinephrine consisted of catecholamine granules with a mean length of 270 nm (100 nm larger than the mean length of granules in the normal adrenal medulla). The majority of the catecholamine granules were of one morphologic type (Figs. 3.17 and 3.18) (965). The electron-dense material was composed of particles varying in diameter from 50 to 100 Å. Mitochondria were greatly increased in these tumors when compared with the normal medullary cells. In addition, rough-surfaced endoplasmic reticulum was prominent and scattered throughout the cytoplasm, and several sets of Golgi apparatus were seen in the juxtanuclear position (Fig. 3.17).

There is no indication that pheochromocytoma cells are richer in endoplasmic reticu-

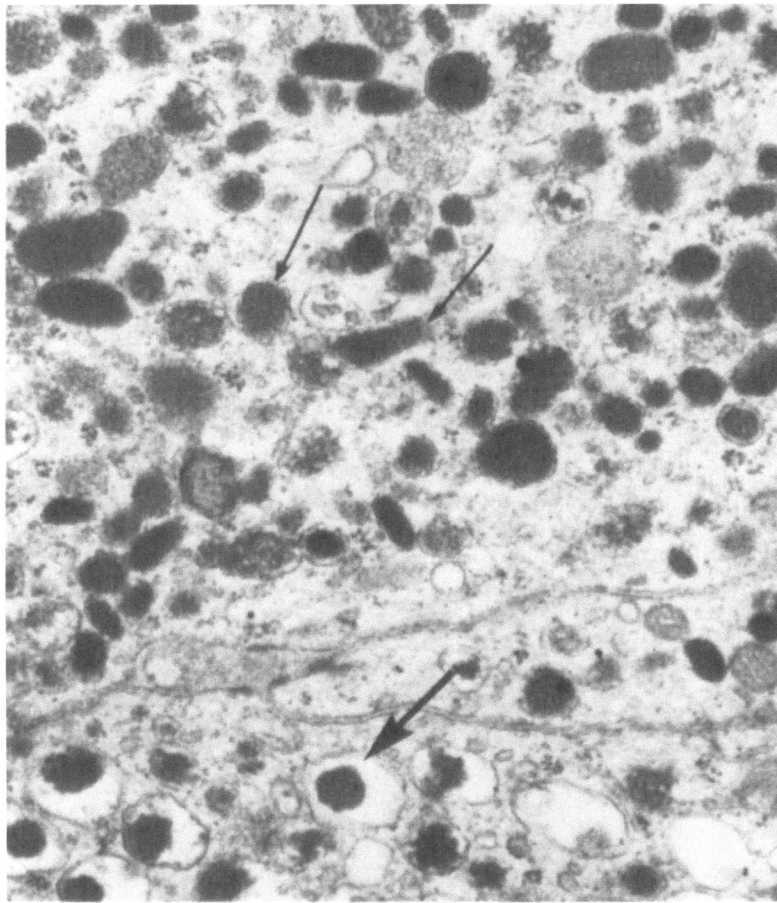

Fig. 3.16 Electron micrograph of two catecholamine-containing cells in normal adrenal medulla. Smaller arrows point to different epinephrine-containing granules. Larger arrow points to norepinephrine granules in a different cell. Note prominence of nonelectron-dense space adjacent to dark granules. (30,000×). From Tannenbaum, M. Ultrastructural pathology of adrenal medullary tumors. In: Somers, C. S., ed. *Pathology Annual.* Courtesy of Appleton-Century-Crofts, 1970, p. 148.

lum than are those of normal tissue (56, 397, 782, 1067). It has been reported to be sparse in cells containing many chromaffin granules, and more abundant when these granules are relatively few (782).

Tannenbaum reported that five pheochromocytomas containing almost entirely norepinephrine were composed of cells with granules of electron-dense material surrounded by a clear space or halo (Fig. 3.19) (965). Some of the norepinephrine granules seen under higher magnification were adjacent to lucent regions but not always distinctly surrounded by halos (Fig. 3.20). The electron-dense material never appeared finely granular and sometimes contained lucent areas (Fig. 3.20). He stated that in seven pheochromocytomas containing 10 times as much norepinephrine as epinephrine, the predominant cell contained granules characteristic of the norepinephrine-storage type, whereas a small percentage of cells contained epinephrine-storing granules (965). It is interesting that catechol-amine-containing granules were detected in cell blocks of plasma (after centrifugation) from some of these patients with pheochromocytoma. These granules were similar to those observed in the vascular spaces adjacent to cells of a normal adrenal medulla (Fig. 3.21). It is worth mentioning, however, that intact catecholamine-containing granules from rat hearts are biologically inert when injected intravenously into rats (768).

Sinusoids have been reported in many pheochromocytomas (178); however, although endothelium invariably lines the sinusoids of the normal adrenal medulla, not infrequently it is lacking in the sinusoids of these tumors (965). Tannenbaum has observed numerous fenestrations in the endothelium lining the capillaries or sinusoids in these tumors as well as in the normal adrenal medulla. Furthermore, he not infrequently observed portions of cells extruding through these fenestrations into the vascular spaces, particularly in pheochromocytomas (Fig. 3.22) (965).

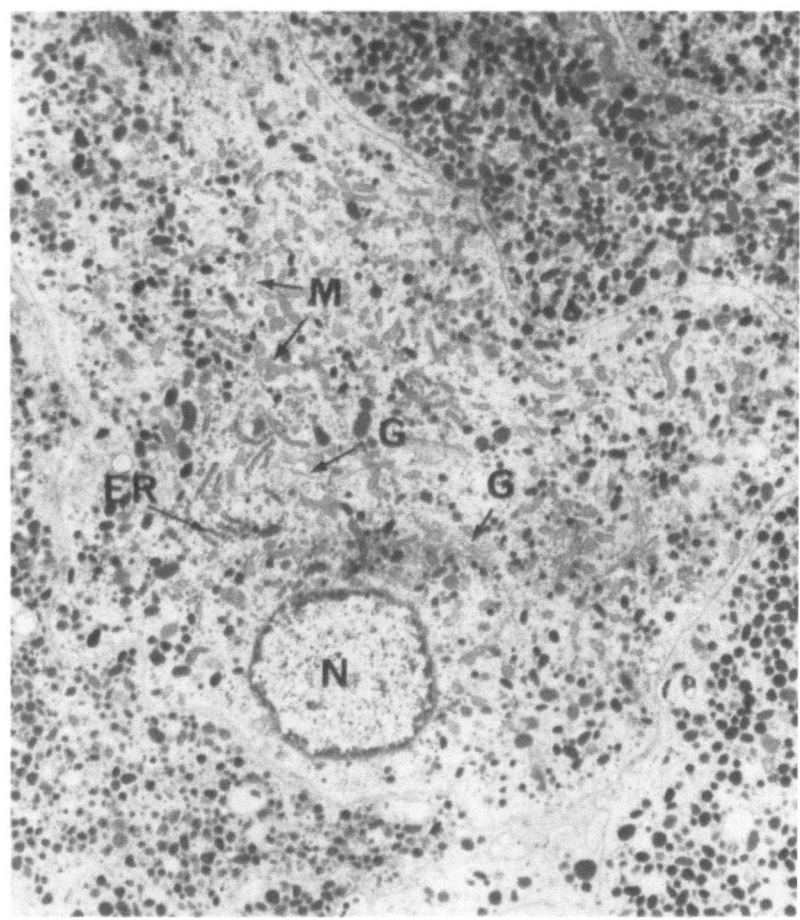

Fig. 3.17 Electron micrograph from a biochemically pure epinephrine-containing pheochromocytoma. There are marked numbers of mitochondria (M), prominent rough-surfaced endoplasmic reticulum (ER), and Golgi apparatus (G). Granules are of a uniform type. N= nucleus (7,000×). From Tannenbaum, M. Ultrastructural pathology of adrenal medullary tumors. In: Somers, C. S., ed. *Pathology Annual.* Courtesy of Appleton-Century-Crofts, 1970, p. 153.

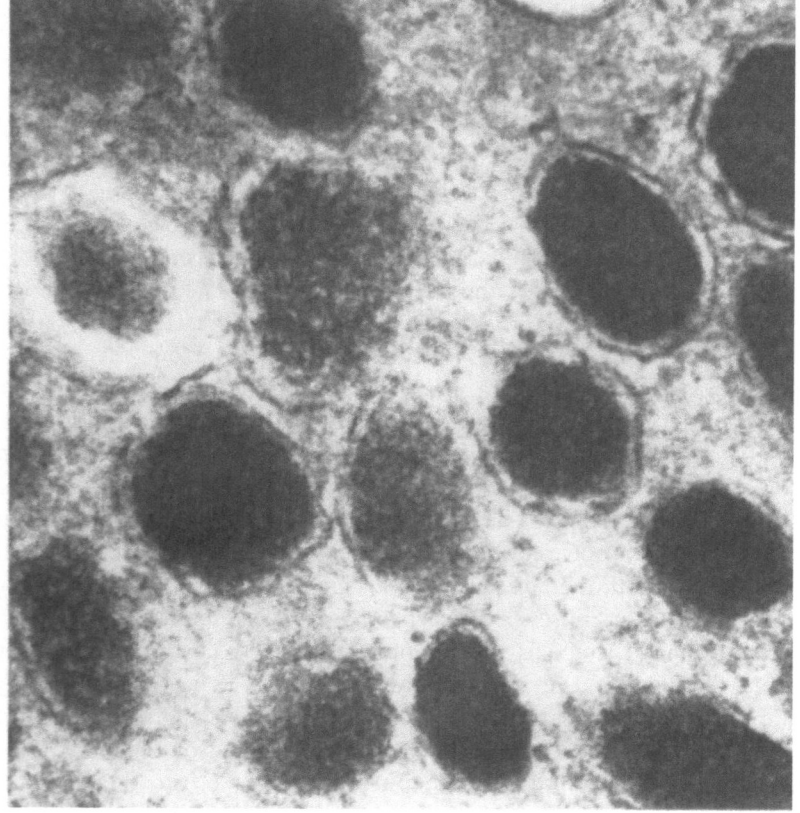

Fig. 3.18 Electron micrograph of "epinephrine" granules at higher magnification demonstrating a finer granular substructure and limiting membrane (150,000×). From Tannenbaum, M. Ultrastructural pathology of adrenal medullary tumors. In: Somers, C. S., ed. *Pathology Annual.* Courtesy of Appleton-Century-Crofts, 1970, p. 154.

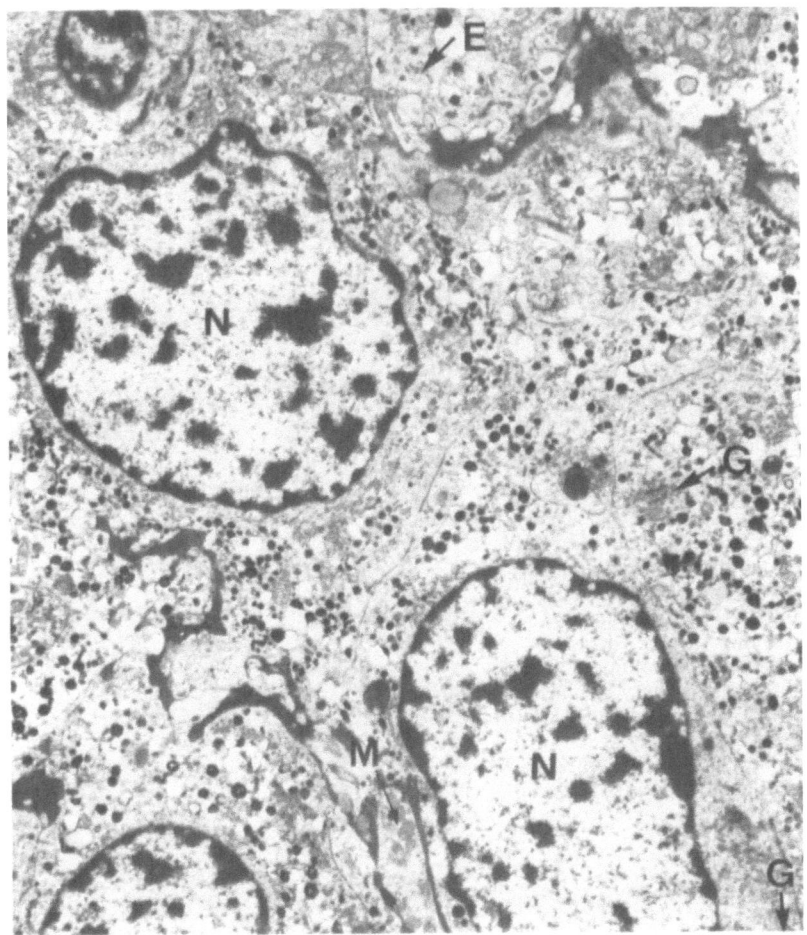

Fig. 3.19 Electron micrograph of several biochemically pure norepinephrine-containing cells from a pheochromocytoma. Note the clear space in the numerous catecholamine-containing granules. Some mitochondria (M), rough-surfaced endoplasmic reticulum (E), and Golgi apparatus (G) are discernable. N= nucleus (10,000×). From Tannenbaum, M. Ultrastructural pathology of adrenal medullary tumors. In: Somers, C. S., ed. *Pathology Annual*. Courtesy of Appleton-Century-Crofts, 1970, p. 157.

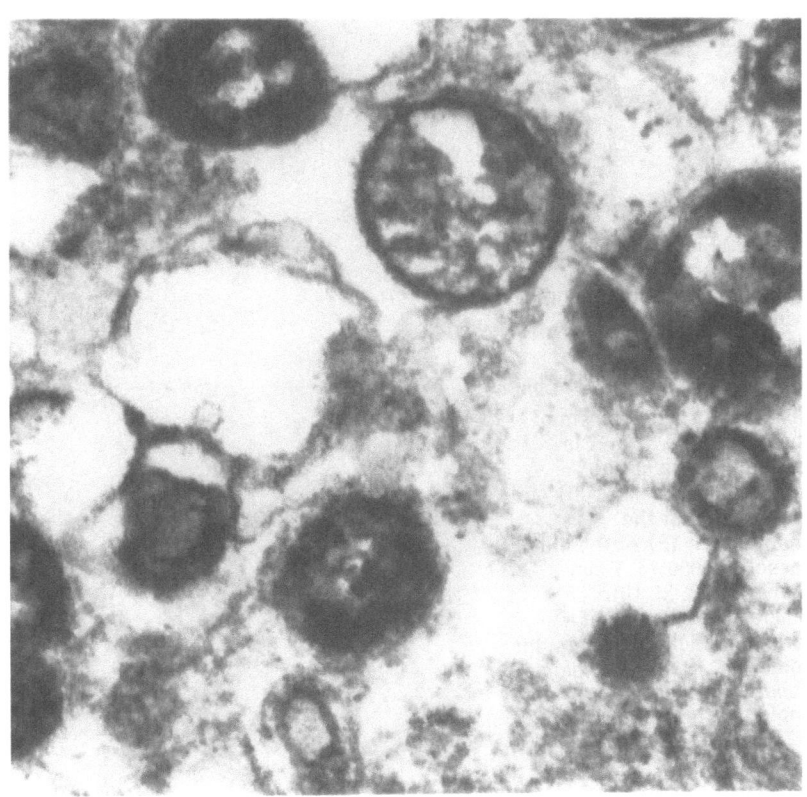

Fig. 3.20 Granules from "norepinephrine" containing cells. Note that substructure is very much different from epinephrine-containing cells in Figure 3.18 (110,000×). From Tannenbaum, M. Ultrastructural pathology of adrenal medullary tumors. In: Somers, C. S., ed. *Pathology Annual*. Courtesy of Appleton-Century-Crofts, 1970, p. 158.

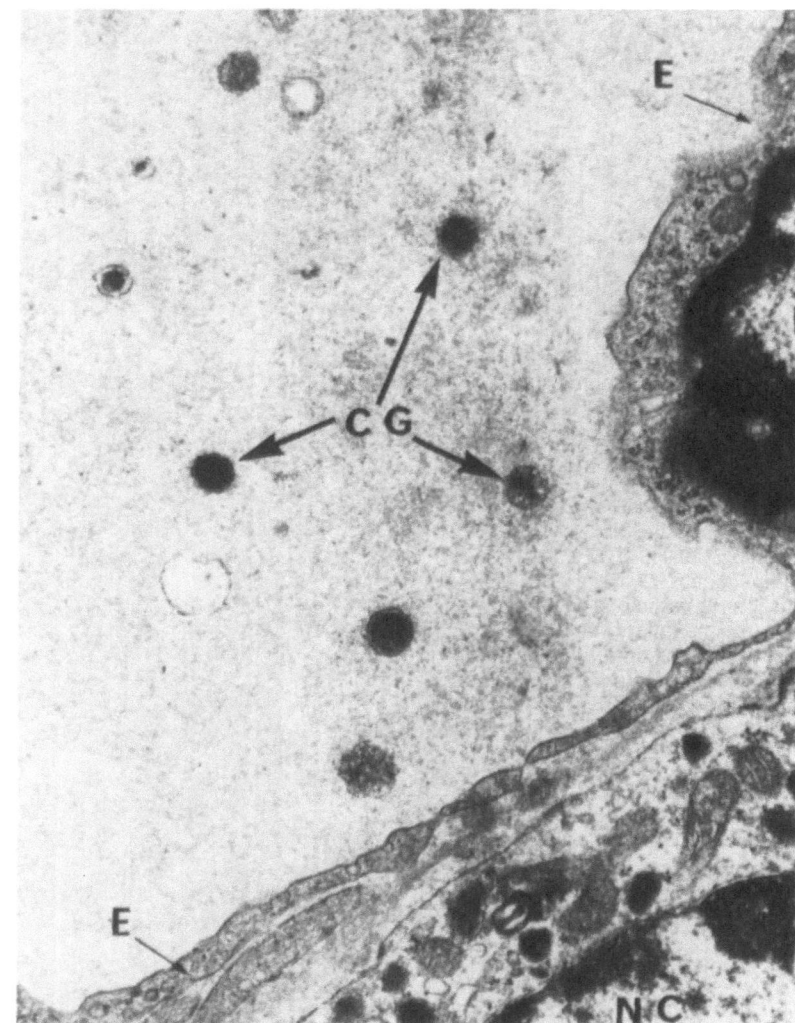

Fig. 3.21 Electron micrograph of intact catecholamine granules (CG) in vascular space adjacent to normal adrenal medullary cell. E= endothelium of blood vessel; NC=nucleus of catecholamine cell (epinephrine-containing cell); N=nucleus of endothelial cell (30,000×). From Tannenbaum, M. Ultrastructural pathology of adrenal medullary tumors. In: Somers, C. S., ed. *Pathology Annual*. Courtesy of Appleton-Century-Crofts, 1970, p. 160.

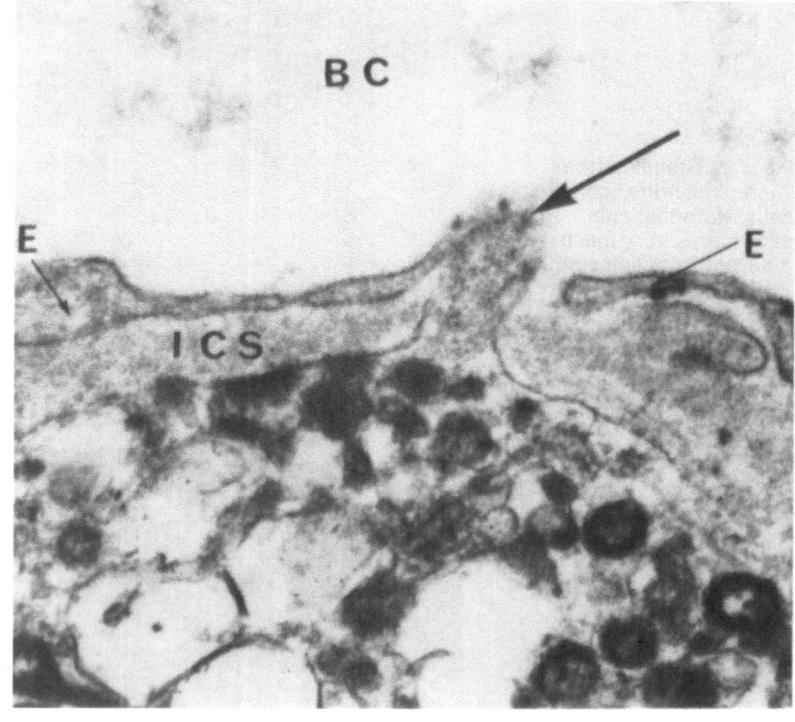

Fig. 3.22 Electron micrograph of a portion of a norepinephrine-containing cell adjacent to a blood capillary (BC) or blood sinusoid in a pheochromocytoma. A portion of the cytoplasm of the cell (large arrow) is extruding through the intercellular space (ICS) and fenestration of the endothelium (E) of the blood vessel (65,000×). From Tannenbaum, M. Ultrastructural pathology of adrenal medullary tumors. In: Somers, C. S., ed. *Pathology Annual*. Courtesy Appleton-Century-Crofts, 1970, p. 159.

Figure 3.23 illustrates the size distribution of chromaffin granules from normal human adrenal medulla and from pheochromocytomas. An excellent correlation between the concentrations of epinephrine and norepinephrine in normal human adrenal medullary tissue and pheochromocytomas, and the morphology of the storage granules, was demonstrated by Tannenbaum (Table 3.9). Winkler and Smith also noted some correlation between the catecholamine content of pheochromocytomas and the number of chromaffin granules (Fig. 3.24).

Misugi and coworkers have reported similar ultrastructural characteristics in a pheochromocytoma, with the exception that many of the mitochondria were vacuolated (669). Yokoyama and Takayasu, on the other hand, reported studies on five pheochromocytomas and found that, although the granules varied in size, they were always round, with a fine grainy structure, and were similar in all tumors despite the fact that one of the tumors was biochemically the reverse of the other four (1067). Furthermore, they reported considerable variability in the tumor cells containing catecholamine granules, and described pheochromocytoma cells which did not contain catecholamine, a finding only rarely observed by Tannenbaum (personal communication, Dr. Myron Tannenbaum, College of Physicians and Surgeons, New York City). Because of an apparent close association of catecholamine granules with the Golgi area in the group of catecholamine-producing

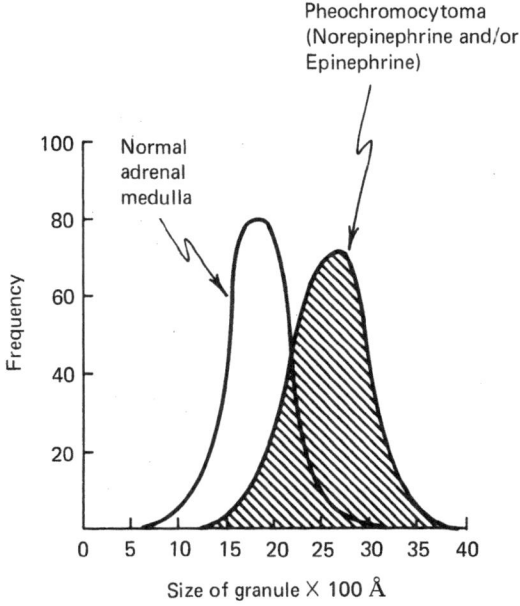

Fig. 3.23 Diagram of the distribution of size of chromaffin granules from normal human adrenal medulla and pheochromocytoma initially fixed in glutaraldehyde (2.5 percent). From Tannenbaum, M. Ultrastructural pathology of adrenal medullary tumors. In: Somers, C. S., ed. *Pathology Annual.* Courtesy Appleton-Century-Crofts, 1970, p. 155.

tumors they studied, Misugi and coworkers speculated that the Golgi complex may be synthesizing these granules (669). Several other studies have suggested that, as is the case in normal chromaffin cells, the Golgi region is responsible for the formation of chromaffin granules in pheochromocytomas (551, 782, 1067).

Table 3.9 *Biochemical and Ultrastructural Comparison of Pheochromocytoma and Normal Human Adrenal Medulla*[a]

	Homogenate (catecholamine mg/g adrenal)		Morphology of granule type	
Normal	Epinephrine	4.05	Epinephrine	(95%)
	Norepinephrine	0.70	Norepinephrine	(5%)
Tumor				
Epinephrine	Epinephrine	8.96	Epinephrine	(>95%)
(2)	Norepinephrine	0.20	Norepinephrine	(<5%)
Norepinephrine	Epinephrine	0.15	Epinephrine	(<1%)
(5)	Norepinephrine	10.20	Norepinephrine	(>95%)
Mixed	Epinephrine	0.96	Epinephrine	(5%)
(7)	Norepinephrine	9.30	Norepinephrine	(95%)

[a] From Tannenbaum, M. Ultrastructural pathology of adrenal medullary tumors. *In:* S. C. Sommers, ed., *Pathology Annual.* Courtesy of Appleton-Century-Crofts, 1970, p. 156.

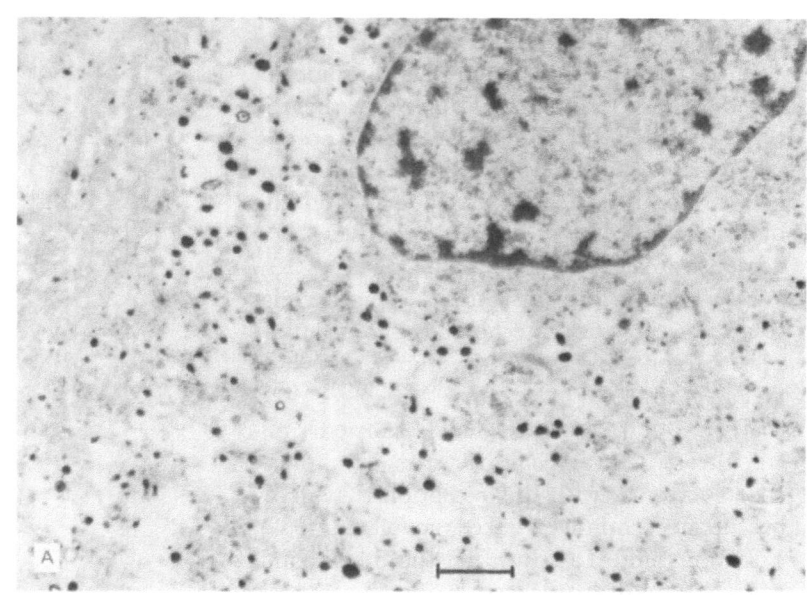

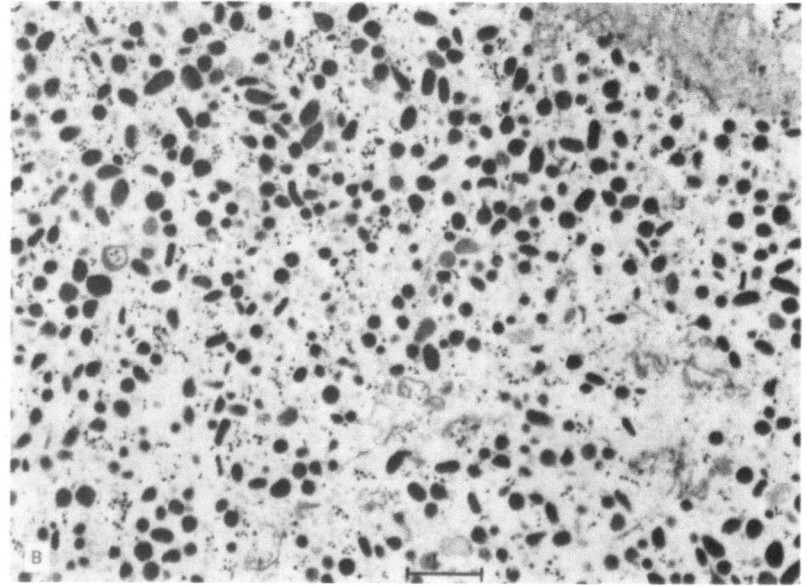

Fig. 3.24 Comparison of catecholamine content of two tumors with the number of chromaffin granules in each. A. Section from a tumor (Blaschko et al., 1968) which contained 1.2 mg catecholamines/g and gave a count of 178 chromaffin granules (mean of four sections). B. Section from a tumor which contained 6 mg catecholamines/g and gave a count of 740 chromaffin granules (mean of six sections). The scale represents 1 μ. From Winkler, H. and Smith, A. D. Pheochromocytoma and other catecholamine producing tumors. In: Blaschko, H. and Muscholl, E., eds. *Catecholamines.* Courtesy of Springer-Verlag, 1972, p. 911.

Electron micrographs of a chromaffin granule fraction isolated from one pheochromocytoma revealed that the shape of granules was quite variable. Apart from the globular granules, elongated, rodlike forms (noted by others in tissue sections from pheochromocytomas and also from normal adrenal medulla) were frequently observed (44a).

Morphologically similar granules have been found in neuroblastoma, ganglioneuroblastoma (669, 965), and tumors of the carotid body and jugular glomus (37), in addition to being found in pheochromocytoma (397, 552, 669, 965, 1067), the normal carotid body (568,

814), the adrenal medulla, and sympathetic nerve endings (790). Lauper and coworkers (552) confirmed the ultrastructural appearance of pheochromocytoma as described by Tannenbaum and by Yokoyama and Takayasu. A number of investigators (175, 669, 965, 1067) have demonstrated that the tumor cells closely resemble those of the normal adrenal medulla. Tannenbaum stated that in pheochromocytomas there were separate cells containing only norepinephrine or epinephrine; on the other hand, Blaschko and coworkers (82) and Lauper and coworkers (552) found that some cells of these tumors contained both epinephrine and norepinephrine granules.

Winkler and Smith have pointed out that in normal medulla of adult animals the granules containing epinephrine and granules containing norepinephrine are confined to separate cells, and that only in the fetal rabbit has a mixture of these granules been reported in the same cell (1053).

The study by Lauper and coworkers also confirmed the finding of Tannenbaum that there was excellent correlation between the morphology of the pheochromocytomas and the biochemically determined concentrations of epinephrine and norepinephrine. However, no correlation between morphology and clinical symptomatology was apparent, and there was no evidence to indicate functionally different tumors (i.e., the fine structure of tumor cells in patients with paroxysmal or sustained hypertension was similar to the structure of those in asymptomatic patients). Normetanephrine and metanephrine concentrations in the pheochromocytomas analyzed by Lauper and coworkers averaged 1 percent (or less) of the concentrations of norepinephrine and epinephrine. The concentrations of these O-methylated metabolites were not appreciably higher in tumors from patients with high catecholamine storage than they were in tumors from patients with low storage. These metabolites were very low in the tumor of one asymptomatic patient. These investigators concluded that the fine structure of pheochromocytomas was compatible with rather uniform function, mainly catecholamine synthesis and storage (552). The findings of Greenberg and coworkers also suggest no major metabolic differences between pheochromocytomas containing large and those containing small stores of catecholamines (397).

MALIGNANT PHEOCHROMOCYTOMA

As mentioned previously, it is impossible to determine from the histologic appearance whether a pheochromocytoma is malignant. This has also been emphasized by others (507, 959). Nuclear atypicality, pleomorphism, and mitosis may exist without malignancy, and

only tumor invasion of adjacent tissues and/or metastases can establish that a pheochromocytoma is malignant. Even capsular invasion and vascular penetration are not proof of malignancy (43, 302, 829), for these latter features can be found in tumors which pursue a benign course (704). One report indicated that seven tumors had histologic or angiographic evidence of capsular invasion or penetration, but none was considered malignant (1070). In a large series of pheochromocytomas studied at Columbia Medical Center, Melicow has observed that invasive malignant cells usually appeared to be smaller than cells of nonmalignant pheochromocytomas (personal communication). Since these tumors may be multicentric in origin, it must be appreciated that the differentiation between a metastatic and a benign pheochromocytoma may not always be clear. As pointed out by Roth, Dockerty, and Hightower, the extraordinary pathologic characteristic of pheochromocytoma is that it displays "one or more of the features which among other species of new growths would be indicative of malignancy" (819). These investigators have also aptly commented that "the pathologist is equally perplexed by the infrequency of metastasis in the face of cellular dedifferentiation and the paradoxical ability of these anaplastic cells to manufacture hormonal principles" (819).

Generally, these malignant tumors are slow growing, quite resistant to x-ray therapy, and usually metastasize to lymph nodes, liver, lung, and bone. Metastatic lesions occur elsewhere less commonly. Metastases to the scalp (875a) and to the brain have been observed, and one patient has been reported who had metastases not only to the usual sites but also to the prostate (649).

This latter case is extraordinarily interesting and instructive, since it serves not only to illustrate the extensive metastases that can occur in a patient with pheochromocytoma but also to emphasize how the "vagaries of metastatic malignancy in clinical practice can astound, baffle and confuse" (649). The details of the pathologic findings in this patient, who was studied at Columbia Medical Center, were reported by Melicow and associates:

This 56-year-old man had complained of recurrent hematuria, backache, and weight loss of 15 to 25 lb for 1.5 years. Five years earlier a Grade I to II papillary urothelial carcinoma (Fig. 3.25) of the bladder was fulgurated. Blood pressure was 120/80 mmHg and physical examination was unremarkable except for a large firm nodule in the right lobe of the prostate and several small nodules in the left lobe. Many red blood cells were present in the urine and on one occasion malignant-looking cells (Class III) were noted. Chest x-ray revealed bilateral interstitial fibrosis and prominence of the hilar markings. IVP demonstrated impaired function and hydronephrosis of the right kidney. Serum acid and alkaline phosphatases were elevated to 1.41 Bessey-Lowry Units and 350 international units, respectively. Blood urea nitrogen was 26 mg/dl and the sedimentation rate was 70 mm in 1 hr. Several bladder irregularities, seen at cystoscopy, were fulgurated. Perineal prostatic biopsy showed "benign prostatic acini and clusters of malignant anaplastic cells" which were interpreted as of prostatic origin or possibly from a bladder tumor, since the biopsy of the bladder had also shown a similar histopathologic pattern of anaplastic cells (Figs. 3.26 and 3.27). Liver scan was normal; however, a bone scan indicated abnormalities in the pelvis and some vertebrae (T1 and L5). X-rays revealed diffuse blastic and lytic lesions, suggesting metastatic malignancy (Fig. 3.28A). Bone biopsy established the presence of

malignant cells (Fig. 3.28B), and it was concluded that the most likely diagnosis was carcinoma of the prostate, with extension into the bladder and metastases to the bones.

Despite orchidectomy, transurethral prostatic resection (to relieve urinary retention), estrogen administration, and rathiotherapy, the patient continued to deteriorate and died in 4 months. Autopsy revealed a pheochromocytoma of the organ of Zuckerkandl (apparently the primary site), with metastases to lymph nodes, prostate, urinary bladder (obstructing the right ureter), liver, lungs, lumbar vertebrae, ribs, and the frontal bone (Fig. 3.29). Microscopic appearance of the tumor of the organ of Zuckerkandl (Fig. 3.30) and of the metastases in the liver and lung (Fig. 3.31) and of those in the vertebrae (Fig. 3.32) and prostate (Fig. 3.33B) was typical of pheochromocytoma. Cell staining did not reveal the presence of chromaffin granules, which suggested that the tumor was nonsecretory. This was consistent with the absence of hypertension and other characteristic manifestations of pheochromocytoma.

The first functioning metastases of a pheochromocytoma were described in 1951 by Allen and coworkers (7). Metastases may be not only functional but also composed of fully differentiated pheochromocytes (208, 507). One patient has been reported who had an adrenal pheochromocytoma which contained

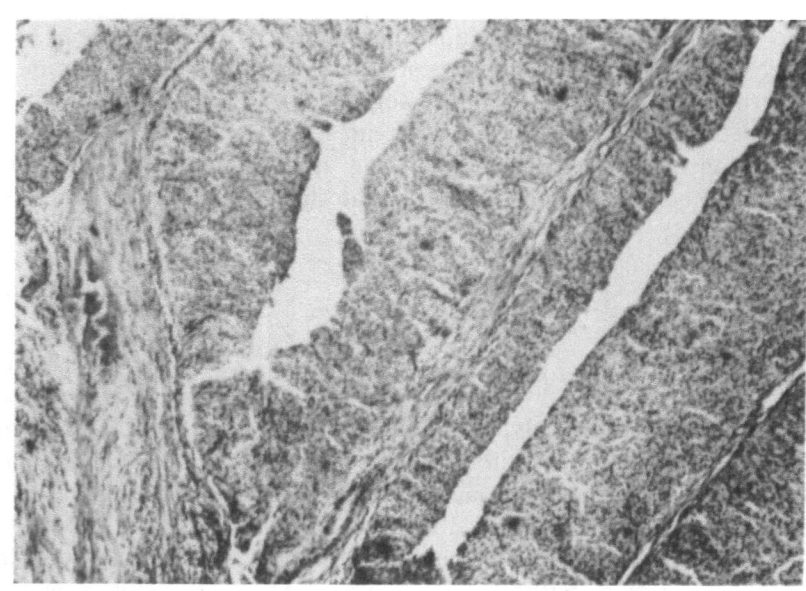

Fig. 3.25 Photomicrograph of biopsy of Grade I to II papillary vesical tumor, fulgurated 5 years before patient's admission to hospital for reported complaint. From Melicow, M. M., Uson, A. C., and Veenema, R. J., *J. Urol. 110:* 97, 1973. By permission of Williams & Wilkins Co.

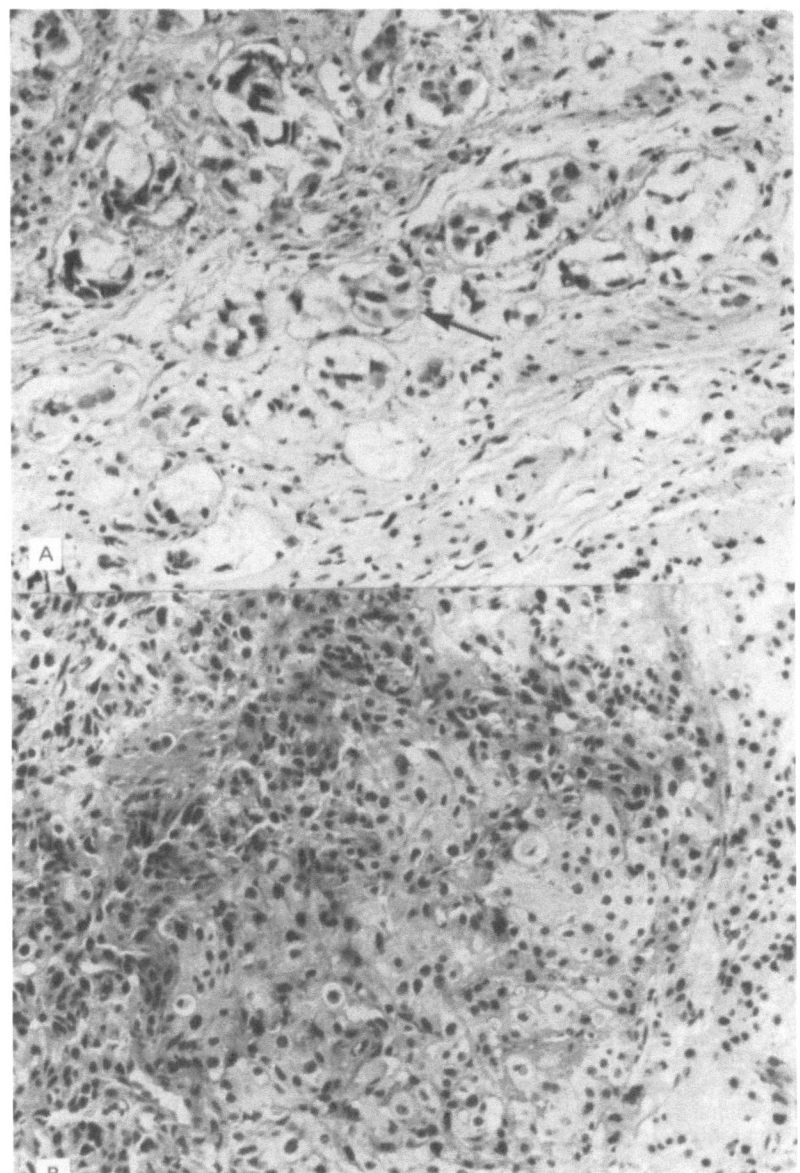

Fig. 3.26 A. Biopsy of prostate shows hyperchromatic cells with irregular nuclei occupying prostatic acini (arrow). Pattern suggests anaplastic carcinoma of prostate gland. B. Another area of same biopsy shows solid sheet of cells resembling those seen in part A. Pattern in both fragments not incompatible with diagnosis of anaplastic carcinoma of prostate with invasion. From Melicow, M. M., Uson, A. C., and Veenema, R. J., *J. Urol. 110:* 98, 1973. By permission of Williams & Wilkins Co.

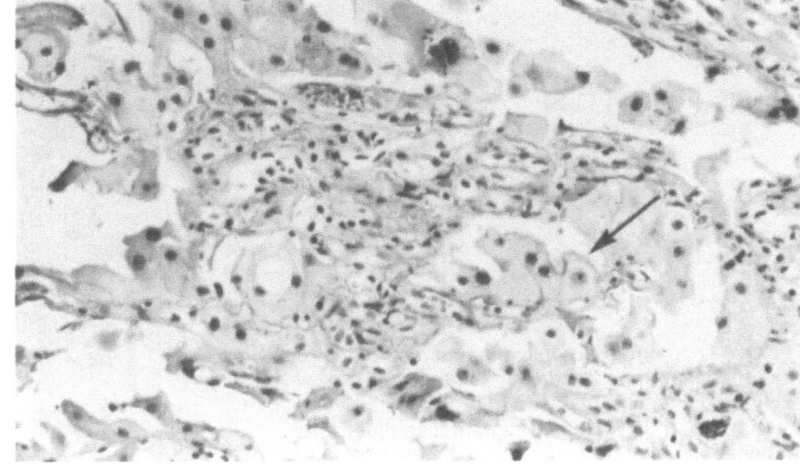

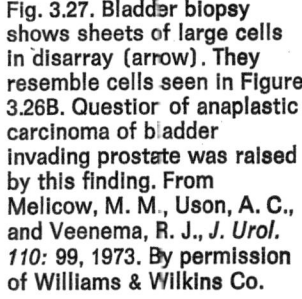

Fig. 3.27. Bladder biopsy shows sheets of large cells in disarray (arrow). They resemble cells seen in Figure 3.26B. Question of anaplastic carcinoma of bladder invading prostate was raised by this finding. From Melicow, M. M., Uson, A. C., and Veenema, R. J., *J. Urol. 110:* 99, 1973. By permission of Williams & Wilkins Co.

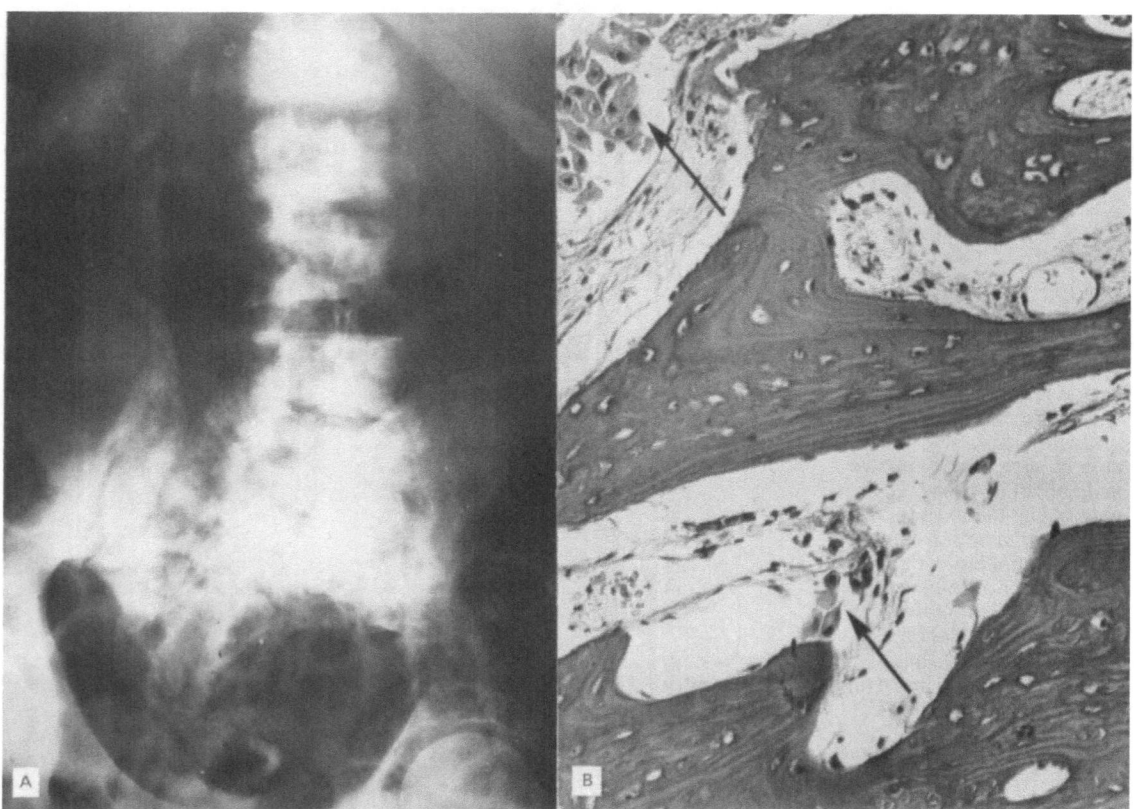

Fig. 3.28 A. Radiograph of lumbosacral spine. Note evidence of osteoblastic and osteolytic lesions. B. Bone biopsy reveals spicules of bone enclosing few clusters of malignant cells (arrows) resembling those seen in prostate. This finding plus slightly elevated serum acid phosphatase and evidence of metastatic bone disease favored diagnosis of carcinoma of prostate with metastases.
From Melicow M. M., Uson, A. C., and Veenema, R. J., *J. Urol. 110:* 99, 1973. By permission of Williams & Wilkins Co.

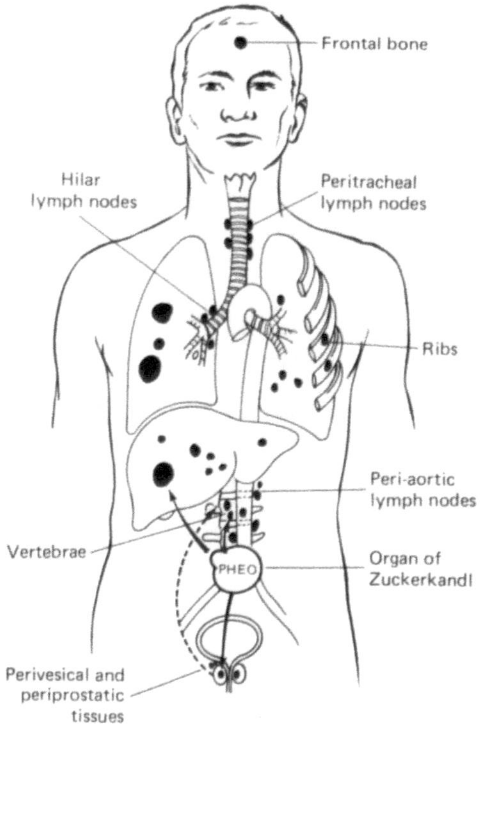

Fig. 3.29 Diagram of autopsy findings depicts spread from malignant pheochromocytoma of organ of Zuckerkandl and metastases to prostate, perivesical, and periprostatic regions. Diagram also illustrates metastases to lymph nodes, liver, lungs, lumbar spine, and frontal bone. From Melicow, M. M., Uson, A. C., and Veenema, R. J., *J. Urol. 110:* 100, 1973. By permission of Williams & Wilkins Co.

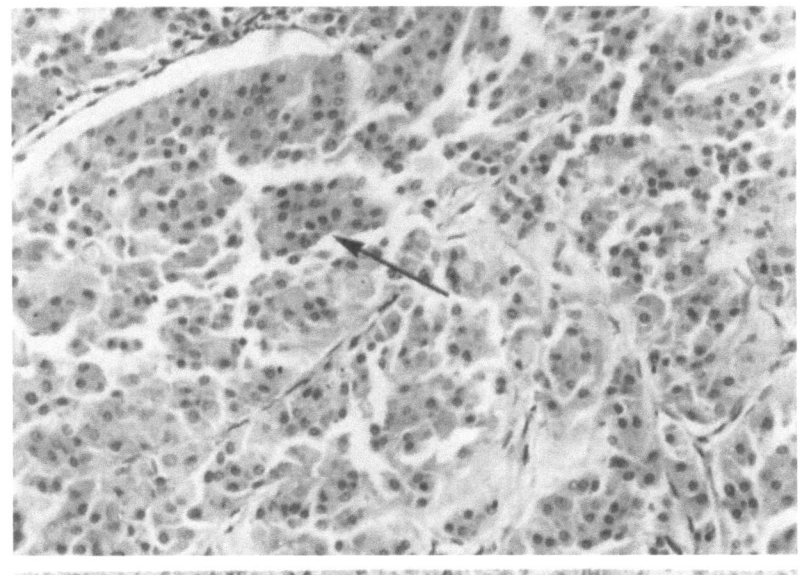

Fig. 3.30 Photomicrograph of section through malignant pheochromocytoma of organ of Zuckerkandl. Note clusters of ova to polygonal compact cells (arrow) with eosinophilic granular cytoplasm. Compartmentalization characteristic of pheochromocytoma. From Melicow, M. M., Uson, A. C., and Veenema, R. J., *J. Urol. 110:* 100, 1973. By permission of Williams & Wilkins Co.

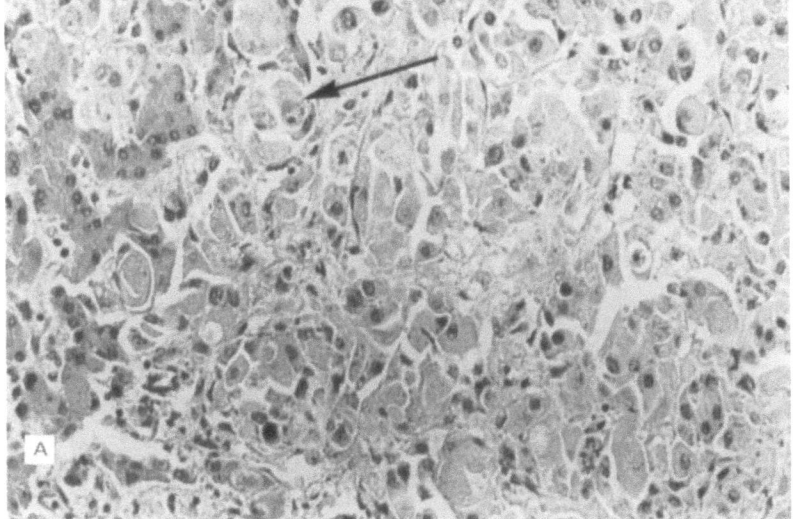

Fig. 3.31 A. Metastasis to liver. Note penetration of malignant cells between liver cell cords (arrow). B. Metatasis to lung. Note large cluster of tumor cells surrounded by alveoli (arrow). From Melicow, M. M., Uson, A. C., and Veenema, R. J., *J. Urol. 110:* 101, 1973. By permission of Williams & Wilkins Co.

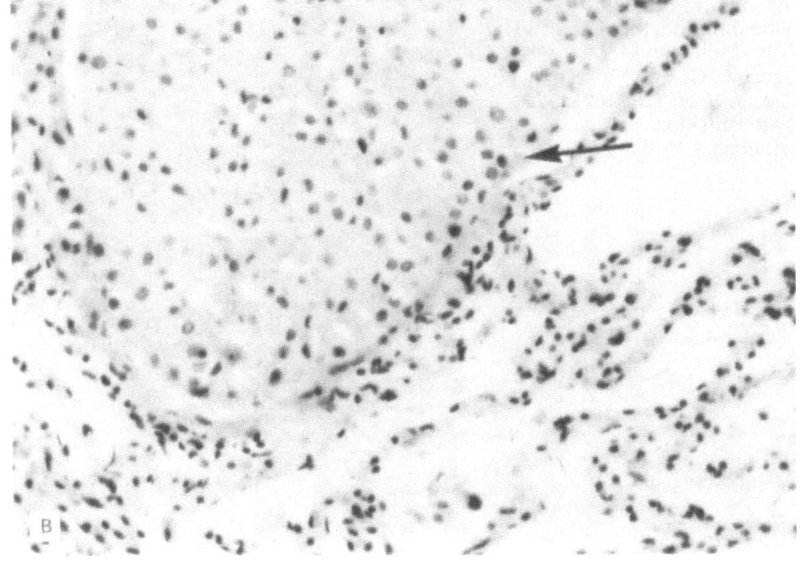

Fig. 3.32 Section through vertebra shows extensive invasion of bone by cells resembling primary focus in organ of Zuckerkandl (arrow). From Melicow, M. M., Uson, A. C., and Veenema, R. J., *J. Urol. 110:* 102, 1973. By permission of Williams & Wilkins Co.

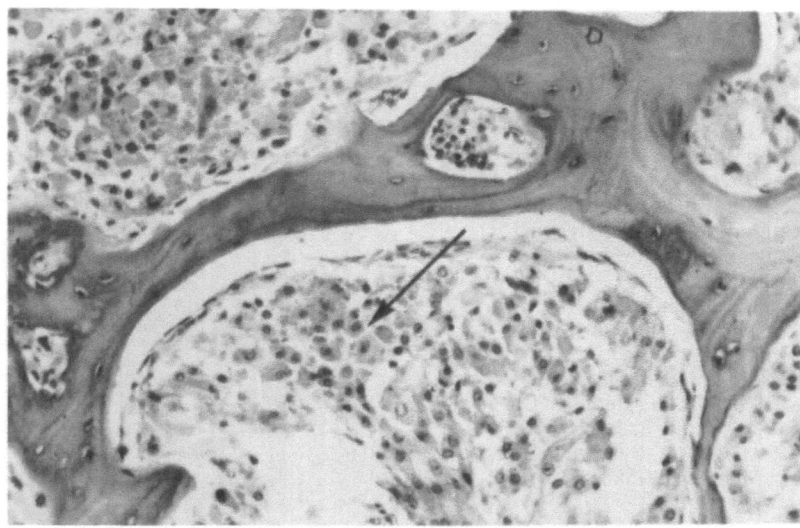

Fig. 3.33 A. Section through prostate shows benign acini, some rather small, without any evidence of primary prostatic malignancy. B. Another area of prostate shows clusters of cells resembling those in pheochromocytoma (arrow). From Melicow, M. M., Uson, A. C., and Veenema, R. J., *J. Urol. 110:* 102, 1973. By permission of Williams & Wilkins Co.

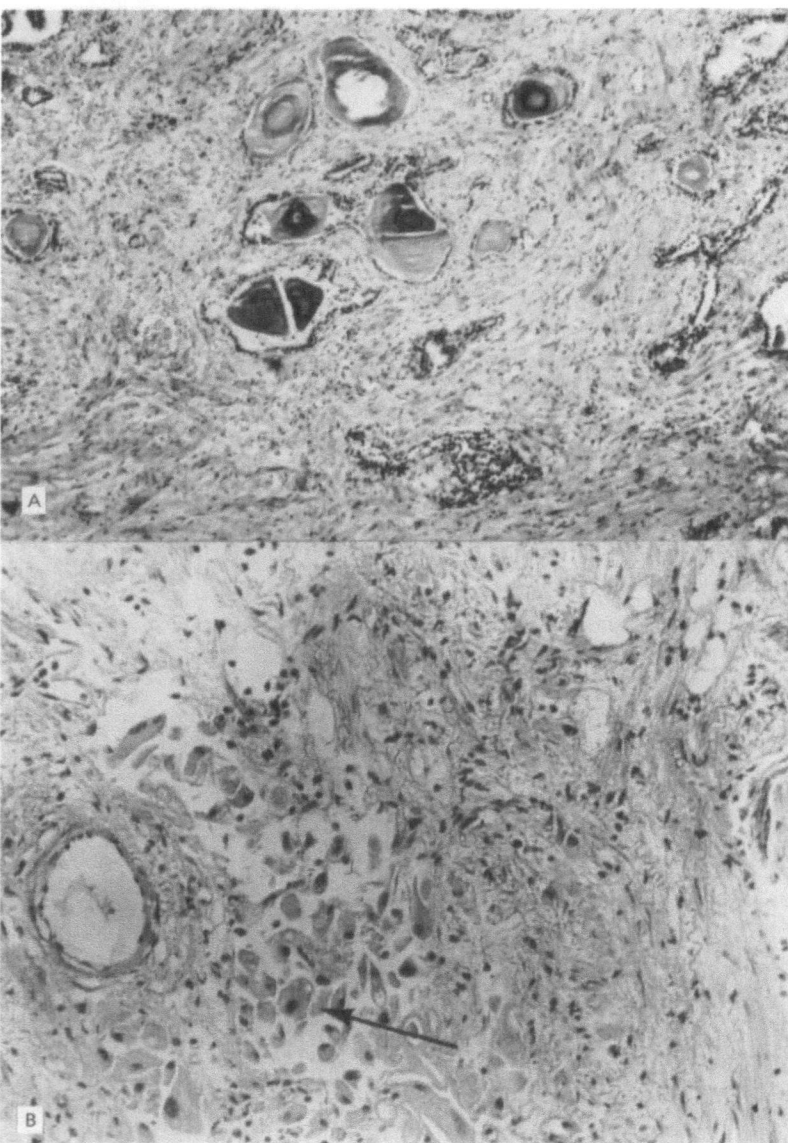

epinephrine and norepinephrine; however, a hepatic metastasis contained only norepinephrine (507). In this patient, the presence of high concentrations of adrenocortical steroids could have accounted for the methylation of norepinephrine to epinephrine in the adrenal pheochromocytoma; furthermore, the metastasis could have been composed of more primitive, fetal-like chromaffin cells, which have little or no ability to methylate norepinephrine (178).

A point of interest is that in a series of 18 patients with malignant pheochromocytoma, 72.3 percent were females whereas only 27.7 percent were males (784). As mentioned previously, estrogen or growth hormone administration has been reported to induce pheochromocytomas in the experimental animal. Whether hormonal influences are important etiologically or in the development of pheochromocytoma and its malignant transformation in the human remains to be seen.

Another point of interest is that tumors producing paroxysmal hypertension are rarely malignant and seldom recur after removal; however, the claim that paroxysms of hypertension and other signs of crisis are lacking in patients with malignant pheochromocytoma (641, 928) is in error. One of our patients with paroxysmal hypertension had a metastatic pheochromocytoma (patient No. 38 in Chapter 7). Another patient with a malignant pheochromocytoma with metastases to the cervical spine, which resulted in a Brown-Sequard syndrome, also had paroxysmal hypertension (184). Still another patient, whose primary adrenal pheochromocytoma had been completely extirpated, had paroxysmal hypertensive episodes (the pressure rising from normal levels to 240/150 mmHg) due to functioning metastases in the skeleton, lungs, pleura, lymph nodes, and liver (208).

In our experience, as well as in that of Symington and Goodall (959), Graham (392), and Scott and associates (875a), approximately 10 percent of pheochromocytomas were found to be malignant, whereas Remine and associates reported malignancy in 13.1 percent of 133 cases seen at the Mayo Clinic (784). On the other hand, Sjoerdsma and coworkers reported the incidence to be roughly 6 percent (909), whereas an analysis by Hume

of pheochromocytomas reported in the literature revealed malignant tumors in only 2.8 percent of adults and 2.4 percent of children (466). The incidence of malignancy appears to be the same whether the tumor site is in the adrenal gland or the organ of Zuckerkandl (319, 426). Remine and associates reported a considerably higher incidence of malignancy in extraadrenal pheochromocytomas (28.6 percent) as compared to that in adrenal pheochromocytoma (11.3 percent). Since the incidence of extraadrenal pheochromocytoma is roughly 10 percent, it is not surprising to find that 11 of 50 malignancies reviewed in the literature by Hermann and Mornex arose from extraadrenal sites (437).

The percentages recorded above refer to the incidence of malignancy in sporadic pheochromocytoma. It is noteworthy that four of 15 patients with familial adrenal pheochromocytoma had malignant tumors (an incidence of 26.6 percent) (135b). The explanation for this higher incidence of malignancy in familial than in sporadic intraadrenal pheochromocytoma remains unclear; however, the fact that six of these 15 patients were normotensive, and the fact that four of the 15 did not have any symptoms suggesting pheochromocytoma, indicates that clinically it is more difficult to detect familial than sporadic pheochromocytoma. A greater delay in the diagnosis of familial than of sporadic pheochromocytoma may partly account for the difference in the incidence of malignancy between these conditions.

Malignant pheochromocytoma with multiple mediastinal and lung metastases has also been described in the thorax (76). In this latter case chyle continued to accumulate in the pleural cavity and required repeated drainage. Another intrathoracic malignant pheochromocytoma, situated at the tip of the left pleural cavity, caused a Horner's syndrome on the left side (749). A number of reports seem to indicate that patients with pulmonary metastases have a particularly poor prognosis (784).

In a review of 21 cases of malignant pheochromocytoma recorded in the literature up to 1959, Bartels found that the longest interval between removal of the primary tumor and its clinical reappearance was 4.5 years (43). However, recurrence, which is usually.

first manifested by excess catecholamine excretion, may not be evident for many years: in 11 of 13 patients followed at the Mayo Clinic, after malignant pheochromocytomas were resected for cure, recurrence developed with a median distribution of 5.6 years postoperatively (784). Remine and associates have emphasized that "recurrence should be viewed with optimism as it is compatible with long survival, even up to 20 years" (784). The experience with 138 cases of pheochromocytoma seen at the Mayo Clinic revealed that recurrence after surgical treatment was 9.8 percent and the 5-year survival was 96 percent for benign tumors (similar to the normal population) and 44 percent for the malignant neoplasms (784). Since pheochromocytoma may arise in multiple sites, a recurrence of symptoms after removal of a tumor may be due to the appearance of another benign pheochromocytoma, rather than to a metastasis. In evaluating this problem of malignancy, Symington and Goodall found that frequently pheochromocytomas thought to be recurrent or metastatic could be explained as of multicentric origin (959). This possibility has also been emphasized by MacKenzie (599).

A malignant pheochromocytoma may be nonfunctional, as was the case in the patient of Melicow and associates reported in detail above. It is possible that, on a rare occasion, a functioning pheochromocytoma may give rise to a nonfunctioning malignant tumor. Scott and associates described one patient with a functioning pheochromocytoma which appeared to be benign and which was excised with the entire left adrenal gland. The patient then remained asymptomatic for 5 years, during which time a nonfunctioning highly malignant pheochromocytoma developed in the left suprarenal fossa. Whether this was a recurrence or a new malignant tumor could not be determined (875a).

There are no biochemical features that identify a pheochromocytoma as malignant. Metastases may (7, 145, 208, 616, 624) or may not be functional, and it appears that they may contain and secrete any of the three catecholamines. One adrenal pheochromocytoma secreted epinephrine, whereas a metastasis secreted norepinephrine (437). The speculation of Anton in 1967 that the presence of dopamine, or its precursor (dopa), indi-

cated a malignant pheochromocytoma (16) has subsequently proved invalid (91, 365, 586, 729, 748, 830, 888). Sato and Sjoerdsma found only one out of five patients with malignant pheochromocytoma to excrete increased concentrations of HVA (855). Yet, from the few reports in the literature of pheochromocytomas containing dopamine, the prevalence of malignancy does appear greater than in those tumors not containing this amine.

Neoplasias exhibit immunologic activity more frequently than do normal tissues. Furthermore, Seegal and associates have reported that malignant tumor cells appear to react with fluorescein-labeled antibodies (i.e., immunoglobulins, complement, and foreign antigens) more often than do benign tumor cells. It is therefore interesting that four out of five pheochromocytomas which were considered benign exhibited a particularly high degree of immunologic activity and showed a higher intensity of fluorescence than most other tumors (877a). It is unclear why this unusual immunologic activity of benign pheochromocytomas occurred; additional studies of this type should be performed in order to determine whether there are any differences between the immunologic activity of cells from benign and malignant pheochromocytomas. Similar comparative studies on cells from sporadic and familial pheochromocytomas are also indicated.

PATHOLOGIC COMPLICATIONS

Complications of pheochromocytomas are primarily those secondary to the hypertension [e.g., *cardiovascular* and *cerebrovascular accidents, neuroretinopathy* (observed primarily with sustained hypertension), *benign* and *malignant nephrosclerosis* and *arteriosclerosis* (668)]. As mentioned earlier, if the tumor is undetected and the hypertension unchecked, the complications will almost invariably cause death. The ravages of severe sustained hypertension (reaching 206/152 mmHg) due to a bilateral pheochromocytoma are well-illustrated in a case report by Kremer (528) of a 14-year-old girl who died of cerebral thrombosis. There was marked myocardial hypertrophy and degeneration, severe coronary

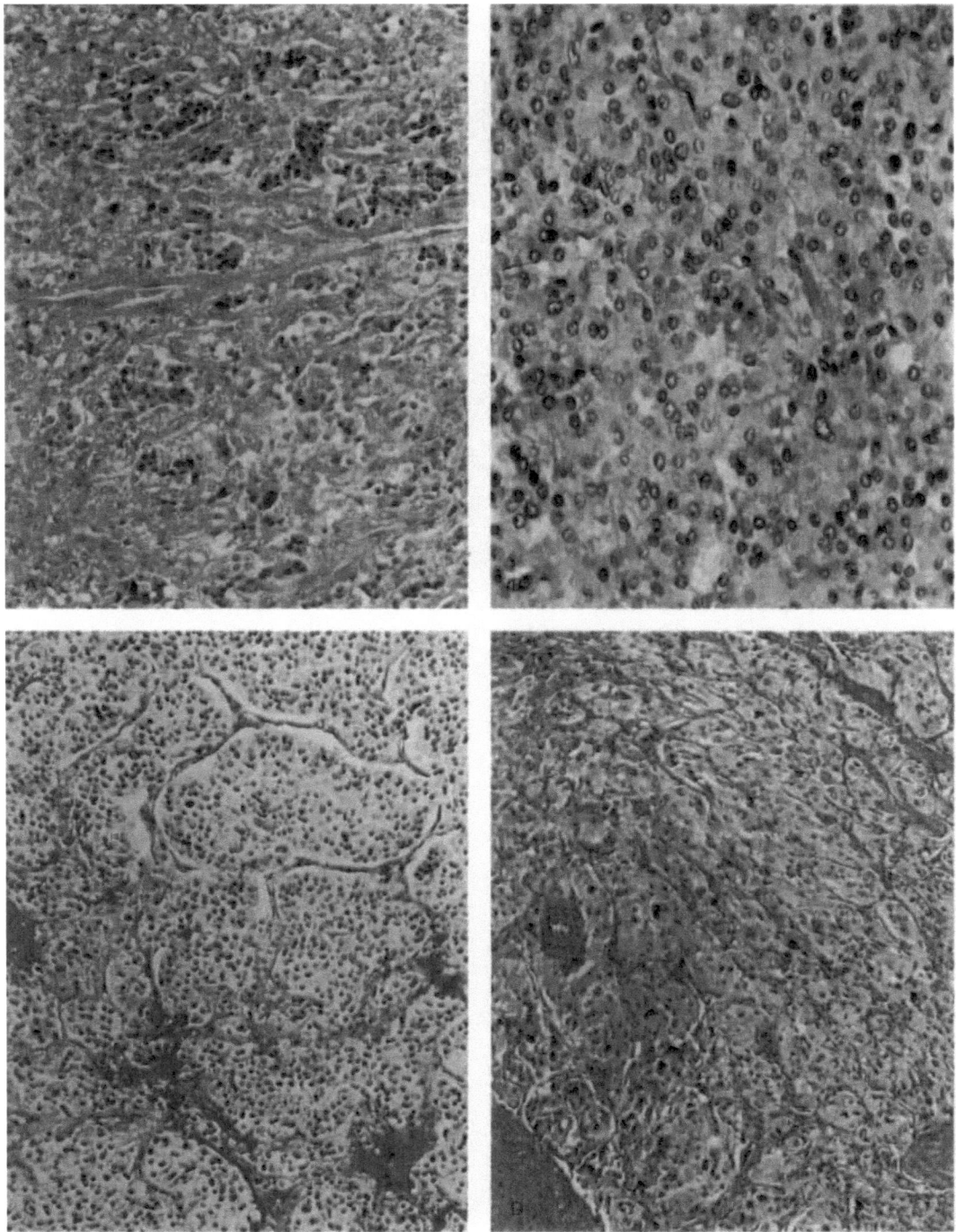

Fig. 3.3 A. Nonfunctional carotid body paraganglioma. This is an area of nonfunctional carotid body paraganglioma showing typical fixation artifact of cellular vacuolization and foci of pyknosis (225×). B. Functional jugular paraganglioma. This illustrates the epitheliomatous appearance of a functional jugular paraganglioma (350×). C. Para-aortic (Zuckerkandl) paraganglioma. This paraganglioma removed from the organ of Zuckerkandl shows an alveolar pattern indistinguishable from that of a carotid body paraganglioma (140×). D. Urinary bladder paraganglioma. This intramural bladder paraganglioma, removed from a 29-year-old man, was present in the midline with symptoms of secretory activity (140×). From Glenner, G. G. and Grimley, P. M. Tumors of the extra-adrenal paraganglion system (including chemoreceptors). In: *Atlas of Tumor Pathology*, second series, fascicle 9. Courtesy of Armed Forces Institute of Pathology, 1974, p. 83.

Fig. 3.4 Formalin-induced fluorescence in jugular paraganglioma. This illustrates the localization of norepinephrine by formalin-induced fluorescence in a jugular paraganglioma. The patient did not have clinical symptoms of a secreting tumor (60×). (Courtesy of Dr. B. Hamberger.) From Glenner, G. G. and Grimley, P. M. Tumors of the extra-adrenal paraganglion system (including chemoreceptors). In: *Atlas of Tumor Pathology*, second series, fascicle 9. Courtesy of Armed Forces Institute of Pathology, 1974, p. 65.

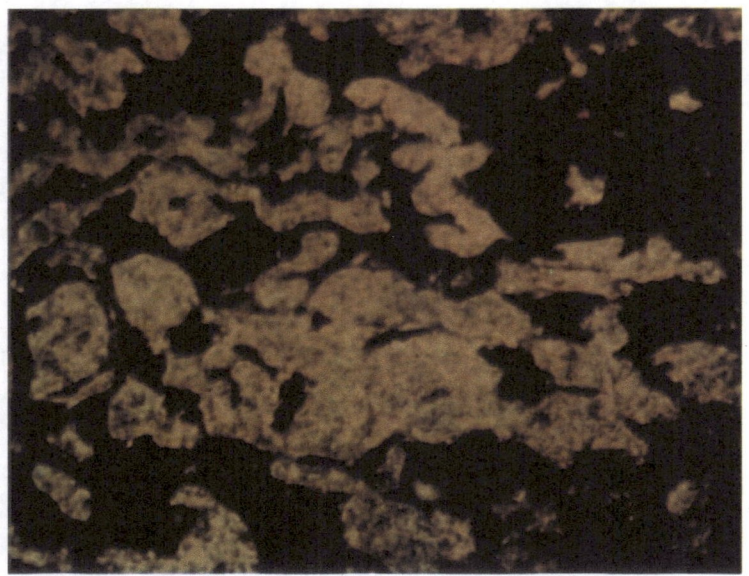

Fig. 3.10 A. An average size (6×6×4.5 cm) encapsulated pheochromocytoma weighing 70 g and occurring in right adrenal area (note wedge-shaped adrenal gland attached to round pheochromocytoma). B. Sectioned tumor reveals reddish-gray appearance with several small hemorrhagic foci.

The patient was a 28-year-old black woman who gave a 4-year history of paroxysmal episodes of hypertension (up to 305/200 mmHg), severe pounding headaches, weakness, blurring of vision, sweating, flushing, nervousness, palpitation, and nausea. Initially attacks had occurred once per month but recently had increased to several times per day and lasted 10 to 20 min. In addition, the patient had experienced a weight loss and epistaxis. Attacks could be provoked by bending to the left side but not to the right and on one occasion an attack occurred 10 min following an enema. Left ventricular strain pattern (on ECG) and elevation of blood glucose from 84 to 145 mg percent were noted with paroxysm of hypertension.

Physical examination revealed a blood pressure that varied from 125/100 mmHg to severely hypertensive levels; a benzodioxane test was positive. Urinary catecholamines were markedly elevated. A presacral pneumogram and IVP were interpreted as revealing a left suprarenal mass when in fact the tumor occurred in the right adrenal area. Postoperative blood pressure normalized. Courtesy of Dr. M. M. Melicow, Dept. of Pathology, Columbia Medical Center, New York, New York.

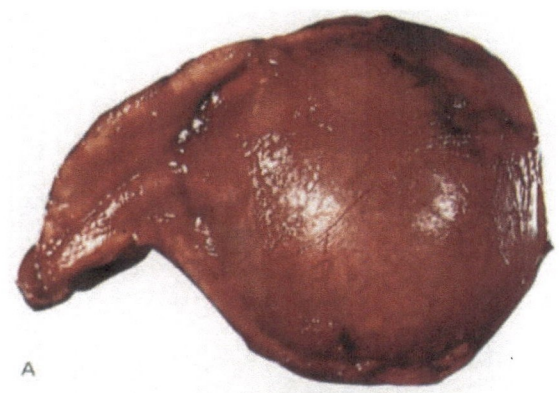

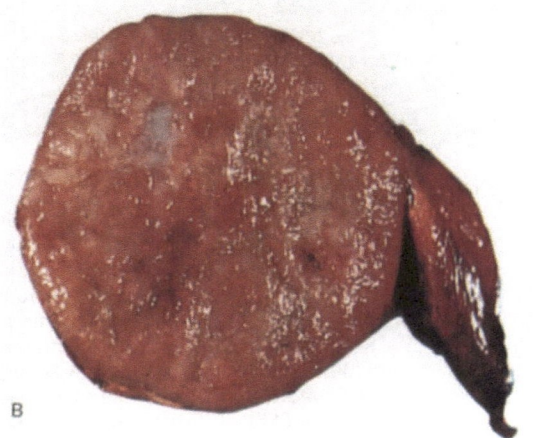

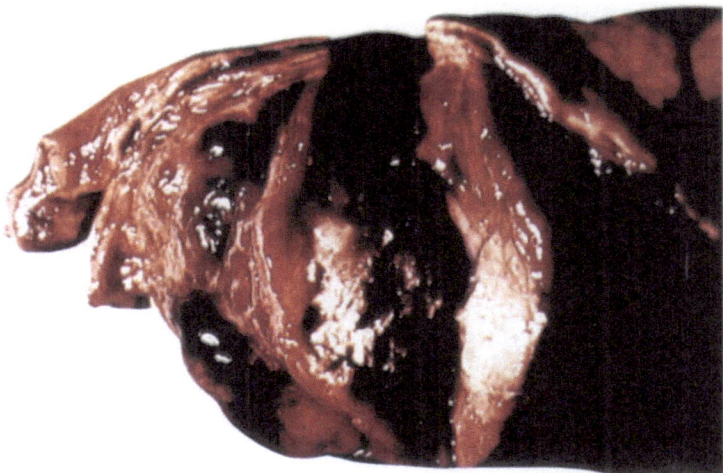

Fig. 3.11 A 28-g pheochromocytoma of the right adrenal gland containing calcium. The patient was a 28-year-old man with sustained hypertension and superimposed paroxysmal elevations. Courtesy of Dr. M. M. Melicow, Dept. of Pathology, Columbia Medical Center, New York, New York.

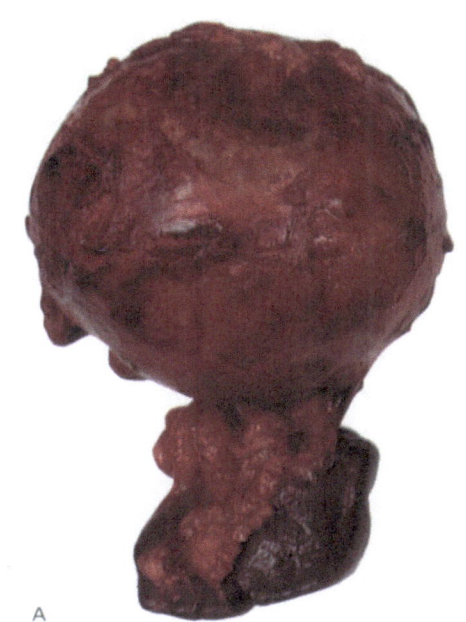

Fig. 3.12 A huge cystic pheochromocytoma measuring about 13 cm in diameter, weighing 1330 g and containing about 1 liter of brownish fluid. This tumor occurred in the left adrenal gland of a 47-year-old woman with paroxysmal hypertension. A. Cystic (round) pheochromocytoma removed with spleen. B. Cystic pheochromocytoma on section. (See patient No. 36, Chapter 7.) Courtesy of Dr. Q. J. Valensi, Dept. of Pathology, New York University Medical Center, New York, New York.

A

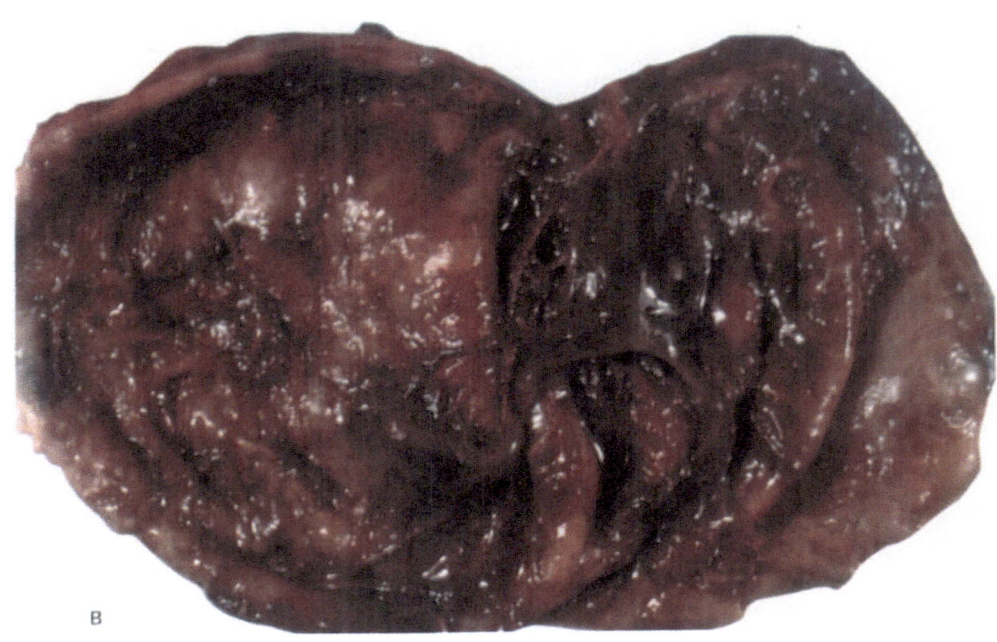

B

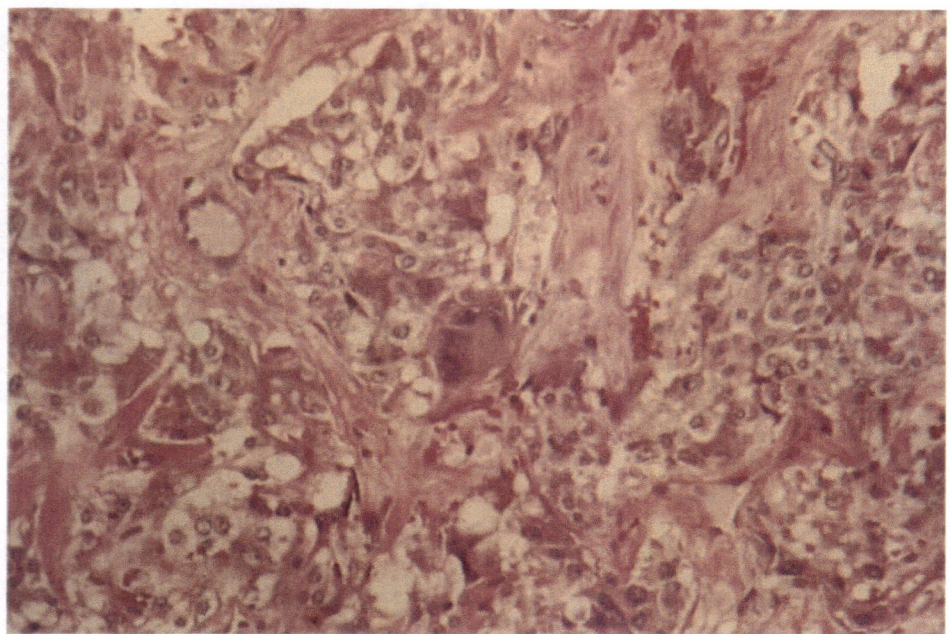

Fig. 3.13 Photomicrograph (medium power 100×) of pheochromocytoma removed from left adrenal area. (Section removed from tumor shown in Fig. 3.12.) Note multinucleated giant cell in center of field and pleomorphic pattern of cells (see patient No. 36, Chapter 7). Courtesy Dr. Q. J. Valensi, Dept. of Pathology, New York University Medical Center, New York, New York.

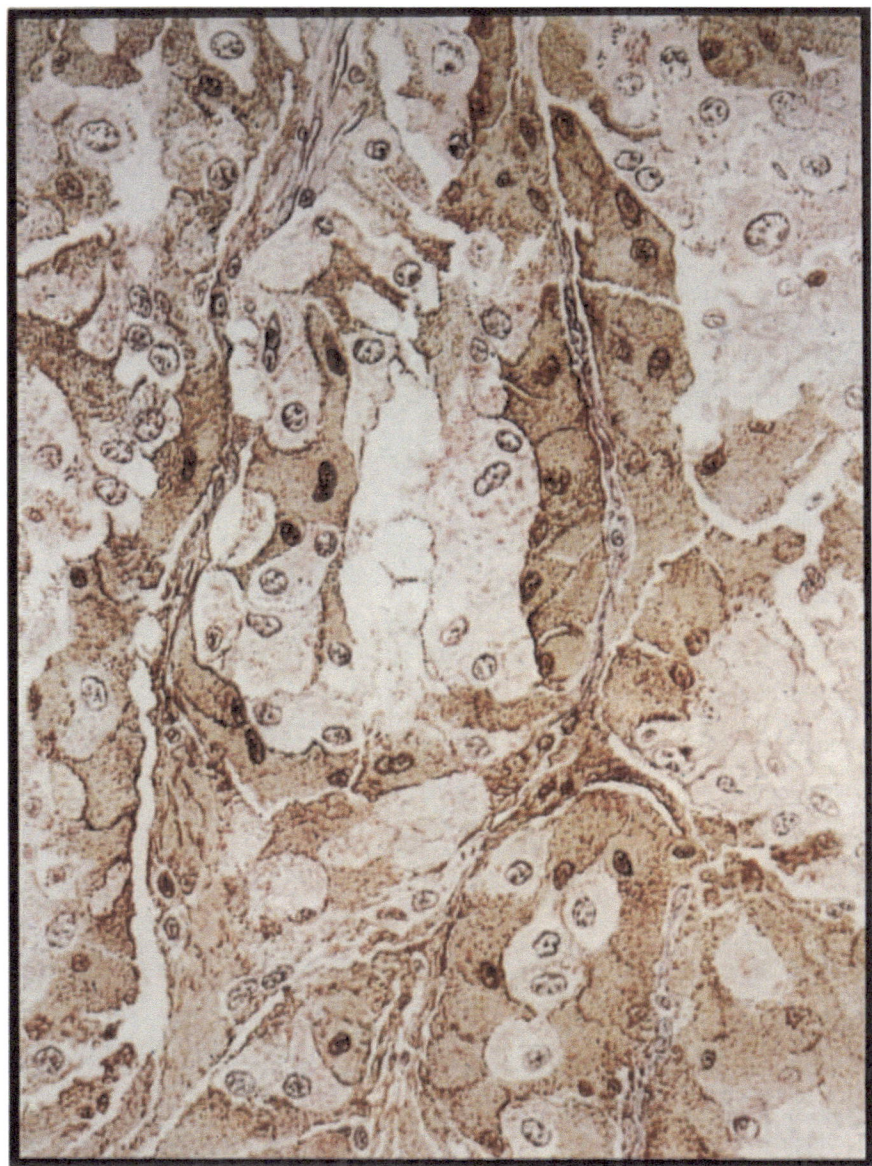

Fig. 3.15 Colored photomicrograph of pheochromocytoma treated with chromate. Note that some cells are not chromated and that the brown granules vary in size and in number in the cytoplasm of the chromated cells. A. F. I. P. Neg. Acc. No. 218755-C6. From Karsner, H. T. Tumors of the adrenal. In *Atlas of Tumor Pathology*, section VIII, fascicle 29. Courtesy of Armed Forces Institute of Pathology, 1950, p. 44. By permission of Williams & Wilkins Co.

Fig. 3.34 A. Right fundus; (a) zone of papilledema, (b) zone of hard and soft exudates, (c) zone of hard exudates (high molecular weight lipoproteins) and B, left fundus of a 22-year-old white male with sustained hypertension (250/150 mmHg) due to a large pheochromocytoma of the right adrenal area. One year previously he had been given electroshock therapy by a psychiatrist. Blood pressure had been normal 5 months ago. Initially he had been admitted to the New York Institute of Ophthalmology because of markedly blurred vision (only able to count fingers) for 3 months. Treatment with cortisone had been started 7 months before admission with little improvement of vision.

Photographs A and B were taken with a wide angle (45°) Nikon camera; they reveal an acute Group 4 hypertensive retinopathy with bilateral papilledema, many hemorrhages, hard and soft exudates (extending along the arcades and involving the macular zones), neovascularization in the peripapillary areas, and severe arteriolar narrowing. The marked degree of retinal edema extended 30° from the optic discs, i.e., even beyond the limits of these funduscopic photographs.

Subsequently, when hypertension was discovered, workup for pheochromocytoma revealed radiologic evidence of a large solid (by ultrasonography) right suprarenal mass depressing the right kidney, and also elevated urinary metanephrines, varying from 16 to 18 mg/24-hr urine (normal range 0.3 to 0.9).

Following extirpation of a 165-g pheochromocytoma, the blood pressure and catecholamine metabolites normalized, although this occurred only a number of days postoperatively. The retinopathy completely resolved within 10 months, leaving only residual fibrous sheathing along some of the arterioles near the discs, pigment epithelial disruption, and glial tissue along former areas of edema. Vision improved to 20/40 OS and 20/80 OD within 1 year but did not return to normal because of residual gliotic changes. Photographs were obtained through the courtesy of Dr. F. A. L'Esperance, Jr., Professor of Ophthalmology, Columbia Medical Center, New York, New York. Dr. L'Esperance stated that the degree of papilledema was the most severe he had ever seen.

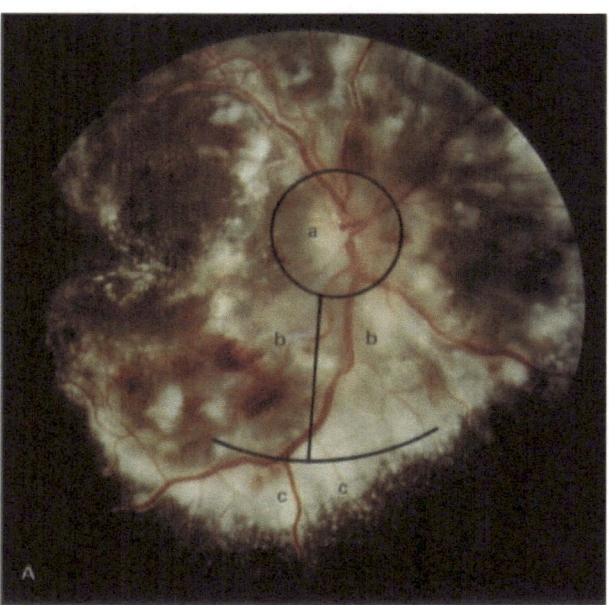

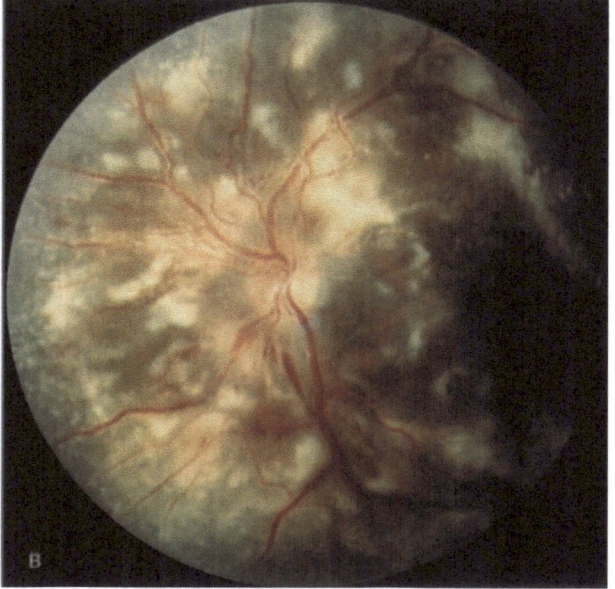

Fig. 4.5 A. Showing facial flushing during a paroxysmal attack of hypertension. B. Normal appearance. This patient was a 45-year-old woman with a 6-week history of hypertension, discovered because she began to have short episodes of nausea, vomiting, and marked facial flushing. These paroxysms lasted 5 to 10 min and were accompanied by mild headache and profuse perspiration especially around the head and neck. Her blood pressure was intermittently elevated, varying from 100/70 mmHg to 240/140 mmHg during attacks. Attacks occurred several times daily. Although the marked flushing was more suggestive of serotoninism than a pheochromocytoma, urinary catecholamines (576 μg/24 hr) and VMA (21 mg/24 hr) were elevated, whereas 5-HIAA excretion was normal. An intravenous urogram revealed a right suprarenal tumor which proved to be a 330-g pheochromocytoma with focal capsular penetration. Removal of the tumor relieved all her symptoms, but she had residual labile hypertension. Postoperatively, the urinary excretion of catecholamines and their metabolites was normal. R. W. Gifford, Jr., Cleveland Clinic, Cleveland, Ohio, unpublished.

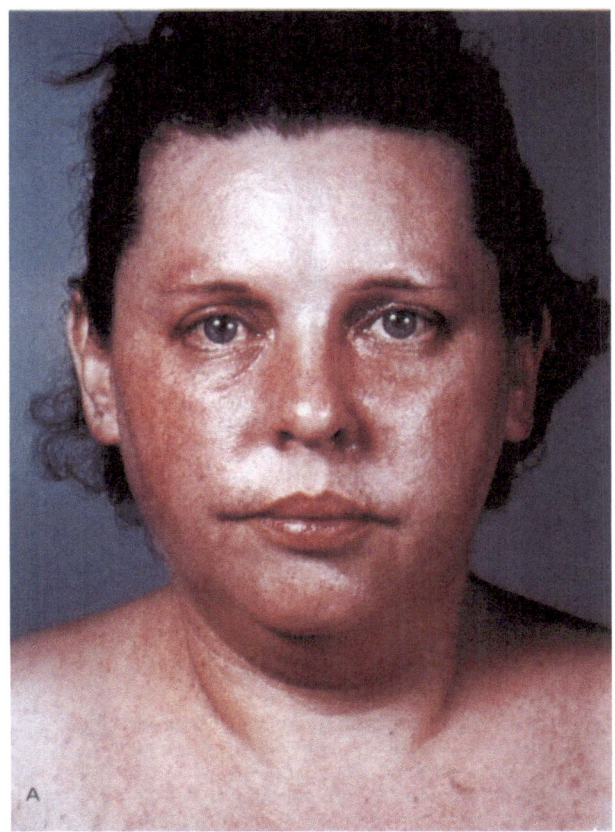

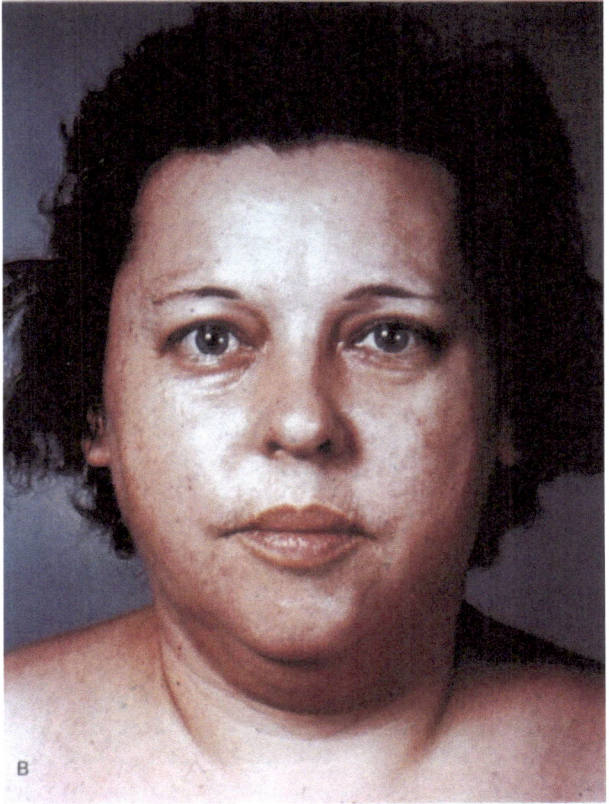

78

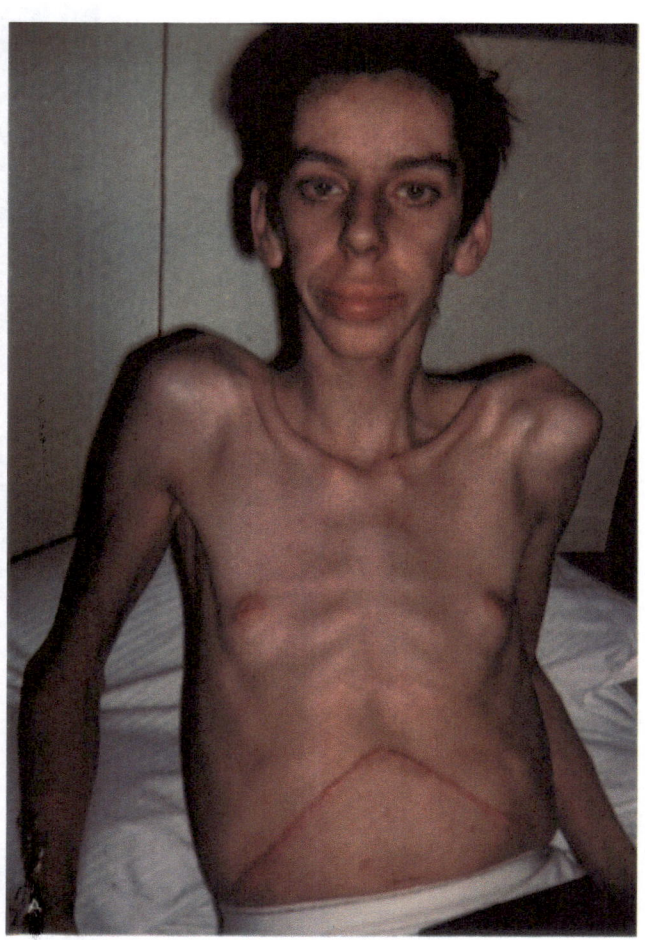

Fig. 4.13 A. Face and body habitus. Note characteristic facies, thick lips, and pectus carinatum. B. Highly visible corneal nerves in right eye seen during slit-lamp examination (present bilaterally).

This 20-year-old white male had a recent history of congestive heart failure and blood pressure and pulse varying from 150/70 to 240/150 mmHg and 70 to 140/min, respectively. Several years earlier tumors of lips were removed to reduce macrocheilia and partial glossectomy was performed to remove tumors of anterior one-third of tongue. Family history unremarkable. *Px:* marfanoid habitus (tall, thin, extremities long in relation to torso, arachnodactyly, pes cavus, pectus carinatum, scoliosis); high arched palate; thickened tarsi of eyelids; yellowish masses (plexiform neuromas) near limbus of each conjunctiva; gynecomastia; absence of beard and axillary hair; palpable thyroid. *Laboratory studies:* elevated VMA (56 mg/24 hr); consistently elevated serum calcitonin; intradermal histamine caused wheal formation but no flare. *Course:* Bilateral benign pheochromocytomas were removed but patient succumbed to metastatic medullary thyroid carcinoma. From Baum, J. L. and Adler, M. E., *Arch. Ophthalmol. 87:* 579, 1972.

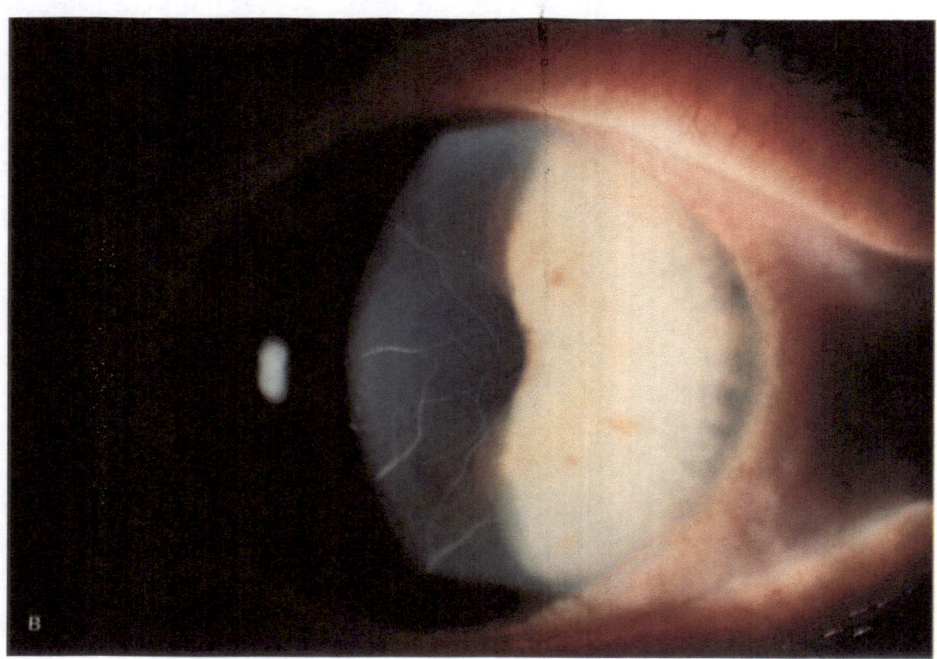

sclerosis, and a history of precordial pain thought to be of cardiac origin. There were also arteriosclerotic changes of the aorta, lungs, spleen, and ovaries, and a pronounced degree of arteriosclerosis in the pancreas, thyroid, and diaphragm. Sclerosis of the retinal arterioles was present in addition to optic atrophy, and considerable retinal degeneration with numerous atrophic areas and exudates. The kidneys contained anemic infarcts, arteriolar and intraglomerular hyaline thromboses, arteriolar proliferation, and a severe tubular hyalinization. There was also an eccentric thickening of the intima of the renal arteries. An erroneous diagnosis of nephritis had been made in this child, but, in retrospect, nephritis seems unlikely, since there was never any evidence of impaired renal function to suggest acute or chronic renal disease.

Cerebral accidents (hemorrhage and/or infarction) and *acute cardiac decompensation* are common causes of death in patients with pheochromocytoma (Table 3.10). Cerebral infarction may sometimes be massive (875a). One patient, whose pheochromocytoma was apparently undetected for 40 years, was reported to have had three *subarachnoid hemorrhages,* each one occurring during a paroxysm of hypertension (267). *Focal embolic nephritis* and necrosis in some of the glomeruli and parenchyma have also been described (464), and severe *arteriolitis* with necrosis and hyalinization may occur in many organs (1007) *Myocardial infarction* and recurrent cardiac pain accompanying episodes of headache, hypertension, and diaphoresis have occurred in the presence of pheochromocytoma (229); myocardial infarction may be the presenting complaint in some patients (498, 817). Gupta indicated that the frequency of myocardial infarction was greater in patients with pheochromocytoma and paroxysmal hypertension than in those with sustained hypertension. He speculated that the sudden stimulation of β-receptors in the heart might cause infarction in man (406). *Dissecting aneurysm,* which occurs rarely, may result in a ruptured thoracic aorta with hemorrhage, shock, and death (137, 467, 938a, 979).

An example of the extreme severity of *retinopathy* that can occur in a patient with sustained hypertension due to pheochromo-

Table 3.10 *Cause of Death in 72 Patients Not Operated upon for Pheochromocytoma[a]*

Cause	No. of cases
Cerebral vascular accident	19
Acute cardiac decompensation	15
Died in "attack"	9
Hyperpyrexia	4
Pneumonia	4
Coronary occlusion	2
Meningitis	2
Intercurrent operation	
Fractured ankle, reduction	1
Extraction of tooth	1
Appendectomy	1
Herniorrhaphy	1
Cecostomy, for fecal impaction	1
On anus	1
Delivery under spinal anesthesia	2
Intercurrent trauma	
Childbirth	1
Injection (intravenous) for cholecystography	1
Perforated duodenal ulcer	1
Hemorrhage from tumor (spontaneous)	1
Dissecting aneurysm	1
Volvulus	1
Uremia	1
Infection of face	1
Unknown, associated with rubor of body and dilated pupils	1

[a] From Graham, J. B. *Int. Abstr. Surg. 92:* 115, 1951. By permission of *Surgery, Gynecology, and Obstetrics.*

cytoma is shown in Figure 3.34 (p. 76). Elevation of blood pressure in retinal arterioles and a significant degree of retinal and choroidal vascular damage in this patient are demonstrated by the appearance of fluorescein-illuminated blood at an inordinately high intraocular pressure, ophthalmodynamometrically induced according to the method of hemobarometry (565) (Fig. 3.35), and by the evidence of considerable extravasation of fluorescein into the retina and choroid adjacent to the "leaky" vasculature (Fig. 3.36).

Circulatory shock may also result from hemorrhage and necrosis within a large pheochromocytoma (59, 219, 355, 468, 485, 564, 923, 990), or even from a retroperitoneal hemorrhage secondary to a ruptured adrenal gland (69, 220). Significant hemorrhage within a pheochromocytoma is rare; a review

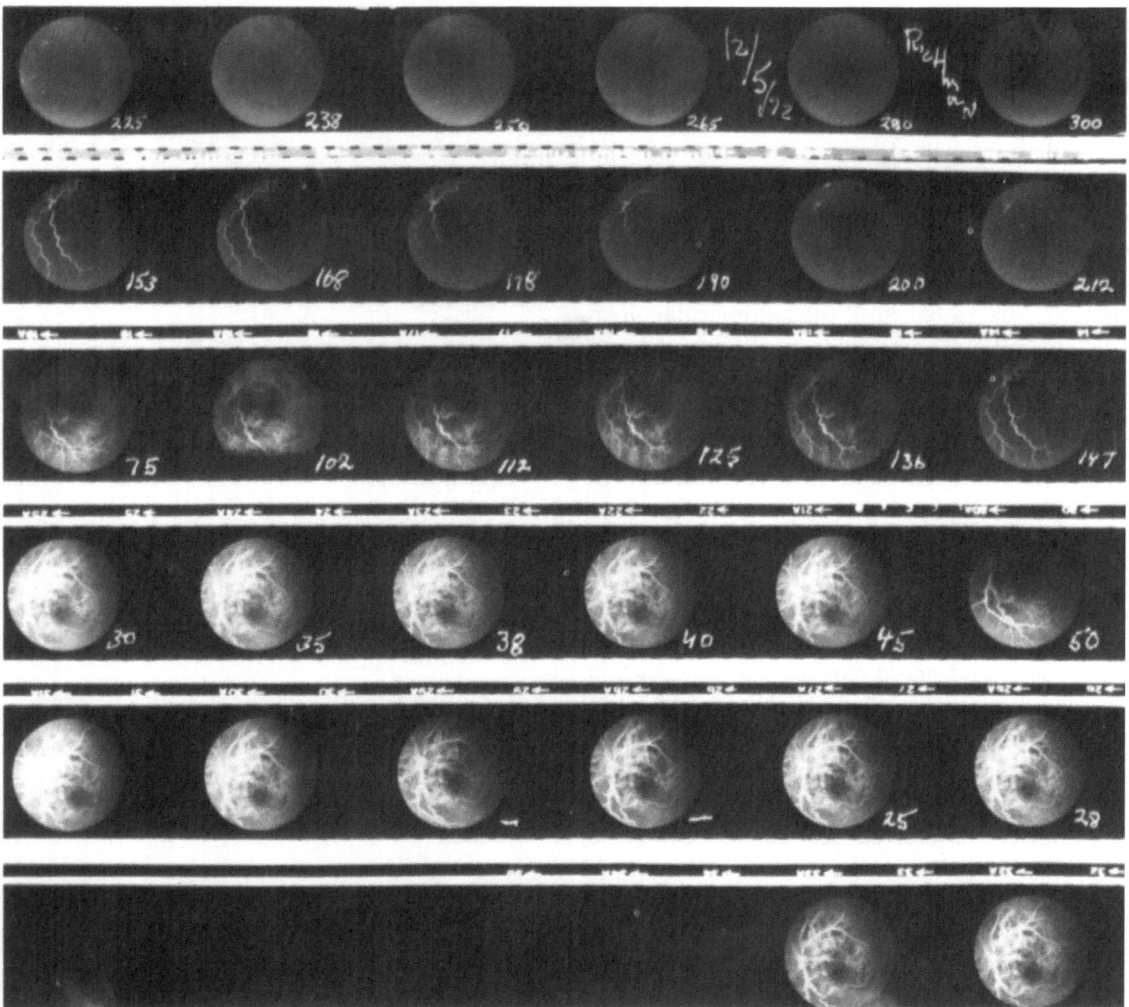

Fig. 3.35 (Same patient as described in Fig. 3.34). A series of photographs of fluorescein-illuminated blood in the vasculature of the left fundus at various intraocular tensions, taken with the hemobarometric technique of L'Esperance. As the intraocular tension was decreased (from frame labeled "300" at top right to bottom left) the first appearance of fluorescein can be seen at frame labeled "225" which corresponded to a markedly elevated pressure in the arteriole. Furthermore, transit of the fluorescein into the macular and paramacular areas was delayed and impaired due to marked edema of the posterior retina.

Hemobarometry "simply balances an external pressure against the pressure of the blood column as it forces its way along the various arterioles and venules." It "combines the features of applanation tonometry, suction ophthalmodynamometry, fluorescein angiography, and fundus photography in order to record the specific intraocular pressure at various points in the chorioretinal vasculature. This technique is useful in determining the degree of pathologic change in various vascular and degenerative chorioretinal diseases" (565). Courtesy of Dr. F. A. L'Esperance, Jr. Columbia Medical Center, New York, New York.

of the literature in 1965 by Huston and Stewart revealed only four such cases in addition to their own patient (468). The occurrence and implications of *hemorrhagic necrosis* in a pheochromocytoma are dis-cussed in detail in Chapter 5, Differential Diagnosis.

Shock has occurred following severe and prolonged hypertensive crises. Engel and co-workers reported a patient with pheochromo-

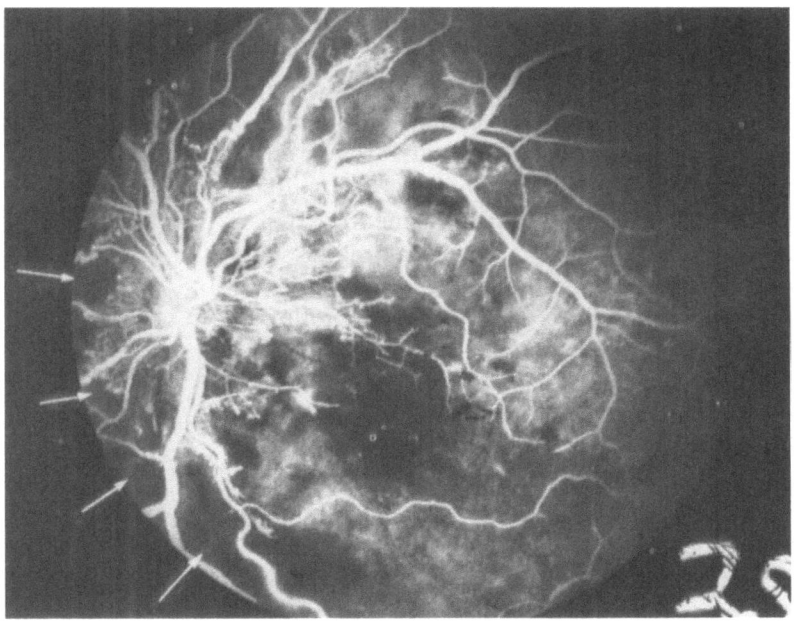

Fig. 3.36 (Same patient as described in Figs. 3.34 and 3.35.) A magnification of frame labeled "28" in Figure 3.35. Note the extensive extravasation (diffuse white patches, especially evident adjacent to vasculature) of fluorescein into the chorioretinal tissue. This degree of extravasation is abnormal and consistent with pathologic changes in the chorioretinal vessels and "leaky" vasculature. Some areas adjacent to the medial rim of this funduscopic photograph appear to be avascular (i.e., no fluorescein or vessels are present) (see arrows), and are probably ischemic and infarcted. Courtesy of Dr. F. A. L'Esperance, Jr., Columbia Medical Center, New York, New York.

Fig. 3.37 Small intestine; necrotic mucosal villi and numerous fibrin thrombi in mucosal capillaries and submucosal venules (phosphotungstic acid-hematoxylin, 105×). From Rosati, L. A. and Auger, N. A., Jr. *Gastroenterology 60:* 583, 1971.

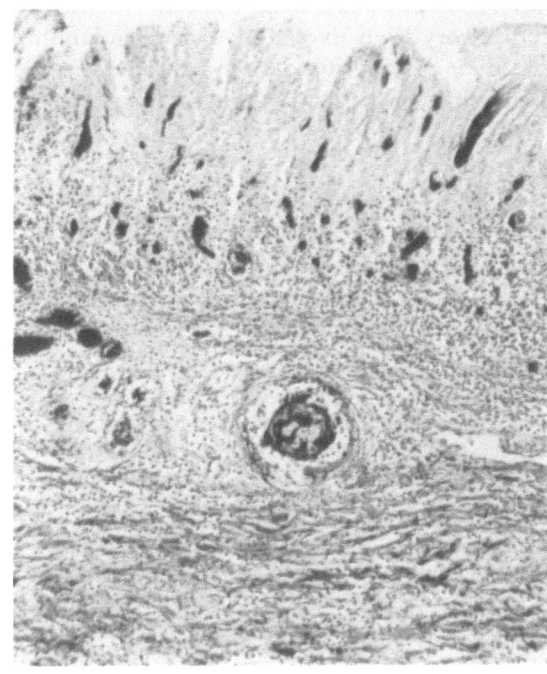

cytoma whose blood pressure fell to 76/60 mmHg and remained at that level for several hours after a severe paroxysm of unusual length (264). Since, in addition, there were hemoconcentration, tachycardia, and torpor in their patient, they suggested that "epinephrine shock" (similar to that seen after prolonged infusions of epinephrine in experimental animals) was a potential manifestation of pheochromocytoma. Another patient was reported to have developed shock following spontaneous hypertensive attacks, and it appeared that the diagnosis was almost certainly pheochromocytoma (366). Shock not infrequently has occurred in patients with pheochromocytoma during anesthesia, operation, or even following relatively minor trauma (3, 19, 44, 79, 123, 125, 160, 511, 528, 628, 668, 734, 984, 1007).

Increased concentrations of circulating catecholamines may inhibit gastrointestinal motility and cause *severe ileus* with *megacolon* and *obstipation*. One patient with megacolon associated with pheochromocytoma developed intestinal obstruction and died during emergency surgery (465). Probably as a consequence of intense splanchnic vasoconstriction due to the massive quantities of circulating catecholamines, *ischemic enterocolitis* has, rarely, occurred (197, 804), and may be accompanied by gastrointestinal hemorrhage and infarction of the ileum (168) (Fig. 3.37). One patient with pheochromocytoma and a very high excretion of catecholamines and their metabolites developed a fatal gastric hemorrhage which was thought to be the re-

sult of severe vasoconstriction with resulting ischemia and necrosis of the gastric mucosa (713).

Another patient with pheochromocytoma of the right adrenal gland and mild attacks

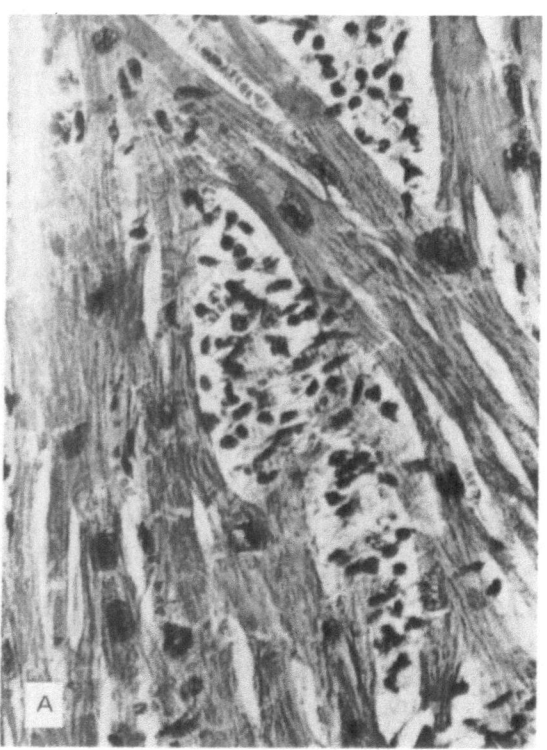

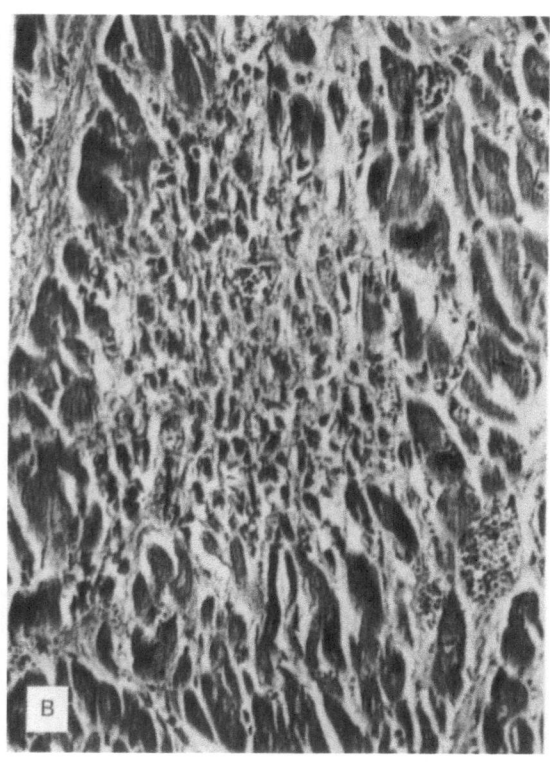

Fig. 3.38 A. Left ventricular myocardium of a 45-year-old man, who died with an unsuspected pheochromocytoma 5 days after removal of the left kidney, showing active myocarditis, with focal degeneration of myocardial fibers and inflammation (hematoxylin and eosin stain, 375×). Delicate collageneous fibers were present in these foci. B. Left ventricular myocardium of a 38-year-old man, who died of congestive heart failure that was thought to be due to myocarditis (hematoxylin and eosin stain, 200×). An unsuspected pheochromocytoma was present. The myocardium showed active myocarditis consisting of foci of degenerated myocardial fibers and inflammation. (Note: This patient's ECG is shown in Fig. 6.2.) From Van Vliet, P. D., Burchell, H. B., and Titus, J. L., reprinted by permission from *N. Engl. J. Med.* 274: 1105, 1966.

of paroxysmal hypertension had recurrent attacks of melena with severe blood loss and anemia; extensive gastrointestinal studies, two laparotomies, and a careful examination at necropsy failed to account satisfactorily for the gastrointestinal bleeding. At the second laparotomy, multiple bleeding areas were found in the jejunum; however, despite resection of four feet of small bowel the gastrointestinal bleeding recurred. Spontaneous nose bleeds and spontaneous ecchymoses were also observed while the patient was hospitalized. During his final attack his blood pressure rose to only 170/110 mmHg and he developed a large retinal hemorrhage with loss of vision in that eye. Several hours later he expired following a cerebral hemorrhage. A blood dyscrasia could not be demonstrated and it was postulated that a constitutional weakness of the vasculature combined with the paroxysmal hypertension may have accounted for the bleeding manifestations (347).

Cardiomyopathy has been noted at autopsy in some patients who died from complications of pheochromocytoma (517, 805, 988). Van Vliet, Burchell, and Titus reported that of 26 patients at the Mayo Clinic who died with pheochromocytoma, 15 (58 percent) had active myocarditis which these authors believed resulted from excessive catecholamines (988). Examples of active myocarditis in two of their patients is evident in Figure 3.38. Focal areas of degeneration and necrosis of myocardial fibers, with foci of inflammatory cells (predominantly histocytes, but some plasma cells and occasional polymorphonuclear leukocytes) were present and most numerous in the left ventricle. In addition, increased fibrosis in these foci and diffuse edema of the myocardium were observed. In a few cases of hearts with active myocarditis, there was thickening of small and medium-sized arteries due to edema of the intima and media, and some fibrous replacement of the media. A moderately severe degree of coronary sclerosis was found in 14 of the 26 patients.

The pathologic changes of active myocarditis were found in patients with pheochromocytoma who had sustained or paroxysmal hypertension; they were similar to lesions seen in the myocardium of some patients who had received therapeutic infusions of norepinephrine, and in lesions found in various laboratory animals after injections of catecholamines. No active catecholamine myocarditis was evident in four patients with pheochromocytomas which were apparently nonfunctioning (988).

Eleven of the 15 patients with active myocarditis had left ventricular failure with pulmonary congestion, which was frequently accompanied by a period of hypotension (refractory to treatment) prior to death. In one patient a diagnosis of active myocarditis had been made on the basis of cardiomegaly, dyspnea, tachycardia, and palpitations. Signs and symptoms had been present for 13 years before a pheochromocytoma was discovered at autopsy (988). Engelman and Sjoerdsma reported a patient whose cardiomyopathy, presumably related to excess catecholamine, subsided after resection of the pheochromocytoma (275). Significant left ventricular failure may occur in the absence of longstanding or severe hypertension (1065).

In rare cases a chromaffin tumor may grow to sufficient size to press on adjacent structures and sometimes impair function of nearby organs. For example, a pheochromocytoma originating in the organ of Zuckerkandl caused *ureteral obstruction* (349). *Oliguria* or *anuria* may occur with shock, no matter what the cause; also, occasionally, renal insufficiency may result from the prolonged periods of hypotension which, in some patients with pheochromocytoma, have followed severe episodes of hypertension (36, 42, 161). Significant renal insufficiency with azotemia only rarely results from *nephrosclerosis* occurring in patients with pheochromocytoma. Howard and Barker reviewed the pathologic findings in eight patients who were autopsied, and observed that nephrosclerosis was uncommon; when present, it was of mild degree, except in one patient where it was severe. The degree of nephrosclerosis did not correlate with the retinal lesions (462). An outline of the pathologic features and complications of pheochromocytoma is presented in Table 3.11.

The cause of death in 72 patients not operated on for pheochromocytoma was reported by Graham (392) and appears in Table 3.10. The tumor may cause sudden death from cardiac arrhythmia (242), which is most likely a common cause of death during a hypertensive crisis.

Table 3.11 *Pathology of Pheochromocytoma*

1. Tumor of chromaffin (ectodermal) cells
   Adrenal
   Paraganglia
   Organ of Zuckerkandl
   Some chemoreceptors
   Sympathetic nerve plexuses
   Ectopic cells
2. Etiology ?
   Occurs in animals (e.g., rats, bulls, dogs, especially Boxers)
   Experimentally produced by irradiation, growth hormone, estrogens
   Familial incidence (?10%) (± medullary thyroid carcinoma, hyperparathyroidism,
       neuromas, thickened corneal nerves, marfanoid habitus, alimentary-tract
       ganglioneuromatosis)
   Occurs at all ages
   No sex predilection except in children (2/3 are males)
3. Location[a]
   Abdomen and pelvic cavity (99%)
   Adrenal
     Adult
        81% Single, more common on right
         7% Bilateral
         8% Multiple, adrenal and extraadrenal
     Children
        49% Single, more common on right
        24% Bilateral
        35% Multiple, adrenal and extraadrenal
     <2.0% Chest, paravertebral
     <0.1% Neck, may be chemodectoma
4. 70% weigh <70 g. Can weigh up to 3,600 g (1,000 g tumor with 10 g catecholamines
   reported)
5. Usually encapsulated, highly vascular, hemorrhagic, necrotic, cystic
   Polygonal, spheroidal, pleomorphic cells + granular cytoplasm; cytoplasm and granules
   stain with chromic acid
   Cannot determine if malignant (10%) from histology—rare mitosis
6. If malignant, usually
   Slow growing
   Quite resistant to x-ray
   Metastasize to lymph nodes, liver, lung, bone
   (If paroxysmal = rarely malignant; rarely recur after removal)
7. Complications
   CVA (infarction or hemorrhage)
   Neuroretinopathy (if sustained hypertension)
   Myocardial hypertrophy ± failure
   Myocardial infarction
   Cardiomyopathy (active catecholamine myocarditis, fibrosis)
   Necrotizing arteriolitis
   Renal vascular lesions (benign or malignant nephrosclerosis ± azotemia)
   Arteriosclerosis
   Dissecting aneurysm ± aortic rupture (hemorrhage)
   Shock (due to hemorrhage, tumor necrosis, catecholamine excess or deficiency)
   Ischemic enterocolitis ± G.I. hemorrhage and infarction
   Ileus + megacolon + obstipation
   Pressure effects on
     Adjacent structures (e.g., ureteral obstruction, spinal cord compression)
     Distant structures by metastasis
   Oliguria or anuria
   Encephalopathy
   Death

Clinical Manifestations

CHAPTER FOUR

FREQUENCY AND OCCURRENCE OF ATTACKS

The clinical manifestations encountered in patients with pheochromocytoma consist of such a large variety of symptoms and signs that they have been described as kaleidoscopic. The pleomorphism of the disease has been emphasized and about 80 manifestations have been reported (215, pp. 105, 106; 437, p. 83). Often symptoms caused by this endocrinopathy occur in a dramatic and explosive fashion when the tumor suddenly releases catecholamines into the circulation. On rare occasions sudden death may occur with the initial attack in a patient with pheochromocytoma who has previously been asymptomatic (984). Also, on rare occasions, patients may present with clinical manifestations of one of the complications of these tumors. An abrupt onset of complaints is extremely common during an episode of paroxysmal hypertension. Rarely, there may be a premonition that an attack is about to occur (927). About 50 percent of patients with persistent hypertension experience a sudden onset of symptoms usually associated with episodic increases in the hypertension; however, in patients with sustained hypertension, symptoms are generally less pronounced than in patients with paroxysmal hypertension. Very rarely a patient with pheochromocytoma and paroxysmal or sustained hypertension may be relatively asymptomatic (938) or even symptomless. Nonfunctioning pheochromocytomas are extremely unusual and may be an incidental finding at autopsy. As mentioned earlier, Melicow and associates reported an interesting case of a patient with a nonfunctioning malignant tumor of the organ of Zuckerkandl (649) (see Chapter 3). The patient complained of symptoms related to the metastatic malignancy, and an erroneous diagnosis of prostatic carcinoma was made prior to autopsy.

Symptomatic intervals have been noted to vary from once every few months to 25 times daily, and in duration from less than 1 min to 1 week. Paroxysms may also occur daily at a set time (942), but they usually occur quite irregularly. About three-fourths of patients with pheochromocytoma experienced one or more attacks weekly, and one-fourth had one or more attacks daily (976). A characteristic feature of the attacks in one patient was that they came, receded, and came again, usually in waves of four or five during each attack. The symptoms experienced and the order of the occurrence remain remarkably similar during each episode, although the duration of attacks may vary, even in the same patient. Attacks last less than 15 min in about one-half the patients, less than 1 hr in 80 percent (976) and invariably subside more slowly than they start. Typically, attacks become more frequent but not necessarily more severe with the passage of time; however, a patient with pheochromocytoma has been reported in whom attacks decreased in frequency, perhaps due to degeneration of the tumor (138). In another patient spontaneous cure apparently resulted from hemorrhage into the tumor (4). Paroxysmal attacks observed for 1.5 years in a patient with pheochromocytoma disappeared when the blood pressure became sustained (464). Attacks occurred in some patients for several years and then subsided for several more years, only to return again (462, 600). Another patient had attacks that ceased for 10 years and then returned (415).

Attacks sometimes occur at night and awaken the patient, and not infrequently the onset of symptoms has been experienced while in bed in the early morning hours (462) or shortly after arising in the morning. It seems likely that when a patient is recumbent and quiet there may be an increase in the stores of catecholamines in the tumor; however, it is also reasonable to speculate that early morning restlessness and frequent changes in body position may trigger the release of catecholamines and thereby induce a hypertensive crisis. Attacks may sometimes be precipitated by any of the following: massage or steady pressure for 1 or 2 min in the area of the tumor, lying in a particular position, postural changes (especially involving flexion and bending of the body), exercise, anxiety, having the blood pressure taken, eating, ingestion of certain foods, certain alcoholic beverages (namely, beer and wine) or fruit juice, hyperventilation, increased intraabdominal pressure, parturition, the valsalva maneuver, tight clothing, laughing, pressure on the carotid sinuses, micturition, bladder distention, dysuria, constipation, straining at stool, defecation, smoking a cigarette, shaving, gargling, sneezing, sexual intercourse, trauma, pain, changes in body temperature, angiography, and the intravenous, intramuscular, or subcutaneous administration of certain drugs [e.g., histamine, glucagon, epinephrine, tyramine, tetraethylammonium, mecholyl, anectine, nicotine, ACTH, corticotropin, phenothiazines, propylthiouracil, amobarbital, saralasin (and other angiotensin II analogs)], intubation, anesthesia, or operative manipulation. [Note: Only Moorhead and coworkers have reported the precipitation of paroxysms in patients with pheochromocytoma following the administration of amobarbital or propylthiouracil (680). We are unaware of any other similar reports.] In some patients attacks seemed worse during menses or they became more frequent and worse just before menses (462).

Occasionally, patients with pheochromocytoma may develop a rapid progression of their disease with acceleration of both the severity and frequency of hypertensive attacks (perhaps alternating with hypotension), and this pattern has been designated "acute pheochromocytoma" (254).

Particularly unusual circumstances which precipitate hypertensive crises in patients with pheochromocytoma have been observed on rare occasions. For example, an attack was induced by administration of an enema to a patient with pheochromocytoma of the organ of Zuckerkandl. A 26-year-old woman gave a history of "pronounced palpitations, profuse sweating and severe agitation during sexual intercourse, particularly at orgasm;" some attacks terminated in syncope, and deep palpation of the lower abdomen could induce an attack. In this latter patient a 6 cm pheochromocytoma was removed from the organ of Zuckerkandl, and she has subsequently remained symptom-free (personal communication from Dr Meyer M. Melicow, Given Professor Emeritus, Uropathology Research, Columbia Medical Center). A patient with an intrathoracic pheochromocytoma pressing against the esophagus at times experienced attacks after swallowing (76). In still another patient, drinking 1000 ml of water for a renal function study caused a fatal paroxysm (462). Occasionally even the slightest excitement, such as application of a blood pressure cuff, may provoke a marked blood pressure rise (229). A 30-year-old housewife sometimes experienced attacks when a letter from home or unexpected company arrived (1024).

Certain diagnostic procedures (e.g., presacral aerograms, renal arteriograms, lumbar puncture, ventriculography, etc.), endotracheal intubation, anesthesia induction, anesthesia, hypoxia, hypercapnia, and abdominal operations may also cause a sudden release of catecholamines from a pheochromocytoma and induce paroxysmal attacks of hypertension. Pheochromocytomas are well-known to cause unsuspected operating room deaths (14, 18, 182, 702, 788, 792, 840). Death in patients with pheochromocytoma has resulted from trauma (121, 352, 466), pregnancy, and delivery (714). Even anesthesia and relatively minor surgery, such as incision of a septic finger, have resulted in the death of patients harboring this tumor (160). It should be emphasized that pregnancy may be accompanied by development of persistent or labile hypertension related to the presence of a pheochromocytoma; severe hypertension and/or hypertensive crises are particularly apt to occur in the third trimester and during or shortly after labor.

The mechanism responsible for a sudden *release of catecholamines* into the circulation may be simply a mechanical action of compressing the tumor, such as massage, postural changes, exercise, defecation, sneezing, or sexual intercourse. Certain foods and alcoholic beverages may contain substances (e.g., tyramine) which cause a displacement and liberation of catecholamines from tumor tissue or from excessive stores in sympathetic nerves. One patient with a pheochromocytoma was reported to experience attacks whenever she drank orange juice. The latter contains synephrine (Sympatol), which can displace and release tissue catecholamines (907).

The mechanism whereby anxiety and hyperventilation sometimes release catecholamines in patients with pheochromocytoma is unclear. Raab cited several reports in which paroxysms of hypertension were attributed to the massaging action of the diaphragm on the tumor; however, he and Smithwick observed one patient with pheochromocytoma in whom a fall of blood pressure from hypertensive to normotensive blood pressures occurred during hyperventilation. This decrease in blood pressure was interpreted as the response of oversensitive vasomotor centers to the lowering of blood CO_2 (776, p. 79). It is noteworthy that in one patient psychic stimulation or massage of a tumor caused an initial decrease in blood pressure, followed by a hypertensive crisis (473). Catecholamines sometimes released by cigarette smoking in patients harboring these tumors may be attributed to the effect of nicotine directly on the tumor or sympathetic nerves. Histamine, glucagon, tyramine, tetraethylammonium, mecholyl, anectine, ACTH, saralasin (and other angiotensin II analogs) diamorphine, and nitroglycerine may cause a release of catecholamines from pheochromocytomas, but it is also possible that some of these drugs liberate catecholamines from sympathetic nerves which have accumulated excess stores of these amines. Any situation which activates the sympathetic nervous system could theoretically induce a hypertensive crisis by liberating catecholamines from sympathetic nerves if the stores of these amines are excessive. Whether certain anesthetic agents and contrast media used in arteriography have a similar action is not clear. Presacral aerography and possibly arteriography may cause a release of catecholamines from these tumors by mechanical pressures, which "flush" catecholamines from the tumor.

SYMPTOMS

Symptoms experienced by patients with pheochromocytoma result from either the pharmacologic effects of excess concentrations of catecholamines in the circulation or from the complications of the hypertension induced by these pressor amines. It is especially important to question carefully patients suspected of having this tumor since symptomatology is protean (i.e., "exceedingly variable and readily assuming different shapes or forms"— *Webster's International Dictionary*). The frequency of occurrence of major symptoms in adults is listed in Table 4.1, which shows that, with few exceptions, symptoms occur more frequently in patients with paroxysmal than persistent hypertension. This finding is not surprising, since the highest concentrations of plasma catecholamines usually occur during a paroxysm of hypertension. The effects of a sudden increase in plasma catecholamines occurring during an attack would be more pronounced and perceptible in patients with paroxysms of hypertension than in patients with sustained hypertension, where the blood pressure and plasma catecholamines change relatively less. As a consequence, symptoms of metabolic and cardiovascular alterations, including the incremental rise in blood pressure, are usually most pronounced in patients during paroxysmal hypertension.

HEADACHES

Headaches are almost always paroxysmal in character, frequently throbbing, bilateral, and usually severe or even violent and "bursting" during a paroxysm of hypertension. They are abrupt in onset and subside as the blood pressure returns to normal. Headaches which sometimes lasted hours or days (543, 971), or which occurred after an attack (462, 1024), have been described, but these headache patterns are most unusual. Not infrequently the headaches are accompanied by nausea and vomiting. Often they are occipital and/or frontal in location, but at times are generalized, and characterized as an intense pressure sensation. Occasionally there is a throbbing in the temporal regions. Some patients were awakened by severe headache in the early hours of the morning. However, though headaches may be severe in patients with sustained

hypertension due to pheochromocytoma, sometimes the headaches are mild to moderate and indistinguishable from tension headaches and those experienced in patients with essential hypertension. In 26 patients with pheochromocytoma seen at the Henry Ford Hospital, headaches were mentioned by 13 but were rarely a prominent symptom (680). The incidence of headache in our series was significantly greater, 92 and 72 percent, respectively, in patients with paroxysmal or sustained hypertension. Rarely, headaches may be accompanied by convulsive seizures, neck stiffness, or a pseudomeningeal state, and loss of consciousness (437, p. 75).

EXCESS SWEATING

Although some have claimed that excess sweating is almost always present in patients with pheochromocytoma (907), this has not been our experience. About two-thirds of our patients complained of excess perspiration (often drenching in nature) which was generalized, more so in the upper body and not confined to one area. Diaphoresis was the main complaint in one patient, who had both a pheochromocytoma and acromegaly (492). The patient also had a persistent tachycardia and an increased excretion of urinary catecholamines but was never found to be hypertensive. The sweating pattern was unusual in that, despite the fact that the patient was bathed in perspiration, his extremities distal to his elbows and knees remained cold and dry. Another patient was described who had such profuse sweating that he had to change his pajamas six times during the night (42). In still another patient the "sweating was so profound that sheets, blankets, and mattresses had to be changed repeatedly every day" (329). It is interesting that in this latter patient profuse sweating was evident when the blood pressure was only 180/90 mmHg. In patients with paroxysmal attacks, we and others (229) have occasionally noted that diaphoresis is not synchronous with the elevation of blood pressure but appears as the crisis recedes and when the pressure has returned toward normal; however, the sweating and hypertension usually appear concomitantly. The most profuse sweating appears in those patients having paroxysmal attacks of hypertension. Peart has observed that sweating is

Table 4.1 Symptoms

	Approximate percent	
	Paroxysmal (37 patients)	Persistent (39 patients)
A. Symptoms presumably due to excess catecholamines and/or hypertension		
Headaches (severe)	92	72
Excess sweating (generalized)	65	69
Palpitations ± tachycardia	73	51
Anxiety or nervousness (± fear of impending death; panic)	60	28
Tremulousness	51	26
Pain in chest and/or abdomen (usually epigastric) and/or lumbar regions and/or lower abdomen and/or groin	48	28
Nausea ± vomiting	43	26
Weakness, fatigue, prostration	38	15
Weight loss (severe)	14	15
Dyspnea	11	18
Warmth ± heat intolerance	13	15
Visual disturbances	3	21
"Dizziness" or faintness	11	3
Constipation	0	13
Paresthesia or pain in arms	11	0
Bradycardia (noted by patient)	8	3
Grand mal	5	3
Miscellaneous		

Pain in the lower back, neck, shoulder, flank, jaw and gums, or extremities; intermittent claudication; tingling of fingers; cold extremities; shivering sensations; hunger; polyphagia; gagging; perioral numbness; piloerection; tightness in the throat; coughing; yawning; sneezing; ptyalism; tinnitus; vertigo; dysarthria; syncope; unsteadiness; photophobia; sensations of neck pressure and swelling, suffocation; depression; delirium; polydipsia and polyuria; nocturia; nocturnal enuresis; oliguria; anuria; obstipation; diarrhea; abdominal distention. NOTE: With pheochromocytoma of the urinary bladder there may be: painless hematuria, frequency, nocturia, and tenesmus

B. Symptoms due to complications
Congestive heart failure
Myocardial infarction
Cerebrovascular accident
Ischemic enterocolitis
Azotemia
Dissecting aneurysm
Encephalopathy
Shock
Hemorrhagic necrosis in a pheochromocytoma

C. Symptoms due to coexisting diseases or syndromes
Cholelithiasis
Medullary thyroid carcinoma ± effects of secretions of serotonin, calcitonin, prostaglandin, ACTH-like substance
Hyperparathyroidism
Neurofibromatosis and its complications
Cushing's syndrome (rare)
Mucocutaneous neuromas
Marfanoid habitus
Alimentary-tract ganglioneuromatosis
von Hippel-Lindau disease (very rare)
Virilism or Addison's disease or acromegaly (extremely rare)

D. Symptoms caused by metastases

only profuse in patients having the severest hypertension and occurs with tumors secreting epinephrine or norepinephrine (798). Smithwick and coworkers felt that sweating might result from a reflex activation of parasympathetic centers of the midbrain in an attempt to maintain homeostasis (particularly body temperature), which had been disturbed by the effects of excess catecholamines (920). Haimovici demonstrated an adrenergic component in the nervous mechanism of sweating in man which he felt could explain the diaphoresis occurring in patients with pheochromocytoma (409).

The mechanism for the diaphoresis is still not clear. The sympathetic nerves supplying the atrichial sweat glands (i.e., those independent of hair follicles and covering most of the body surface) are cholinergic, and sweating results from the liberation of acetylcholine from these nerves and may be induced by the administration of parasympathomimetic drugs. The epitrichial sweat glands (i.e., those associated with hair follicles in the axillary, inguinal, circumanal, and circumareolar regions) in man have a nerve supply and α-receptors. At first glance, it may seem confusing and parodoxical that increased concentrations of circulating catecholamines in patients with pheochromocytoma can cause profuse and generalized sweating. In a review of the mechanisms of sweating and the role of catecholamines in the control of sweat glands, Robertshaw pointed out that all cholinergic sweat glands can be stimulated by catecholamines but that there was no firm evidence that this was physiologically significant (798). Prout and Wardell found that parasympathetic blockade by hyoscine prevented sweating attacks in two patients with pheochromocytoma (771). Robertshaw has suggested that in some patients with pheochromocytoma small amounts of epinephrine and norepinephrine may conceivably pass the blood-brain barrier in the region of the hypothalamus and centrally stimulate heat loss mechanisms (798). However, it is possible that increased concentrations of circulating catecholamines, especially epinephrine, may directly stimulate the sweat glands or in some way activate their nerve supply. The latter possibility seems all the more reasonable in view of evidence suggesting that there may also be a β-receptor

component in the response of human sweat glands to catecholamine stimulation (8).

Watanabe and Morita have demonstrated a reduced sensitivity of eccrine (atrichial) sweat glands following the intracutaneous injection of epinephrine or norepinephrine in patients with pheochromocytoma; extirpation of the tumor restored sensitivity in each patient (1008). They pointed out that their findings were consistent with previous reports that patients with pheochromocytoma appear to have a decreased responsiveness of their cardiovascular system to catecholamines (392, 893, 1068).

It has been pointed out that sweating is one of the few symptoms occurring continuously in patients who have persistently secreting tumors (976). Smithwick and coworkers stated that 90 percent of their patients with pheochromocytoma whom they questioned on this point had excess sweating, whereas in the literature this symptom was mentioned in only 52 percent of 107 cases of pheochromocytoma. They emphasized that unless specifically questioned some patients could easily omit including excess sweating as a complaint (920).

PALPITATIONS, TACHYCARDIA, AND BRADYCARDIA

Palpitations, the third most common symptom, are usually accompanied by tachycardia, although sometimes there may be a reflex bradycardia due to the increase in blood pressure. Frequently the patient complains of a pounding of the chest, sometimes severe enough to be described as "like a sledge hammer," or as if the heart were going to burst through the ribs. It is noteworthy that infusions of epinephrine are accompanied by palpitations (42), whereas comparable doses of norepinephrine rarely cause this symptom (42, 617).

ANXIETY, TREMULOUSNESS, NAUSEA, VOMITING, AND FAINTNESS

The anxiety, which is sometimes associated with a sense of impending death, and the nervousness, tremulousness, nausea (with or without vomiting), and the "dizziness" and faintness may result in part from the marked apprehension caused by the multitude of unpleasant symptoms; some of the latter may, however, be primarily manifestations of an overactive vegetative (sympathetic) nervous system. Occasionally patients have found that they gain some relief from nausea by inducing vomiting (355). Vomiting every few days or nightly has been reported as the presenting symptom in some patients with pheochromocytoma (355). It seems unlikely that any one of the symptoms is due to a direct effect of the catecholamines on the brain, if, as demonstrated by some, these pressor amines do not cross the blood-brain barrier. Hermann and Mornex cite evidence that epinephrine and norepinephrine cause intensification of electrical activity in the cerebral cortex of the cat; the effect caused by norepinephrine is considerably less than that caused by epinephrine. It appears that these catecholamines do not exert a direct effect on the cerebral cortex; the effect on the cortex has been attributed to stimulation of the ascending activating mesencephalic reticular system (437, p. 17).

CHEST AND ABDOMINAL PAIN

The mechanisms of chest and abdominal pain are frequently uncertain but on some occasions are due to ischemia (e.g., typical angina pectoris with radiation down the left arm, compatible with myocardial ischemia). Some have suggested that pain in the upper abdomen may occasionally be due to hepatic congestion (417, 462, 791) or perhaps spasm of the pyloric sphincter (417). Likewise, pain in the region of the symphysis pubis might result from spasm of the bladder sphincter (417). Usually there is no sharp pain but rather a pressure, tightness, or constriction in the epigastrium and substernal area; however, a crushing chest pain may be experienced (1034). Rarely, abdominal pain and vomiting have simulated cholecystitis and led to cholecystectomy (417, 556). Occasionally, of course, pain, nausea, and vomiting may be related to an associated cholelithiasis, the incidence of which is markedly increased in patients with pheochromocytoma. One patient with pheochromocytoma experienced severe abdominal pain and vomiting as a result of hemorrhage into the tumor (355). This serious complication, which can cause an acute abdomen, is discussed in detail in Chapter 5. Of 26 patients analyzed by Moorhead and coworkers, abdominal pain was the presenting complaint in five and a prominent complaint in eight

others; however, six of these patients gave either a history of peptic ulcer or evidence of an active duodenal ulcer (680). One of their patients also had a hiatus hernia and another developed a massive gastrointestinal hemorrhage of unknown etiology (680).

WEAKNESS, FATIGUE, AND PROSTRATION

Toward the end of an attack, weakness, fatigue, and prostration occur and persist for a while. Following an attack, some patients find it necessary to go to bed for several hours because of extreme weakness and fatigue. Extreme fatigue and prostration, lasting for 5 min to a whole day, were experienced in 10 of 18 patients following paroxysms of hypertension (462). These symptoms appear to be correlated with subsidence of the metabolic and cardiovascular stimulation caused by the excess catecholamines; however, some patients have complained of constant weakness (680).

WEIGHT LOSS

We have particularly stressed that it is unusual for a patient with pheochromocytoma, especially if the hypertension is sustained, to maintain his weight (352, 534, 535). This weight loss, which occurs despite a normal or even increased appetite, is probably related to increased metabolism caused by excess catecholamines. Patients are not anorexic (except in the presence of extensive metastases), and occasionally they may have a voracious appetite (543). It is only rarely that the patient is obese (392, 466, 560) (the so-called "fat-pheo") and gives no history of weight loss when the hypertension is sustained (352). This rare situation occurs principally in patients with paroxysmal hypertension. Some patients have been observed to have significant weight gain over a prolonged period despite the presence of a functioning tumor (680, 971). Lee and Rousseau reported a weight gain of 10 percent in eight of 22 patients with pheochromocytoma (560). Deviations from standard body weights in 64 patients with pheochromocytoma seen at the Mayo Clinic are recorded in Table 4.2. About 67 and 47 percent of those with paroxysmal and persistent hypertension, respectively, were within ±10 percent of their standard body weight. However, about 41

Table 4.2   *Deviations from Standard Body Weight of 64 Patients with Pheochromocytoma at Time of Diagnosis at Mayo Clinic[a]*

Deviation from standard weight (%)	Paroxysmal function		Persistent function	
	Patients	%	Patients	%
−30 to −39.9	1	3.3	2	5.8
−20 to −29.9	2	6.7	6	17.7
−10 to −19.9	4	13.3	6	17.7
0 to − 9.9	13	43.4	10	29.4
+ 0.1 to +10	7	23.3	6	17.7
+10.1 to +20	1	3.3	3	8.8
+20.1 to +30	2	6.7	0	—
>+30	0	—	1	2.9
Total	30	100.0	34	100.0

[a] From Gifford, R. W., Jr., Kvale, W. F., Maher, F. T., Roth, G. M., and Priestley, J. T. *Mayo Clinic Proc. 39:* 286, 1964.

and 23 percent of those with persistent and paroxysmal hypertension, respectively, were 10 percent or more below standard body weight. The only patient who was more than 30 percent above standard weight was felt, on the basis of clinical and postmortem findings (352), to have essential hypertension and a nonfunctioning pheochromocytoma.

DYSPNEA

The slightly greater incidence of dyspnea in patients with persistent hypertension is probably explained by the sustained strain of high blood pressure on the left ventricle, with some degree of left ventricular failure and pulmonary congestion. Acute pulmonary edema in this condition may occur in the absence of cardiac enlargement or coronary artery disease. One patient, who had marked cardiac enlargement and electrocardiographic evidence of coronary artery disease, repeatedly developed pulmonary edema and cardiac asthma during paroxysms of hypertension (229). Pulmonary edema occurred during one or more episodes of paroxysmal hypertension in nine of 18 patients reviewed by Howard and Barker; three of these patients died in their first attack of pulmonary edema (462). A point worthy of mention is that the combination of dyspnea, sinus tachycardia, and cardiomegaly with nonspecific electrocardiographic changes may result from active catecholamine myocarditis (988).

WARMTH AND HEAT INTOLERANCE

Warmth, with or without heat intolerance, may be partly related to hypermetabolism. One patient described a sensation of "burning up" during an attack (415). In addition to hypermetabolism, intense vasoconstriction and pyrexia can contribute to the heat intolerance experienced by some patients.

VISUAL DISTURBANCE

It is noteworthy that visual disturbance (e.g., blurred vision and/or patchy loss of vision) occurred much more frequently in patients with persistently functioning tumors, this being due to retinopathy or neuroretinopathy produced by the sustained hypertension. Papilledema may occur and result in decreased visual acuity and central scotomata. Paroxysmal visual symptoms have been noted in 11 percent of patients with this tumor. During attacks, complete and almost complete loss of vision have occurred (778, 976); some patients have experienced scintillating scotomata synchronously with each heart beat and others have complained of "snowy vision," wavy lines, or black spots before the eyes (976). One patient reported by Rodin experienced pain in the eyes (especially on looking upward) during paroxysms of hypertension. In addition she had transitory decrease in vision for near and far objects and a sensation of light coming from all directions during attacks (800). In another patient, blurring of vision in one eye occurred immediately after an attack and 2 weeks later the opposite eye was similarly affected (927). In still another patient, who was 8 months pregnant and had sustained hypertension up to 210/150 mmHg, therapeutic termination of the pregnancy (without removal of the pheochromocytoma, which was unrecognized) was followed by loss of sight for 2 months (196).

CONSTIPATION

As might be anticipated, marked constipation was noted only in the presence of persistent hypertension since it was undoubtedly related to impaired intestinal motility induced by prolonged elevation of plasma catecholamines.

PARESTHESIAS AND PAIN IN EXTREMITIES

The fact that paresthesias and arm pain were complaints of some patients—but only when the hypertension was paroxysmal—suggests that these symptoms might result from the transitory effects of severe vasoconstriction and ischemia produced by a sudden massive increase of plasma catecholamines. In one patient the onset of paroxysmal attacks was ushered in by prickly sensations in the extremities, followed by cramps. The cramps then shifted from the legs to the abdomen and this was followed by precordial pain and oppression, and later by "terrific headaches" (462). It is possible that with a prolonged elevation of plasma catecholamines, as in patients with sustained hypertension due to pheochromocytoma, peripheral vasoconstriction is less intense and ischemia less marked, so that paresthesias and pain are not experienced. It has been reported that paresthesias and numbness—almost always bilateral—may affect the hands, face, perioral region, and scalp, and that in some instances a secondary hyperventilation may be responsible for some of these phenomena (976). A sensation of "pins and needles" in the arms following attacks has also been noted (927). One patient reported his arms and legs felt heavy and powerless during attacks (832). Another patient was unable to appreciate temperature differences with his right hand during an attack, and occasionally burned his right fingers with his cigarette (42).

Rarely, pain may occur in the lower extremities and may result from ischemia caused by catecholamine-induced vasoconstriction. Moorhead and associates have reported ischemia of the toes and intermittent claudication in some patients with pheochromocytoma (680). They also cited somewhat similar experiences by Scharf and coworkers (who observed two patients with intermittent claudication and leg ulcers), and by Engelman and associates (who observed a patient with peripheral cyanosis, ulceration, and sloughing of the skin). Intense vasoconstriction caused by circulating catecholamines was apparently responsible for the ischemia and ulceration in these patients (269).

Radtke and colleagues at the Mayo Clinic recently reported a fascinating case of a 41-year-old white woman who experienced painful tingling in both feet and in the right hand and subsequently developed infarctive and purpuric skin lesions of the feet and ankles (Fig. 4.1A) (778). Excessive circulating catecholamines, resulting from an adrenal pheochromocytoma, caused severe arterial spasm (Fig. 4.1B) and probably accounted for the symptoms and signs in her extremities.

Rarely, pain in the extremities may result from compression of adjacent nerves by a pheochromocytoma. In one patient, a tumor of the sacral concavity which eroded the sacrum and iliac bone caused sciatic pain (756).

GRAND MAL

The cause of grand mal reported in patients with pheochromocytoma is unclear. Thomas and coworkers found that in one of their patients, generalized convulsions occurred at the time of the paroxysmal symptoms, whereas in four other patients experiencing similar seizures, the blood pressure was persistently and markedly increased (976). Another patient developed a jerking of his right middle and ring fingers; immediately thereafter a convulsive seizure occurred which was followed by 2 hr of unconsciousness (942). Seizures may occur once or several times per month and may increase in frequency and severity (1024). In one patient typical grand mal seizures and an abnormal electroencephalogram were observed before surgery; one seizure occurred 6 months after extirpation of the pheochromo-

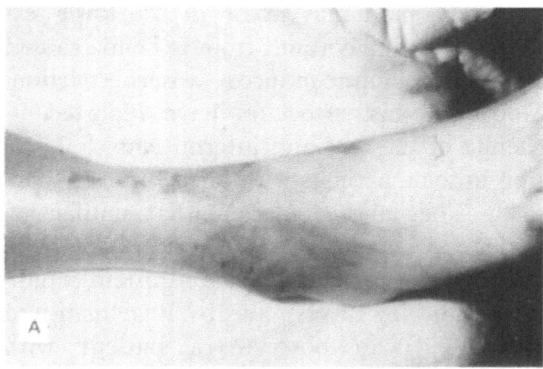

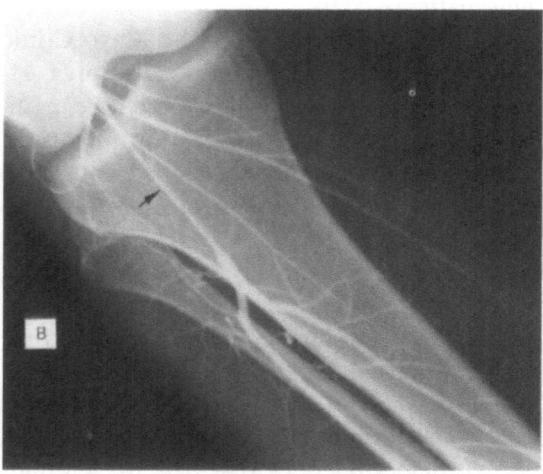

Fig. 4.1 A. Infarctive and purpuric skin lesions. B. Right femoral arteriogram revealing narrowing of the popliteal artery by spasm over a distance of 5.5 cm (arrow). This 41-year-old white woman complained of pain and tingling in both feet and the right hand; extremities were cool. Livedoreticularis was observed in several fingers and there was pallor and mottled cyanosis of the feet; voluntary toe movements were limited. Femoral and popliteal pulses were present and equal but posterior tibial and dorsalis pedis pulses were absent bilaterally. "No thrombus could be retrieved by means of a Fogarty embolectomy, and bilateral femoral arteriography in the operating room revealed diffuse spasm" (B). Following this procedure, the right dorsalis pedis pulse was Grade 4 and blood pressure was 130/110 mmHg; however, infarctive and purpuric skin lesions developed over feet and ankles during the following 2 days (A). Subsequently an adrenal pheochromocytoma was successfully removed and peripheral pulses remained normal. From Radtke, W., Kazmier, F. J., Rutherford, B. D., and Sheps, S. G., *Am. J. Cardiol. 35:* 703, 1975.

cytoma, at which time the EEG was again abnormal. However, during a 4-year follow-up period, no additional seizures were noted (320).

MISCELLANEOUS

An array of miscellaneous symptoms (listed in Table 4.1) has sometimes been reported in patients with pheochromocytoma, but frequently their relationship to excess circulating catecholamines is not apparent. Polydipsia, which is much more commonly observed in children, has been noted in adult patients with paroxysmal or sustained hypertension and may possibly be related to marked diaphoresis and dehydration. Conceivably, increased circulating catecholamines may suppress the antidiuretic hormone and thereby cause a diuresis. Urine production may be suppressed during a prolonged episode of paroxysmal hypertension whereas polyuria may occur for 1 hr or more following a paroxysm (462). Dysarthria, which has been rarely noted, may have resulted from a hyperventilation state (976).

SIGNS

HYPERTENSION (SUSTAINED AND/OR PAROXYSMAL)

The signs that may occur in patients with pheochromocytoma are listed in Table 4.3. At least one-half of adult patients with this tumor have sustained hypertension, whereas the remaining 40 to 50 percent have paroxysms of hypertension with relatively normal intervals. In 138 patients with pheochromocytoma seen at the Mayo Clinic, 91 percent had hypertension; in 42 percent the hypertension was paroxysmal, whereas in 49 percent it was sustained (784). A small percentage of pheochromocytomas apparently cause no signs or symptoms, either because they are nonfunctioning or because they release relatively small amounts of catecholamines into the circulation. These tumors may be found accidentally by x-ray or at operation or autopsy (668). It has been emphasized that some patients may be symptom-free and then suddenly die after some mild trauma or operative procedure (18, 20). Howard and Barker reported a patient with paroxysmal hypertension who usually became symptomatic during attacks; however, occasionally pronounced blood pressure elevations occurred while the patient remained asymptomatic (462). Finally, as Hume has mentioned, some patients with pheochromocytoma may

Table 4.3 *Signs*

A. Blood pressure changes
  ± Hypertension ± wide fluctuations (rarely paroxysmal hypotension or hypertension alternating with hypotension)
  Hypertension induced by
    Physical maneuver
    Palpation and massage (of flank or mass elsewhere)
  Orthostatic hypotension ± postural tachycardia
  Paradoxic response to antihypertensive drugs and induction of anesthesia
B. Other signs of catecholamine excess
  Hyperhydrosis
  Tachycardia or reflex bradycardia; very forceful heart beat; arrhythmia
  Pallor of face and upper part of body (rarely flushing)
  Anxious, frightened, troubled appearance
  Hypertensive retinopathy
  Dilated pupils (very rarely exophthalmos, lacrimation, scleral pallor or injection; may not react to light)
  Leanness or underweight
  Tremor (± shaking)
  Raynaud's phenomenon and/or livedo reticularis (occasionally puffy, red, cyanotic hands in children)—skin of extremities ± wet, cold, clammy, pale; ± goose-flesh (occasionally cyanotic nail beds)
  Fever
C. Mass lesion
  Palpable tumor in abdomen (rare)
  Neck
    Pheochromocytoma or chemodectoma
    Thyroid carcinoma
    Thyroid swelling (very rare)
D. Miscellaneous
  Heart murmurs; apnea; tachypnea (respirations may be deep and rapid); swelling of neck veins, epistaxis; gingival bleeding; abdominal bruit; barely perceptible pulse; growth defects
E. Signs of complications
  Cardiomegaly and/or congestive heart failure
  Myocardial infarction
  CVA
  Shock
  Arrhythmias
  Dissecting aneurysm
  Azotemia
  Encephalopathy
  Ischemic enterocolitis with megacolon and hemorrhage
  Very rarely, gastric ulceration; infarctive, purpuric skin lesions
F. Signs of associated conditions
  Neurofibromatosis (± café-au-lait spots)
  Cholelithiasis
  Medullary thyroid carcinoma ± effects of secretions
    Serotonin
    Calcitonin
    Prostaglandin
    ACTH-like substance
  Hyperparathyroidism
  Mucocutaneous neuromas with characteristic fascies
  Thickened corneal nerves (seen only by slit lamp)
  Marfanoid habitus
  Alimentary-tract ganglioneuromatosis
  Cushing's syndrome (rare)
  von Hippel-Lindau disease (very rare)
  Virilism or Addison's disease or acromegaly (extremely rare)
G. Signs caused by metastases

have some clinical and metabolic manifestations of excess catecholamines without either sustained or paroxysmal hypertension (466). Pheochromocytoma without hypertension has been mentioned by others (122, 492, 517, 535, 760, 971) and it appears that at least some of these tumors were functioning.

At this point it is relevant to remark that on extremely rare occasions a tumor which is actively secreting catecholamines may cause minimal or no clinical manifestations. Taubman, Pearson, and Anton reported a 40-year-old woman with bilateral pheochromocytoma detected radiographically. She was asymptomatic and they emphasized the important point that the diagnosis of pheochromocytoma should be considered when an unexplained mass is demonstrated in the vicinity of the kidneys, even in the asymptomatic patient (971). Their patient did, however, give a two-year history of dull headaches over the left hemicranium which occurred about once monthly (usually in the morning, but occasionally severe enough to awaken her at night) and lasted 1 to 3 days. They were frequently accompanied by dizziness, nausea, and vomiting. She had no other symptoms and she had gained 23 kg over the past 4 years. Other than obesity, the physical examination was negative except for two mild blood pressure elevations (150/100 mmHg on admission and 124/96 mmHg during hospitalization) on more than 50 recordings. Unfortunately her blood pressure was apparently unknown during her episodes of headache. Since headaches have not recurred since the removal of her tumors, it seems likely that they resulted from the effect of increased circulating catecholamines.

Taubman and coworkers ascribed the paucity of symptoms and signs in their patient to minimal secretory activity of the tumors, significant inactivation of norepinephrine within the tumor, and tolerance of tissues to circulating catecholamines. Although the mechanism for this tolerance is unknown, they pointed out that many patients with pheochromocytoma have circulating catecholamine concentrations at a level reported to be fatal in man following the accidental injection of excessive doses of catecholamines (592). Finally, they indicated that similar tolerance can exist in children with neuroblastoma who show no manifestations of cardiovascular abnormali-

ties despite the excretion of relatively large amounts of norepinephrine (399).

An asymptomatic catecholamine-secreting carotid body tumor has also been reported (60).

Usually, but not invariably, there is a marked increase of both systolic and diastolic pressure in patients having paroxysmal attacks. Several patients were found to have elevations as high as 300/240, 325/200, 290/185, and 300/180 mmHg during paroxysmal attacks (462). Wavelike variations of the blood pressure have been noted in some patients during paroxysmal attacks. In one patient the blood pressure rose to 300/200 mmHg for about 5 min; this cycle then recurred repeatedly during the attack, which sometimes lasted several hours. Similarly, another patient had a blood pressure which would rise to about 280/160 mmHg and then fall to 65/40 mmHg at approximately 15-min intervals (462).

Strickler reported a patient as having a blood pressure which reached over 330 mmHg systolic and 150 mmHg diastolic. An unusual feature in this patient was the recurrent daily pattern of blood pressure elevation. A relatively normal value was observed in the early morning, but then the blood pressure rose gradually throughout the remainder of the morning to very high levels, only to return to fairly normal levels in the evening (Fig. 4.2) (942). An example of the frequent fluctuations in blood pressure which may occur in a patient with paroxysmal hypertension due to pheochromocytoma is given in Figure 4.3.

A patient reported by Ross and coworkers is an example of how unimpressive the presenting symptoms and hypertension may sometimes be in a patient with pheochromocytoma (813). This 56-year-old man at a routine medical examination had a blood pressure of 145/90 mmHg; he was symptom-free except for tiredness and occasional night sweats. The electrocardiogram, however, revealed left ventricular strain, and an alert physician found the urinary VMA to be excessive. Subsequently, blood pressures under observation in the hospital were found to range from 160/100 to 200/110 mmHg and a pheochromocytoma was demonstrated at operation.

Very rarely there may be an elevation of the systolic and a simultaneous lowering of the diastolic pressure. Bauer and Belt reported a patient with pheochromocytoma who had ex-

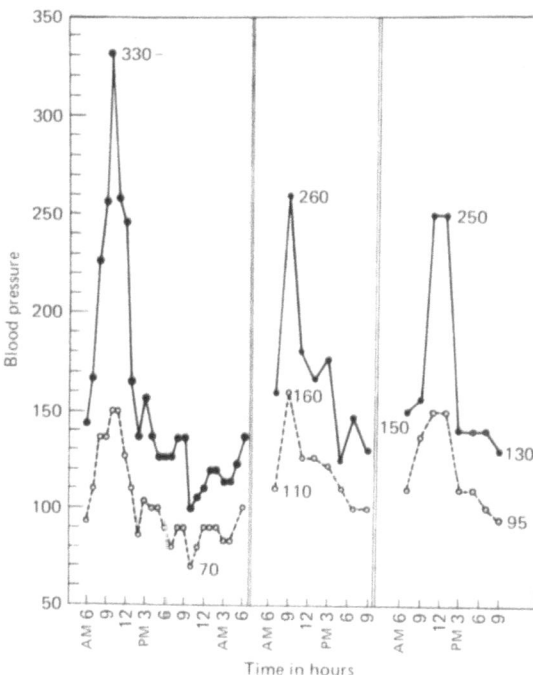

Fig. 4.2 Typical paroxysms of hypertension which occurred regularly at about the same time each day. From Strickler, C. W., Jr., *Southern Surgeon 11:* 196, 1942.

140/80 mmHg between attacks, but only a few months later he developed persistent hypertension of 210/130 mmHg (462).

Not infrequently the blood pressure of the patients with sustained hypertension will fluctuate widely, due to variations in the secretion of catecholamines into the circulation. One patient with sustained hypertension varying between 180/120 and 220/140 mmHg became transiently normotensive when she was treated with bed rest and sedation (856). Although the sustained hypertension is generally of considerable magnitude, occasionally the hypertension is rather mild. An abrupt onset of sustained hypertension has been well-documented (147).

Paroxysmal hypertension, usually of a marked degree, is the hallmark of pheochromocytoma, yet episodes of symptoms suggestive of increased circulating catecholamines but without hypertension have occasionally been described (492, 517, 640, 760, 832)— especially in patients with familial pheochromocytoma (938). A particularly unusual finding was the case of a 19-year-old woman whose blood pressure was variable, but in whom the variability had no relationship to her attacks of hotness, dizziness, profuse sweating, trembling, palpitations, and cold extremities; blood pressure was repeatedly

treme variations of blood pressure during an attack, on one occasion the pressure changing from 120/80 to 230/40 mmHg (47). It is of interest that intermittent hypertension may become persistent (393). One 45-year-old man experienced two or three daily attacks which lasted 1 to 10 hr; the blood pressure was

Fig. 4.3. Systolic and diastolic blood pressure monitored by an arteriocorder (an automatic sphygmomanometric instrument devised by Roche) at 2 or 5 min intervals for about 16½ hr. This patient had paroxysmal hypertension due to a right adrenal pheochromocytoma (patient No. 35 in Chapter 7).

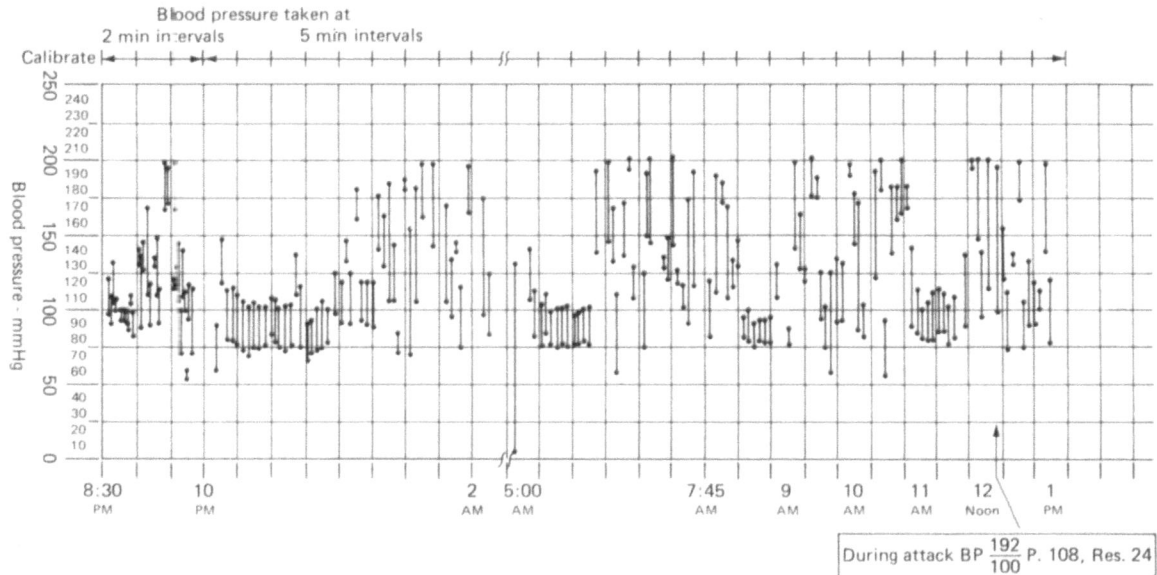

During attack BP $\frac{192}{100}$ P. 108, Res. 24

normal during attacks, and high on several occasions when she was symptom-free (640). It is noteworthy and intriguing that the hypertension in members of a family afflicted with pheochromocytoma tends to be consistent [i.e., either all members of a family having this tumor will have sustained hypertension, or all will have paroxysmal hypertension (938)]. However, patients from a kindred having familial pheochromocytoma, medullary thyroid carcinoma, and parathyroid adenoma may have either paroxysmal or sustained hypertension (144).

Finally, a patient with profound paroxysmal hypotension and tachycardia due to an epinephrine-secreting pheochromocytoma has been reported (791). This patient was occasionally observed to have hypertension (mainly systolic) which was followed by hypotension. The first patient reported as having an epinephrine-secreting tumor remained normotensive for 6 years despite recurrent symptomatic attacks (833). Other patients with this tumor have developed hypotension or have had periods of hypotension alternating with hypertension (36, 141, 229, 329, 366, 417, 436, 459, 556, 780, 974). This "manic-depressive" behavior of the blood pressure should immediately suggest pheochromocytoma.

It should always be kept in mind that during a paroxysm of hypertension in a patient with pheochromocytoma the blood pressure may, rarely, be unobtainable with a sphygmomanometer because of severe peripheral vasoconstriction rather than because of hypotension. Usually the intraarterial pressure in such patients is markedly elevated. However, one patient in whom the blood pressure was unobtainable on auscultation had an intraarterial pressure of 130/70 mmHg [right atrial pressure was 0 to 1 mmHg and pulmonary artery pressure was 32 (systolic) and 20 (diastolic) mmHg], while the peripheral pulses were absent (carotid and femoral pulses were forceful) (778).

It is of particular interest, and of value diagnostically, to ascertain whether any physical maneuver may mechanically squeeze the tumor and cause a liberation of catecholamines, thereby producing symptoms and signs experienced by a patient during a spontaneous attack. For example, one of our patients had noted that attacks were induced by shoveling snow. When this patient performed a shoveling motion in his hospital room, his blood pressure rose markedly and he experienced a typical attack; simultaneously his plasma catecholamines became markedly elevated.

Rolling over in bed may cause sufficient pressure in the region of a pheochromocytoma to liberate catecholamines into the circulation and produce symptoms which awaken the patient. With tumors located in the adrenal area, palpation and massage in the flank may sometimes cause liberation of catecholamines and a characteristic attack. Gitlow has noted that paroxysmal episodes can be produced by abdominal massage in 12 percent of patients (personal communication from Stanley E. Gitlow, Professor of Clinical Medicine, Mount Sinai Hospital, New York, New York). However, it should be mentioned that paradoxical results have, rarely, been produced by maneuvers causing pressure in the flank. For example, one of our patients with a pheochromocytoma the size of a large grapefruit in the left adrenal area could only precipitate attacks by rolling on her right side; another patient with a pheochromocytoma the size of a tangerine in the region of the right adrenal developed an elevated blood pressure when pressure was applied to the right or left loin (229). It is noteworthy that we and others (462) have observed that patients who experience attacks induced by bending motions usually have relatively large tumors.

ORTHOSTATIC HYPOTENSION

Orthostatic hypotension occurring in a hypertensive patient who is not being treated with antihypertensive medications suggests pheochromocytoma (107, 108, 158, 392, 459, 639, 722, 934, 952, 1009, 1050). Smithwick and coworkers first emphasized the diagnostic value of this observation in differentiating patients with pheochromocytoma from those with essential hypertension (919). Some have claimed this occurs in 70 percent of patients (267, 907). The mechanism for this hypotensive response is not certain but may be related to a depression, by excessive circulating catecholamines, of the sympathetic reflex which maintains blood pressure in the upright position. Engelman and coworkers believe this hypotensive phenomenon in some patients is due to a functional autonomic blockade resulting in a defect in sympathetic vasomotor reflexes (276); in other patients they felt orthostatic hypotension might result from a diminished blood volume. It is, of course, conceivable that in some patients both a reduced blood volume and a diminished sympathetic reflex may play a role. Whether decreased blood volume may occasionally be a contributing factor in causing postural hypotension has not been settled. Some have claimed blood volume is normal in the majority of patients with this tumor (909); others have demonstrated hypovolemia in most of their patients, especially those with sustained hypertension (223, 489, 966). The blood pressure in both the sitting and standing position may be much lower than when the patient is recumbent (107). Occasionally, hypotension has been observed in some patients with pheochromocytoma even when they are sitting (329, 856), or recumbent (212, 310).

The postural hypotension is observed primarily in patients with pheochromocytoma who have sustained hypertension, and not in those who are normotensive or have paroxysms of hypertension. Very rarely, orthostatic hypotension may be the presenting complaint. The drop in blood pressure is usually to normotensive levels or slightly below (Fig. 4.4), but a decrease to shock levels has, on rare occasions, been reported (329).

The presence of postural hypotension is best elicited by having the patient remain in the recumbent position until the blood pressure stabilizes, and then recording the effect of standing erect for about 3 min. We believe (as taught by Dr. I. H. Page) that it is worthwhile to record the blood pressure of all hypertensives in the seated, the standing, and the recumbent positions. Such blood pressure recordings will not only enable the physician to better control a patient's antihypertensive therapeutic regimen, but it may occasionally detect postural hypotension in the untreated patient with pheochromocytoma.

POSTURAL TACHYCARDIA

Postural tachycardia is almost invariably associated with the orthostatic hypotension, yet it may occur in the absence of hypotension. Smithwick reported that five out of nine patients with pheochromocytoma had an increase in heart rate of 20 beats or more per min when changing from a recumbent to a standing position (920).

It has been stressed that even a slight reduction of diastolic blood pressure when a hypertensive subject assumes an erect position, especially when associated with an unusual rise in heart rate, should make one suspect pheochromocytoma (920).

PARADOXIC BLOOD PRESSURE RESPONSE

Paradoxic blood pressure response to antihypertensive drugs or induction of anesthesia appear related to the liberation of catecholamines by these agents. It is especially important to recall this point in the hypertensive patient whose blood pressure fluctuates widely and whose hypertension is poorly controlled during treatment with antihypertensive drugs.

GENERALIZED SWEATING

As discussed above, sweating is a very common symptom in patients with pheochromocytoma; it is also a very helpful diag-

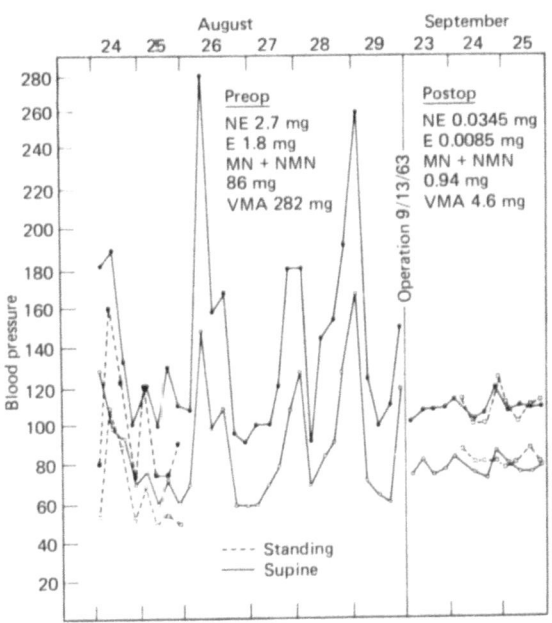

Fig. 4.4 Typical blood pressure pattern in a patient with pheochromocytoma. Note the orthostatic hypotension and the paroxysmal pressor episodes during the preoperative period. Twenty-four-hour urinary catecholamines and their metabolites pre- and postoperatively are also recorded. From Engelman, K. Bull., *N. Y. Acad. Med.* **45**: 852, 1969.

nostic sign. In some patients with either sustained or paroxysmal hypertension caused by pheochromocytoma, generalized sweating (primarily of the upper body, neck, and face) is very pronounced, whereas in others it is inconspicuous or absent. The abrupt onset of drenching sweats is associated with paroxysms of hypertension. Sometimes profuse diaphoresis appears as an attack ends. In one patient sweating occurred every 3 to 5 min as the blood pressure declined following a paroxysm (462). No sweating was observed in about one-third of our patients. The occurrence of diaphoresis and hypertension, particularly in a patient who is at rest and in a relatively cool environment, immediately suggests pheochromocytoma as a possible cause.

TACHYCARDIA AND REFLEX BRADYCARDIA

The myocardium of patients with pheochromocytoma is stimulated by increased circulating catecholamines, frequently resulting in tachycardia (of atrial or rarely ventricular origin) and/or premature contractions (242). Furthermore, the increased free fatty acids occurring in some patients with pheochromocytoma may also possibly augment myocardial irritability, since an increase in myocardial oxygen consumption is caused by the utilization of free fatty acids as the major energy substrate (720). Sometimes with the sudden paroxysms of hypertension occurring with these tumors, there is a reflex bradycardia with escape of lower pacemakers (116, 281). It has been demonstrated that the reflex bradycardia occurring during norepinephrine infusion is of vagal origin since it can be blocked by atropine administration (42, 378). One patient was observed during an attack to have a decrease of his heart rate from 52 to 36 beats per min (42). Furthermore, during marked bradycardia, the beats may come in pairs (42). One of us (W.M.M.) has observed two patients with pheochromocytoma who developed reflex bradycardia and nodal escape rhythm when their blood pressures rose from normal to markedly hypertensive levels in association with marked increases in plasma catecholamines (322). In some patients with pheochromocytoma, tachycardia may occur initially during an attack but then be followed by reflex bradycardia. Not infrequently the pulse may

become weak. During very severe and prolonged hypertensive crises, Aranow (personal communication from Dr. Henry Aranow, Professor of Medicine, Columbia Medical Center, New York) and others (920) have observed patients whose pulses became absent, but this is very rare. This latter finding could be confusing during operative removal of a pheochromocytoma and might be misinterpreted as circulatory shock instead of intense vasoconstriction.

PALLOR AND FLUSHING

Pallor of the face and upper part of the body has been observed in about 60 and 28 percent of patients having paroxysmal and sustained hypertension, respectively (351). Occasionally, generalized pallor has been reported, or only blanching of the distal portion of the extremities may be evident (338). This pallor, or ashen-gray appearance, may, rarely, precede an attack (42) but usually occurs at the time of an episode of increased blood pressure, and is undoubtedly due to the intense vasoconstriction in the face caused by the circulating catecholamines. During an attack one patient had a heliotrope cyanosis affecting the face, hands, and feet which would alternate with pronounced pallor in the circumoral region (942). Purplish mottling or ashen cyanosis of the face may, rarely, appear and sometimes extend to the chest during a paroxysm. Two patients were described as developing blanching and flushing intermittently coincident with the rise and fall of blood pressure, respectively (462). During a paroxysmal attack associated with marked pallor, the skin temperature has been reported to have decreased as much as 10° to 15°F (303).

Owing to vasomotor instability with vasodilation, flushing of the face may, very rarely, be observed alone, or following the pallor. A patient observed by one of us (R.W.G.) became markedly flushed during paroxysmal attacks caused by her pheochromocytoma (Fig. 4.5, p. 77). In some patients the face was described as being flushed even between attacks (462).

An increased blood flow to the extremities has been noted in some patients and may be a reaction to the elevated temperature and BMR (920). A history of manifestations of peripheral vasoconstriction was elicited in 47 percent of the cases in the literature reviewed by Smithwick and coworkers, whereas 90 percent of their own patients had evidence of vasoconstriction (920). They stressed the importance of specifically questioning patients for signs of peripheral vasomotor phenomena, since patients may not mention these as complaints.

ANXIETY

Frequently during a severe paroxysmal attack patients may appear anxious and frightened because of a sense of impending death. Furthermore, they may appear uncomfortable because of palpitations and exquisitely painful headaches.

RETINOPATHY

Retinopathy associated with pheochromocytoma is indistinguishable ophthalmologically from that seen in primary hypertension. Retinopathy of Group III or IV (504) classification occurred in about 53 percent of our patients with persistent hypertension due to pheochromocytoma. About 40 percent of our patients with sustained hypertension had Group I or II changes, and only 5 percent had normal fundi. Of the patients with paroxysmal hypertension, about 50 percent had Group I or II changes, and the remaining ones had normal ophthalmoscopic findings.

After analyzing the ocular findings in 38 cases of pheochromocytoma reported in the literature up to 1947, Bruce stated that 88 percent showed ocular pathology (107). In this latter group 35 percent had retinopathy and 100 percent had vascular constrictions; however, he did not divide the groups into sustained and paroxysmal hypertension. He also reported the findings in three children with sustained hypertension seen at Columbia Medical Center. Two of these children had Group IV retinopathy, whereas the third had arteriolar narrowing with banding, tortuosity, increased light reflexes, and a beginning retinal edema. He indicated that the findings in the patients with pheochromocytoma could not be differentiated from those with "essential hypertension." Furthermore, Bruce pointed out that the ophthalmologist may be consulted initially before the internist, since the ocular manifestations may be the first or only symptoms.

In 1948 Hollenhorst reported the ocular changes associated with pheochromocytoma in patients seen at the Mayo Clinic and cases recorded in the literature (453). He divided his 70 patients into three groups: Group A, 24 patients with paroxysmal hypertension but with normal blood pressure between attacks; Group B, 37 patients with paroxysmal hypertension but sustained hypertension (>150/90 mmHg) between attacks; and Group C, nine patients with sustained hypertension but with no paroxysms.

Although 41.6 percent of Group A had normal fundi, two of the 24 patients had retinopathy. One of these latter patients had paroxysms in which the blood pressure rose repeatedly from 140/70 up to 290/200 mmHg over a period of 8 months. Twenty-five percent of Group A had minimal to moderate sclerosis of the retinal arterioles. Only 10.5 percent of Group B had normal fundi, whereas 62.2 percent had either Group III retinopathy or, more commonly, Group IV neuroretinopathy, and 43.2 percent had retinal arteriolar sclerosis. In Group C, 11 percent had normal fundi, 66.7 percent had retinopathy, and 55.5 percent had retinal arteriolar sclerosis varying from mild to severe.

The retinal lesions in some patients with pheochromocytoma reported by Hollenhorst consisted of papilledema, hemorrhages, exudates (cotton wool patches), macular stars, arteriolar narrowing of various degrees, mild to severe arteriolar spasm with focal constrictions, and arteriolar sclerosis of varying severity. Even retinal and optic nerve atrophy (perhaps secondary to neuroretinitis) with loss of central vision has occurred in a child with severe sustained hypertension due to bilateral adrenal medullary tumors. Some patients with pheochromocytoma have been studied during an attack of hypertension without a detectable change in the caliber or appearance of the retinal vessels. Sometimes there was slight narrowing and expansile pulsation of the arterioles. In reviewing the reports of others, Hollenhorst mentioned that rather striking changes were occasionally observed in the fundi of patients with pheochromocytoma during paroxysmal attacks of hypertension. Some patients had very definite spasms of the arterioles, with considerable narrowing and irregularity. The diastolic pressure of one patient rose to 300 mmHg, the pupils became widely dilated, the arterioles further constricted, and there was an increase in the papilledema, hemorrhages, exudation, and arteriovenous nicking. In another patient the retinal arterioles and veins became dilated and the diastolic blood pressure in the central artery rose from 45 to 75 mmHg during an attack (453).

Nearly always there is progressive improvement in the retina following the lowering of blood pressure after removal of pheochromocytomas. Photographs of the retina at intervals after surgery in one patient revealed gradual disappearance of papilledema, hemorrhages, exudate, macular stars, and narrowing of the arterioles, until the occular fundi appeared normal 3.5 years later (800). The apparent diminution in degree of arteriolar sclerosis in the retina postoperatively may indicate that in severe hypertension with marked narrowing of retinal arterioles, a heightened arteriolar light reflex may simulate severe sclerosis (453). Hollenhorst has pointed out that a clue to the diagnosis of pheochromocytoma exists in recognizing a hypertensive retinopathy, without associated retinal arteriolar sclerosis. This is especially true if the retinopathy is of the acute hypertensive type and particularly if seen in a child (453). It must be appreciated that a similar acute hypertensive retinopathy may be seen in some patients with renovascular disease. However, sclerosis of the retinal arterioles (some resembling white lines) has been observed in a 12-year-old child who apparently had sustained hypertension due to bilateral pheochromocytoma for only 2 years (528).

Most reports indicate that lacrimation and dilation of the pupils occur during attacks of paroxysmal hypertension. In one patient marked salivation and lacrimation during attacks was reported (462). Exophthalmos was observed coincident with a marked rise in blood pressure in patients with pheochromocytoma (970). The exophthalmic stare and marked pupillary dilatation were observed in one patient in the presence of normotension (462). The pupillary dilation is probably due to the effect of epinephrine, since no change was noted during infusions of norepinephrine or during instillation of 1:1000 norepinephrine into the conjunctival sac (42). A homolateral

Horner's syndrome was described in a patient with a paraganglioma involving the left first thoracic ganglion. Impairment of efferent sympathetic nerve impulses to the left eye would explain the Horner's syndrome (453).

Pupillary dilation may occur transiently during attacks accompanying liberation of catecholamines into the circulation. Widely dilated pupils were described in some patients even between attacks (462). One report concerns a patient in whom anesthesia and minor surgery apparently triggered release of catecholamines and produced widely dilated pupils which did not react to light. Even 10 min after the anesthetic was discontinued, this pupillary status persisted (160). Widely dilated pupils not reactive to light during an attack have also been reported in another patient (927). This physical finding must be kept in mind, since its presence during a hypertensive paroxysm, if not pathognomonic for pheochromocytoma, should strongly suggest the diagnosis. In this connection, one patient with tabes dorsalis and miotic Argyll-Robertson pupils was observed to have widely dilated pupils (not reactive to light) during a paroxysm of hypertension. A pheochromocytoma was suspected in this patient but no tumor was found on laparotomy (58). Bilaterally dilated pupils were observed during an episode of autonomic hyperreflexia in a patient with a posttraumatic incomplete transection of the spinal cord below the level of the fifth cervical segment (977).

WEIGHT LOSS

As mentioned previously, the majority of patients with pheochromocytoma give a history of mild to moderate weight loss. This is more usual in the patients with the persistent form of hypertension, where the constant secretion of catecholamines by the tumor results in sustained elevation of the basal metabolic rate. About 41 and 23 percent of patients with persistent and paroxysmal hypertension, respectively, are 10 percent or more below their standard weight (Table 4.2) (352). Weight loss may also be associated with malignancy per se if metastatic pheochromocytoma is present; very rarely, weight loss in the extremities may be observed if Cushing's syndrome also occurs.

TREMOR

Tremor occurred in about half the patients during episodic hypertension, and in approximately one-fourth of patients with sustained hypertension. This was a fine tremor and similar to that seen in hyperthyroidism; however, there may be, rarely, a coarse tremor of the hands (42). Rarely, shaking has been reported during an attack (144); one patient shivered and his teeth chattered (42), and another patient shivered so violently that the bed shook (366). Conspicuous trembling can be produced by epinephrine infusions but is not evident with comparable norepinephrine infusions (42, 617).

RAYNAUD'S PHENOMENON

Raynaud's phenomenon (and/or livedo reticularis and/or mottled cyanosis and/or pallor), which was frequently observed, probably resulted from altered circulation of the extremities induced by the catecholamines. The extremities may appear wet, cold, and clammy, occasionally with goose flesh and cyanotic nailbeds. Obliteration of the nailbed capillaries has been observed during a paroxysm of hypertension (462).

FEVER

Fever may be a manifestation of pheochromocytoma, but when it is present the temperature is usually only slightly elevated. Smithwick and coworkers stated that fever has not been emphasized sufficiently in connection with the diagnosis of pheochromocytoma, since approximately 76 percent of their patients and 70 percent of cases in the literature (where the temperature was recorded) had unexplained elevations of temperature (1°F or more) (400, 920). They observed that the fever was not necessarily related to paroxysmal symptoms, but occasionally the temperature could become elevated to 105°F during a paroxysmal attack; therefore, it has been recommended that frequent rectal temperatures be recorded for 48 hr in patients suspected of having pheochromocytoma (920). Chills do not accompany the fever. Elevation of the temperature apparently results from impaired heat elimination due to peripheral vasoconstriction and an increased BMR caused by the catecholamines. Some patients seriously ill with pheochromocytoma have been re-ported to have had fevers up to 107°F (462, 938).

NEUROFIBROMATOSIS

The characteristic manifestations of neurofibromatosis are described in detail later in this chapter. Because of the increased incidence of pheochromocytoma in persons with neurofibromatosis, all persons with this latter condition who have paroxysmal or sustained hypertension should be screened for the presence of a chromaffin tumor.

PALPABLE MASS IN THE ABDOMEN OR NECK

Graham has stated that about 14 percent of pheochromocytomas are palpable. This is quite similar to the experience of Moorhead (680) and of Gitlow, who claim that these tumors are palpable in about 10 percent of patients (personal communication from S. E. Gitlow, Professor of Clinical Medicine, Mount Sinai Medical Center, New York City). MacKeith found that an abdominal tumor (sometimes a displaced kidney) is palpable in about one-third of cases (598). Eight of 18 patients reviewed by Howard and Barker had a mass palpable on the side of the abdomen in which the tumor was found. The other masses palpated were kidneys which had been displaced downward by the tumors. The liver was found pushed down to the level of the umbilicus by one tumor (462). On the other hand, our experience has been that only rarely is it possible to palpate a mass in the abdomen, since pheochromocytomas are usually deep-seated and relatively small. A huge cystic pheochromocytoma which fills the entire abdomen may, rarely, be found (469). Pheochromocytomas or chemodectomas occurring in the neck are frequently detectable on palpation, and massage may cause a release of catecholamines and a rise in blood pressure.

Rarely, an associated thyroid carcinoma may be felt in the neck. Since it has been demonstrated that some of the medullary thyroid carcinomas occurring in association with pheochromocytoma secrete prostaglandin, calcitonin, and serotonin (844, 907), conceivably some of these secretions, if present in sufficient amount, might also produce additional signs. For example, serotonin excess could theoretically cause signs and symptoms of bronchial asthma, hypermotility of the intestine, and vasomotor phenomena in the skin (e.g., flushing of the face) as seen in patients with carcinoid. However, these signs caused by excess serotonin would probably be observed only—if at all—in patients at a time when the circulating catecholamines were not elevated, since increased concentrations of epinephrine and norepinephrine would tend to counteract these effects of serotonin. Calcitonin and prostoglandin may also be involved in the causation of diarrhea seen in some patients with medullary thyroid carcinoma.

SWELLING OF THE THYROID GLAND

Paroxysmal hypertension due to pheochromocytoma with concomitant swelling of the thyroid gland has been reported (47, 208, 416, 944). During paroxysmal attacks in one patient with pheochromocytoma, the neck veins became engorged up to 5 cm above the manubrium, the thyroid became enlarged, and on one occasion a bruit was heard over it. His neck at times became so swollen (by as much as 1.5 inches in circumference) that he had to remove his collar and tie (208). Others have reported remarkable neck vein distention and an increase in cervical distention during attacks (462). Some have suggested that thyroid swelling results from pronounced hyperemia of the thyroid induced reflexly by sudden increased pressure in the carotid sinus. Norepinephrine infusion has also been reported to have caused soft swelling in the region of the thyroid gland, which in one patient persisted for 6 hr after the infusion ended (42).

MISCELLANEOUS

Apnea or Tachypnea A number of miscellaneous signs have, rarely, been noted and are listd for completeness (Table 4.3). For example, with a severe paroxysmal attack, an initial apnea or tachypnea may be seen, and the heart action may be "tumultuous" and forceful enough to shake the whole body or the bed or chair (462, 598). Despite an extremely forceful cardiac impulse, the radial pulse may, on occasion, be barely perceptible or even unobtainable (927), because of intense peripheral vasoconstriction. The respiratory rate in five patients was recorded as increasing to 36 per min during paroxysmal attacks, with

the patients becoming dyspneic (462); as mentioned above, pulmonary edema may accompany these attacks. Tetany was reported in one patient, but it is likely that this was alkalotic in origin; hyperventilation and vomiting were prominent features of the attacks and, furthermore, the blood calcium concentration was normal (462).

Heart Murmurs and Bruits Of additional interest is the fact that a number of patients with pheochromocytoma have been reported with harsh systolic and/or soft diastolic murmurs (15, 102, 262, 326, 485, 598, 730, 791), which probably resulted from hemodynamic alterations caused by the increased circulating catecholamines. For example, an 18-year-old girl with severe hypertension due to a pheochromocytoma was found to have a loud split second pulmonic sound and a harsh systolic murmur, accompanied by a thrill, heard at the second left parasternal space; subsequently, when she was normotensive, the intensity of the murmur diminished (102). Another patient, a 39-year-old man with a pheochromocytoma which was causing alternating episodes of hypertension and hypotension (ranging between 200/100 and 80/40 mmHg), had a harsh Grade 3 systolic murmur which fluctuated in intensity for 12 hr and then disappeared (730). In still another patient, the appearance of a Grade 1/6 precordial ejection murmur (heard best at the left sternal border in the fourth intercostal space), which within 24 hr increased in intensity to Grade 3/6, suggested an erroneous diagnosis of bacterial endocarditis (326).

Fred and associates pointed out that reports in the literature have indicated that loud murmurs in the apical, pulmonic, and aortic areas have appeared during or shortly after paroxysmal attacks; however, no pathologic lesions have been demonstrated to account for any of these murmurs (326).

Very rarely, there may be pronounced engorgement of the neck veins during an attack (208, 462), and in one patient an aortic diastolic murmur was heard at the height of a paroxysm (64). Another patient had a palpable cystic pheochromocytoma in the left adrenal area over which a bruit was heard (856). It should be kept in mind that, if a pheochromocytoma or a coexisting intraabdominal neurofibroma compresses a renal artery, a bruit may be heard which may erroneously suggest that a primary renal aterial lesion is responsible for the hypertension.

Growth Defects Isolated instances of growth defects, retarded appearance of ossification centers, and sexual precosity have also been reported (437, p. 76).

SIGNS OF COMPLICATIONS

Signs of complications of pheochromocytoma consist mainly of hypertensive *cardiovascular* and *cerebrovascular* derangements, with their characteristic manifestations. Also, as mentioned previously, *arrhythmias* and *congestive heart failure* may result from *catecholamine cardiomyopathy.*

CIRCULATORY SHOCK

Circulatory shock may result from significant cardiovascular or cerebrovascular complications. In addition, shock may result from a severe hemorrhage from any source, including bleeding within the tumor itself. In some patients, shock may follow a hypertensive crisis without any obvious explanation. Howard and Barker cited the report of a 35-year-old woman who experienced weight loss and marked asthenia, and who developed episodes of shock during the latter part of her illness prior to operation; these episodes sometimes lasted 2 to 3 days and were of "such severity that diagnosis of internal hemorrhage and adrenal insufficiency were seriously considered" (462). It is possible that a marked decrease in circulating catecholamines at the termination of a paroxysm of hypertension may result in a state of inadequate vasoconstriction, as occurs, for example, following removal of a pheochromocytoma. Infusion of moderately high concentrations of catecholamines in experimental animals will initially cause a rise in arterial blood pressure; however, with prolonged administration the blood pressure will eventually fall to shock levels and result in death (567, 679). The exact mechanism for this latter sequence of events is not clear, but Lever and coworkers have presented evidence that the hypotension following cessation of norepinephrine infusion might be due to the re-

lease of a vasodilator (567). Prolonged infusions of epinephrine in dogs can produce sufficient vasoconstriction with consequent oligemia to induce shock (327).

The hypotension occurring in the presence of excess circulating catecholamines might also be related to a reduced cardiac output (546) due to arrhythmias (242), myocardial damage (710), or low plasma volume (780). Loss of peripheral sensitivity to catecholamines may also play a role. Coggin and coworkers have stated that the hypotensive phase may be associated with cardiac, peripheral, or central nervous mechanisms, depending on the conditions and the species (161).

Hypotension has occurred in man following infusions of epinephrine (394, 518). Also, as mentioned previously, hypotension has, rarely, been reported in patients with pheochromocytoma following hypertensive attacks, or it may occur spontaneously, particularly in patients with predominantly epinephrine-secreting tumors.

GASTROINTESTINAL DISTURBANCES

Severe constipation occurring in some patients with pheochromocytoma can result in a grossly distended tympanitic abdomen without peristalsis (69). Catecholamines relax intestinal smooth muscle (with a decrease in frequency and intensity of peristalsis), and cause a contraction of the pyloric and ileocecal sphincters and a vasoconstriction of splanchnic arterioles. Constipation occurred in 13 percent of patients with sustained hypertension but it was not experienced by those with paroxysmal hypertension. In one patient harboring a pheochromocytoma episodes of diarrhea occurred (586); however, this manifestation is most unusual and atypical in patients with pheochromocytomas unaccompanied by other pathology. It is interesting that in one patient with pheochromocytoma who developed severe constipation which simulated acute intestinal obstruction, administration of phentolamine inhibited the action of the catecholamines and promptly resulted in a simultaneous drop in blood pressure and in profuse fecal incontinence. This patient had not had a stool for 8 days (69). Laparotomy was performed on one patient with progressive abdominal distention caused by pheochromocytoma in the mistaken belief that the patient might have peritonitis

(166). Another patient with severe substernal and epigastric pain, followed by extreme abdominal tenderness and gaseous distention, was thought to have coronary thrombosis and mesenteric infarction, but necropsy revealed only a pheochromocytoma of the left adrenal gland (485). The rare occurrence of megacolon in patients with pheochromocytoma could also contribute to the constipation.

Rarely, ischemic enterocolitis may occur and result in obstipation, and ultimately ileus, colonic distention, hemorrhage, necrosis, and even perforation of the small and large intestine (69, 105, 106, 804).

It is noteworthy that pallor of the mucosa of the ileum and rectum have been observed during norepinephrine infusion (42). Further, gastrointestinal disturbances and pathologic lesions identical to those observed in some patients with pheochromocytoma have been described in patients administered infusions of norepinephrine (78, 106, 797). One of the patients reported by Brown and Borowsky was found to have a proliferative arteritis of the splanchnic arterioles and widespread venous and capillary thrombi (105).

MISCELLANEOUS

Compression of adjacent structures may result in complications of urinary tract obstruction (728), and even spinal cord compression due to extension of a thoracic pheochromocytoma has been described (605). Although relatively uncommon, signs of medullary thyroid carcinoma, mucocutaneous neuromas, alimentary-tract ganglioneuromatosis, Cushing's syndrome, hyperparathyroidism, cholelithiasis, and von Hippel-Lindau disease occur in both familial and sporadic pheochromocytoma. Even signs of virilism, Addison's disease, or acromegaly have occurred.

Finally, it should be mentioned that signs and symptoms can, of course, result from metastases of a malignant pheochromocytoma, e.g., bone pain. Pulmonary metastases may result in hemoptysis (218), pleural effusion or chylothorax (76), cough and dyspnea, etc.

ATYPICAL MANIFESTATIONS

When pheochromocytoma occurs in childhood or in pregnancy, or when the tumor arises in the urinary bladder, certain atypical mani-festations and unusual characteristics are frequently evident. The importance of recognizing how manifestations in these special circumstances may differ considerably from manifestations usually occurring in adults with pheochromocytoma deserves particular attention. These three situations will therefore be discussed below in some detail.

PHEOCHROMOCYTOMA IN CHILDREN

In 1904 Marchetti first reported finding pheochromocytomas (involving both adrenals) in a 15-year-old boy who had died of typhoid fever (629). Although pheochromocytoma is considered a rare tumor, in children it is one of the most common endocrine tumors (1048, pp. 886, 887). Of 100 consecutive patients with pheochromocytoma seen at Columbia Medical Center, 11 were children (Table 3.8).

It is important to emphasize that the clinical manifestations of pheochromocytoma in children may differ in a number of ways from those in adults with this tumor. Several extensive reviews of the occurrence of this tumor in children have been made (310, 466, 933, 975), and it appears to have a broad racial and geographic distribution (933). When in 1960 Hume (466) reviewed the world literature on pheochromocytoma, he found that only 8 percent of the children (16 years and younger) with this tumor had paroxysmal hypertension. Almost two-thirds of the children were males. The average age of these children was 9.8 years (varying from 5 months to 16 years), with a maximum incidence of pheochromocytoma at 13 years of age. The average duration of symptoms was 1.5 years, and varied between 2 weeks and 9 years. It has been emphasized that it is doubly important to measure the blood pressure routinely during a physical examination of children, since over 90 percent of those with pheochromocytoma have sustained hypertension (466). [It has been recommended that muffling (IV Karotkoff sound), as well as the disappearance of the sound (V Karotkoff sound), be recorded when estimating diastolic blood pressure, since recording only the point of disappearance could cause gross underestimation of the diastolic pressure. Furthermore, it has been reported that in some children the diastolic sound may not disappear until the mercury is almost at zero (670).] A high incidence of sustained hypertension (88 percent) was confirmed by Stackpole and associates in 100 cases of pheochromocytoma in children up to 15 years of age (933). Bradley and associates have suggested (96) that the higher incidence of sustained hypertension in children than in adults with pheochromocytoma may reflect the capacity of children to elaborate considerably greater percentages of norepinephrine in the adrenal medulla than can adults (1029). Our experience and that of Cahill (122) and of Kvale (533, 535) indicated that paroxysmal hypertension occurs in about 50 percent of adult patients with pheochromocytoma, although some investigators have reported the incidence to be only about 25 to 50 percent (377, 393, 920). Table 4.4 can be a helpful guide for the pediatrician, or for the physician who occasionally examines children, since it reveals "normal" standards of systemic blood pressure in children. Tabulated, by age groups, are the 50th and 95th percentiles for systolic and diastolic pressures for children and teenagers. Since the data represent a composite of several studies, it is felt that repeated blood pressure values above the 95th percentile should be considered abnormally elevated (670).

Hume tabulated the findings in 71 children with pheochromocytoma (Table 4.5), and stated that *sweating* and *visual complaints* were more common than in adults. The frequency of visual complaints was undoubtedly related to the high incidence of eyeground changes (77 percent) occurring in the children with sustained hypertension. *Nausea, vomiting* (occasionally projectile), and *weight loss* also occur more frequently in children with pheochromocytoma than in adults. In general, the

symptoms and signs caused by catecholamine release from a pheochromocytoma in a child or in an adult are quite similar. It is noteworthy, however, that *polydipsia* and *polyuria* occurred in 25 percent of the children with pheochromocytoma, whereas we observed these symptoms only rarely in adults. One 8-year-old boy with a pheochromocytoma of the right adrenal gland and sustained hypertension was mistakenly diagnosed and treated as a case of diabetes insipidus for 18 months before the correct diagnosis was recognized. His daily fluid intake ranged from 5 to 7 liters, and there was an inability to concentrate urine above a specific gravity of 1.005. In addition to polyuria and polydipsia, which diminished with vasopressor administration, the patient experienced excessive diaphoresis (975). Urea clearance was normal (89.5 ml/min) and nonprotein nitrogen was 46 mg/dl. It seems reasonable to believe the polyuria might be related to an increased renal blood flow. The latter could result from an increased cardiac output (which occurs in many patients with pheochromocytoma) and the sustained hypertension —provided that vasoconstriction within the kidney caused by the circulating catecholamines was not sufficiently intense to counterbalance this effect and reduce renal blood flow. Polydipsia could then be related to the polyuria, and perhaps also in some degree to severe diaphoresis. Alternately, one might speculate that the antidiuretic hormone is suppressed by excessive circulating catecholamines in patients with pheochromocytoma, yet an antidiuretic action of epinephrine and norepinephrine administered intravenously has been demonstrated in the dog (213). However, why polyuria and polydipsia are less frequently observed in adults with pheochromocytoma remains unclear.

Polyphagia was also noted in two children but not in adults (466). (Significant weight loss may occur despite a ravenous appetite.) *Convulsions* were reported in 23 percent of the children (466), but in only 3 to 5 percent of the adults (352, 976). Finally, a *reddish-blue mottling of the skin* has occasionally been described in children (728), and a *puffy, red, cyanotic appearance of the hands* was reported in 11 percent of children with pheochromocytoma (466) but was not observed in adults. The incidence of symptoms and signs in the children with

Table 4.4 *Percentile Values for Blood Pressure by Age*[a]

	Systolic Pressure		Diastolic Pressure	
Age	50%	95%	50%	95%
0 to 6 mo	≤ 80	≤110	≤45	≤60
3 yr	≤ 95	≤112	≤64	≤80
5 yr	≤ 97	≤115	≤65	≤84
10 yr	≤110	≤130	≤70	≤92
15 yr	≤116	≤138	≤70	≤95

[a] From Mitchell, S. C., Blount, S. G., Jr., Blumenthal, S., Hoffman, J. I. E., Jesse, M. J., Lauer, R. M., and Weidman, W. H. *Pediatrics 56:* 3, 1975.

Table 4.5 *Symptoms, Signs, and Diagnosis of Pheochromocytoma in Children*[a,b]

A. Hypertension[c]
   Sustained: 64 cases
   Paroxysmal: 5 cases
   Normal between attacks: 1 case (not determined during attack)
   Of 64 sustained, 1 previously had paroxysmal hypertension and 14 had further elevation with attacks

B. Symptoms	No.	Percent
Headache	55 of 68	81
Sweating	48	68
Nausea	40	56
Visual changes	29 of 66	44
Weight loss	31	44
Abdominal pain	25	35
Nervousness, palpitation	24	34
Weakness, fatigue	19	27
Pallor	19	27
Polydipsia	18	25
Polyuria	18	25
Convulsions	16	23
Dyspnea	11	16
Puffy, red, cyanotic hands	8	11
Constipation (sometimes severe)	6	8
Epistaxis	3	4
Polyphagia	2	3

C. Signs and laboratory findings		
Eyeground changes	51 of 66	77
Basal metabolic rate over +20%	19 of 23	83
Fasting blood sugar over 120 mg%	6 of 15	40
Glycosuria	2	3
Neurofibromatosis	1	1.4

D. Diagnosis

Catecholamines	Mean	Range
Urine, μg/liter	1800	(300–3500)[d]
Plasma norepinephrine, μg/liter	31	(6.1–65)[d]

   Intravenous pyelogram: 25 negative, 11 positive
   Presacral air pyelogram: 12 negative, 14 positive
   Calcified tumor on x-ray film: 4 cases
   Aortogram: 1 positive, 1 negative
   17-ketosteroids: normal in 4 of 4
   17-hydroxycorticosteroids: normal in 3 of 3

[a] Adapted from Hume, D. M. Reproduced with permission of the publisher of *Am. J. Surg. 99:* 461, 1960.
[b] Based on 71 cases with adequate information unless otherwise indicated.
[c] Average normal blood pressures: In the newborn: 80/46 mmHg
   At 1 year of age: 90/66 mmHg
   At 14 years of age: 118/60 mmHg
[d] Values invariably elevated above normal.

pheochromocytoma reported by Hume and coworkers (467) was very similar to the findings of Stackpole and coworkers, except that the latter found a significantly higher occurrence (22 percent) of acrocyanosis (933). What the explanation is for the differences between the manifestations in children and those in adults with these tumors is not clear. According to Page and Copeland, *an obstructive uropathy or obstruction of a renal artery* may occasionally be the presenting manifestation of a pheochromocytoma in children (728).

Congenital cyanotic heart disease has been reported in six children with pheochromocytoma (786), and it has been speculated that hypoxemia might cause adrenal medullary hyperplasia and ultimately an autonomously functioning pheochromocytoma (786).

Page and Copeland have pointed out that a severe and stormy course is characteristic of pheochromocytoma in children and that frequently these tumors are bilateral, multiple, and ectopic (728). Reviewing the cases of pheochromocytoma reported up to 1968, these authors found that the ratio of males to females before puberty was 2 to 1; but after puberty there was a marked increase in the incidence of pheochromocytoma in females, the overall occurrence of this tumor in children being, then, only slightly greater in males (728).

Stackpole reported that in a series of 100 children there were 140 pheochromocytomas; about one-third of these children had multiple tumors, most of them bilateral. Also, in about one-third of cases the tumors were extra-adrenal. Nine children had more than two tumors and one had as many as six (see Fig. 3.9). Others have also reported multiple tumors in children, e.g., two boys, 10 and 11 years of age, had four pheochromocytomas each (96, 464), and one 10-year-old boy was found to have multiple pheochromocytomas involving 10 para-aortic ganglia and both adrenal glands (956). We were involved with Drs. Cobin, Pertsemlidis, Gitlow, and Krieger (at Mount Sinai Medical Center) in studying a most interesting case of a 19-year-old woman who, during the course of her 4-year illness (see patient No. 19 in Chapter 7) had 15 benign pheochromocytomas (one in the neck, one in the thorax, five para-aortic in the abdomen, two in the wall of the urinary bladder, one in the vaginal wall, three on the anterior surface of the aorta, and one on each side between the aorta and the adrenal gland)! To our knowledge this is the largest number of benign pheochromocytomas ever found in a patient.

In Stackpole's series the tumors were usually small but six were palpable. The appearance of a second pheochromocytoma after surgical removal of one tumor occurred in five children. The distribution of 140 pheochromocytomas in 100 children reviewed by Stackpole and associates is indicated in Figure 3.9 (933). In 76 cases of pheochromocytoma in children reported by Hume, 39 percent of the tumors were multiple (either bilateral adrenal, single adrenal plus extraadrenal, or multiple extra-adrenal) and 14 percent were single extra-adrenal tumors (Table 3.4). Hume has stressed the importance of the upper transverse abdominal incision in children, since a very thorough search for the presence of more than one tumor is mandatory. The majority of deaths from pheochromocytoma in children resulted from the presence of a second tumor which had been missed when the first pheochromocytoma was removed (466).

PHEOCHROMOCYTOMA IN PREGNANCY

Kawashima first reported a fatality in a pregnant patient who was found to have a pheochromocytoma at autopsy (502). In 1927 Oberling and Jung reported the occurrence of pheochromocytoma in pregnancy (714). Their patient was a 28-year-old woman who had paroxysmal hypertension and died following delivery in unexplained shock. Autopsy revealed a pheochromocytoma of the left adrenal gland. It was not until 1955 that there was reported (by Maloney) the first case of pheochromocytoma in which the diagnosis was made antepartum (608). That year, Keir reported a pheochromocytoma (discovered at a previous cesarean section) which was successfully removed antepartum and followed by delivery of a normal baby at another cesarean section (503). Bennett and Mather first described a case in which the diagnosis and removal of a pheochromocytoma was made in the antenatal period and was followed by spontaneous delivery of a normal baby (59). The intraabdominal pressure changes accompanying pregnancy may account for the increased release of catecholamines from a pheochromocytoma which may previously have been relatively quiescent. Labor may further compress a pheochromocytoma and increase the release of catecholamines from the tumor.

Paradoxically, complete disappearance of a typical syndrome of pheochromocytoma during pregnancy (506) and transient relief of symptoms with the onset of pregnancy (116) have been reported. There is no clear explanation of why, in some patients, attacks appear to be aggravated by pregnancy, whereas in others attacks do not occur during the entire course of pregnancy (462).

Peelen and De Groat in 1955 pointed out the seriousness of this tumor complicating pregnancy, noting that the maternal and fetal mortality was 45 and 32 percent, respectively. Death usually occurred in the women within 72 hr of delivery. Symptoms generally appeared in the third trimester, and the hypertension was paroxysmal in at least 80 percent of their series of 20 pregnancies accompanied by pheochromocytoma (739). The tumor involved the left or right adrenal with equal frequency in 18 cases and was bilateral in two. Gemmell reviewed 35 cases of pheochromocytoma occurring during pregnancy and observed that symptoms developed in almost one-third of the patients between the onset of labor and 24 hr after delivery. On the other hand, he noted that symptoms were as likely to develop during the puerperium (346). Symptomatology was quite similar to that observed in children and adults with pheochromocytoma (466), although occasionally manifestations similar to fulminating preeclampsia developed and the patients died (346). Two patients reported in Gemmell's series had pheochromocytomas removed before their first pregnancies and the deliveries were normal. It is intriguing that these same two patients were found to have pheochromocytomas during their second pregnancies (346).

In a series of 32 pregnancies complicated by pheochromocytomas reported by Dean in 1958, maternal mortality occurred in 16, but in 13 of these cases the diagnosis was not made until autopsy (212). This latter finding emphasizes the vital importance of suspecting the possibility of pheochromocytoma as the underlying cause of hypertension in any pregnancy. When Hume reviewed the literature in 1960, he found that there were at least 37 cases in which symptoms of pheochromocytoma were experienced during pregnancy (466). He noted that manifestations of pheochromocytoma during pregnancy could appear as (1) severe preeclampsia; (2) paroxysmal hypertension with typical symptoms; (3) typical symptoms without hypertension (98, 754); (4) sudden shock and death in the antepartum period (59); (5) hyperpyrexia (754) after delivery; or (6) shock after delivery (with or without previous apparent symptoms) occurring spontan-

eously, or induced by anesthesia or delivery. Hume pointed out that pregnancy complicated by pheochromocytoma may be confused with (a) toxemia, when sustained hypertension is present during the early stages of pregnancy; (b) preeclampsia, when headache, edema, tachycardia, and hypertension are present in late pregnancy; or (c) a ruptured uterus, when the patient goes into shock during or immediately after labor (466). Hume has indicated that patients with toxemia of pregnancy, preeclampsia, or unexplained attacks should be screened for the presence of pheochromocytoma. We would further reemphasize that, unless the cause of an elevated blood pressure is very obvious, any pregnant patient with paroxysmal or sustained hypertension should be carefully evaluated for the presence of pheochromocytoma.

A final point of particular fascination is that clinical manifestations (e.g., attacks of sweating, pallor, tingling of the hands and feet, headaches, palpitations, and hypertension) suggesting excess circulating catecholamines have been observed during the last weeks of pregnancy in six mothers whose fetuses developed neuroblastoma (759, 1000). It was presumed that the signs and symptoms exhibited by the mothers resulted from catecholamines secreted by these congenital neuroblastomas. In a pregnant patient with manifestations of excessive circulating catecholamines, it is always mandatory to consider the diagnosis of a neural crest tumor in the mother; however, one should consider the remote possibility that the mother's manifestations may result from a neural crest tumor in the fetus. (There have been no reports of manifestations of excessive circulating catecholamines in the mother caused by a pheochromocytoma in the fetus. We know of only one case of congenital pheochromocytoma.)

PHEOCHROMOCYTOMA OF THE URINARY BLADDER

Since the first instance of pheochromocytoma of the urinary bladder was noted by Zimmerman and coworkers in 1953 (1073), these tumors, situated in the wall of the bladder, have been reported in a number of patients. They frequently produce a characteristic syndrome (440, 561), in that a typical paroxysmal attack usually occurs during or shortly after micturition or with distention of the bladder (e.g., by retained urine or cystography) due to liberation of catecholamines by compression of the tumor. Attacks have also been precipitated by defecation (963). Other symptoms of a bladder tumor are usually present, and painless hematuria has been reported to occur in from 50 (728) to 65 percent of patients (561). At times, focal ulceration of the mucosa may cause gross hematuria with expulsion of blood clots (5). In addition, urinary frequency, nocturia, and tenesmus on urination may occur (5). Page and Copeland pointed out that the urinary metabolites of catecholamines may be within the normal range in patients with these tumors, perhaps because there is a release of catecholamines for only brief periods during bladder contraction. Furthermore, cystoscopy and cystograms may sometimes be normal since the tumors are usually small and located in the muscular wall of the bladder (728). Cystoscopy may be normal even when the tumor is malignant (484). Elevation of the blood pressure during micturition or bladder distention, or with massage of the bladder area, is of particular diagnostic value.

In an excellent study in 1971, Leestma and Price (561) reported 24 cases of paraganglioma (pheochromocytoma) involving the urinary bladder and compared these with 34 similar tumors referred to in the literature. It would appear that the frequency of occurrence in the bladder of this relatively rare tumor suggests that it probably does not arise from "ectopic" chromaffin cells. These pheochromocytomas occurred with equal frequency in males and females (age range, 11 to 78 years), and account for 0.06 percent of all bladder tumors.

Dr. M. M. Melicow has reviewed the world literature (April, 1976, unpublished data), including the recent reports by Takahashi (963) and Lindsey (578), on the frequency and age distribution of pheochromocytoma of the bladder, and found reports on 76 patients. The age and sex distribution of these cases is given in Figure 4.6. As can be seen in the figure, pheochromocytoma of the bladder was somewhat more common in females than in males. Particularly interesting is the finding that tumors occurred most frequently in patients between 10 and 19 years of age. Up to 1975, six patients with malignant pheochromocytoma of the urinary bladder were reported (484); this suggests an incidence of malignancy similar to that in adrenal pheochromocytomas.

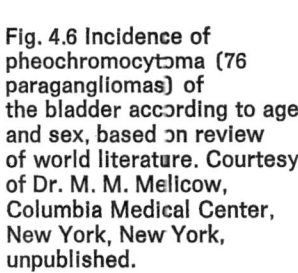

Fig. 4.6 Incidence of pheochromocytoma (76 paragangliomas) of the bladder according to age and sex, based on review of world literature. Courtesy of Dr. M. M. Melicow, Columbia Medical Center, New York, New York, unpublished.

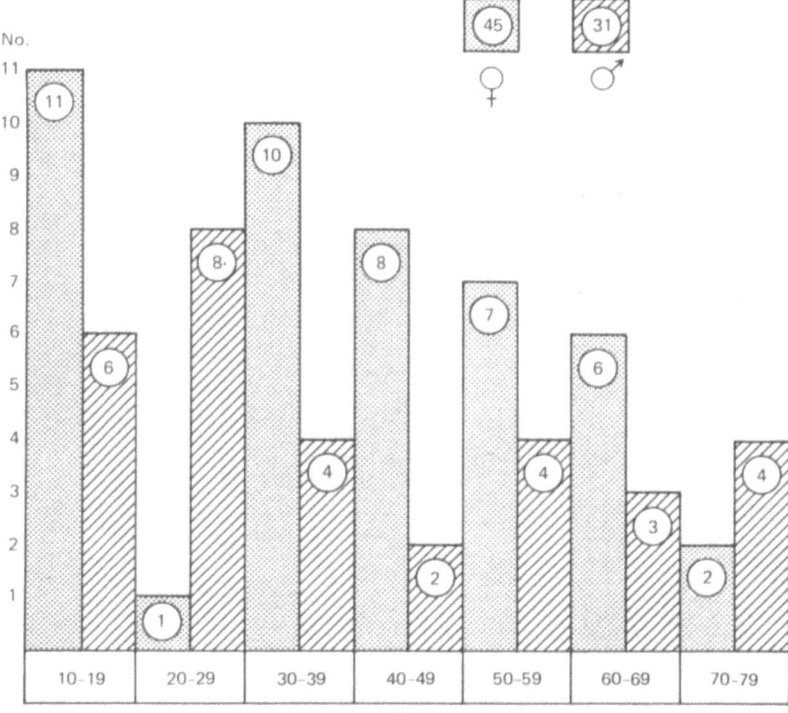

Fig. 4.7 Gross photograph of paraganglioma (pheochromocytoma) of urinary bladder illustrating the usual protruding cauliflower appearance (3×, A.F.I.P. Neg. 68-8287). From Leetsma, J. E. and Price, E. B., Jr. Reproduced from *Cancer 28:* 1065, 1971, by permission of the American Cancer Society.

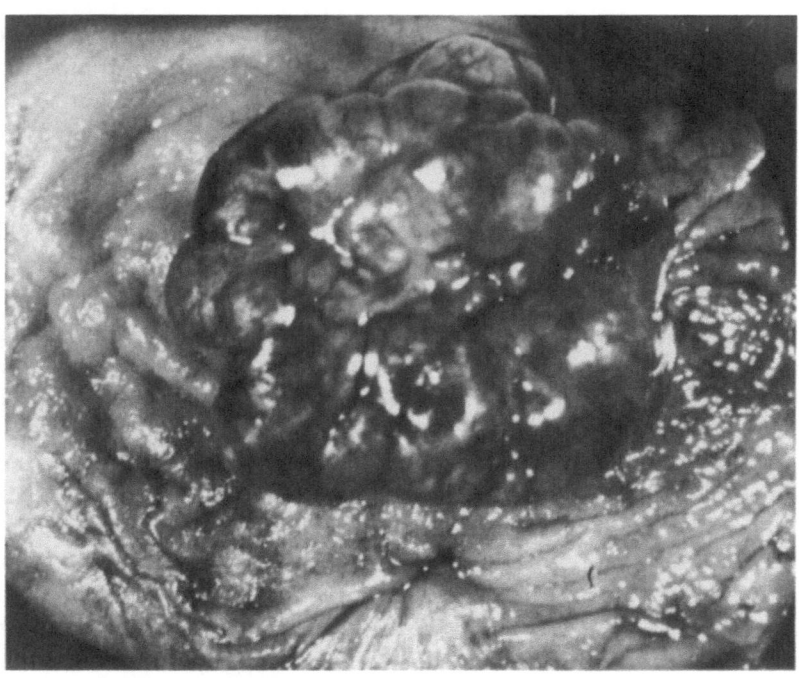

Fig. 4.8 A. Typical "zellbalen" pattern of paraganglioma (pheochromocytoma) illustrating septations and central clear vacuoles resembling collections of fat (hematoxylin and eosin stain, 135×, A.F.I.P. Neg. 69-560). B. An island of paraganglioma (pheochromocytoma) separating bundles of smooth muscle in the bladder wall and having a close relationship to what appear to be small vascular channels (hematoxylin and eosin stain, 235×, A.F.I.P. Neg. 69-562.) From Leetsma, J. E. and Price, E. B., Jr. Reproduced from *Cancer 28:* 1065, 1971, by permission of the American Cancer Society.

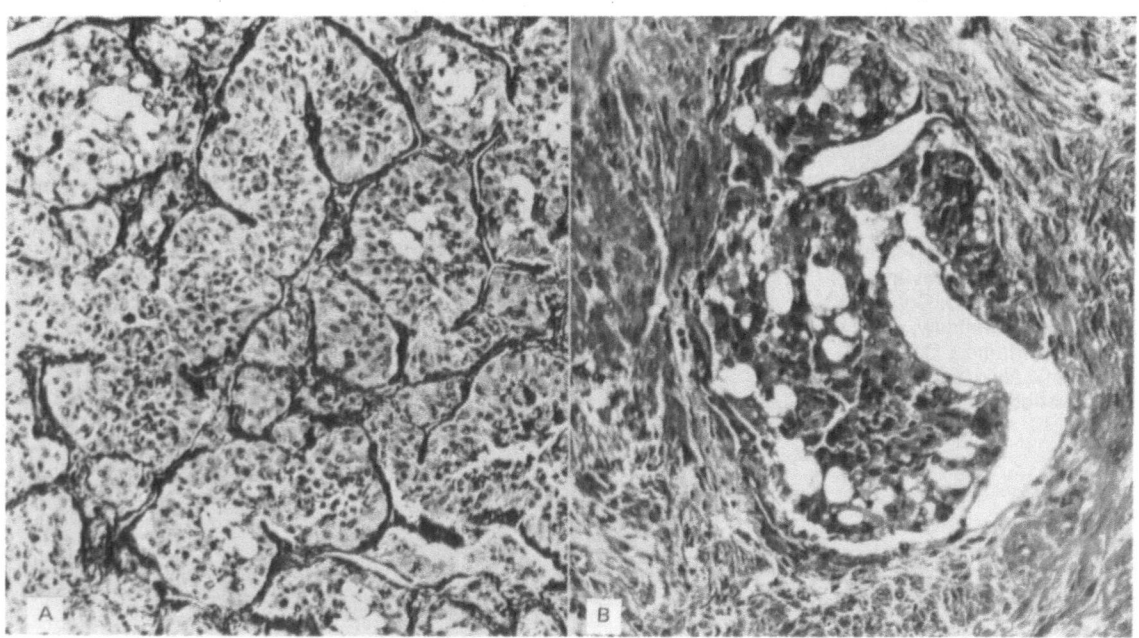

In the 24 cases reported by Leestma and Price, tumors varied in size from 0.3 to 5.5 cm in greatest diameter, were usually located submucosally, and bulged into the bladder lumen, became ulcerated, and bled. Figures 4.7 and 4.8 illustrate the characteristic gross and microscopic features of these tumors. Some tumors were relatively separate from surrounding tissue and appeared circumscribed (Fig. 4.8), but the majority were intermingled with adjacent muscle bundles of the bladder wall. The cells, which were polyhedral and acidophilic, contained central or eccentrically placed ovoid nuclei with peripherally situated chromatin. The nuclei contained one or more nucleoli and were sometimes distorted; however, mitoses were rarely seen. Cells were arranged in balls or cords which were delimited from each other by connective tissue and vascular septation. Less than 7 percent of these bladder tumors become malignant and, as pointed out by Leestma and Price, multifocality is not uncommon and may be mistaken for evidence of metastasis (561).

It has been proposed that the origin of these urinary bladder pheochromocytomas are small nests of chromaffin paraganglia which migrate with sympathetic ganglia and become located in the wall of the bladder. It is noteworthy that Coupland has identified multiple chromaffin bodies associated with sympathetic nerve fibers in the perivesical and periprostatic tissues of the newborn child (178). Paraganglia related to autonomic nerves are located mainly in the muscular layer of the bladder wall (95). The most common presenting complaint in 65 percent of these 24 patients was gross, intermittent, but painless terminal hematuria. No incidence of thyroid neoplasm was detected in these patients.

Table 4.6 summarizes the pertinent findings in the cases reported in the literature and those reported by Leestma and Price, and also the frequency of findings when all cases were combined. These investigators suggested that the smaller mean size of the tumors in their series, and the smaller percentages of their patients having hypertension or some sort of micturitional attack, might be due to the fact that many of the tumors in their cases were

Table 4.6 *Comparison of Cases of Paraganglioma (Pheochromocytoma) of the Urinary Bladder Reported in the Literature with Those Reported by Leestma and Price[a]*

Category	Literature cases	Leestma and Price	Combined cases
No. cases	34	24	58
Mean age	38 years	43 years	41 years
Sex	16 male	12 male	28 male
	18 female	12 female	30 female
Location			
Dome	11	4	26%(15/58)
Trigone	10	9	33%(19/58)
Anterior wall	8	4	21%(12/58)
Posterior wall	2	2	7%(4/58)
Bladder neck	1	1	3%(2/58)
Not stated	3	3	10%(6/58)
Mean size	4 cm	2 cm	3 cm
Hypertension	85%	35%	65%
Hematuria	53%	65%	58%
Micturitional attacks	76%	13%	51%
Chromaffinity	8+, 2—[b]	6+, 1—[b]	14+, 3—[b]
Catecholamines and/or VMA elevated in urine	8 of 16	3 of 5	11 of 21
Multifocality	8	2	18%(10/58)
Metastases	3	0	5%(3/58)

[a] Modified from Leestma, J. E. and Price, E. B., Jr. Reproduced from *Cancer* 28: 1069, 1971, by permission of the American Cancer Society.
[b] + = positive; — = negative.

found incidentally, either at autopsy or during a urologic procedure for some other condition. Hence, the tumors in their cases may not have had time to develop fully and produce symptoms (561). Most urinary bladder tumors occur in the submucosa and about 80 percent can be seen on cystoscopy. About 20 percent, however, cannot be visualized because of their deeper location. One pheochromocytoma, arising from the intravesical portion of the ureter, caused a filling defect in the bladder and presented as a ureterocele (119).

The clinical triad of (1) hypertension, often paroxysmal, (2) gross, intermittent, terminal hematuria, and (3) attacks typical of pheochromocytoma which occur on micturition, was present in about one-half of the combined series of patients analyzed.

It should be mentioned that one patient with a pheochromocytoma of the urinary bladder has been reported who developed oliguria and renal failure, probably secondary to the effects of a hypotensive period following a paroxysm of hypertension (161). Urinary retention and azotemia have been reported in patients with pheochromocytoma in locations other than the urinary bladder (36, 42). It has been suggested that excess circulating norepinephrine may occasionally lead to urine retention by causing excessive contraction of the internal vesical sphincter and possibly relaxation of the bladder muscles (36).

The diagnosis of pheochromocytoma can almost invariably be confirmed by the presence of excess urinary excretion of catecholamines and/or their metabolites which occurs during and following a paroxysm of hypertension. Very rarely, however, the chemical assays of the urine may be normal. In one patient, with a small tumor in the bladder wall, only the catecholamine concentration in plasma sampled at the junction of the common iliac veins increased significantly at the time of postmicturition hypertension (85).

PATHOLOGIC ENTITIES SOMETIMES ASSOCIATED WITH PHEOCHROMOCYTOMA

There are several conditions which occur in patients with pheochromocytoma more frequently than they do in the general population. The physician must be acutely aware of disease entities and familial syndromes which may be associated with pheochromocytoma since these may be important in the diagnosis and management of these patients. We feel this important point has not been adequately emphasized, and undoubtedly associated pathology has been overlooked in a significant number of cases. Also, only very rarely is the initiative taken to screen any members of a patient's family in an attempt to exclude a familial link.

CHOLELITHIASIS

At the Mayo Clinic cholelithiasis has occurred in about 30 percent of patients having paroxysmal hypertension and in about 10 percent of those having persistent hypertension caused by pheochromocytoma. Kirkendall and associates reported an incidence of about 18 percent in 17 patients with pheochromocytoma (513). Prospective surveys indicate that the prevalence of cholelithiasis in white adults (30 to 62 years of age) in the United States is roughly 6 percent for females and 1.3 percent for males (913a). Approximately 96 percent of all gallstones are composed essentially of cholesterol to which bilirubin, calcium, cellular debris, and glycoprotein have been added. Whether catecholamines can significantly influence the physiology of bile formation, secretion, and excretion in a manner that augments the formation of gallstones is unknown. Serum cholesterol elevations of 450 mg/dl and 400 mg/dl were reported in two patients with paroxysmal hypertension and pheochromocytoma. After tumor removal the cholesterol in one of these patients was found to be normal (229). Serum cholesterol is almost invariably within the normal range in patients with pheochromocytoma and sustained hypertension or when quantitated between attacks in patients with paroxysmal hypertension; however, one of our patients with moderately severe sustained hypertension had a preoperative serum cholesterol level of 356 mg/dl with normal triglycerides. One week following tumor removal serum cholesterol concentration was 306 mg/dl, whereas 7.5 months later it was 247 mg/dl. It is noteworthy that cholesterol levels may become elevated in normal subjects during emotional stress, which activates the sympathetic nervous system (331, 1028). It should be stated, of course, that there is no good evidence that hypercholesterolemia alone can cause cholelithiasis. The composition of gallstones occurring in patients with pheochromocytoma has not been studied.

MEDULLARY THYROID CARCINOMA

An increased incidence of thyroid carcinoma in patients with pheochromocytoma was first suggested in 1952 (215). Sipple in 1961 reported thyroid carcinoma to occur 14 times more frequently in patients with pheochromocytoma than ordinarily expected (897). Within the next few years the association of these tumors was reported by a number of investigators (232, 453, 711, 849, 864, 913, 1043). The simultaneous occurrence of these tumors has become known as Sipple's syndrome, and by 1975 more than 200 patients with this syndrome had been reported (136). Thyroid carcinoma is found with both familial and nonfamilial (sporadic) pheochromocytoma and, when these tumors occur simultaneously, the chromaffinomas are said to occur bilaterally in the adrenals in 70 percent of patients (144, 849, 938, 1042).

In 1968 Steiner and coworkers reviewed the literature and made the interesting observation that when pheochromocytoma occurred in families not afflicted by medullary thyroid carcinoma 32 of 51 patients (i.e., 63 percent) had sustained hypertension. On the other hand, when pheochromocytoma occurred in families afflicted by thyroid carcinoma, sustained hypertension occurred in only five of 35 patients (i.e., 14 percent). They also observed that none of 14 patients with sporadic pheochromocytoma and an associated thyroid carcinoma had sustained hypertension (938). It appears that for some unknown reason the pheochromocytomas occurring in patients afflicted with thyroid carcinoma frequently do not constantly liberate adequate concentrations of catecholamines into the circulation to cause sustained hypertension; however, although purely speculative, it is conceivable that the secretion of vasodilating substances from the thyroid carcinoma might occur in some of these patients and could in part counterbalance the hypertensive effect of circulating catecholamines. These thyroid carcinomas had originally been classified as anaplastic, papillary, adenocarcinoma, or medullary carcinoma (not infrequently calcified) with amyloid struma (938).

Medullary thyroid carcinoma was described as a pathologic entity in 1959 (428); more recently it has been stated that thyroid carcinoma occurs in association with familial pheochromocytoma in about 23 percent of cases (938). This type of thyroid carcinoma, which is a nonfollicular tumor consisting of polyhedral, round, and spindle cells, and which usually has amyloid in the struma (428, 461, 864, 1043), may secrete calcitonin (198, 653, 664), prostaglandin (1045), serotonin (471, 581, 672), and ACTH-like substances (231). This tumor may also elaborate other monoamines (307). Histaminase (50) and dopa decarboxylase (24, 503a) have also been found in these tumors. Baylin and coworkers have suggested that abnormal histaminase activity in the serum may prove valuable in detecting the development of metastatic medullary thyroid carcinoma. Periodic determinations of serum histaminase may also prove helpful in evaluating effectiveness of chemotherapy (e.g., with aminoguanidine) on the tumor cells (50). Subsequent experience has, however, indicated that the absence of elevated levels of serum histaminase in no way excludes the presence of medullary thyroid carcinoma, even when the neoplasm is extensive and has metastasized (83a).

Medullary thyroid carcinoma, which occurs at all ages but most often between 40 and 50 years (580), is composed primarily of parafollicular calcitonin-producing C cells. The latter contain secretory granules which are 100–200 nm in diameter and it is thought that these cytoplasmic granules represent stored calcitonin; however, there is evidence that calcitonin cannot be exclusively assigned to secretory granules or microsomes (657). The accompanying hypercalcitonemia and consequent hypocalcemia may cause the development of parathyroid hyperplasia or adenoma, which not infrequently is discovered in association with medullary thyroid carcinoma (144).

The amyloid which may be produced by the tumor cells (657) differs histologically from the usual immunoamyloid. Yet it exhibits the characteristics of all amyloids, such as affinity for congo red and green birefringence when studied in polarized light (913b). It appears to be nonimmunoglobulin-related and probably has no light chains. Antiserum to protein of the amyloid from medullary thyroid carcinoma does not cross-react with any other type of amyloid so far observed (913b). Meyer and associates observed that secretory granules were intimately associated with amyloid fibrils of the medullary thyroid carcinoma and they suggested that the granules may play a role in the formation of the amyloid, perhaps providing a protein or polypeptide precursor (657). More recently Sletten and coworkers have characterized the amyloid fibril protein. They determined that the amino acid composition of the major component of the total amyloid material was only slightly different from calcitonin. Since the molecular weight of the amyloid (5680 daltons, indicating about 53 amino acid residues) was considerably larger than that of calcitonin (3380 daltons), and since the amino acid composition was similar, but with differences, it was felt that the major component of the amyloid may represent a prohormone for calcitonin or a fragment of a precursor (913b).

It is interesting that the cells of some medullary thyroid carcinomas tend to form an alveolar pattern remarkably similar to pheochromocytomas and carotid body tumors (90). As with familial pheochromocytoma, the familial form of medullary thyroid carcinoma appears to be transmitted through an autosomal dominant gene with a high degree of penetrance (144, 580, 864, 938); however, chromosomal abnormalities apparently do not occur in Sipple's syndrome (566). Evidence has been presented which suggests that C cell hyperplasia precedes development of familial medullary thyroid carcinoma (340, 1058).

One patient with a pheochromocytoma and an associated medullary thyroid carcinoma had elevated urinary 5-hydroxyindole acetic acid and, in addition, the thyroid tumor cells developed a yellowish fluorescence when exposed to vaporized formaldehyde, probably due to excessive amounts of serotonin (221). The presence of catecholamines and serotonin has been demonstrated histochemically and biochemically in the cells of familial medullary thyroid carcinoma and pheochromocytoma (307). It is significant that argentaffin cells have been identified among the parafollicular C cells of the thyroid (90), and may account for the secretion of serotonin by some of these

thyroid carcinomas. The C cells, some of which apparently show an argentaffin or chromaffin staining, appear to be of neural crest origin (557). As mentioned earlier, secretion granules have been observed in the cells of both pheochromocytomas and medullary thyroid carcinomas (463). Since chromaffin cells in the adrenal medulla contain catecholamines and traces of serotonin in secretory granules (922), and since parafollicular cells also contain serotonin (482) and probably calcitonin (323), it was suggested about 10 years ago that these tumors may reflect the biochemistry of the normal cells from which they originate (581).

It is of interest that up to 30 percent of patients with medullary thyroid carcinoma not infrequently experience chronic, moderately severe diarrhea (68, 471, 871, 1045), which may result from stimulation of intestinal motility by excess serotonin and/or prostaglandins (871). In the light of the demonstration that calcitonin itself can cause increased jejunal secretion of water and electrolytes in normal subjects, it is possible that this hormone could be a cause of, or contribute to, the diarrhea experienced by some patients with medullary thyroid carcinoma (392a). Explosive diarrhea may occur with loss of 10 to 25 liters per day and with a marked electrolyte depletion. The ACTH-like substances secreted by some medullary thyroid carcinomas may on rare occasions cause Cushing's syndrome (231).

Medullary thyroid carcinoma is a rare type of tumor, but it is almost invariably the type of thyroid carcinoma occurring in cases of Sipple's syndrome (144, 1043). In this syndrome it involves both lobes of the thyroid and tends to be multicentric with frequent metastatic involvement of cervical and mediastinal lymph nodes (144). It accounts for only about 6 to 10 percent of all thyroid malignancies (317), occurring about 1.3 times more commonly in males than in females (144, 317, 1044). Only about 3 percent of all patients with this type of thyroid carcinoma have an associated pheochromocytoma (1044); and, as mentioned above, pheochromocytomas are bilateral in about 70 percent of cases (144, 849, 938, 1043). Hill found that when pheochromocytomas occurred in patients with medullary thyroid carcinoma, they were always located in the adrenal (441).

In patients with Sipple's syndrome, the

diagnosis of medullary thyroid carcinoma may precede that of pheochromocytoma, since, as pointed out by Catalona and associates, symptoms of pheochromocytoma may often be overlooked (144). A high incidence of simultaneous occurrence in one kindred emerged from a routine diagnostic screening of family members (144). About 80 percent of patients with medullary thyroid carcinoma have a 5-year survival rate (144), but some patients have survived with recurrences for 25, 28, 30, and 36 years (90, 144, 501a). Usually the course is indolent but it may be aggressive in some patients (501a).

As mentioned previously, medullary thyroid carcinomas secrete calcitonin (217, 340, 903, 968); however, some have claimed that perhaps one-third of patients with familial forms of this malignancy have normal plasma concentrations of calcitonin under basal conditions (479, 652). It has been reported that in asymptomatic patients who have normal basal concentrations of plasma calcitonin, administration of pentagastrin, calcium, or glucagon will almost always significantly increase the calcitonin level if a medullary thyroid carcinoma is present; however, no remarkable change in calcitonin concentration occurs in normal subjects (902). It has been claimed that these stimulation tests may be of value in detecting an occult medullary thyroid carcinoma occurring in association with pheochromocytoma (902). Dr. Glen W. Sizemore recently stated that by screening 50 patients whose pheochromocytomas had been considered sporadic (nonfamilial) for evidence of increased serum thyrocalcitonin* they were able to detect unsuspected medullary thyroid carcinomas in 7 percent of these patients (personal communication from Dr. Glen W. Sizemore, internist at the Mayo Clinic). This important finding indicates that the prevalence of the combination of pheochromocytoma and medullary thyroid carcinoma (Sipple's syndrome) is probably greater than previously reported in patients with familial pheochromocytoma (i.e., greater than 23 percent); establishing whether tumors are familial or not may sometimes be very difficult or impossible. The combination of pheochromocytoma and medullary thyroid carcinoma may, of course, occasionally occur in sporadic (nonfamilial) cases (938). The finding of Sizemore

is also a compelling argument to screen practically all patients with pheochromocytoma for evidence of medullary carcinoma and for the presence of hyperparathyroidism. (The occurrence of multiple endocrine neoplasia is discussed later in this chapter.)

Pentagastrin stimulation used conjointly with selective catheterization of the inferior thyroid vein has proved especially accurate in detecting elevations of thyrocalcitonin in patients with medullary thyroid carcinoma (1025). Usually the level of serum calcitonin correlates well with the extent of the thyroid malignancy.

Using a highly specific and sensitive radioimmunoassay, Almquist and associates found the measurement of serum calcitonin to be highly accurate in the detection of histologically verified medullary carcinomas of the thyroid (9). In their experience no false negative or false positive results were noted. Primary and metastasizing medullary thyroid carcinomas invariably produced increased serum concentrations of calcitonin; therefore, it was possible to determine postoperatively whether the tumor had been completely removed. They acknowledged the uncertainty of calcitonin levels near the upper limit of normal, and they suggested that in these cases measurement of calcitonin during a 4-hr calcium infusion test might be of value.

Diagnosis of medullary thyroid carcinoma by fine needle aspiration biopsy has also been successfully employed (925). Gagel and associates found that provocative testing with pentagastrin or calcium infusion was also of value in detecting the premalignant condition of C-cell hyperplasia in the thyroid. These investigators have presented evidence to support the intriguing concept that in Sipple's syndrome pheochromocytomas develop upon a background of diffuse adrenal medullary hyperplasia, a situation analogous to C-cell hyperplasia preceding medullary thyroid carcinoma (340). Their findings support the hypothesis and pathologic findings of Carney and coworkers, that diffuse hyperplasia of the adrenal medulla may be the precursor of pheochromocytoma in Sipple's syndrome (135b, 136).

---

* Note: Thyrocalcitonin = calcitonin.

Familial medullary thyroid carcinoma is almost invariably bilateral, whereas the non-familial (sporadic) form of this malignancy is unilateral. Hence, one should always exclude the possibility that a patient with bilateral disease of the thyroid may also have a pheochromocytoma and/or hyperparathyroidism. Total thyroidectomy with resection of regional lymph nodes is the only effective treatment since these thyroid tumors and their metastases are unresponsive to [131]I. Unless extensive bilateral metastases to lymph nodes in both tracheo-esophageal grooves require extensive dissection, preservation of parathyroid function on at least one side of the neck should be possible in most patients (83a). The incidence of regional lymph node metastases has been reported to be 50 to 60 percent, and hematogenous spread to the lung, liver, and bone is also common (144). If a pheochromocytoma is also present, thyroidectomy should never precede extirpation of the pheochromocytoma.

Menof has reported acute enlargement of the thyroid in man after the intravenous infusion of norepinephrine (656). The speculation was made that thyroid carcinoma may result from repeated stimulation of the thyroid gland by the catecholamines from a preexisting pheochromocytoma (976); however, Steiner and coworkers have stated that this hypothesis seems unlikely for two reasons: (1) a number of patients have been observed in whom medullary thyroid carcinoma appeared before symptoms of pheochromocytoma; and (2) in families reported to have some members with coexistent pheochromocytoma and medullary thyroid carcinoma, there have been nine instances of individuals having thyroid carcinoma without pheochromocytoma (938).

As mentioned by Manning and coworkers, the occurrence of multiple endocrine neoplasia raises some fascinating questions regarding etiology and may at times pose formidable diagnostic problems (627). Cushman first reported the coexistence of pheochromocytoma, metastatic thyroid carcinoma, and a parathyroid adenoma (199), whereas the occurrence coincidentally of familial pheochromocytoma, hyperparathyroidism with multiple parathyroid adenomas, and medullary thyroid carcinoma was first reported by Manning and associates in 1963. Their patient was 18 years

of age when seen at the Mayo Clinic because of palpitations (5 months) and persistent tachycardia (4 months), followed by markedly impaired vision, headaches, and detection of hypertension (154/120 to 240/180 mmHg). She had bilateral Grade 4 retinopathy with severe vasospasm and an area of retinal detachment in her right eye. Excretory urogram was normal but pharmacologic testing was positive for pheochromocytoma. Bilateral multilobular pheochromocytomas (35 g on right; 55 g on left) were removed with their capsules intact, preserving normal adrenal tissue in both glands. Blood pressure and histamine stimulation test were normal postoperatively.

Except for rare bouts of palpitation and a history of "preeclampsia" in one of four pregnancies, she remained well for 10 years, when she returned to the clinic because of vertiginous attacks and burning facial paresthesias of 3 weeks' duration and recurrence of hypertension (190/115 mmHg supine; 145/100 mmHg standing). Both siblings, a brother and sister, had had bilateral pheochromocytomas removed since the patient's first operation (821), and her father had died, supposedly of Bright's disease and a cerebrovascular accident. Some scarring and pigmentation of both retinas were present but no retinopathy. The right kidney was palpable but examination was otherwise negative. Plasma catecholamines rose significantly to 11.9 μg/liter from a normal level of 2.1 μg/liter (fluorometric method modified by Manger), and urinary catecholamines increased following a histamine stimulation test. Excretory urogram, with adequate visualization of the pelvocalyceal systems, revealed bilateral nephrocalcinosis (Fig. 4.9). A recurrent pheochromocytoma (27 g) (Fig. 4.10A) and numerous satellite tumors were removed from the right adrenal area. During tumor palpation, cardiac arrest occurred but responded to resuscitation.

One month postoperatively, because of persistent elevations of serum calcium to between 12.8 and 14.1 mg/dl (inorganic phosphate varied from 3.0 to 3.6 mg/dl, and alkaline phosphatase was slightly elevated), three parathyroid glands were removed, and subtotal resection of the remaining gland was performed. Pathologic diagnosis of two enlarged resected glands (weighing 500 mg and 1250 mg) was chief-cell adenoma (Fig. 4.10B),

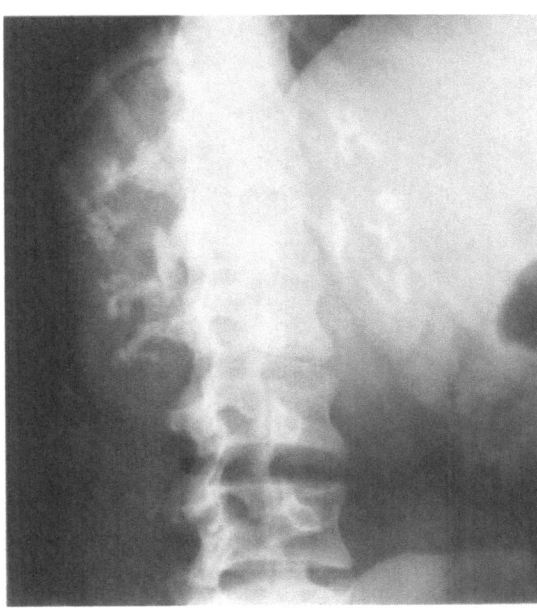

Fig. 4.9 Excreto-y urogram (oblique view) showing bilateral nephrccalcinosis. From Manning, P. A., Jr., Molnar, G. D., Black, B. M., Priestley, J. T., and Woolner, L. B. Feprinted by permission from *N. Engl. J. Med. 268:* 69, 1963.

designated chief-cell hyperplasia by some (171). Subtotal thyroidectomy was performed because of an enlarged right lobe; thyroid carcinoma with amyloid stroma (Fig. 4.10C and D) was found in both lobes. Postoperatively, she was maintained on replacement therapy (calcium lactate, levothyroxine, and hydrocortisone). In hyperparathyroidism, multiple parathyroid adenomas have been reported to occur in 4.3 to 7.3 percent of cases, and nephrocalcinosis in 5 to 7 percent of cases (627).

It is interesting that the sister of the patient reported by Manning and coworkers (627) developed evidence of medullary thyroid carcinoma and hyperparathyroidism 15 years after bilateral adrenalectomy had been performed for bilateral pheochromocytoma (732). Functioning metastatic pheochromocytoma had manifested itself 7 years postadrenalectomy, and paroxysmal hypertension had been controlled medically. It is particularly intriguing that amyloid was demonstrated not only in the thyroid carcinoma but also in the pheochromocytoma. Furthermore, some of the thyroid carcinoma cells resembled some of the pheochromocytoma cells. Morphology of the thyroid carcinoma cells varied from large granular eosinophilic polyhedral cells with large vesicular nuclei (resembling cells of the pheochromocytoma), to small ovoid cells with scanty pale to hypereosinophilic cytoplasm and a small oat-shaped hyperchromatic nucleus.

In support of the hypothesis that Sipple's syndrome results from a defect in neuroectoderm, Paloyan and coworkers (732) cite the following: (a) the report by Ljungberg that medullary thyroid carcinomas have the staining characteristics of chromaffin tissue (581); (b) the identification by Kaplan of a calcitonin-like substance in the adrenal medulla (495); and (c) the striking similarity in morphology between some cells of the thyroid carcinoma and the pheochromocytoma in the patient they reported (732).

Associated adenoma or hyperplasia of the parathyroid glands, which were usually thought to be of endodermal origin, may possibly be explained, as mentioned below, on the basis of a compensatory response to the hypocalcemia resulting from thyrocalcitonin excess. Hyperplasia of parathyroids has been observed to develop within 8 weeks in response to hypocalcemia resulting from prolonged administration of glucagon (732); it has also been observed in cows with parturient paresis and hypocalcemia (134a).

Wilkie and Krook have reported the occurrence of ultimobranchial tumors of the thyroid (equivalent to medullary thyroid carcinoma) and pheochromocytoma in the bull (1040). These tumors may occur alone or coexist, indicating that other vertebrates are affected with spontaneous multiple endocrine neoplasia.

A Hurthle cell tumor of the thyroid has been observed in one patient with bilateral pheochromocytoma (69); however, some believe this thyroid tumor to be a variation of an adenoma and possibly a premalignant lesion (302, 1047).

Very rarely, enlargement of the thyroid occurs concomitantly with paroxysmal crises of hypertension due to pheochromocytoma (42, 47, 414, 462, 944). This may cause a sensation of swelling in the neck. During a hypertensive attack in one patient, the thyroid became markedly enlarged and was bulging so that its contours were clearly visible. In addition, the skin over the anterior neck region became hyperemic (47).

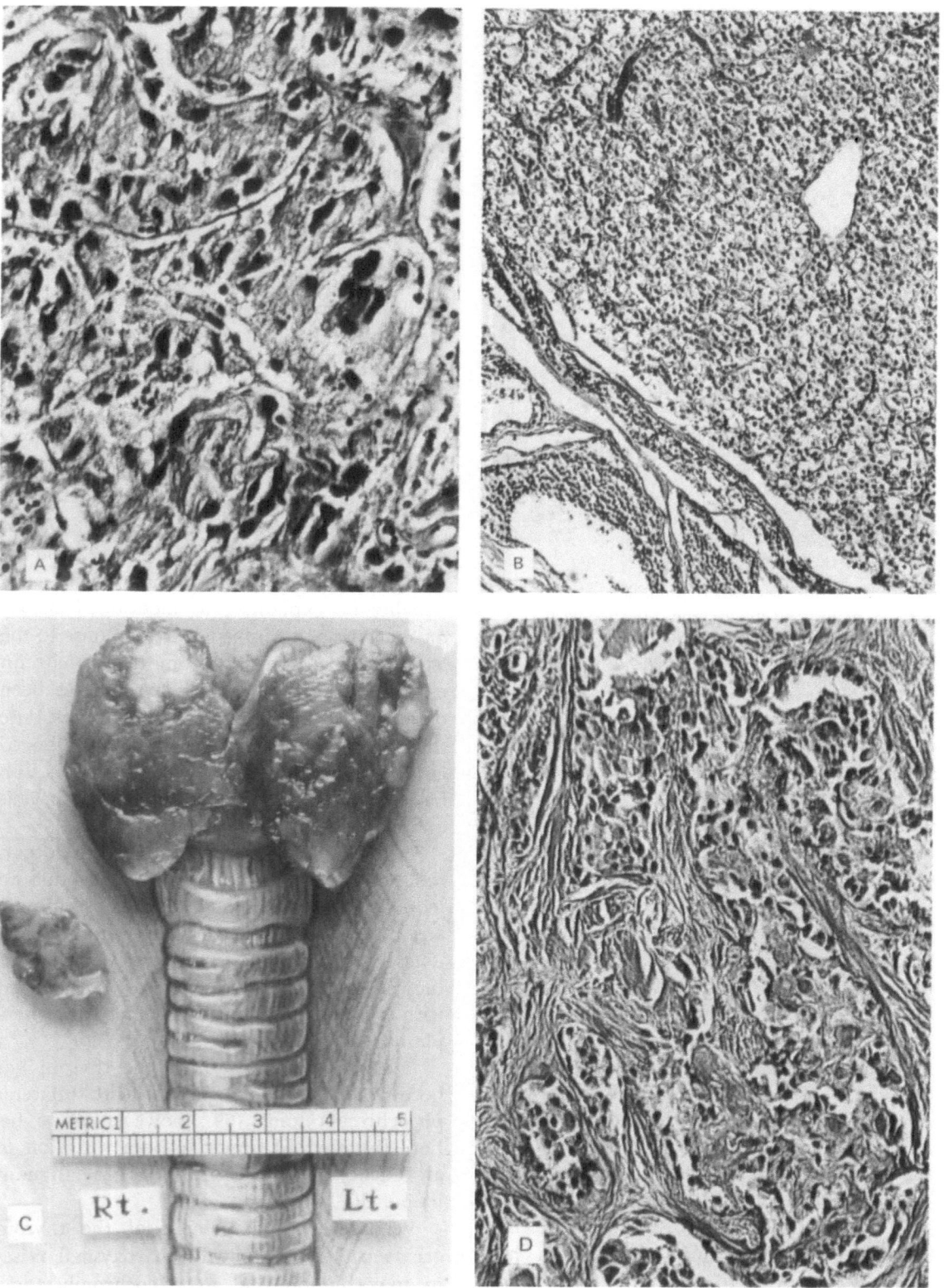

Fig. 4.10 A. Section of recurrent pheochromocytoma, showing marked variations in the size of cells and organoid pattern (hematoxylin and eosin stain, 285×). B. Section of one enlarged parathyroid gland, showing a tumor composed entirely of chief cells (hematoxylin and eosin stain, 125×). C. Gross appearance of resected thyroid gland, showing solid carcinomas in each upper pole (one of the enlarged parathyroid glands appears on the right side). D. Section, showing carcinoma of the thyroid gland with amyloid stroma (hematoxylin and eosin stain, 180×). From Manning, P. C., Molnar, G. D., Black, B. M., Priestley, J. T., and Woolner, L. B. Reprinted by permission from *N. Engl. J. Med. 268:* 70, 1963.

HYPERPARATHYROIDISM

In addition to the case of Manning and coworkers cited above, hyperparathyroidism due to adenoma or chief-cell hyperplasia has been reported in a small number of patients with familial pheochromocytoma and medullary thyroid carcinoma (144, 850, 864). The true incidence of parathyroid disease in patients with Sipple's syndrome is not known. A survey of the literature by Steiner and coworkers in 1968 revealed that parathyroid adenomas, or chief-cell hyperplasia, was reported in five of 85 familial cases of pheochromocytoma (an incidence of 6 percent), and in five cases that appeared to be nonfamilial (938). On the other hand, Catalona and associates reported that six of 12 patients with familial pheochromocytoma and/or medullary thyroid carcinoma had parathyroid adenoma or hyperplasia; five of these were associated with both pheochromocytoma and medullary thyroid carcinoma, whereas the sixth was associated only with the latter (144).

Hyperparathyroidism occurs both with familial and, much less frequently, with sporadic pheochromocytoma. However, when parathyroid tumors or hyperplasia occur in association with pheochromocytoma, there is usually also a medullary thyroid carcinoma, which may elaborate thyrocalcitonin and cause hypocalcemia by inhibiting resorption and release of calcium from the bone, thereby inducing a compensatory hyperparathyroidism (653, 865, 969). This concept, that hyperparathyroidism is induced by hypocalcemia, is purely speculative, and it is quite possible that the hyperparathyroidism is simply another manifestation of a genetic aberration; this seems all the more likely since evidence has been presented that the parathyroid (at least in the frog) is derived from neuroectoderm, as are chromaffin cells and the parafollicular cells of the thyroid (personal communication, Dr. Antony G. E. Pearse, Royal Postgraduate Medical School, London). It is of course, conceivable that in some instances of familial pheochromocytoma the coexistence of hyperparathyroidism may be caused by thyrocalcitonin-induced hypocalcemia, whereas in other instances the parathyroid hyperplasia or adenomas may be genetically determined.

Medullary thyroid carcinoma is the only tumor known to elaborate calcitonin, and the concentration of this hypocalcemic agent in this carcinoma has been found to be 2000 times greater than in normal thyroid tissue (653, 969). The fact that hypocalcemia occurs only rarely may be due to the ability of the parathyroids to compensate adequately (144).

Although hypercalcemia has been reported in Sipple's syndrome (850), it is interesting that clinical hyperparathyroidism is rare in this condition. In a study of six patients with familial pheochromocytoma with medullary thyroid carcinoma and parathyroid adenoma or hyperplasia, the following were occasionally noted: hypercalcemia with hypophosphatemia and hypercalciuria, renal stones, peptic ulcer, and pseudogout (144). Two-thirds of patients with parathyroid involvement had clinical or chemical evidence of hyperparathyroidism (144).

It has been shown that parathyroid hormone secretion may be increased by catecholamine stimulation of β-adrenergic receptors (315). This mechanism was proposed in two patients whose hypercalcemia and hypophosphatemia returned to normal after removal of pheochromocytomas (530, 958). Parathyroid hormone, measured in only one of these patients, fell from an elevated preoperative level to a normal value postoperatively. Keiser and associates reported that two of three normocalcemic patients who underwent selective venous catheterization preoperatively had elevated levels of parathormone in venous effluent from one or both sides of the neck (501a). From an evaluation of parathyroid function in patients with pheochromocytoma, Miller and associates concluded that (1) hypercalcemia occurs infrequently; (2) an excess of circulating catecholamines does not cause increased secretion of immunoreactive parathyroid hormone or calcitonin; and (3) parathyroid disease in pheochromocytoma is a genetically determined component of multiple endocrine neoplasia–type 2 (667).

If the presence of hyperparathyroidism is established and the patient also harbors a pheochromocytoma, surgical exploration of the parathyroids should be delayed until the pheochromocytoma is removed. Following pheochromocytoma extirpation, a thorough evaluation of the patient for evidence of a thyroid carcinoma and hyperparathyroidism can be performed at a later date without any risk of inducing a hypertensive crisis. An additional point of value with this approach is that the detection of intraabdominal thyroid metastases during removal of the pheochromocytoma may have some bearing on subsequent treatment of the patient (144). In the event that familial medullary thyroid carcinoma and hyperparathyroidism coexist, total thyroidectomy, regional lymphadenectomy, and exploration and resection of the parathyroid glands may be performed at the same operation. Keiser and associates believe that parathyroid glands should not be excised unless they are grossly abnormal or unless the patient is hypercalcemic (501a); usually more than one parathyroid gland is involved (665a). Steiner and associates pointed out that, in contrast to familial hyperparathyroidism, a single adenoma occurs in 80 percent of patients with nonfamilial hyperparathyroidism and chief-cell hyperplasia is evident in only 10 percent of patients (938).

In 1973 Keiser and associates at the National Institutes of Health recommended that relatives of patients with familial pheochromocytoma be screened. Their diagnostic screening procedure included taking a history; measuring blood pressure; palpating the neck; determining serum levels of calcium, phosphorus, alkaline phosphatase, histaminase, and calcitonin (during a calcium infusion test in those with normal basal levels); and determining 24-hr urine catecholamine metabolites. If thyroid nodules were detected, or if either serum calcitonin or histaminase were elevated, thyroid function tests, radiographic scans of the thyroid, venography, appropriate venous blood sampling in the neck, and arteriography were done prior to neck exploration. It is noteworthy that they found palpable thyroid nodules in two of 16 patients with medullary thyroid carcinoma; nine of 10 nodules could be seen on radioisotopic scans of the thyroids (501a). The radiographic features of medullary thyroid carcinoma are discussed in Chapter 6 under Radiographic Techniques.

Currently, as mentioned previously, it is generally agreed that the determination of histaminase is not highly reliable in determining the absence, or even the presence, of a medullary thyroid carcinoma (83a). Experience also indicates that pentagastrin is probably the most reliable thyrocalcitonin-stimulating agent (340, 903a); however, the performance of the pentagastrin test and the calcium infusion test (in those patients having a negative response to pentagastrin) is more reliable in detecting medullary thyroid carcinoma than either test alone (340). Serum calcitonin assays are valuable not only in screening patients for the presence of medullary thyroid carcinoma but also in postoperative assessment (83a).

It is recommended that preoperative determination of parathyroid hormone (when possible) be performed, in addition to serum calcium and phosphate measurements (83a). Rarely, determination of parathyroid hormone may be particularly helpful in detecting the presence of hyperparathyroidism, since the hormone elevation may antedate serum calcium elevation in some patients with familial medullary thyroid carcinoma. Usually, however, plasma parathyroid hormone levels are elevated in patients who have coexistent hyperparathyroidism with elevated serum calcium. Peripheral serum parathyroid hormone levels have generally been within the normal range (less than 0.3 ng/ml), whereas blood obtained from thyroid veins are almost invariably elevated (737a). It is noteworthy that an abnormally low serum phosphate level has been of greater value than the serum calcium level in indicating the presence of hyperparathyroidism in some patients (83a). From the experience of screening 88 members of a family with Sipple's syndrome Hamilton and co-workers concluded that hyperparathyroidism was not reliably predicted from serum calcium and parathormone levels. Furthermore, nine of these subjects had elevated serum parathormone without hypercalcemia or other evidence of Sipple's syndrome; significance of this isolated abnormality was unknown (414).

MULTIPLE ENDOCRINE NEOPLASIA, TYPE 2 AND TYPE 3*

The triad of tumors (or hyperplasia) of the adrenal medulla, thyroid, and parathyroid glands is thought to be genetically distinct from "multiple endocrine adenomatosis" or "polyadenomatosis," in which there may be coexistence of tumors, or hyperplasia of sev-

---

* Some have suggested that multiple endocrine neoplasia (MEN) type 2 be designated type 2A and that type 3 be designated 2B or 2b.

eral endocrine glands, and sometimes peptic ulcerations (1026a). In multiple endocrine adenomatosis lesions occur in the anterior pituitary, parathyroids, pancreatic islet cells, and adrenal cortex; occasionally adenomatous goiters are evident in the thyroid gland (1026a). Steiner and associates suggested that familial pheochromocytoma in association with multiple endocrine tumors be classified as "multiple endocrine neoplasia (MEN), type 2," whereas "multiple endocrine adenomatosis" be renamed "multiple endocrine neoplasia, type 1" (938). In "multiple endocrine neoplasia (MEN), type 2" pheochromocytomas are much more often bilateral or multiple than in sporadic cases (144, 732). Today the terms "multiple endocrine neoplasia, type 1" and "multiple endocrine adenomatosis, type 1" are used interchangeably; the same applies to the "type 2" familial endocrinopathy. The term "multiple" is somewhat confusing since a neoplasm may be present in only one endocrine organ when the patient is first seen. However, the subsequent development of neoplasms in other endocrine glands and/or the presence of multiple endocrine neoplasia in relatives establishes the diagnosis of multiple endocrinopathy.

In the 1960's a number of patients were reported who had *multiple mucosal neuromas* (neuromatous masses on the eyelids or conjunctivae, lips, or tongue), bilateral pheochromocytoma, and medullary thyroid carcinoma (Fig. 4.11) (267, 390a, 865, 1046). Gorlin and coworkers reviewed the literature up to 1968 and found reports of 17 patients (11 female and six male) with multiple mucosal neuromas. Some of these patients also had medullary thyroid carcinomas (diagnosis established in seven and probable in two) and/ or pheochromocytomas (diagnosis established in seven and probable in three). In addition, three patients had a marfanoid habitus, two had diverticulosis, one had diffuse ganglioneuromatosis of the intestinal tract, and eight had medullated corneal nerves (390a). Previously, Braley had observed plexiform (i.e., resembling a plexus or network) neuromas of the eyelids and myelinated corneal nerve fibers in patients with pheochromocytoma (97). (This will be discussed below.) Gorlin and Merkin have hypothesized that this multiple mucosal neuroma syndrome may result from a defec-

tive gene which normally represses the growth of cells capable of synthesizing biologically active substances (i.e., the APUD cells, described later in this chapter) (390).

Within the past 5 years evidence has been accumulating that the coexistence of mucosal neuroma, pheochromocytoma, medullary thyroid carcinoma, and sometimes a marfanoid habitus may constitute still another distinct familial entity with an autosomal dominant mode of inheritance. This familial endocrinopathy has been designated "multiple endocrine neoplasia, type 3" (510a) and "multiple endocrine neoplasia, type 2B or 2b" (135a, 150a). The term "MEN–type 2" has continued to designate patients with this familial endocrinopathy without the mucosal-neuroma phenotype, although some have suggested the term be changed to "MEN–type 2A." Since the nomenclature has varied and is unsettled, we prefer to use the designation "MEN–type 2" in those patients without mucosal neuromas; in those with the mucosal neuroma phenotype the designation MEN–type 3 will be used hereafter.

Apparently, the association of mucosal neuromas and a marfanoid habitus with pheochromocytoma and thyroid carcinoma has not been noted even in large families with MEN–type 2 of the usual variety. On the other hand, in several other families, essentially all individuals with a pheochromocytoma and/or a medullary thyroid carcinoma also had mucosal neuromas and/or a marfanoid habitus. Furthermore, the incidence of hyperparathyroidism in MEN–type 2 is thought to be about 54 percent, whereas it occurred in only one patient of a series of 41 (2.4 percent) with MEN–type 3 (510a).

The characteristic features of MEN–type 3 have been clearly described by Khairi and coworkers (510a). Aside from the manifestations of pheochromocytoma, medullary thyroid carcinoma, and very rarely, hyperparathyroidism, the following are considered hallmarks of MEN–type 3:

(a) *Neuromas* (having a dense neurofibrillary structure), especially of the lips, tongue, buccal mucosa, eyelids, conjunctivae, and corneas. (Thickened corneal nerves may be seen with a slit lamp.) Less commonly, there may be impaired pupillary dilation and decreased lacrimation.

(b) *Characteristic facial appearance* with "bumpy lips." Occasionally there is an associated prognathism and an "acromegalic" facial appearance.

(c) *Gastrointestinal tract abnormalities* with symptomatology (diarrhea, or constipation with megacolon) and/or neuromatomous involvement (diffuse intestinal ganglioneuromatosis). Certain radiographic findings (abnormal haustral markings, thickened mucosal folds, diverticula, and dilation) have occasionally been misdiagnosed as ulcerative colitis, Crohn's disease, or congenital megacolon.

(d) *Marfanoid habitus* with "asthenic build," sparcity of body fat and poorly developed musculature, with extremities appearing long and thin (dolichostenomelia and arachnodactyly), muscular hypotonicity, increased laxity of joints, dorsal kyphosis, pectus excavatum, pes cavus, and decreased upper to lower body segment ratio. (However, none of these patients had ectopia lentis or the aortic abnormalities frequently seen in typical Marfan's syndrome.)

(e) *Muscular wasting* may suggest a clinical myopathy (510a).

(f) *Abnormal intradermal histamine test*, i.e., indradermal injection is followed by the appearance of a wheal but without the subsequent development of a flare (which is observed in normal subjects). [It is noteworthy that in patients with familial dysautonomia the flare response is usually absent (914a).]

Recently, Carney and associates have emphasized that alimentary-tract ganglioneuromatosis is a major component of MEN–type 3 (135). They reported 16 patients (nine female and seven male) with this syndrome. Ninety-four percent had bilateral medullary thyroid carcinoma, 31 percent had bilateral adrenal medullary disease (ranging from nodular medullary hyperplasia through diffuse medullary hyperplasia with superimposed pheochromocytoma to pheochromocytoma with metastasis), 81 percent had skeletal anomalies (marfanoid habitus, pes cavus, slipped femoral capital epiphysis, pectus excavatum, and scoliosis), and 100 percent had alimentary-tract manifestations (pathologic or clinical or both). Nine patients had diffuse ganglioneuromatosis

extending from the lips to the rectum, and constipation or diarrhea or both were present in six of these patients. Similar symptoms were present in six of the seven remaining patients from whom alimentary-tract tissue was not obtained. Megacolon was present in five of the 16 patients and led to operation in four. Colectomy was performed on a sixth patient for diverticulitis which was complicating diverticulosis. "Mega-appendix" was found at operation in two patients.

Microscopic studies in some of these patients revealed proliferation of nerves and nerve plexuses in the lips, tongue, esophagus, stomach, small intestine, large intestine and appendix. "The plexuses-mucosal, submucosal, myenteric and serosal, according to location, were replaced by large, irregular conglomerations of Schwann cells, neurites and ganglion cells, constituting ganglioneuromatosis. Nerve trunks exhibited tortuosity, increased diameter and branching, and occasional internal structural disarray, constituting neuromatosis; numerous ganglion cells were encountered in these nerves. The microscopic picture was that of diffuse proliferation of the peripheral autonomic system, nerves and ganglions" (135). The entire group of neural changes was referred to as ganglioneuromatosis. Pancreatic ganglioneuromatosis (but without islet involvement) was found in all autopsied cases and ganglioneuromatosis of the gallbladder was also present in one case where this organ was examined.

Carney and associates have stressed the importance of recognizing alimentary-tract manifestations in the MEN–type 3 syndrome since in 14 of the 16 patients they studied such manifestations were present before endocrine neoplasms were detected; 10 of the patients had symptomatic alimentary-tract involvement present at birth or shortly thereafter. They further pointed out that alimentary-tract ganglioneuromatosis should not be confused clinically or pathologically with involvement of the alimentary tract in von Recklinghausen's neurofibromatosis; in the latter condition symptoms are delayed until adulthood and are usually different from those in alimentary-tract ganglioneuromatosis. The neural and myomatous tumors which occur in neurofibromatosis differ from the diffuse non-tumorous hyperplasia of the autonomic nervous system seen in MEN–type 3 (135). Rectal biopsy may be helpful in establishing the diagnosis of alimentary-tract ganglioneuromatosis (47a). In von Recklinghausen's disease (neurofibromatosis) the most common manifestations caused by tumors (neurofibromas, leiomyomas, or sarcomas) of the gastrointestinal tract are melena, pain, and hematemesis; less commonly, there may be constipation or symptoms suggesting peptic ulcer. Occasionally an abdominal mass may be palpable and intestinal obstruction and perforation have been reported (517a).

The types of lesions of the lips and tongue which may be seen in patients with MEN–type 3 are illustrated in Figures 4.11 and 4.12A, B, and C. Carney and associates at the Mayo Clinic emphasized that mucosal neuromas "constitute a valuable marker of the syndrome, since they are present in childhood and generally antedate clinical presentation of the thyroid and adrenal neoplasms" (135a). In addition to mucosal neuromas of the lips, tongue, and eyes, there may be involvement of the nasal, laryngeal, and gingival

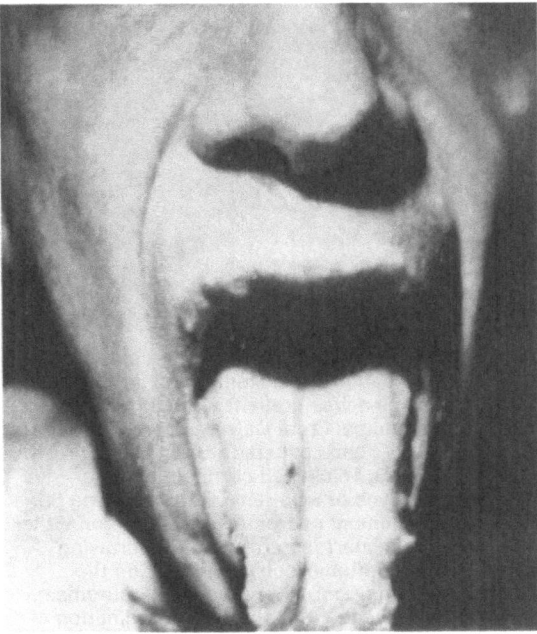

Fig. 4.11 Neurocutaneous lesions of the tongue and lips in a patient with multiple adrenal pheochromocytomas and medullary carcinoma of the thyroid. The patient also had soft tissue tumors of the conjunctivae and autonomic dysfunction of visceral organs. From Engelman, K., *Bull., N. Y. Acad. Med. 45*: 853, 1969.

mucosa (390a). The oral lesions are asymptomatic, benign, and their growth appears to be self-limited late in the second decade.

Carney and coworkers have further stressed the early endocrine evaluation of patients with abnormal facial and oral appearance—particularly measurement of serum calcitonin and urinary excretion of epinephrine, VMA, and the metanephrines. The importance of early diagnosis was evident from the finding that among 51 patients with the syndrome, 40 (78 percent) had medullary thyroid carcinoma and 16 (31 percent) had pheochromocytoma. In 22 of those with thyroid carcinoma the tumor had metastasized or was locally invasive at the time of diagnosis; nine died subsequently. The deaths of three patients and possibly two others were caused by pheochromocytoma. Of 15 additional patients with MEN–type 3 seen at the Mayo Clinic, 10 had metastatic or locally invasive medullary thyroid carcinoma; one died of metastatic thyroid carcinoma; and three were alive with metastatic disease. Two died of pheochromocytoma. Two of their patients were siblings, aged 5 and 2 years, with characteristic mucosal findings but with no evidence of abnormality of the thyroid glands on palpation. Both, however, had high immunoreactive serum calcitonin concentrations. Operation revealed thyroid carcinoma in the older child, whereas foci of parafollicular cell (C-cell) hyperplasia, the probable precursor of medullary thyroid carcinoma, were present in both lobes of the younger sibling (135a).

Cunliffe and coworkers reported a most unusual case of MEN–type 3 in a 19-year-old girl with a calcitonin-secreting medullary thyroid carcinoma associated with mucosal neuromas, marfanoid features, myopathy, and pigmentation. The pigmentation, which proved to be melanin, and which occurred on the skin around the mouth and on the hands and feet, was aggravated by sunlight. Since it disappeared after thyroidectomy, it was felt that the carcinoma may have elaborated a humoral agent which affected melanin synthesis. The myopathy particularly involved the proximal muscles; there were scattered areas of myopathic degeneration, and the normal differentiation of muscle fibers into two types, on the basis of histochemical and ultrastructural examination, was absent. An additional

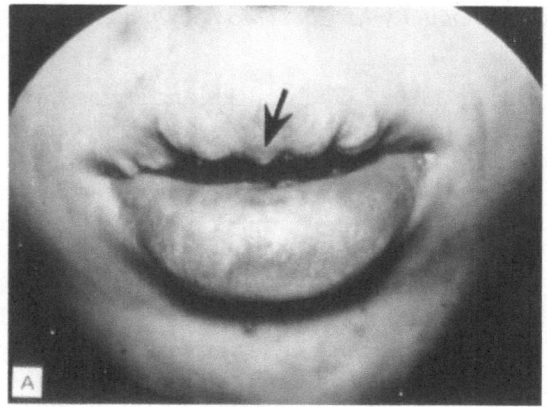

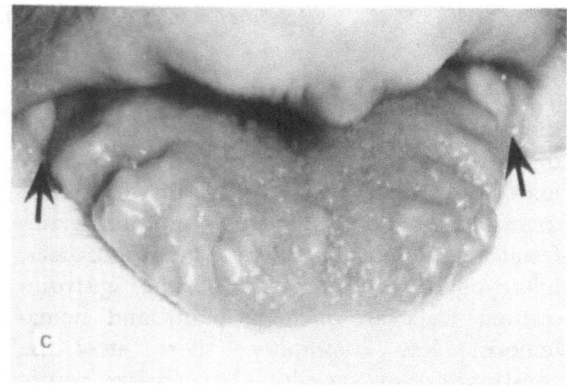

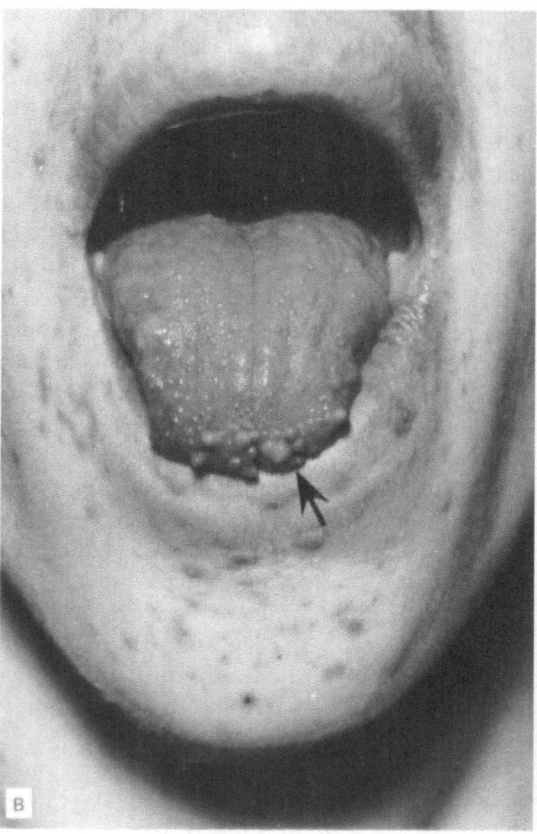

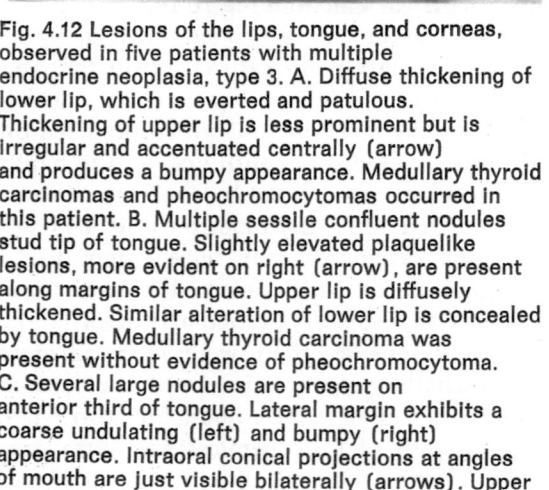

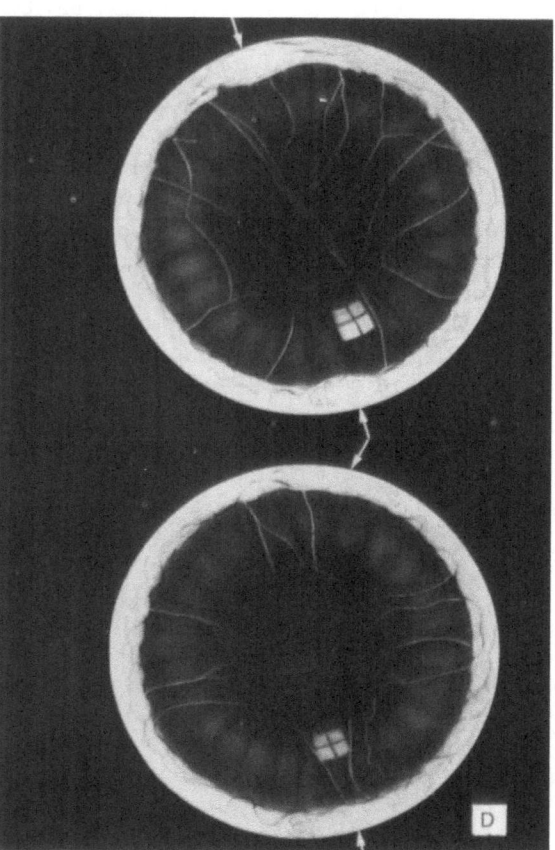

Fig. 4.12 Lesions of the lips, tongue, and corneas, observed in five patients with multiple endocrine neoplasia, type 3. A. Diffuse thickening of lower lip, which is everted and patulous. Thickening of upper lip is less prominent but is irregular and accentuated centrally (arrow) and produces a bumpy appearance. Medullary thyroid carcinomas and pheochromocytomas occurred in this patient. B. Multiple sessile confluent nodules stud tip of tongue. Slightly elevated plaquelike lesions, more evident on right (arrow), are present along margins of tongue. Upper lip is diffusely thickened. Similar alteration of lower lip is concealed by tongue. Medullary thyroid carcinoma was present without evidence of pheochromocytoma. C. Several large nodules are present on anterior third of tongue. Lateral margin exhibits a coarse undulating (left) and bumpy (right) appearance. Intraoral conical projections at angles of mouth are just visible bilaterally (arrows). Upper lip is diffusely thickened and exhibits characteristic central accentuation of thickening. Medullary thyroid carcinoma was present without evidence of pheochromocytoma. From Carney, J. A., Sizemore, G. W., and Lovestedt, S. A., *Oral Surg. 41:* 746, 747, 1976. D. Thickened corneal nerves of right and left eyes of a patient with MEN–type 3. Thickened perilimbal neuromas are visible on either side of each limbus (see arrows). This drawing by Dr. Dennis M. Robertson was based on the precise location of corneal nerves and neuromas determined by sequential slit-lamp examination of the entire cornea. From Robertson, D. M., Sizemore, G. W., and Gordon, H., *Trans. Acad. Ophthalmol. Otolaryngol. 79:* 773, 1975. E. Drawing of the white medullated corneal nerves in a patient with MEN–type 3 examined with a slit-lamp by Dr. A. E. Braley. From Braley, A. E., *Trans. Am. Ophthalmol. Soc. 52:* 190, 1954.

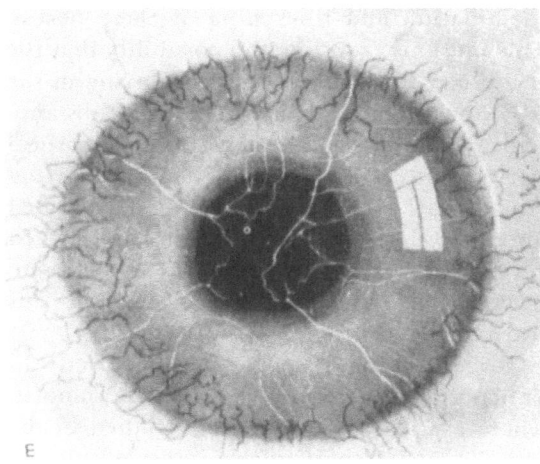

E

point of interest was that the patient had experienced spontaneous attacks of facial flushing, associated with sweating, which lasted about 30 min despite the fact that there was no evidence of a coexisting pheochromocytoma. Furthermore, periods of hypotension (with systolic blood pressures of 60 mmHg persisting for several minutes) recurred during thyroidectomy, and it was concluded that some pharmacologically active agent released by the carcinoma might have caused the hypotensive episodes and the flushing attacks. The patient was thought to represent a complex developmental disorder of mesodermal, ectodermal, and neuroectodermal origin (198a).

The importance of recognizing the eye manifestations in patients suspected of having MEN–type 3 should be stressed; some investigators have recently indicated that the presence of thickened corneal nerves in a clear stroma is virtually diagnostic of this syndrome (Fig. 4.12D, E) (799a). Therefore, a brief review of this subject is presented.

The first report of the presence of thickened corneal nerves in a patient (a 28-year-old white male) with pheochromocytoma was made in 1940 by Koke and Braley (cited in 97); a marfanoid habitus was also evident. In 1954 Braley reported the findings in this original patient, plus similar findings in two additional patients (a 36-year-old white male and a 37-year-old white female) (97). All three patients had thickened corneal nerves (seen by slit-lamp examination) and plexiform conjunctival neuromas (which in some instances resembled coiled, gelatinous masses similar to the coils of medullated nerve fibers of "amputation

neuromas"). None of these patients had von Recklinghausen's neurofibromatosis. All had adrenal pheochromocytomas which caused attacks of palpitations, excessive sweating, and heat intolerance; in one patient the hypertension was sustained whereas in the other two the hypertension was paroxysmal. All three patients had elevated basal metabolic rates, hyperglycemia, and some flattening of the T waves in their electrocardiograms.

Biomicroscopic examination of the corneas of the 28-year-old man revealed grayish-white anastomotic and interlacing fibers situated in the stroma. Several of the main trunks (5 to 6 mm in length) could be seen without magnification and the limbal vessels were prominent and superficial (Fig. 4.12E). The grayish-white fibers branched dichotomously—some branches arched backward while others extended into the more superficial stroma. Small bulbous enlargements were seen at a few of the bifurcations. Following removal of an adrenal pheochromocytoma in each of the two men, symptoms subsided and subsequently the white fibers in the corneas and the plexiform neuromas disappeared.

The 37-year-old woman had had paroxysmal attacks for 24 years, sometimes accompanied by palpitations, swelling of the neck, prominence of the eyes, dizziness, and rapid breathing. Her blood pressure became markedly elevated during paroxysms from about 165/90 mmHg to as high as 240/140 mmHg. Two pheochromocytomas were removed from the left adrenal area; however, attacks continued and became more frequent and pharmacologic tests suggested the presence of additional pheochromocytomas. The medullated corneal nerves and plexiform neuromas remained unchanged. Approximately 6 months later she expired during what appeared to be an episode of ventricular tachycardia. Postmortem examination revealed residual tumors in the left adrenal area and also a right adrenal pheochromocytoma.

Braley commented that although medullated corneal nerves may be observed with the biomicroscope in some normal subjects, they rarely extend beyond the limbus for more than a millimeter. He also cited observations by others of the occurrence of thickened or medullated corneal nerves in patients with neurofibromatosis who had extensive involvement of the face, lids, or other areas; some had elephantiasis of the lids and face (97). However, it has been suggested that some of these cases associating thickened corneal nerves with neurofibromatosis were probably patients with MEN–type 3 (799a). Baum and Adler have stated that corneal nerves, which are visible on slit-lamp examination, have been described in keratoconus, Refsum's syndrome, primary amyloidosis, and "colloidin skin" syndrome; however, they pointed out that the nerves in these conditions are thinner and much less visible than in MEN–type 3 (47a).

The fact that the corneal nerves lost their myelin sheaths and disappeared in two patients in whom pheochromocytomas were removed but did not change in the patient who had residual tumors following operation, suggested that some factor elaborated by the pheochromocytoma might have been responsible for the medullation of the corneal nerves (97). More recent studies seem to indicate that the thickened corneal nerves occur only in MEN–type 3 or, rarely, in the MEN–type 2 syndrome. Disappearance of thickened corneal nerves was not observed following total pheochromocytoma extirpation in a patient with MEN–type 3 studied for 2.5 years postoperative by Robertson and associates (799a). On the other hand, Baum and Adler reported a decrease in the prominence of the corneal nerves following removal of bilateral pheochromocytomas in their patient with MEN–type 3 (47a). (The facial and chest appearance and the highly visible corneal nerves prior to removal of the pheochromocytomas in the patient reported by Baum and Adler are seen in Fig. 4.13A and B, p. 78). The cause of the thickened corneal nerves is unclear. Whether or not a humoral or neurotropic substance may account for medullation of corneal nerves in some patients with pheochromocytoma remains uncertain. Since the thickened corneal nerves may occur only as a manifestation of the MEN–type 3 (or very rarely, MEN–type 2) syndrome it is conceivable that they represent still another expression of a genetic aberration in this syndrome. The fact that some patients with thickened corneal nerves and MEN–type 3 have no detectable evidence of a pheochromocytoma (799a) seems to almost exclude the possibility that a substance secreted by a pheochromocytoma may be responsible for the

medullation and thickening of these nerves. One must also consider the possibility that the medullary thyroid carcinoma occurring in the MEN syndromes might elaborate a substance which causes medullation of the corneal nerves; however, one would then have to conclude that such a substance is elaborated almost exclusively by the medullary thyroid carcinomas occurring in the MEN–type 3 syndrome. Further studies are needed on this intriguing problem.

Robertson and coworkers reported 15 patients with the MEN–type 3 syndrome in whom eye manifestations were studied in detail (799a). This particularly indicated the importance of slit-lamp examination of the cornea in patients suspected of having this syndrome. As mentioned above, they consider the presence of thickened corneal nerves, occurring in a clear stroma, as pathognomonic for the presence of multiple endocrine neoplasia, usually MEN–type 3 but occasionally MEN–type 2. Robertson and coworkers have stressed the importance of prompt recognition of this syndrome by the ophthalmologist since early diagnosis and treatment may be life-saving, not only for the patient, but for the patient's first-degree relatives. Thickened corneal nerves are not visible with the naked eye but are abnormally prominent on slit-lamp biomicroscopy.

Other ophthalmic findings were neuromas of the conjunctiva and lid, prominent vessels, and dryness of the eyes. Paralimbal neuromas were usually associated with dilated perilimbal conjunctival blood vessels, in which case the eyes may appear chronically red. Decreased tear flow may produce symptoms of keratoconjunctivitis sicca; the cause of the dry eyes is unclear. Calcific deposits may be seen in the conjunctiva of patients with hypercalcemia; however, although hyperparathyroidism occurs in about one-half of the patients with MEN–type 2, it rarely occurs in patients with MEN–type 3.

Fourteen of the patients reported by Robertson had medullary thyroid carcinoma and the 15th patient had thyroid C-cell hyperplasia. Eight of the patients were known to have metastases of the thyroid carcinoma. None of the parathyroid glands that were examined macroscopically and microscopically were abnormal.

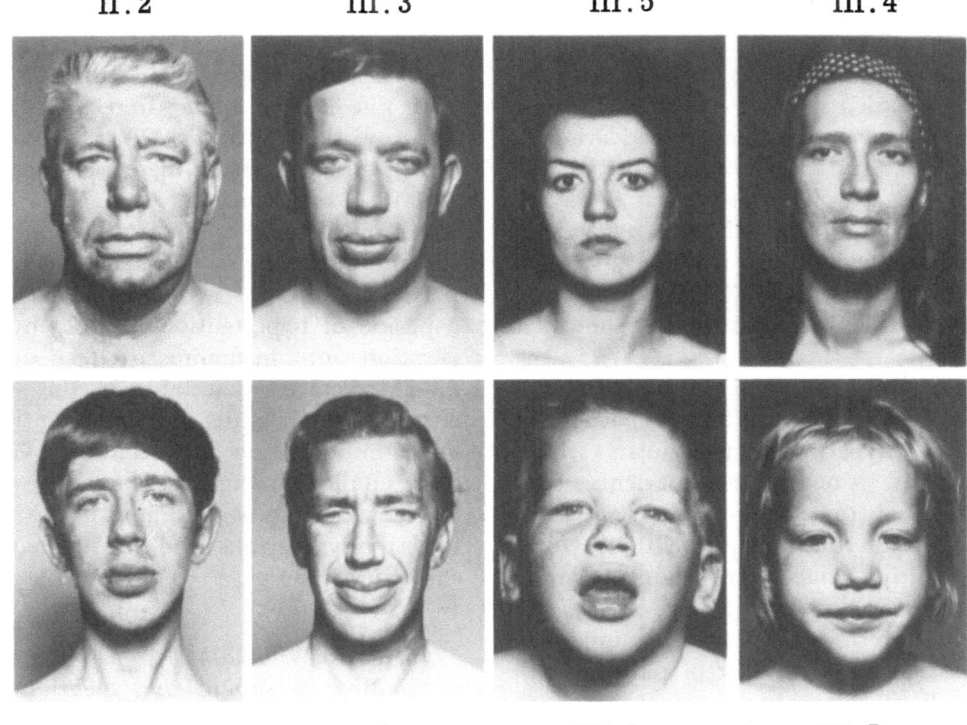

II.2   III.3   III.5   III.4

III.7   III.2   IV.4   IV.5

Fig. 4.14A Facial features in members of the pedigree reproduced in Figure 4.14B. Each panel, reading from left to right: II.2, III.3, III.5 (normal), III.4, III.7, III.2, IV.4, and IV.5. Normal facial characteristics of III.5 are in striking contrast with those of other affected members.

Fig. 4.14B Pedigree of family, seven of whose members had multiple endocrine neoplasia, type 3 [index member II.2 (arrow)]. Note autosomal dominant pattern of inheritance. (N=normal; diagonal stroke indicates death of family member.) From Robertson, D. M., Sizemore, G. W., and Gordon, H., *Trans. Am. Acad. Ophthal. Otolaryngol. 79:* 772–787, 1975.

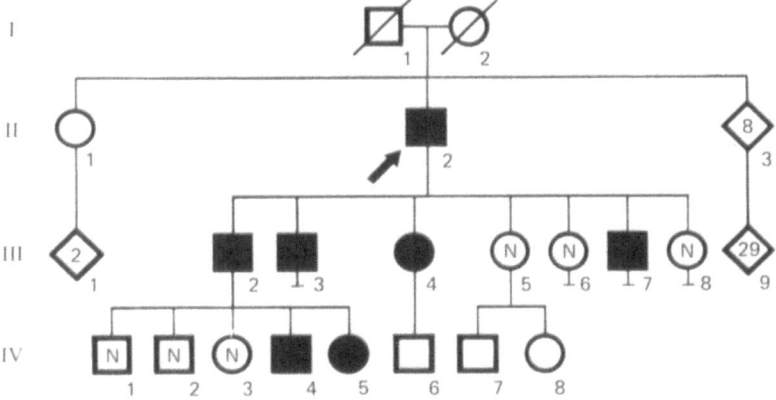

Four of the 15 patients were known to have pheochromocytomas, which in all cases were bilateral. It is noteworthy that extensive testing for evidence of a pheochromocytoma in one of these patients was negative, and bilateral adrenal medullary tumors were only discovered at autopsy. The point to be kept in mind is that in patients with pheochromocytoma associated with multiple endocrine neoplasia clinical and laboratory findings are not infrequently normal, and every effort must be made to eliminate the presence of this tumor.

In this series of MEN–type 3 reported by Robertson, a marfanoid habitus, tongue neuromas, and thickened lips were present in almost all patients. Since occasionally somewhat thickened corneal nerves and even the marfinoid habitus were seen in patients with MEN–type 2, it was suggested that there may be a phenotypic overlap of MEN–type 2 and MEN–type 3. The facial features and pedigree of a family with MEN–type 3 reported by Robertson and coworkers are shown in Figure 4.14.

In addition to the usual features of MEN–type 3, Giroux and associates reported the presence of hyperplastic para-aortic sympathetic ganglia in one of their patients. They also estimated that when medullary carcinoma of the thyroid and pheochromocytoma coexist, multiple mucosal neuromas occur in about 10 percent of cases (356a).

It is noteworhy that, for some unknown reason, a significant number of patients with familial pheochromocytoma are normotensive and asymptomatic—40 and 26.6 percent, respectively, in one series of 15 patients (135a). Contrariwise, patients with sporadic pheochromocytomas almost always have clinical manifestations suggesting functioning tumors.

CUSHING'S SYNDROME
Cushing's syndrome, which has occasionally been observed in patients with either sporadic or familial pheochromocytoma, may result from excess elaboration of ACTH-like substance from the pheochromocytoma and/or from an associated thyroid carcinoma, or from excess secretion of an accompanying pituitary adenoma. Steiner and coworkers (938) have also pointed out that in some patients with pheochromocytoma and Cushing's syndrome, the tumor may produce an excess of cortisol, since it has been claimed that a pheochromocytoma can synthesize cortisol in vitro (232, 688). It is also noteworthy that the surgically removed specimen showed a patient with Cushing's syndrome to have adrenal cortical hyperplasia in addition to a pheochromocytoma (469). On the other hand, although a large amount of cortisol was found in an extract of a pheochromocytoma from another patient, there was no evidence of Cushing's syndrome (780). In one series of eight patients with pheochromocytoma, two had increased cortisol secretion; no mention was made as to whether or not these patients were cushinoid (992a).

It is interesting that two of our patients with pheochromocytoma were found by Paris and coworkers to have ACTH in their serum (624, p. 109). In one of these patients who had sustained hypertension, ACTH was detected in all blood samples obtained preoperatively; in the other patient, who had borderline hypertension, ACTH was detected only during a period of hypertension induced by administration of histamine. After operation, ACTH was not detectable in the serum of either of these patients, even after intravenous administration of histamine. With the assay employed when these studies were performed, ACTH was not found in the serum of hypertensive persons who did not have pheochromocytoma.

ADRENAL VIRILISM
Finally, it should be mentioned that adrenal virilism, which regressed after removal of a pheochromocytoma (700), and a case of malignant pheochromocytoma which simulated an adrenal cortical carcinoma (641), have been reported.

ADDISON'S DISEASE
Hume has noted that adrenal cortical activity, with respect to the glucocorticoids, is almost always normal in patients with pheochromocytoma except for the rare reports of these tumors associated with Addison's disease (598, 793). However, he stated that in some cases adrenal androgen secretion is reduced, although the explanation for this reduction is unclear (466). Excessive amounts of catecholamines can reduce the response of the adrenal cortex to corticotropin (330, 843). One patient with a pheochromocytoma had no increase in 17-ketosteroids and corticoids following corticotropin stimulation (330). It is interesting that ACTH administration to the latter patient caused a marked elevation of blood glucose and a striking decrease in serum calcium. Although catecholamines were not studied in this patient, it is possible that the elevation in blood glucose resulted from a release of catecholamines into the circulation, which was induced by the effect of ACTH on the pheochromocytoma. The response of serum calcium to ACTH remains unclear. In another patient the corticotropin response returned after the removal of the tumor

(705). Nevertheless, Ramsay and Langlands agree with Hume that patients with pheochromocytoma have normal glucocorticoid activity (780). Contrariwise, Mulrow and associates have reported two patients with diminished adrenocortical activity preoperatively who, following pheochromocytoma removal, developed hypotension, which responded only to a combination of pressor amines and adrenocorticosteroids (688). Cortisol was isolated from the tumors of both patients. Mulrow and coworkers postulated that removal of pheochromocytomas which elaborate large amounts of cortisol, thus inhibiting corticotropin secretion, can result in circulatory collapse, since the adrenal cortices are unable to respond adequately to the stress of surgery.

It is believed that corticosteroids sensitize cells to the action of norepinephrine, and that the steroids are required for norepinephrine to exert its vasoconstrictor effect (333, 779, 995). Following removal of a pheochromocytoma, it is not uncommon for patients to require infusions of relatively high concentrations of norepinephrine for several days in order to maintain blood pressure. Peart reported a patient who required 100 μg per min of norepinephrine (738), and Smithwick had a patient who required an infusion containing more than 50 ml of 1/1000 epinephrine in the first 48 hr following removal of a pheochromocytoma (918). Whether this insensitivity to norepinephrine infusion, sometimes observed postoperatively, is related even in part to a temporary deficiency of corticosteroids is not certain.

As pointed out by Ramsay and Langlands, in patients with pheochromocytoma the corticomedullary relationship is complex and may vary from patient to patient (780). In one of their patients corticotropin administration precipitated a fatal hypertensive crisis, with a blood pressure elevation to 300/190 mmHg and a marked rise in the concentration of urinary catecholamines. There was also a slight increase in the urinary concentration of 17-oxysteroids (17-hydroxycorticosteroids) and a slight decrease in 17-hydroxysteroids over a 4-hr period accompanying corticotropin stimulation. They also extracted cortisol from the pheochromocytoma removed at autopsy (780).

In three other patients with pheochromocytoma, the injection of ACTH for diagnostic purposes caused hypertensive crises, which resulted in pulmonary edema and death in two of the cases (680). Page and associates reported a patient with a predominantly epinephrine-secreting pheochromocytoma who developed a severe paroxysm (with hypertension, profuse sweating, palpitations, cramping pains in the upper abdomen, anxiety, nausea, and vomiting) several hours after receiving hydrocortisone, ACTH, and prednisone (730). Steiner and coworkers have suggested that a rapid increase in intraadrenal cortisol might cause an increase in catecholamine secretion by a pheochromocytoma (938). This latter concept is based mainly on evidence presented by Wurtman that ACTH-induced stimulation of adrenal glucocorticoid secretion can result in excessive intraadrenal cortisol, which in turn increases catecholamine synthesis by activating phenylethanolamine-N-methyltransferase (PNMT), the enzyme which converts norepinephrine to epinephrine (1060, 1063). It is important to reemphasize that Steiner and coworkers have properly stressed the *danger of using the ACTH stimulation test* in any patient who might possibly have a pheochromocytoma (938). Critchley and associates have also presented findings which highlight the dangers of administering corticotropin and metyrapone when investigating patients with pheochromocytoma (181). [We have recently heard of a 46-year-old man who, except for a chronic dermatitis of his hands, had apparently been in good health until he received steroids. Several hours after receiving an injection of steroid for his dermatitis he developed severe chest pain, hypertension (200/130 mmHg), tachycardia (190/min) with premature ventricular contractions and atrial fibrillation, and pyrexia (105°F). Ultimately he expired, and a pheochromocytoma in the right adrenal gland was found at autopsy (personal communication, Dr. James A. Pitcock, Pathologist, Baptist Memorial Hospital, Memphis, Tennessee). It is conceivable that the injection of steroid precipitated the hypertensive crisis in this patient; however, we are unaware of similar reports in the literature.]

Steiner and associates have raised the possibility that excessive intraadrenal cortisol in some patients could increase PNMT activity, which in some way might induce adrenal medullary hyperplasia or neoplasia. However, they have pointed out that in patients with coexisting Cushing's syndrome and pheochromocytoma, who had been cured of Cushing's syndrome by resection of the pheochromocytoma, it appeared that the tumor was the cause of the hyperadrenocorticism, rather than vice versa (938).

Finally, despite some claims to the contrary, it is doubtful that pheochromocytomas are capable of synthesizing cortisol, since there is no evidence that these tumors have the necessary enzymes for synthesis of steroids. It seems conceivable that extracts of pheochromocytoma reported to contain large amounts of cortisol may have been contaminated by adjacent adrenal cortisol-containing tissue.

NEUROCUTANEOUS LESIONS

Neurofibromatosis The first report of the coexistence of neurofibromatosis and pheochromocytoma appears to have been made by Suzuki in 1910 (957). Neurofibromatosis (von Recklinghausen's disease), with or without café-au-lait spots, occurs in about 5 percent of patients with pheochromocytoma, either sporadic or familial; others have reported an incidence varying between 4 and 23 percent (206a, 420, 829). On the other hand, the incidence of pheochromocytoma in von Recklinghausen's disease may be less than 1 percent (99). A report from the Mayo Clinic in 1972 indicated that neurofibromatosis occurred in three of 132 patients with pheochromocytoma (i.e., 2.3 percent of these patients); since approximately 600 patients with neurofibromatosis had been seen, the incidence of hypertension due to pheochromocytoma occurring in all patients with neurofibromatosis was only 0.5 percent (596a). They cited the findings of Schlegel (437, pp. 68–73), who reported 23 cases of pheochromocytoma and 15 cases of neurofibromatosis in 25,274 autopsies. In this latter study pheochromocytoma and neurofibromatosis coexisted in two patients (2 out of 15) i.e., a coexistent incidence of 8 percent (2 out of 23) in patients with pheochromocytoma and 13 percent (2 out of 15) in patients with neurofibromatosis. Re-

view articles on the association of these lesions have appeared (147, 371, 866).

Neurofibromatosis is a form of congenital dysplasia, an autosomal dominantly inherited disease without sex linkage. It occurs in all races throughout the world at a rate of 1 per 2000 to 3000 births; about 50 percent of relatives are also afflicted. It is easily recognized when it appears (usually after puberty) with characteristic multiple flat or pedunculated subcutaneous nodules (neurofibromas of the peripheral nerves) (Fig. 4.15) and typical café-au-lait spots. Sometimes a generalized hyperpigmentation, vascular nevi, hairy moles, and sacral hypertrichosis may also be present; however, in some patients there may be only a few inconspicuous nodules. Page and Copeland have pointed out that axillary freckling is almost always present and that café-au-lait spots greater than 2 cm in diameter and numbering more than five should suggest the disease (728). Café-au-lait macules are composed of melanin located deep in the epidermis. Patients and their relatives from a kindred with Sipple's syndrome were noted to have café-au-lait spots without fibromatosis or mucosal neuromas (144).

Neurofibromatosis may appear in three main forms (90, 420): (1) peripheral neuro-

Fig. 4.15 Neurofibromatosis in a patient without pheochromocytoma. These lesions, which probably arise from neurilemma of peripheral nerves, are subcutaneous, freely mobile, and may be tender. They seldom interfere with nerve function. Rarely, sarcomatous degeneration occurs. Courtesy of Dr. A. Domonkos, Professor of Dermatology, Columbia Medical Center, New York, New York.

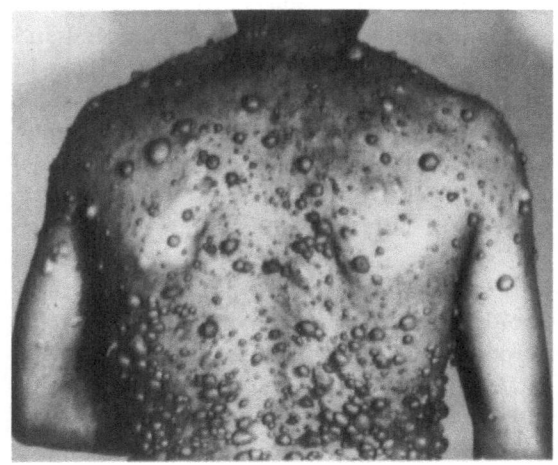

fibromatosis involving primarily the peripheral nerves, (2) central neurofibromatosis, involving primarily the central nervous system [central neurofibromatosis may be associated with combinations of gliomas, meningiomas, and schwannomas; also patients with von Recklinghausen's disease appear to have an increased incidence of brain tumors (526, 829)]; and (3) visceral neurofibromatosis, mainly an involvement of visceral and autonomic ganglia with neurofibromas, schwannomas, and ganglioneuromas. Neurofibromatosis of the myenteric plexus and multiple mucosal ganglioneuromas may occur (829).

Others have found that meningiomas and gliomas may frequently involve the nervous system (147), and that bilateral acoustic neuromas are more common in patients with neurofibromatosis. Also, a case of familial pheochromocytoma in association with ependymoma of the spinal cord has been described (408).

It should be kept in mind that vascular anomalies (e.g., coarctation, renal artery stenosis, and/or renal artery aneurysm) may occur with neurofibromatosis and may result in hypertension (118, 174, 410, 596a, 654, 874, 917a). These vascular lesions are thought to represent neurofibromatosis involvement in the wall of the artery. Lynch and associates reported a 22-year-old white male with neurofibromatosis and hypertension who had a tight fibrous stenosis of the superior mesenteric artery and both renal arteries. Small plexiform neurofibromas were spread over the aorta and located particularly in the region of the celiac ganglion and renal vessels. Neurofibromas and café-au-lait spots had been noted when this patient was 2 years old, and a neurofibroma had been removed from the posterior mediastinum when he was 5 years old. Their review of the literature up to 1972 revealed 14 other cases of neurofibromatosis with renovascular abnormalities which apparently caused hypertension. Of these 15 patients, all had renal artery stenosis or aneurysms, five had bilateral renal vascular abnormalities, and five had coarctation of the aorta. They further reported that "seven had microscopic evidence of neurofibroma or ganglioneuroma in the arterial wall, and three had the pathologic findings of intimal fibrosis, disorganization of the media, and fibrotic

changes of the adventitia referred to as vascular neurofibromatosis" (596a).

A 3.5-year-old patient was reported to have hypertension, neurofibromatosis, and stenosis of one renal artery, due to pressure from a ganglioneuroma (410). Ganglioneuromas have, rarely, been reported in other patients with pheochromocytoma (1070). Coexistence of ganglioneuroma, neuroblastoma, and neurofibromas has also been observed (767). It is important, therefore, to keep in mind that the above mentioned lesions, which sometimes coexist in patients with pheochromocytoma, may cause hypertension by their involvement of the renal arteries and/or the aorta.

The incidence of pheochromocytoma originating in the left adrenal gland or bilaterally appears greater when von Recklinghausen's disease occurs concomitantly. Neurofibromas may cause bone lesions and may occasionally compress spinal nerves and result in paralysis. They may arise from the spinal cord or intercostal nerves and present as mediastinal tumors in patients with von Recklinghausen's disease, and they may undergo malignant sarcomatous degeneration (847). It has been stated that in 13 to 29 percent of patients with von Recklinghausen's disease this type of malignant transformation may occur in peripheral neurofibromas by the age of 40 (99); however, we and Domonkos (personal communication from Dr. A. N. Domonkos, Clinical Professor of Dermatology, College of Physicians and Surgeons) have never encountered this malignant transformation in any of our patients with neurofibromatosis. The possible association of a mediastinal neurofibroma in a patient with multiple neurofibromatosis and pheochromocytoma should be kept in mind, since the tumor in the chest might erroneously be considered the pheochromocytoma.

It is intriguing that increased nerve growth-stimulating activity has been identified in disseminated neurofibromatosis (862). Administration of this growth factor causes enlargement of spinal and sympathetic ganglions in vivo (570); however, there appears to be no information on whether it has any effect on chromaffin cells.

One patient with pheochromocytoma was reported who had multiple soft, mobile, nontender, subcutaneous nodules on the arms, back, and abdomen which proved to be angiolipomas (322).

Mucosal Neuromas Association of the neurocutaneous lesions (phacomatoses) with pheochromocytoma is best explained by the fact that all these lesions are of neuroectodermal origin. The occurrence of mucosal neuromas in "multiple endocrine neoplasia type 3" has been discussed above. Association of pheochromocytoma with neurofibroma, aganglionic megacolon, and megaloureter had suggested to Shocket and Tehoh in 1957 that several neural abnormalities may be related and coexist in the same patient (870).

von Hippel-Lindau Disease Rarely, pheochromocytoma occurs in association with von Hippel-Lindau disease [cerebellar hemangioblastoma (146, 687, 706) with regional angioma (371)]. Furthermore, neurofibromatosis has been reported in association with mucosal neuromas and/or von Hippel-Lindau disease in addition to pheochromocytoma (978). Hume reported one patient with neurofibromatosis and cerebellar hemangioma, and another patient with multiple hemangiomas of the brain stem and a family history of von Hippel-Lindau disease and neurofibromatosis (466). von Hippel's disease consists of angiomatous malformations of the retina (angiomatosis retinae), and in 20 percent of patients, signs of intracranial tumor develop (783). Lindau found that the lesion of the central nervous system was a cystic hemangioblastoma involving the cerebellum (576), and this became known as Lindau's disease. This cerebellar tumor is highly vascular and often multicystic. von Hippel-Lindau disease may produce symptoms of cerebellar dysfunction (especially incoordination, ataxia, and intention tremor) and/or visual disturbance (e.g., field defects, blurred vision, diplopia, and nystagmus). In one family afflicted with pheochromocytoma and a high incidence of café-au-lait spots, two members were found to have von Hippel-Lindau disease as well (978). Retinal angiomatosis, which is usually peripheral, is accompanied by edema, hemorrhages, and exudates. It occurs bilaterally in 50 percent of patients and frequently leads to retinal detachment and secondary glaucoma.

ACROMEGALY

Four patients with pheochromocytoma in association with acromegaly have been reported (348, 492, 665, 717). In one of these patients pheochromocytoma was detected 20 years following hypophysectomy, whereas in another patient pheochromocytoma was recognized 13 years after pituitary irradiation. In the other two cases, both tumors occurred concurrently and in addition, one of these patients had a toxic goiter, diabetes mellitus, and endometriosis (665). The association of pheochromocytoma and acromegaly is particularly intriguing since, as mentioned previously, adrenal medullary tumors (in addition to neoplasms of the lungs and reproductive organs) have been induced in rats by prolonged administration of growth hormone (595, 675–678). Kahn has stated that clinically the occurrence of tumors (especially pheochromocytoma) has not been observed more commonly in acromegalics than in the random population (492). However, it has been suggested that since 37 percent of acromegalics have hypertension, the small reported incidence of pheochromocytoma may indicate that this association is rarely considered (665).

One teenage girl we aided in studying at Mount Sinai Medical Center (N.Y.C.) (see Chapter 7, patient No. 19) had 15 benign pheochromocytomas and hyperparathyroidism, and ultimately developed signs of acromegaly and an enlarged sella turcica due to a predominantly acidophilic cell tumor. Since in this case the pituitary tumor appeared to follow the manifestations of pheochromocytoma, it was speculated (Drs. Cobin, Pertsemlidis, Gitlow, and Krieger, case report, in press) that excessive concentrations of circulating catecholamines might have induced an overproduction of growth hormone and ultimately an autonomous pituitary tumor.

In support of this speculation, it is noteworthy that infusions of phenylsynephrine or methoxamine have been reported by Imura and coworkers to increase growth hormone in some normal subjects (472). Furthermore, Nakano and associates have found elevated basal growth hormone levels, a poor suppression of this hormone by glucose, and an exaggerated rise following insulin injection in two of three patients with pheochromocytoma (699). However, there was no correlation between the growth hormone levels and the concentration of urinary catecholamines in these two patients.

Cobin and coworkers (case report, in press) have suggested that the coexistence of pheochromocytomas, acromegaly, and hyperparathyroidism in this patient might indicate an "overlap" between multiple endocrine adenomatosis, type 1 (Wermer's Syndrome) (313, 983, 1026), and multiple endocrine neoplasia, type 2 (Sipple's Syndrome) (763, 850, 897, 938). The pituitary tumor would fit with MEN–type 1, and the pheochromocytomas with MEN–type 2, whereas the hyperparathyroidism would be common to both types. MEN–type 1 is a familial disease with autosomal dominant transmission and, as mentioned above, is characterized by hyperplasia or neoplasia, usually involving the parathyroids, pancreatic islets, pituitary, and occasionally the adrenal and thyroid. It is also rarely associated with a carcinoid neoplasm. The potential overlap of MEN–types 1 and 2 seems reasonable and probable, especially in view of the similar genetic transmission and the neural crest ancestry of many of these endocrine cells. The suggestion of these investigators is in keeping with Bolande's classification of multiple endocrine neoplasia (MEN–type 1 and 2) under the heading of "neurocristopathic syndromes and complex neurocristopathies" (90).

MISCELLANEOUS

In addition to conditions mentioned above, pheochromocytomas have been reported in patients with carcinoid (41), hypernephroma (419), neurolemmoma (1070), multiple hepatic hamartomas (721), hepatic hemangioma (347), neuroblastoma (209), ependymoma (987a), astrocytoma (633a), meningioma (398a), spongioblastoma (20a), chemodectoma (761), and Down's syndrome (531). In one patient a pheochromocytoma occurred in one adrenal and a cortical adenoma in the other (769). It is interesting that Glushien and coworkers have predicted 10 percent of patients with pheochromocytoma may also have neurocutaneous manifestations such as neurofibromatosis, von Hippel-Lindau disease, tuberous sclerosis or Sturge-Weber disease (encephalotrigeminal angiomatosis) (371). The increased association of hamartoma and neurofibromatosis with tuberous sclerosis is well recognized (542); however, to our knowledge, tuberous sclerosis has not been observed in patients with pheochromocytoma (542, 633) and only one patient with both hamartoma and pheochromocytoma has been reported (721). Megacolon may, rarely, occur in patients with pheochromocytoma, neurofibromata, and multiple mucosal neuroma. Apparently the megacolon may be due to neurofibromatosis of the myenteric plexus or aganglios is (90). It is important to appreciate the association of pheochromocytoma with cholelithiasis, thyroid carcinoma, mucosal neuroma, alimentary-tract ganglioneuromatosis, marfanoid features, hyperparathyroidism, Cushing's syndrome (and, extremely rarely, adrenal virilism or Addison's disease), neurofibromatosis and von Hippel-Lindau disease, and even acromegaly, since manifestations of these conditions may be superimposed on the symptoms and signs of pheochromocytoma, and may be extremely confusing to the clinician.

Undoubtedly, pheochromocytoma has occurred in association with a number of disease entities; however, whether some of these associations have been simply coincidental or whether they have relevance to pathogenetic mechanisms involved in their genesis is at times difficult—or impossible—to determine. A significantly increased incidence of pheochromocytoma, occurring particularly in association with a neoplasm which shares a similar primitive cell of origin, suggests that the stimulus for these neoplasms may be similar, if not identical.

In an interesting review in 1974, Bolande presented a unifying concept of disease arising from neural crest maldevelopment (90). He coined the term "neurocristopathies" to designate the constellation of embryogenetically related disease entities such as pheochromocytoma, neuroblastoma, neurofibromatosis, medullary thyroid carcinoma, carcinoid tumors, Hirschsprung's disease, nonchromaffin paragangliomas (chemodectomas), melanotic progonoma, multiple endocrine neoplasia, and neurocutaneous melanosis. He also discussed combinations and permutations of these diseases and suggested that the pathogenetic common denominator in all these

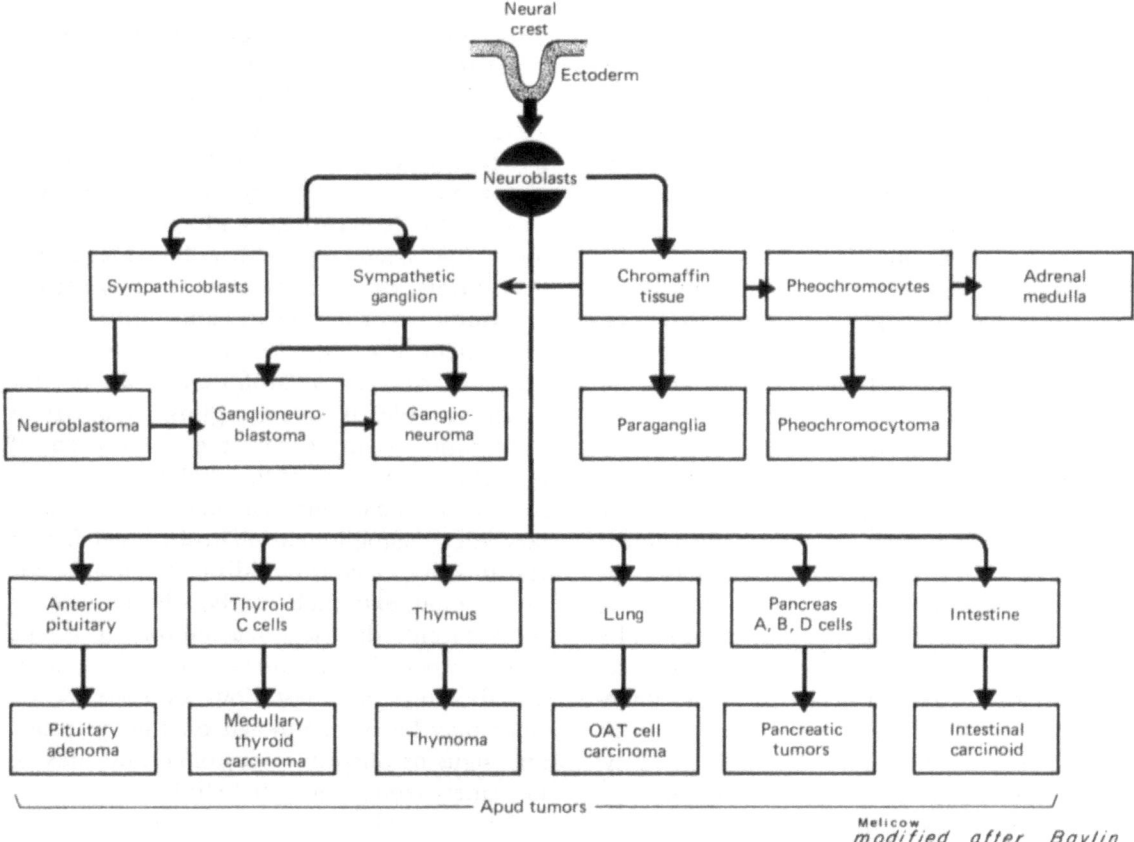

Fig. 4.16 Ectodermal origin of APUD tumors. From Baylin, S. B., *Hospital Practice 10:* 124, 1975. Modified by Dr. M. M. Melicow, Columbia University Medical Center, New York, New York.

conditions appeared to be aberrant neural crest development (90). The fact that some of these conditions are associated with the elaboration of catecholamines supports this latter concept. It is intriguing that increased urinary VMA excretion has been reported in one patient with retinoblastoma (519a) and in another patient with a melanotic progonoma (melanotic neuroectodermal tumor of infancy) in the anterior maxilla (93).

Citing the studies of Weston (1032), Bolande stated that "neural crest cells seem unusually labile in terms of their ultimate destinations and cyto-differentiated end points. This might well predispose these cells to teratogenic, mutagenic, and oncogenic influences. In this regard it is important to emphasize the prevalence of genetic factors in this group of diseases" (90).

In keeping with the hypothesis of Bolande is the concept of the "APUD" cell system, proposed originally by Pearse in 1968 (735,

737). Pearse has delineated a group of cells which have certain cytochemical and ultrastructural features in common. These cells, which are present in a variety of endocrine as well as nonendocrine tissues, appear to have a neuroendocrine function and probably arise from the neural crest. They elaborate low molecular weight polypeptide hormones or hormone precursors. The term "APUD" is derived from the initial letters of the most characteristic cytochemical behavior of these cells [i.e., *a*mine (amino acid) and amine *p*recursor *u*ptake and *d*ecarboxylation.] Thus, these cells elaborate amines by taking up amine precursors, which they decarboxylate. Pearse has proposed that the APUD cell system constitutes "a peripheral neuroendocrine system, analogous to the central neuroendocrine system of the hypothalamus" (736). As pointed out by Bolande, the "APUD" classification of Pearse encompasses and supersedes the earlier chromaffin and argentaffin cell groupings (90). (In personal conversation, Pearse has cautioned that the acronym "APUD" should not be misconstrued to mean "Anthony Pearse's Ultimate Dogma!")

Endocrine polypeptide-producing tumors have been linked together comprehensively under the title of "Apudomas" (962); some of these (including medullary thyroid carcinoma, pheochromocytoma, bronchial carcinoids, insulinomas, and carotid body tumors) produce amyloid (apudamyloid), which, unlike secondary immunoamyloid, lacks tryptophan and tyrosine (737). Pearse has postulated that most likely the amyloidogenic polypeptide in endocrine tumors is either the nonhormone residue of the prohormone or perhaps a polypeptide elaborated, for some reason, concomitantly with the hormone (737). He suggested that chromogranin may play a key role in the occasional production of amyloid in pheochromocytomas. Pearse has stated (in a recent communication) that "an Apudoma is an 'endocrine' tumor possessing the A-P-U-D and associated chemical qualities of its presumptive precursor cell, characterized cytologically and ultrastructurally by the presence of specific storage granules and containing a peptide component with or without an associated catecholamine or indolalkylamine." It is noteworthy that, recently, Pearse has described a *v*asoactive (vasoconstrictor) *i*ntestinal *p*eptide (VIP) which has been identified in a number of locations, including sympathetic nerves, adrenal medulla, and some pheochromocytomas.

A clear display of the potential ramifications of the neuroectodermal cell is indicated in Figure 4.16, which was prepared by Dr. M. M. Melicow from Baylin's review of APUD tumors (50). Parathyroid adenomas should also be included in the list of apudomas if it is established that the parathyroid glands in the human are derived from neuroectoderm.

Differential Diagnosis

CHAPTER FIVE

GENERAL REMARKS

Because of the great variety of symptoms and signs occurring in patients with pheochromocytoma, this tumor has been called the "great mimic" among hypertensive disorders (215). It is no wonder then that the differential diagnosis includes a long list of unrelated disease entities (Table 5.1). No tumor or disease process is capable of causing a more diversified constellation of manifestations than pheochromocytoma and its associated pathologic entities. The extraordinary overlap of many symptoms and signs of the conditions listed is indeed fascinating, though often a frustrating challenge to the physician's diagnostic acumen. It is important to emphasize and reemphasize that in the final analysis the preoperative diagnosis of this tumor must be confirmed by demonstrating significant elevations of catecholamines and/or their metabolites in the urine or plasma. Since many of the conditions included for the sake of completeness in the differential diagnosis (Table 5.1) can be immediately excluded on clinical grounds by careful attention to the history and physical examination, a detailed discussion of most of them has been presented only in order to point out *dis*similarities which will be of particular aid to the

Table 5.1 *Differential Diagnosis*[a]

All hypertensives (sustained and paroxysmal)
Anxiety, tension states, psychoneurosis, psychosis
Hyperthyroidism
Paroxysmal tachycardia
Hyperdynamic β-adrenergic circulatory state
Menopause
Vasodilating headache (migraine and cluster headaches)
Coronary insufficiency syndrome
Acute hypertensive encephalopathy
Diabetes mellitus
Renal parenchymal or renal arterial disease with hypertension
Focal arterial insufficiency of the brain
Intracranial lesions (with or without ↑ intracranial pressure)
Autonomic hyperreflexia
Diencephalic seizure and syndrome
Toxemia of pregnancy (*or eclampsia with convulsions*)
Hypertensive crises associated with monoamine oxidase inhibitors
Carcinoid
Hypoglycemia
Mastocytosis
Familial dysautonomia
Acrodynia
Neuroblastoma; ganglioneuroblastoma; ganglioneuroma
Acute infectious disease
Rare causes of paroxysmal hypertension (*acute porphyria*; *lead poisoning*; tabetic crisis; encephalitis; *clonidine withdrawal*; hypovolemia with inappropriate vasoconstriction; pulmonary artery fibrosarcoma; pork hypersensitivity; dysregulation of hypothalamus; *tetanus*; *Guillain-Barré syndrome*; *factitious*)
Fortuitous circumstances simulating pheochromocytoma

Conditions sometimes associated with pheochromocytoma
   Coexisting diseases or syndromes
      Cholelithiasis
      Medullary thyroid carcinoma
      Hyperparathyroidism
      Mucosal neuromas
      Thickened corneal nerves
      Marfanoid habitus
      Alimentary-tract ganglioneuromatosis
      Neurofibromatosis
      Cushing's syndrome
      von Hippel-Lindau disease
      Polycythemia
      Virilism, Addison's disease, acromegaly
   Complications
      Cardiovascular disease[b]
      Cerebrovascular disease
      Renovascular disease
      Circulatory shock
      Renal insufficiency
      Hemorrhagic necrosis of pheochromocytoma[b]
      Dissecting aneurysm[b]
      Ischemic enterocolitis with or without intestinal obstruction[b]

---

[a] Conditions in italics may have increased excretion of catecholamines and/or metabolites.

[b] May present as an abdominal or cardiovascular catastrophe.

clinician in making the correct diagnosis. Of course, one should never lose sight of the possibility that certain conditions (Table 5.1) may be *associated with* pheochromocytoma, and their presence should alert the physician to consider their coexistence.

Above all else, it is mandatory that the physician maintain a high index of suspicion, since the secret in making the diagnosis of pheochromocytoma obviously lies first in suspecting it. It is a tragic and shocking fact that prior to 1964 two-thirds of the pheochromocytomas reported in the world literature were not discovered until postmortem examination (437). The extreme importance of recognizing the presence of a pheochromocytoma before any operative procedure is performed is underscored by the report of Kirkendall and associates which revealed that nine of 11 patients known to have pheochromocytoma survived tumor removal, whereas only one of seven patients survived operations for other diseases when the tumor was present but unsuspected (513). Currently, with expertise and highly skilled teamwork, one can anticipate an operative survival rate of greater than 97 percent in those patients in whom the diagnosis of pheochromocytoma has been established preoperatively (784). As Gitlow aptly remarked during a recent lecture, it is mandatory for those involved with the treatment of hypertension, that every effort be made to find this needle in the haystack of hypertensive patients!

HYPERTENSION

It is strongly urged that all symptomatic patients with sustained or paroxysmal hypertension be screened for pheochromocytoma unless the cause of their hypertension is known. Since the diagnosis of essential hypertension is made primarily by excluding other causes, the overwhelming majority of patients with hypertension must be considered pheochromocytoma suspects. Because pheochromocytoma produces symptoms in the vast majority of patients, and is itself only a rare cause of hypertension, it is probably not cost effective to screen all asymptomatic hypertensive patients for pheochromocytoma routinely. Certainly, patients who are symptomatic, no matter how minor the symptoms, and patients whose hypertension is severe (Groups 3 or 4) or resistant to treatment or responds paradoxically to treatment, should have screening tests for pheochromocytoma. Pheochromocytic hypertension notoriously responds poorly to conventional antihypertensive therapy; consequently, the diagnosis is not likely to be overlooked if appropriate tests are made for patients whose hypertension is not well controlled by antipressor therapy. Even asymptomatic hypertensive patients who have diseases known occasionally to coexist with pheochromocytoma, or patients with laboratory abnormalities which may be caused by increased circulating catecholamines, should be screened.

The only objection to routine tests to exclude the diagnosis of pheochromocytoma in all hypertensive patients is an economic one, because there is no risk whatsoever involved in collecting and submitting a 24-hr urine specimen. Pharmacologic tests, which do carry a small but definite risk, are not necessary when hypertension is sustained. The cost for individual determinations of catecholamines or their metabolites in the urine is not exorbitant, but when this is applied to 23 million hypertensive patients it becomes a very significant figure with a very low potential yield.

At the present time no physician can be criticized for routinely obtaining tests to rule out pheochromocytoma on every hypertensive patient, and likewise, no physician can be criticized for omitting such tests for asymptomatic patients whose hypertension has responded appropriately to therapy.

A lengthy history of hypertension in no way excludes the presence of this tumor, since we have had patients whose hypertension existed for two to three decades before a pheochromocytoma was detected. Very rarely, a patient may have paroxysms of hypertension for over forty years before the tumor is discovered (266, 745).

Subjects with a hyperlabile blood pressure (not infrequently a forerunner of essential hypertension) and patients with essential hypertension do not have attacks or vasomotor phenomena. Furthermore, excess sweating and an elevated temperature are distinctly unusual features in patients with essential hypertension (920), and postural hypotension or postural tachycardia is an extremely rare occurrence in these patients unless they are on certain antihypertensive medication. Actually, upright untreated patients with essential hypertension almost invariably have blood pressures which are equal to or higher than their pressures in the recumbent position.

ANXIETY OR PSYCHIATRIC DISORDER

Since anxiety is associated with increased activity of the sympathoadrenal system, it is understandable that tense and apprehensive persons may periodically develop slight or even moderate hypertension, headache, palpitations, tachycardia, diaphoresis, a fine tremor, and decreased salivation. Furthermore, the pupils may be dilated. Hyperventilation may ensue, with giddiness, tingling in the finger tips, and carpopedal spasm. Usually one can detect that these patients are psychologically disturbed and emotionally unstable. Complaints of neurotic patients are frequently chronic, and generally there is a typical psychoneurotic personality. Patients with severe anxiety and sustained essential hypertension present an even more perplexing problem in differential diagnosis. Some patients, in whom the diagnosis of pheochromocytoma has been missed, have been inappropriately treated with psychotherapy.

As pointed out previously by Poutasse and Gifford (769), hyperventilation, although not uncommon in patients who are tense and anxious, may also precipitate a typical paroxysm in some patients with pheochromocytoma.

Patients with pheochromocytoma not infrequently have attacks of severe throbbing headaches, marked elevations of their blood pressures, and pronounced sweating. Patients with pheochromocytoma do not exhibit the personality manifestations of prolonged emotional instability and chronic anxiety unless they are also neurotic. During an attack of hypertension with release of catecholamines into the circulation, as occurs abruptly in patients with pheochromocytoma, apprehension usually appears suddenly but will sub-side significantly as the attack ends and symptoms regress. Sometimes a sense of panic or impending death may be episodically experienced (but only for a brief period) in patients with pheochromocytoma.

It is noteworthy that a 34-year-old woman who had complained of weak spells and depression for 5 years was thought to have an anxiety reaction with depressive features associated with psycholepsy (because of the suddenness of severe headaches). Following her first electroconvulsive treatment, she became unusually restless and apprehensive, with slightly dilated pupils, cold and clammy hands and feet, and an ashen appearance of her face. Shortly thereafter cardiorespiratory arrest occurred and the patient expired. A 128 g pheochromocytoma of the left adrenal gland was found at autopsy. The patient had never been found to have sustained or paroxysmal hypertension; however, her unusually severe and sudden headaches, unexplained low-grade fever, weak spells, nausea and vomiting ("the dry heaves"), tachycardia out of proportion to the degree of manifest anxiety, and electrocardiographic abnormalities were consistent with the presence of excessive circulating catecholamines (236). This case report should serve as a warning to physicians who may elect to administer electroconvulsive shock for the treatment of depression. We know of another patient with pheochromocytoma who was given electroshock therapy, fortunately without fatality (see Chapter 3, patient described for Figs. 3.34–3.36).

A fascinating recent comment by Jackson was that he and his associates know of 12 patients with Sipple's syndrome who developed depressive psychosis. Some of these patients had normal catecholamine metabolites and in several the depression was relieved by thyroidectomy; two patients (who had irresectable thyroid lesions) were markedly improved by administration of imipramine. Whether psychosis resulted from some of the hormonal or other abnormalities occurring in Sipple's syndrome remains to be elucidated. The psychic abnormalities did not correlate with the levels of serum calcitonin (personal communication from Dr. Charles E. Jackson, Henry Ford Hospital, Detroit).

Depressive psychosis has also occasionally been observed in patients with nonfamilial (sporadic) pheochromocytoma, and in some the psychosis disappeared after extirpation of the pheochromocytoma. One patient seen at the Mayo Clinic developed a paranoid psychosis in the presence of metastatic pheochromocytoma (personal communication from Dr. Sheldon Sheps, Internist, Mayo Clinic).

HYPERTHYROIDISM

Symptoms and signs of thyrotoxicosis closely resemble those caused by overstimulation of the sympathoadrenal system (i.e., anxiety, tremor, tachycardia, palpitations, excess sweating, heat intolerance, hypermetabolism, hyperglycemia, and weight loss). It is not surprising that, before more sophisticated methods of detecting excess catecholamines and their metabolites in plasma or urine became available, thyroidectomies were sometimes inadvertently performed on patients with pheochromocytoma (44, 788, 1001). It is important to stress that hyperthyroidism, whether due to Grave's disease or to toxic nodular goiter, can cause diastolic as well as systolic hypertension. In 81 patients with hyperthyroidism and hypertension studied at the Mayo Clinic (478), about two-thirds had systolic and diastolic hypertension and one-third had systolic hypertension only. About two out of three of these patients developed relatively normal blood pressures after the establishment of euthyroidism. Papilledema with retinal hemorrhages and exudates may occur in patients with thyrotoxicosis and hypertension (478).

When present, characteristic eye signs of Grave's disease (e.g., proptosis, lid lag, chemosis), weight loss in the presence of polyphagia, marked diarrhea, and a symmetrically enlarged thyroid gland will help establish a diagnosis of hyperthyroidism; however, many patients with thyrotoxicosis have none of these classical manifestations.

Thyroid function tests (e.g., PBI, T3, T4, and uptake by the gland of radioactive iodine) are normal in patients with pheochromocytoma. Only one patient has been reported who had an elevated uptake of radioactive iodine similar to that occurring in hyperthyroidism (338); therefore, an elevated BMR in a patient with a normally functioning thyroid gland should make the clinician suspect pheochromocytoma. If accurately determined, the presence of a markedly elevated BMR (e.g., $>+50$ percent) without thyrotoxicosis is pathognomonic for pheochromocytoma, if excessive activation of the sympathoadrenal neurosecretory system by other causes (e.g., concussion, poliomyelitis) is excluded. In a series of 76 patients with pheochromocytoma studied at the Mayo Clinic, 60 percent had a BMR above $+13$ percent (the upper limit of normal) and 10 percent had values greater than $+50$ percent, the highest value being $+261$ percent (976). However, it should be noted that the BMR may occasionally be significantly elevated in patients with essential hypertension. Smithwick reported that in 100 consecutive patients with essential hypertension 5 percent had elevations of $+20$ percent or more (920). Since the BMR is now only very rarely determined, its elevation in some patients with pheochromocytoma is practically obsolete as a diagnostic tool.

PAROXYSMAL TACHYCARDIA (ATRIAL AND NODAL)

Supraventricular paroxysmal tachycardia may recur spontaneously or may be precipitated by emotional or physical stress or by the use of coffee or tobacco. Palpitations and breathlessness are frequently noted and may suggest recurrent attacks of excess catecholamine release in patients with pheochromocytoma.

In paroxysmal supraventricular tachycardia the heart rate is >150 beats per minute. The very abrupt onset and abrupt termination of the tachycardia is usually quite apparent to the patient and may be documented by recording the heart rate and by electrocardiogram. Termination of this type of tachycardia may occur spontaneously or can be brought about by having the patient strain or by pressure on a carotid sinus or by various medications. Headache, diaphoresis, and hypertension are not manifestations of paroxysmal supraventricular tachycardia; in fact, hypotension and, occasionally, syncope are more likely to occur with this type of tachycardia.

HYPERDYNAMIC β-ADRENERGIC CIRCULATORY STATE

The hyperdynamic β-adrenergic circulatory state has been defined as a condition in which a hyperkinetic circulation with increased cardiac output (with or without hypertension) results from β-receptor hyperresponsiveness (334, 335). Usually there is mild tachycardia at rest; however, these patients periodically have substantial increases in their heart rates [even up to 170 beats per minute (334)] with palpitations and, not infrequently, attacks of apprehension, sometimes with severe anxiety and dyspnea. These attacks may be precipitated by emotional excitement, standing, physical exertion, or administration of isoproterenol (335). Chest and abdominal discomfort and orthostatic hypotension have been noted (334). Sustained systolic and/or diastolic hypertension of mild to moderate severity may be present. Frequently the blood pressure may be labile and become elevated during episodes of tachycardia.

We have treated a 27-year-old mother of four children whose usual blood pressure and heart rate had been, respectively, about 120/78 mmHg and 78 beats per minute until she developed the hyperdynamic β-adrenergic circulatory state. She had not been on any medication and began to have attacks of tachycardia (sometimes up to 165 beats/min), marked palpitations, elevations of blood pressure (at times to 162/110 mmHg), apprehension, faintness, hot flashes, dull headaches, and the sensation of marked exhaustion. These attacks occurred during the day, particularly in the morning, and occasionally awakened the patient from sleep. Frequently these episodes were precipitated by exertion and sometimes by the ingestion of alcohol. There had been some weight gain (due to increased caloric intake), and no tremor, diaphoresis, or bowel habit changes. Except for a brief period of unexplained galactorrhea just prior to the onset of her symptoms, endocrine and cardiovascular evaluation were within normal limits. She was hyperreactive to the cold pressor test but the blood pressure and plasma catecholamine response to glucagon were within normal limits. Symptomatology was largely eliminated by propranolol. [Subsequently, at 33

years of age, this patient developed angina, frequently experienced at rest and during minimal exertion. A successful coronary bypass procedure was performed at the Cleveland Clinic and a localized atheromatous segment (95 percent occluded) of the right coronary artery was removed; the remaining coronary arteries appeared normal.] The case of this patient is reported to indicate how closely this syndrome of a hyperkinetic β-adrenergic circulatory state can resemble the signs and symptoms of persons with pheochromocytoma. However, diaphoresis and very severe headaches, which are common in patients with pheochromocytoma, have not been observed frequently in patients with the hyperdynamic circulatory state. The symptoms of patients with this latter condition respond dramatically if β-adrenergic blockade is induced with propranolol (335), whereas symptomatology in patients with pheochromocytoma is not dramatically influenced by this drug.

MENOPAUSE

In women with sustained or labile hypertension, superimposed symptoms of the menopause may suggest pheochromocytoma. There may be repeated paroxysms of flushing (hot flashes), sweating, and increases in blood pressure during the day, and the patient may be awakened at night by these symptoms. Not infrequently these patients experience some emotional lability and sometimes complain of symptoms of atrophic vaginitis and vulvitis. Signs and symptoms of the menopause are relieved dramatically by administration of estrogens, whereas no benefit occurs in patients with pheochromocytoma. Pallor is not a manifestation of the menopause; however, although unusual, severe palpitations may be experienced.

VASODILATING HEADACHES

MIGRAINE HEADACHE

Severe migraine headaches, which are said to occur most often in anxious, striving, perfectionistic, rigid, order-loving individuals, may be accompanied by elevations in blood pressure, pallor and/or blushing, irritability, excess sweating, prostration, nausea, vomiting, constipation or diarrhea, photophobia, and phonophobia (203). Tachycardia is not a feature of migraine. Paroxysmal episodes of migraine equivalents (e.g., pain in the chest, abdomen, and extremities or symptoms of pelvic, eye, and cerebral cortex involvement) may replace the headaches in 20 percent of patients (203). Tyramine in certain foods can evoke migraine in susceptible individuals, and recently it has been noted that oral contraceptives may precipitate migraine and will increase the severity and frequency of these headaches. Although the headaches are usually unilateral in onset, they may become bilateral or generalized. Typically, migraine headaches occur less abruptly, less frequently, and last longer than do headaches produced by pheochromocytoma; however, occasionally migraine headaches may last only a few minutes.

Of value in identifying migraine as the cause of the periodic headaches is a family history [perhaps 55 percent (1005)] of this disorder. Furthermore, prodromes, which occur in 10 to 15 percent of patients with migraine and usually take the form of visual and neurologic abnormalities (sometimes associated with electroencephalographic changes), are almost pathognomonic for migraine but never occur as a prodrome to attacks in patients with pheochromocytoma. In contrast to the usual aura of migraine, the transitory loss of vision and scotomata reported in a few patients with pheochromocytoma have occurred during rather than preceding the headache. Also, the paresthesias experienced by patients with pheochromocytoma are bilateral (976). Patients with migraine headaches become subdued and depressed; patients with pheochromocytoma and significant increase in circulating catecholamines are almost always anxious and restless.

Finally, patients with migraine generally respond to treatment with ergotamine tartrate or methysergide, whereas the headaches and other symptoms in patients with pheochromocytoma are not prevented by this medication. We had one patient with pheochromocytoma who also had migraine headaches (see Chapter 7, patient No. 28). Coexistence of these conditions has been reported previously (160, 778). Two patients with recurrent headaches for 10 and 20 years were erroneously considered to have migraine before the headaches were discovered to be a manifestation of pheochromocytoma (199).

CLUSTER HEADACHE

During attacks of cluster headache the systolic and diastolic blood pressure can become significantly increased (258). This type of headache closely resembles a paroxysmal disorder but its unique characteristics and tempo of attacks should easily differentiate it from the paroxysmal headaches associated with pheochromocytoma. It is unilateral, anterior (frequently in the region of the eye), intense, brief, and occurs almost always on the same side; many attacks may occur in quick succession. Typically, headaches occur daily for a period of days or weeks with symptom-free intervals of months or years between clusters. There is conjunctival congestion, rhinorrhea and nasal obstruction, and increased perspiration and vasodilatation on the same side of the face as the headache. It is repetitious in duration, location, and sequence of symptoms (976). Occasionally there is an ipsilateral partial Horner syndrome, but nausea, vomiting, and scotomata are almost always absent. The attacks, which very frequently occur during sleep, may be precipitated by alcohol, nitroglycerine, and histamine. It is of importance that when histamine causes a response in patients with pheochromocytoma, it is immediate, whereas cluster headaches occur usually 20 to 60 min after administration of this drug (976). Treatment with methysergide or ergotamine tartrate may be effective, and prophylaxis with serotonin antagonists may be of value (257).

It is noteworthy that since both migraine and cluster headaches may be relieved partially or completely by intravenous infusions of norepinephrine (203), patients with either type actually might note improvement of their headaches if they have also developed a continually secreting pheochromocytoma.

CORONARY INSUFFICIENCY SYNDROME

In some patients with chest pain due to coronary insufficiency, a sudden marked rise of blood pressure accompanied by sweating, tachycardia, and flushing may suggest a paroxysmal attack due to pheochromocytoma (460). This may be particularly confusing since the release of catecholamines by this tumor may also result in coronary insufficiency and chest pain, particularly in patients with coexisting coronary atherosclerosis.

It appears that in some patients with coronary insufficiency due to atherosclerosis, spontaneous chest pain may occur at rest and may precede the rise in blood pressure. Although the chest pain, per se, may be responsible for these elevations in blood pressure, it has been proposed that these pressor episodes may be reflexly triggered by temporary reductions in coronary flow (460). There is evidence in some patients that angina at rest may be precipitated by a spontaneous rise in blood pressure.

In patients with pheochromocytoma who develop chest pain, the hypertension precedes the pain; furthermore, narcotics, sedatives, and nitrates which relieve the chest pain may result in a reduction of blood pressure in patients with coronary insufficiency, whereas hypertension due to pheochromocytoma will not be affected or may even be augmented. Some of our colleagues have observed hypertensive crises following the administration of morphine whereas some investigators have even used nitroglycerine to provoke the release of catecholamines from pheochromocytomas (218).

ACUTE HYPERTENSIVE ENCEPHALOPATHY

Acute hypertensive encephalopathy usually occurs in association with severe hypertension which has been present for a prolonged period; however, it may occur with sudden severe rises of blood pressure. Headaches, nausea, vomiting, fleeting episodes of blindness (amaurosis), convulsive seizures, stupor, and coma may occur. Transient focal neurologic defects (e.g., transient motor paralysis and sensory disturbances) may appear, and funduscopic examination may reveal retinal arterial spasm and papilledema with or without hemorrhages and exudates. Cerebrospinal fluid pressure and protein are often elevated.

Pheochromocytoma is capable of causing malignant hypertension and hypertensive encephalopathy, but a prolonged history of episodes of sudden onset of headaches, palpitations, tachycardia, diaphoresis, and pallor —so frequently noted in patients with pheochromocytoma—is not typical in patients with hypertensive encephalopathy from other causes.

DIABETES MELLITUS

Because of the presence of hyperglycemia in some patients with pheochromocytoma (65 and 56 percent of patients with sustained and paroxysmal hypertension, respectively), an erroneous diagnosis of diabetes mellitus may be made. Not infrequently one can elicit a family history of diabetes mellitus in diabetic patients. Hypertension is not uncommon in patients with diabetes mellitus. This is usually essential hypertension but sometimes it may be attributed to renal disease resulting as a complication of diabetes. The hypertension of the Kimmelsteil-Wilson syndrome in diabetes mellitus is accompanied by proteinuria and edema, and by characteristic microscopic renal alterations known as the Kimmelsteil-Wilson lesions. Diabetes mellitus is usually present for at least 5 years before renal lesions appear.

Diabetic retinopathy with characteristic microaneurysms is readily distinguished from the retinopathy of pure hypertensive disease, although in the Kimmelsteil-Wilson syndrome there may be a combination of diabetic and hypertensive retinopathy.

Patients with pheochromocytoma may have an abnormal glucose tolerance curve. In some patients with pheochromocytoma, extreme variations in blood glucose may be observed during a glucose tolerance test (e.g., hyperglycemia may be followed by hypoglycemia). One patient was reported who actually had a slight decrease in blood glucose following a glucose tolerance test (47); however, fasting hyperglycemia and glycosuria are usually not very marked. The highest fasting blood glucose concentrations in the series of patients with pheochromocytoma seen at the Mayo Clinic were 226 mg percent (976) and 274 mg percent (822); however, one patient with pheochromocytoma and paroxysmal hypertension, who was thought to have diabetes mellitus, had a fasting blood sugar of 400 mg percent (229). This patient was found to have severe acidosis with very high blood glucose levels and glycosuria (up to 60–80 g per day) which required large amounts of insulin. Following tumor removal, there was no evidence of diabetes mellitus (229). Ketoacidosis is almost never seen in patients with pheochromocytoma.

There is no correlation between the degree of hypertension and the presence of hyperglycemia. The occurrence of paroxysmal hyperglycemia concomitantly with paroxysms of hypertension should immediately suggest pheochromocytoma; furthermore, during periods of normoglycemia and normotension, the glucose tolerance test may be within normal limits in patients with pheochromocytoma and paroxysmal hypertension.

It has been shown that the diabetic oral glucose and intravenous tolbutamide tolerance tests noted in some patients with pheochromocytoma usually return to normal after removal of the tumor. Hyperglycemia in patients with pheochromocytoma results not only from glycogenolysis provoked by the catecholamines but also, apparently, from other factors. For example, the resistance to the hypoglycemic action of insulin that occurs may be related to elevated plasma free fatty acids which may directly impair carbohydrate metabolism and peripheral sensitivity to insulin (930). Also, the catecholamines exert an inhibitory effect on insulin release (764, 1035). Suppression of the insulin response to glucose and tolbutamide, which appears to be mediated through a pancreatic α-adrenergic receptor mechanism, can be reversed by phentolamine (930). It has been reported that during an infusion of glucose, administration of phentolamine to a patient with pheochromocytoma causes an increase in plasma insulin concentration and a decrease in blood glucose, in addition to the characteristic drop in blood pressure (930). These responses to phentolamine (described in Chapter 6) are not observed in the patient with diabetes mellitus, or in patients with hypertension secondary to conditions other than pheochromocytoma (931). In conclusion, it is well to recall in the differential diagnosis that the presence of a family history of diabetes

mellitus, the presence of diabetic retinopathy, and/or Kimmelsteil-Wilson nephropathy, and/or a history of ketoacidosis are found in patients with diabetes mellitus but are not typical of patients with pheochromocytoma.

RENAL PARENCHYMAL OR RENAL ARTERIAL DISEASE WITH HYPERTENSION

Urinary abnormalities and altered renal function are not infrequently noted in patients with pheochromocytoma. In 1937 Howard and Barker reported proteinuria in nine out of 18 patients (462), and in 1946 Green found 24 of 37 patients with pheochromocytoma to have altered renal function, which improved after tumor removal (393). Proteinuria may be produced transiently with infusions of epinephrine (935) or it may result from reflex renal vasoconstriction induced by cold pressor stimulation of the sympathetic nervous system (150). Of 76 patients studied by Gifford and coworkers at the Mayo Clinic (352), 35.1 and 64.1 percent with paroxysmal or persistent hypertension, respectively, had a Grade 1 or higher proteinuria (Table 6.3).

In addition, hyaline and granular casts and occasionally red blood cells may be seen in urinary sediment of patients with pheochromocytoma (556); however, severe renal insufficiency with uremia is uncommon. Death in uremia was reported in only three out of 207 cases reviewed by Graham (392). In 69 patients studied by Gifford and associates (352), blood urea elevation occurred in 18.7 and 24.3 percent of those with paroxysmal or persistent hypertension, respectively; values of 60 mg/dl or more were found in only 3.1 and 5.4 percent of these patients (see Table 6.3). L'Abbé and coworkers first described episodes of proteinuria, oliguria, and renal failure following hypertensive attacks in their patients with pheochromocytoma (536). Leather and coworkers, in their report on two patients whose oliguria and azotemia occurred during hypertensive crises due to pheochromocytoma, expressed the belief that interference with renal function resulted from the renal effects of the catecholamines released from tumors (556). Blood urea in one of their patients rose to 290 mg/dl and returned toward normal after the tumor had been removed. A decrease in renal plasma flow (1041), a fall in urea clearance from 90 to 53 percent (987), and suppression of urine formation (462), have been demonstrated during hypertensive attacks in patients with pheochromocytoma.

As pointed out by Leather and associates, uremia in patients with pheochromocytoma and persistent hypertension can result from nephrosclerosis (556); in acute hypertensive attacks, dehydration associated with vomiting may be a contributory cause (752). However, episodes of reversible renal failure occurring during hypertensive crises may be explained by the derangement of renal function caused by the excessive concentrations of norepinephrine and/or epinephrine in the circulation reaching the kidney. It has been demonstrated that infusion of epinephrine causes efferent arteriolar constriction and increases perfusion pressure, with a fall in renal plasma flow and a rise in filtration fraction (66, 148, 157, 481, 685, 781, 787). Norepinephrine infusions also reduce renal plasma flow; however, in a series of six normal men the glomerular filtration rate was not altered (774). Increasing the rate of catecholamine infusion can cause a progressively greater fall in renal plasma flow, and reduce glomerular filtration rate and maximal tubular reabsorption of glucose, which Moyer and Handley attributed to exclusion of nephrons from the circulation (685). Renal "shut-down" has been induced by catecholamine infusion in dogs (173), and with prolonged renal vasoconstriction, tubular necrosis may occur.

From the foregoing, it is not surprising that pheochromocytoma may be mistaken for renal disease with hypertension. Any one of the conditions of bilateral renal parenchymal disease listed in Table 1.1 and some types of unilateral renal disease may be accompanied by hypertension. Furthermore, wide swings of blood pressure several times each day may be observed in some types of nephritis; however, the elevation and decline in blood pressure are almost never as abrupt as that observed in patients with paroxysmal attacks due to pheochromocytoma. Differentiation between pheochromocytoma and renal hypertension should not be difficult if certain points are kept in mind. For example, pro-

teinuria greater than 3 g daily almost always indicates glomerular disease. Furthermore, the nephrotic syndrome (heavy proteinuria, hypoalbuminemia, and generalized edema) has not been reported in patients with pheochromocytoma. Red blood cells or hemoglobin casts, fat-laden foam cells, and "glitter" cells may be seen in the urine of some patients with certain types of renal disease. Also, there may be bacilluria, pyuria, impaired urinary concentration, a decreased glomerular filtration rate, and sometimes oliguria or anuria. These findings are not characteristic of patients with pheochromocytoma. Of course, it must be kept in mind that some pheochromocytomas of the urinary bladder may present with hypertensive episodes accompanied by gross or microscopic hematuria (see Chapter 4). Some pheochromocytomas may displace the ureter and interfere with its function and thereby cause pyelonephritis, pyuria, hydronephrosis, and suppression of the excretory function of the kidney (437, p. 46).

Aside from the history and physical examination, which may be extremely valuable in identifying the presence of bilateral renal disease as listed in Table 1.1, pyelography and renal biopsy may be diagnostic. Also, very marked elevations of renin or angiotensin in peripheral or renal venous blood can occur in patients with renal hypertension but practically never in those with pheochromocytoma; however, modest elevations of plasma renin in patients with pheochromocytoma have been reported (see Chapter 6, under Renin). Pheochromocytoma may compress and narrow the renal artery and may thereby contribute to the hypertension on the basis of a renin-angiotensin mechanism. Neurofibromatosis, when it coexists with pheochromocytoma, may on rare occasions be associated with vascular anomalies involving the renal arteries (see Chapter 4, under Neurofibromatosis), and this can further confuse the differential diagnosis.

Rarely, renal disease and pheochromocytoma may coincidentally coexist. A 24-year-old man with blood pressures ranging between 150/100 and 190/135 mmHg and with fairly classical symptoms of pheochromocytoma was erroneously thought to have hypertension due to renal disease, because intravenous and retrograde pyelography failed to outline the pelvis of his left kidney. Since at operation the kidney was found to be fibrosed and shrunken, it was thought to be responsible for the hypertension and was accordingly removed. During operation circulatory shock and pulmonary edema developed, and the patient died. At necropsy a pheochromocytoma of the right adrenal gland was discovered (196).

The diagnosis of pheochromocytoma, of course, must be established or excluded by the demonstration of elevated urinary or plasma catecholamines or their metabolites. It should be mentioned that by some fluorometric methods a significant degree of azotemia may interfere with the accurate quantitation of plasma catecholamines (620, 624); however, urinary catecholamines and their metabolites have not been reported elevated in renal disease in patients not harboring a pheochromocytoma. It is conceivable that the excretion of catecholamines and their metabolites may actually be decreased in some patients with pheochromocytoma in the presence of marked impairment of renal function. Although speculative, this latter statement gains some support from the special case report described at the beginning of Chapter 7.

FOCAL ARTERIAL INSUFFICIENCY OF THE BRAIN

Focal intermittent cerebral ischemia (impending stroke or cerebrovascular insufficiency) results in brief transient episodes of focal cerebral dysfunction with neurologic manifestations which depend on the area of the brain affected (976). Cerebrovascular insufficiency may occur several times daily or as rarely as once every few months. The episodes are usually quite similar and may vary in duration from 1 min to 1 hr or more (976). Most patients with focal arterial insufficiency of the brain have essential hypertension. Furthermore, during episodes of vertebral basilar artery insufficiency, the blood pressure can rise transiently and suggest a diagnosis of pheochromocytoma. The differentiation of these attacks from those in patients with pheochromocytoma should not be difficult since focal cerebral ischemia causes deficits (e.g., weakness and/or numbness of an ex-

tremity, aphasia, diplopia, ataxia, visual defects). These deficits are unilateral, which would be most unusual in a patient with pheochromocytoma. Further, some phenomena (palpitations, tachycardia, sweating, pallor) observed in patients with pheochromocytoma are usually absent in patients with focal arterial insufficiency. Although occasionally severe head pain is experienced on the side of the involved artery, headache is not usually a prominent symptom in patients with cerebrovascular insufficiency (976).

INTRACRANIAL LESIONS (WITH OR WITHOUT INCREASED INTRACRANIAL PRESSURE)

Periodic ventricular obstruction by an intracranial tumor may be accompanied by hypertension and severe headache of sudden onset. Such episodes may be precipitated by a change in body position or by the valsalva maneuver, both of which have also been noted to provoke attacks in patients with pheochromocytoma (976). Brain tumors which cause a significant increase in intracranial pressure and compromise the circulation to centers of the central nervous system involved in cardiovascular regulation may produce hypertension. The hyperglycemia and glycosuria sometimes occurring in patients with increased intracranial pressure and other brain lesions are also manifestations of activation of the sympathetic nervous system and its effect on carbohydrate metabolism.

Undoubtedly the elevation of blood pressure in association with brain tumor results from intracranial pressure effects, which activate the sympathetic nervous system and thereby cause an increased peripheral resistance. We have demonstrated that marked increases in intracranial pressure in the dog result in significant elevation of plasma catecholamines (624). However, in the patients we studied who had developed hypertension related to intracranial pressure effects from brain tumor, plasma catecholamines were usually normal, but some values were at the upper limit of normal or slightly elevated (624). Gitlow and associates reported that they have observed patients with increased intracranial pressure and coma who excreted increased quantities of catecholamines and their metabolites (358). Posterior fossa neoplasms can produce paroxysmal hypertension and increased urinary catecholamine excretion, and they may mimic the clinical features of pheochromocytoma (128, 301). Recently a patient was reported with a supratentoreal meningioma which produced clinical manifestations (e.g., headache, vomiting, episodic hypertension, and tachycardia which were responsive to α- and β-adrenergic blockade) which mimicked pheochromocytoma (339). In addition, repeated urinary VMA concentrations were elevated; however, neurologic deficits were consistent with the presence of an intracranial neoplasm.

Usually the hypertension occurring in patients with pheochromocytoma is much greater than that in patients with increased intracranial pressure. Also, in the latter condition, bradycardia is frequent, whereas in patients with pheochromocytoma bradycardia is only rarely noted, tachycardia with palpitations being much more characteristic (976). Sudden pallor and profuse diaphoresis, so frequently seen with pheochromocytoma, would be most atypical in patients with brain tumors and increased intracranial pressure.

Choked discs and hemorrhages may be seen on funduscopic examination both in patients with increased intracranial pressure and in those with pheochromocytoma; however, only in the latter condition should hypertensive retinal arteriolar changes and exudates be present. Finally, sudden astatic or "drop attacks" (momentary weakness in the legs or falling to the knees without apparent reason), or brief episodes of unconsciousness, are suggestive of periodic ventricular obstruction due to a brain tumor (976).

Neurologic deficits are frequently found in patients with a brain tumor, but are absent in patients with pheochromocytoma, unless there is a complicating cerebrovascular accident or the rare involvement of the CNS by a pheochromocytoma. Skull x-rays, EEG, computerized tomographic brain scan, pneumoencephalographic abnormalities, etc., may help establish a diagnosis of brain tumor.

A variety of other intracranial lesions will sometimes cause paroxysmal or even sustained hypertension. Raab reviewed the etiology of primary "centrogenic" hypertension (i.e.,

hypertension whose underlying pathogenic mechanism involves the brain or spinal cord) and mentioned the following causes: (1) cerebral concussion or direct brain injury, (2) cerebral hemorrhage, (3) intracranial tumors, (4) inflammatory lesions, (5) carbon monoxide poisoning, (6) sensory or emotional shocks, and (7) lesions of the spinal cord (776). Some of these conditions sould be mentioned, at least briefly, since they may occasionally evoke manifestations of "sympathetic storm" (e.g., paroxysmal hypertension, pallor or flushing, perspiration, anxiety, tachycardia, palpitations, fever, epigastric pain, headaches, hypermetabolism, hyperglycemia) which closely resemble the manifestations of pheochromocytoma.

One patient with concussion presented clinical features resembling those of diencephalic autonomic epilepsy and of pheochromocytoma. This patient experienced violent attacks (which occurred almost daily for 4 months) of systolic and diastolic hypertension, tachycardia, hyperpyrexia, hypermetabolism (BMR as high as +90 percent), profuse sweating, muscle pains, prostration, and mental confusion. Sustained rather than paroxysmal hypertension is seen more frequently after concussion, and the rise in blood pressure may be delayed for days or weeks after the injury (776, pp. 320–326). The intriguing speculation was made that a concussion 4 months previously may have been causally linked to hypertensive paroxysms in one patient with a pheochromocytoma (1007).

Mazey and coworkers have recommended caution in making the diagnosis of pheochromocytoma within several months of a cerebrovascular accident (637). This recommendation was based partly on their findings in a 38-year-old man who gave a seven-year history of hypertension, intermittent epistasis, periods of flushing and generalized sensations of warmth. Blood pressure remained labile despite antihypertensive drugs. On hospital admission he was obtunded and the blood pressure was 240/170 mmHg; a right hemiparesis was present and there was evidence of an infarct in the left temporal lobe. Urinary VMA and catecholamines were elevated. An aortogram caused elevation of the blood pressure from 140/90 to 190/150 mmHg which was lowered by intravenous phentolamine to 140/105 mmHg. Plasma epinephrine was modestly elevated in blood from the left adrenal and renal veins, although radiography suggested an enlarged right adrenal gland. Phenoxybenzamine was required to supplement antihypertensive medication to control the blood pressure. Six weeks after admission VMA and catecholamine excretion remained elevated but lower than on admission. Exploratory laparotomy failed to reveal a pheochromocytoma and, subsequently, urinary VMA and catecholamine concentrations returned to normal.

To further support their viewpoint they cited by findings reported by Meyer and associates, namely, that increased total catecholamine concentrations may occur in both peripheral venous plasma and cerebrospinal fluid in hypertensive but not normotensive patients within 2 weeks of a cerebral infarction (657a).

Temporary elevations of blood pressure and hypertensive crises have been observed after direct cerebral injury or spontaneous hemorrhages in the cerebrum or medulla oblongata. Intracranial neoplasms or cysts of the thalamus, and especially tumors involving the vasoconstrictor centers, may cause sustained or paroxysmal hypertension. Encephalitis, meningitis, and poliomyelitis (especially when it ascends to involve the medulla oblongata) may result in hypertensive episodes and occasionally marked elevations of the BMR (up to $+180$ percent in one postencephalitic case) (776, pp. 320–326).

Carbon monoxide poisoning may cause hypertension. Sensory or emotional shocks have induced hypertension in humans as well as experimental animals. Functional disorders or injuries of the spinal cord (especially transverse spinal cord lesions and tabes dorsalis), which apparently involve sympathetic centers, may also cause hypertensive syndromes that resemble manifestations of pheochromocytoma. These spinal lesions are considered in more detail below.

AUTONOMIC HYPERREFLEXIA

With transverse spinal cord lesions, adequate stimulation of any receptive surface whose afferent fibers enter the distal stump of the cord may evoke a massive response which overflows widely into regions of the spinal cord normally associated with other reflexes (203). Such mass discharges occurring spontaneously or induced by an appropriate stimulus may be due to loss of inhibiting influences from the higher centers (63), perhaps above the midbrain (203).

When the lesion is high enough (at or above the thoracic level) to include the upper thoracic segments in the distal stump of the cord, distention of a hollow viscus (e.g., the bladder or rectum) and even sudden changes in position may result in sweating (especially on the head and neck), pilomotor reaction, severe bitemporal, occipital, or frontal headache, nasal congestion, flushing of the face and neck (but pallor with vasoconstriction and decreased skin temperature elsewhere), shivering and blurring of vision, marked hypertension (sometimes up to 230 mmHg systolic and 195 mmHg diastolic), and bradycardia with a forceful and sometimes irregular beat. If the stimulus and hypertension persist, convulsions and unconsciousness may ensue (203, 977). Vasodilation, with heat and redness of the face and neck result from vasomotor reflexes induced by stimulation of intact pressor receptors in the aortic arch, carotid sinus, and cerebral vessels, caused by the hypertension. It is thought that afferent impulses (e.g., from a wall of a stretched pelvic viscus) are conveyed by sacral roots to the sacral portion of the cord. Excitation then spreads in a cephalad direction in the cord to preganglionic autonomic effector neurons in the lateral horns of the thoracolumbar segments, which results in a mass outflow from these segments and stimulation of sympathetic nerves (203).

The absence or curtailment of inhibition from higher centers and/or the spinal cord (below the level of the lesion) permits activation of the intact sympathetic chain to become excessive and to continue unimpeded (693). Although it is known that at least 85 percent of quadriplegic patients develop autonomic hyperreflexia characterized by paroxysmal hypertension (532), the remote possibility may have to be eliminated that a pheochromocytoma might coexist with spinal cord transection and account for recurrent episodes of hypertension. Excluding the presence of a functioning pheochromocytoma should not be difficult. The presence of diaphoresis and flushing only in the face and neck occurring concomitantly with pallor and evidence of vasoconstriction elsewhere is characteristic in autonomic hyperreflexia but would be totally atypical for pheochromocytoma. Furthermore, any increase of plasma catecholamines during autonomic hyperreflexia is relatively minor compared to that occurring during hypertensive crises in patients with pheochromocytoma.

In contrast to the usual responses to pharmacologic tests (see Chapter 6) observed in patients with pheochromocytoma, Sizemore found that the rapid intravenous injection of 5 to 10 mg of phentolamine in two patients with quadriplegia had no effect on an attack of autonomic hyperreflexia, and that histamine provocative tests were negative in both patients (904).

Some have reported normal concentrations of urinary catecholamines and VMA in patients with quadriplegia (904); others have found significantly elevated urinary concentrations of VMA, HVA, TMN (total metanephrines), and MHPG in quadriplegics in the chronic phase of injury (6 months or longer), but significant elevations of only HVA and MHPG during the acute phase of injury (<6 months) (692). Paroxysmal hypertension due to mass sympathetic crisis may also occur in high level paraplegics (977), and one of our colleagues at the Mayo Clinic (using a catecholamine assay modified by Manger) found elevated plasma catecholamines in a paraplegic patient during and following a hypertensive episode (820). Paraplegic patients in the chronic phase also had significant elevations in urinary concentrations of VMA, HVA, and MHPG (692). Naftchi and coworkers also have found elevations of urinary catecholamine metabolites and serum DBH during and following induction of hypertensive crises in patients with quadriplegia (693). Since DBH does not become markedly elevated in patients with pheochromocytoma (342, 587, 940a), very pronounced elevations of plasma DBH during a hypertensive crisis in a quadriplegic patient would tend to exclude pheochromocytoma as the cause of the crisis.

At the Institute of Rehabilitation Medicine we have quantitated venous plasma catecholamines in 51 patients with quadriplegia at rest, when the blood pressure was normal, and occasionally during hypertensive crises. All patients were recumbent, and samples were obtained under relatively basal conditions shortly before breakfast. Cervical spinal cord transection was physiologically complete in most but not all of these patients. It is interesting that basal blood pressures tended to be lower in quadriplegic patients than in normal subjects at rest; none of the quadriplegic patients had sustained hypertension. In the great majority of these cases plasma catecholamines (particularly norepinephrine) were slightly lower than in normal subjects and were not remarkably elevated even during the hypertensive crisis (W. M. Manger, S. W. Davis, and D. S. Chu, unpublished data). Mathias and coworkers have also found that the mean resting concentration of plasma norepinephrine was significantly less in quadriplegic patients than in normal subjects (635).

More recently, Mathias and associates reported studies on 16 quadriplegic patients with physiologically complete cervical spinal cord transection above the level of the sympathetic outflow (635a). The average systolic and diastolic pressure and the concentrations of plasma norepinephrine and epinephrine were significantly lower than the levels in normal subjects under relatively basal conditions. They also demonstrated that during paroxysmal neurogenic hypertension (induced by bladder and muscle stimulation) in the quadriplegic patients the average blood pressure rose from 109/60 to 168/87 mmHg and the average plasma norepinephrine concentration increased consistently about threefold; however, the levels of plasma norepinephrine during this type of neurogenic hypertension did not exceed the levels in normal subjects. In addition, these investigators determined that an *l*-norepinephrine infusion required to raise pressures to levels comparable to those occurring during neurogenic hypertension resulted in concentrations of plasma norepinephrine about 21 times higher than concentrations occurring during neurogenic hypertension. They therefore concluded that the neurogenic hypertension occurring in quadriplegic patients was not due to a rise in circulating catecholamines. Since hypertensive crises caused by pheochromocytomas are due, almost invariably, to markedly increased concentrations of circulating catecholamines, the differentiation between hypertensive crises caused by pheochromocytoma and those resulting from autonomic hyperreflexia should be possible by determining whether or not plasma catecholamines are markedly elevated.

DIENCEPHALIC SEIZURE (AUTONOMIC SEIZURE OR EPILEPSY; VISCERAL SEIZURES) AND SYNDROME

Diencephalic seizure is a rare form of epilepsy which may be accompanied by almost any of the manifestations observed during attacks in patients with adrenergic tumors (e.g., headache, flushing, or, rarely, pallor of the face, profuse diaphoresis, fluctuating hypertension, tachycardia, palpitations, fever, abdominal cramps, nausea, vomiting, weakness, yawning, hiccuping, paresthesia) (743). Explosive diarrhea has also been occasionally noted. A "hypertensive diencephalic syndrome" described by Page (727) also resembles diencephalic epilepsy and crises due to pheochromocytoma. In this syndrome neurovegetative and emotional outbursts occur mostly in women. It has been stated that these attacks are accompanied by a high basal metabolic rate and that they can be provoked by intradermal injections of histamine and that they are amenable to treatment with barbiturates (776, p. 274).

Symptoms and signs in these conditions apparently result from bursts of diencephalic activity, the precipitating cause of which is usually unknown (727). A marked elevation of blood pressure, severe headache, and marked variation in the duration of spells are distinctly unusual in patients with autonomic seizures. However, Engel and Aring reported the case of an 18-year-old male dwarf with recurrent autonomic seizures in whom the blood pressure varied from day to day, the highest being 220/160 mmHg and the lowest 88/40 mmHg. At autopsy this patient was found to have a small cystic lesion of the thalamus. Usually autonomic seizures are relatively benign, with a strong tendency for

symptoms to fade with the years. Engel and Aring have pointed out that a case of autonomic epilepsy with a pathologic lesion demonstrable at autopsy is a rarity (265); nevertheless, a number of cases of autonomic seizures which resulted from tumors or cysts in the region of the thalamus or hypothalamus have been reported. Penfield reported in detail a particularly interesting case of a woman with diencephalic autonomic epilepsy caused by a brain tumor which periodically obstructed the foramina of Monro and exerted pressure on the thalamus (743).

Loss of consciousness during an attack suggests an epileptic cause, but occasionally a patient with pheochromocytoma will have a seizure and lose consciousness at the height of a hypertensive attack (976). Some patients with diencephalic epilepsy occasionally experience astatic episodes (inability to stand because of muscular incoordination); such episodes have not been observed in patients with pheochromocytoma. A beneficial therapeutic response to antiepileptic agents, of course, points to autonomic seizures as the underlying etiology. The presence of electroencephalographic changes (e.g., high-voltage, slow-wave discharge) may be diagnostic, but only rarely does one have the opportunity of recording the EEG during a seizure. However, it has been pointed out that EEG abnormalities found during attacks may have no causal relationship to the seizures (976).

TOXEMIA OF PREGNANCY (PREECLAMPSIA AND ECLAMPSIA)

Late in pregnancy (usually after the 32nd week but sometimes earlier) toxemia of pregnancy may occur, manifested by edema, hypertension, and proteinuria, in that order of appearance. In severe cases, convulsions (eclampsia) may occur. Typically the edema occurs in the periorbital areas and also in the ankles and hands. Patients with toxemia of pregnancy not infrequently experience headache, midepigastric pain, and visual disturbances. Funduscopic examination frequently reveals arteriolar narrowing with an increased light reflex and tortuosity, but rarely are hemorrhages or exudates observed (265, 312). A particularly valuable biochemical alteration in patients with preeclampsia is the elevation of blood uric acid, which occurs almost invariably. The absence of hyperuricemia should make one suspicious that hypertension during pregnancy is not due to preeclampsia.

Severe diastolic hypertension, palpitations, tachycardia, diaphoresis, tremor, anxiety, pallor, and severe headaches are typical of attacks in patients with pheochromocytoma, but are not characteristic in patients with toxemia of pregnancy. Magnesium sulfate is usually effective in the management of toxemia of pregnancy but is ineffective in controlling the hypertension of patients with pheochromocytoma. *Of extreme importance is the fact that the symptoms and signs of pheochromocytoma may first become manifest during pregnancy.* The close similarity of the clinical manifestations of pheochromocytoma and toxemia of pregnancy are well known (260, 434). The seriousness of pheochromocytoma in a pregnant patient cannot be overemphasized, since without appropriate treatment these tumors may result in the death of the mother and fetus. A mortality rate of 50 percent or more has been reported in the pregnant patient with unrecognized pheochromocytoma (212) and also in the fetus (863). In addition to persistent or labile hypertension and severe headaches, patients with pheochromocytoma may have a spontaneous abortion, develop hyperpyrexia, or suffer sudden shock. It has been pointed out that shock at delivery may be mistaken for a ruptured uterus (728). It has further been emphasized that subsidence of hypertension and symptomatology following pregnancy do not exclude the presence of a pheochromocytoma (728). Pickles reported a patient who had symptoms of pheochromocytoma develop during three pregnancies and who died immediately after the third delivery (754).

Most studies, including our own observations (624), have not revealed any significant elevation of catecholamine excretion in patients with toxemia of pregnancy. As pointed out by Griffin and associates, the finding by Zuspan (1074) of elevated urinary catecholamines in some patients with eclampsia appeared related to stress (e.g., convulsion).

HYPERTENSIVE CRISES AND MONOAMINE OXIDASE INHIBITORS

Monoamine oxidase (MAO) inhibitors (e.g., tranylcypromine, phenelzine, pargyline, iproniazid, nilamide, isocarboxazid) (632) have been used in the treatment of tuberculosis and in the management of patients with hypertension or psychiatric disorders, particularly in patients who are seriously depressed.

Occasionally hypertensive attacks have occurred (with systolic pressures of 200 mmHg or more) in some of these patients receiving MAO inhibitors, and the cardiovascular manifestations may simulate hypertensive crises seen in patients with pheochromocytoma (80, 228, 632). The patients suddenly experience palpitations with, or followed by, the abrupt onset of very severe throbbing occipital or temporal headaches which become generalized. They may complain of photophobia, stiff neck, and an itchy skin. These patients may appear pale, feel flushed, frequently perspire profusely, and become nauseated and vomit. Tachycardia, pulsus bigeminus, atrial fibrillation, and reflex bradycardia associated with the blood pressure elevation have been described (632). Patients sometime develop anginal-type chest pain and acute heart failure with pulmonary edema. Unfortunately, these hypertensive crises occasionally cause subarachnoid or cerebral hemorrhage, with resultant neurologic deficits or coma and death. The length of attacks has been noted to vary from 10 min to 6 hr during which the severity of the hypertension and headaches fluctuates (80). Rarely, these attacks may be followed by hypotension (systolic blood pressure less than 90 mmHg) for 1 or 2 days (80).

It has been determined that certain foods which contain relatively high concentrations of tyramine [e.g., cheddar, camembert, stilton, and certain other cheeses, Chianti wine, sherry, beer, yeast extracts, and pickled herring (632)] are capable of provoking marked elevations of blood pressure accompanied by the symptomatology described. Even the ingestion of bean pods containing L-dopa by patients being treated with pargyline resulted in hypertensive crises due to the conversion of L-dopa to the pressor amine, dopamine (80, 632); however, no instances of adverse reactions attributable to serotonin (5-hydroxytryptamine, 5-HT) in foods eaten by patients on MAO inhibitors have been reported (632).

About 30 percent of hypertensive crises in patients taking MAO inhibitors cannot be attributed to interaction with foods ingested. Apparently some MAO inhibitors have sympathomimetic effects which become manifest once MAO is inhibited. This phenomenon has been termed "autopotentiation" of MAO inhibitors (632).

Finally, the use of various sympathomimetic agents (e.g., the amphetamines, ephedrine) by a patient being treated with MAO inhibitors can induce hypertensive crises with "devastating" headaches, palpitations with a slow or rapid pulse, profuse sweating, chest pain, pulmonary edema, nausea, vomiting, and intracranial hemorrhage (80, 632). Mydriasis, extrasystoles, pulsus bigeminus, hyperreflexia, extensor plantar responses, opisthotonus, hemiplegia, and hyperpyrexia have been reported (632). The blood pressure in one patient given *N*-methylamphetamine rose from 120/80 to 280/150 mmHg and had not returned to normal 24 hr later (632).

Interactions betwen iminodibenzyl compounds (e.g., imipramine or amitriptyline) and MAO inhibitors have resulted in marked hyperpyrexia, agitation, delirium, coma, extreme generalized muscular rigidity, and, sometimes, convulsions. Although a pressor response to interaction of MAO inhibitors and iminodibenzyl compounds has not yet been reported in humans, experimental studies have demonstrated that interaction of these compounds can produce hypertension in the rat (80).

Fundamental in establishing that a hypertensive attack is due to the interaction of MAO inhibitors and some amine is knowledge that the patient is being treated with these inhibitors. It is noteworthy that in contrast to patients with pheochromocytoma, patients developing hypertensive crises related to the use of MAO inhibitors excrete normal concentrations of catecholamines and vanillylmandelic acid (VMA) in urine collected for 24 hr following an attack (80). Presumably these hypertensive crises resulting from drug interaction are not due to the release of significant quantities of catecholamines into the circulation, as occurs in pheochromocytoma.

CARCINOID TUMORS

The carcinoid syndrome consists of a constellation of signs and symptoms which appear to result from the effects of a variety of biologically active agents elaborated by carcinoid tumors and very rarely, by carcinomas [e.g., serotonin, kallikrein (which leads to the production of bradykinin), histamine (which may be released from normal tissue stores or gastric carcinoids), 5-hydroxytryptophan, and prostaglandin].

Carcinoids usually originate in the argentaffin (Kultschintzky) cells of the gastrointestinal tract and, rarely, in the tracheobronchial tree, pancreas, gallbladder, biliary tract, parotid, ovary, testis, or thymus (766). These tumors almost always have extensively metastasized to the liver before the carcinoid syndrome appears. On the other hand, bronchial carcinoids (usually adenomas without argentaffin cells) and carcinoids in ovarian teratomas may produce similar manifestations without metastases. Carcinoids arising from the primitive foregut appear to have a particularly varied endocrine potential in that they may secrete not only serotonin, but also insulin, glucagon, gastrin, ACTH, melanophore-stimulating hormone, kinins, histamine, and even catecholamines (1012).

Recurrent episodes of flushing are characteristic. The flush may be pink, violaceous, or an intense brick-red erythema, frequently with white blotches and patchy cyanotic areas (427). This patchy "geographic" flush may involve only the face and neck but may extend to the trunk and extremities. Episodes, which frequently last only a few minutes, may occur as often as 30 times per day, and some patients may assume a chronic rubicund appearance (427). With the variant bronchial carcinoid syndrome, the flushing is usually more prolonged and may last days or weeks (650). Piloerection, sensation of warmth, tachycardia, palpitations, and mild hypotension may accompany episodes of flushing. Ultimately telangiectasia and small angioma may appear on the skin.

The following are other commonly observed manifestations of the syndrome: diarrhea (sometimes explosive), hyperperistalsis, steatorrhea, wheezing, chest discomfort, dyspnea, giddiness, anxiety, irritability, headache, tremulousness, diaphoresis, nausea, vomiting, abdominal pain, an enlarged liver (sometimes nodular), lacrimation, rhinorrhea, excess salivation, periorbital and peripheral edema, weakness, debility, oliguria, temperature elevations, and weight loss. Hyperglycemia has also been reported (650). Cushing's syndrome and hyperpigmentation have been observed, though rarely, in association with the carcinoid syndrome; this association suggests that these tumors may secrete adrenocorticotropic and melanocyte-stimulating peptide hormones (650).

With a prolonged history of the carcinoid syndrome, there may appear pellagrous skin lesions and dementia (due to niacin deficiency), malnutrition, hypoalbuminemia, and cardiac lesions (consisting of endocardial fibrosis and valvular damage). When secretions from carcinoid tumors drain into the right side of the heart, tricuspid stenosis and/or insufficiency and/or pulmonic stenosis may occur. With drainage from the tumor into the left side of the heart, stenosis and/or insufficiency of the mitral and/or aortic valves have been reported. These valvular lesions frequently lead to right- or left-sided heart failure, with the usual manifestations. Tricuspid insufficiency is usually accompanied by marked venous distention in the neck with a large V wave and systolic liver pulsations.

Attacks of the carcinoid syndrome occur spontaneously but may sometimes be precipitated by emotion, physical exertion, eating, tea, alcohol, defecation, manipulation of the tumor, or by administration of insulin, lysergic acid diethylamide, or catecholamines.

Because of the episodic nature of the carcinoid syndrome, and because of the similarity of many of the manifestations caused both by this tumor and by pheochromocytoma, some confusion in the differential diagnosis may occur. However, flushing is only rarely seen in patients with pheochromocytoma and is always very brief. Furthermore, explosive diarrhea, steatorrhea, wheezing, telangiectasia, pellagrous skin changes, and valvular heart lesions occur in patients with carcinoid tumors but do not result from secretions of a pheochromocytoma.

Although the blood pressure is usually normal or hypotensive during the carcinoid syndrome, marked increases in blood pressure have, rarely, been reported during spontaneous attacks (1, 67) or during an episode pre-cipitated by the intravenous injection of 10 μg of epinephrine (806). A review of the literature in 1968 revealed that at least 22 patients with the carcinoid syndrome had been reported to have had sustained or episodic hypertension (806). Also, in patients with gastrointestinal carcinoids plus renal disease, the incidence of sustained hypertension is significantly greater than would be expected in renal disease alone, suggesting the possibility of potentiation of renal hypertension by serotonin (875).

There have been reports of patients with the carcinoid syndrome who had a modest elevation of urinary catecholamines or VMA (358, 360, 650, 949); however, we and others have not found the plasma catecholamines or urinary VMA to be elevated in patients with the carcinoid syndrome (427, 621). It is, of course, conceivable that in the presence of a significant *hypotensive* reaction in the carcinoid syndrome, plasma catecholamines may become elevated through reflex activation of the sympathoadrenal system.

The diagnosis of the carcinoid syndrome when suggested clinically can be established by biopsy and by the presence of hyperserotonemia and increased urinary excretion of 5-hydroxyindole acetic acid (5-HIAA), a metabolite of serotonin.

Intravenous administration of small doses of epinephrine (5 μg) (or norepinephrine), which will characteristically induce flushing in patients with the carcinoid syndrome, has been used diagnostically. We have also noted that in a patient with this tumor intravenous histamine (0.05 mg) provoked a flush suggestive of the carcinoid syndrome and caused hyperserotonemia without any remarkable change in blood pressure (205).

In contrast, patients with pheochromocytoma show no remarkable response to the administration of catecholamines, whereas histamine very frequently provokes an attack of characteristic symptoms and marked hypertension. It is noteworthy that carcinoid associated with malignant pheochromocytoma and hypotensive crises has been reported (41).

HYPOGLYCEMIA

Hypoglycemia (i.e., blood glucose less than 50 mg/dl) usually causes CNS abnormalities and adrenergic discharge. Evidence of CNS dysfunction is frequently manifest by confusion, lethargy, inappropriate affect, hallucinations, focal signs, incoordination, unsteadiness of gait, tonic spasms, inconjugate ocular deviation, diplopia, convulsions, and coma. Hypothermia may occur in patients during hypoglycemia. The electroencephalogram may reveal slow regular waves during the period of hypoglycemia. Furthermore, with prolonged hypoglycemia, permanent cortical damage may occur. Sympathoadrenal discharge occurs when the development of hypoglycemia is rapid and is evidenced by anxiety, tremulousness, tachycardia or bradycardia, palpitations, pallor, sweating, and a transient rise in blood pressure. Patients may feel faint and complain of nausea and, rarely, vomit; however, inappropriate hunger is frequently experienced, which may result in weight gain.

Although headaches are often experienced during hypoglycemia, the severe headaches commonly experienced by patients with pheochromocytoma are not a feature of low blood glucose. Furthermore, patients with chromaffin tumors are normoglycemic or hyperglycemic. A rapid and dramatic reversal of symptoms due to hypoglycemia occurs after administration of glucose or glucagon, whereas in patients with pheochromocytoma there is no beneficial therapeutic effect noted following administration of glucose. Glucagon, which is sometimes used diagnostically to precipitate attacks in patients with pheochromocytoma, will usually aggravate symptoms in these patients by increasing liberation of catecholamines from the tumor. The diagnosis of hypoglycemia is, of course, established by the demonstration of a low blood glucose, which in patients with spontaneous hypoglycemia may be induced by prolonged fasting (sometimes up to 72 hr), or, in patients with functional hypoglycemia, by ingestion of carbohydrate (e.g., 5 hr after ingesting 100 g of glucose). In patients with recurrent hypoglycemia due to an insulinoma, hypoglycemia may also be precipitated by the intravenous administration of 1 g of tolbutamide. Patients with insulin-secreting tumors sometimes eat excessively and gain weight.

It is noteworthy that, toward the end of an attack of hypoglycemia, convulsions may cause the blood glucose to rise to normal levels (92).

Finally, it should be mentioned that plasma catecholamines are significantly increased in response to hypoglycemia (132, 382), which as we have shown apparently activates the sympathoadrenal system by its effect on the medulla oblongata (132). An elevation of catecholamines ,and/or their metabolites in plasma or urine could confuse the differential diagnosis between hypoglycemia and pheochromocytoma.

MASTOCYTOSIS

Mastocytosis has been classified as "cutaneous mastocytosis" (urticaria pigmentosa) and "systemic mastocytosis." Characteristic skin lesions (e.g., those which redden and urticate with rubbing or other irritation) may make the diagnosis relatively simple. However, skin lesions may be absent in systemic mastocytosis, and then the symptomatology may become a diagnostic challenge.

In cutaneous macular or maculopapular urticaria pigmentosa, pruritus is frequently the only symptom; however, in both cutaneous and systemic mastocytosis there may be episodic flushing, sense of warmth, tachycardia, palpitations, apprehension, irritability, headache, tinnitus, generalized weakness, dyspnea, abdominal pain, nausea, vomiting, weight loss, and sometimes hyperpyrexia (834). Attacks of flushing may occur spontaneously but sometimes are provoked by irritation of the skin, a change in temperature [e.g., a hot bath or application of cold (carbon dioxide) to the skin], anxiety, ingestion of alcohol or spicy foods, use of aspirin, codeine, or polymixin B, or by exercise (834).

Similarities in the symptomatology of patients with mastocytosis or pheochromocytoma are remarkable; however, differentiation should not be difficult, since hypertension is not produced during attacks in patients with mastocytosis. On the contrary, hypotension and shock with pale, cold, clammy extremities may occur due to liberation of histamine from mast cells. Hepatomegaly and splenomegaly have been noted in about 12 percent of patients with mastocytosis, and edema of the face, hands, and ankles sometimes occurs.

Flushing is rare in patients with pheochromocytoma and is brief in duration. On the other hand, rather characteristic flushing episodes have been reported in more than one-third of patients with cutaneous or systemic mastocytosis. Usually these episodes, which are associated with severe pruritus, last for 15 to 30 min, although sometimes they persist for several hours (834). The flush, typically a uniform pink or bright red (without any cyanotic element), primarily involves the face and upper chest but may extend to the rest of the trunk and limbs.

The diagnosis of mastocytosis is based on the presence of characteristic skin lesions and/or the demonstration of excessive numbers of mast cells in biopsy specimens, and/or increased concentrations of histamine and sometimes pathologic amounts of acid mucopolysaccharides in the urine.

FAMILIAL DYSAUTONOMIA (RILEY-DAY SYNDROME)

Dysautonomia is a familial disease with manifestations of disturbance of the central nervous system and impaired autonomic function. Of unknown etiology, it is a disease which occurs almost exclusively in Ashkenazi Jews and is probably the expression of an autosomal recessive gene.

Anxiety, transient episodes of hypertension (especially precipitated by excitement), postural hypotension, and excessive perspiration are almost constant findings, and sometimes gagging, vomiting, abdominal pain, and constipation occur. Hence, it is not surprising that dysautonomia has ben mistakenly diagnosed as pheochromocytoma. Riley reported that five older children with dysautonomia had undergone laparotomy (with negative adrenal exploration) since their symptoms were thought to be due to catecholamine release from pheochromocytoma (794).

If one is aware of the array of unusual signs characteristic of patients with dysautonomia, the diagnosis can be made on a clinical basis and the differentiation from a diagnosis of pheochromocytoma should be simple. For example, in addition to the findings mentioned above, the following signs are almost invariably present in dysautonomia: reduced lacrimation, disturbed swallowing, poor motor coordination, dysarthria, relative indifference to pain, corneal anesthesia, and markedly decreased taste discrimination with

absence of fungiform papillae (probably pathognomonic). Other signs frequently seen are hyporeflexia, impaired temperature regulation, erythematous blotches on the skin, impaired growth, decreased intellectual capacity, irascible disposition, and electroencephalographic abnormalities (794).

Patients with dysautonomia have been found to have a reduced VMA excretion (204), and an increased pressor responsiveness to infusion of norepinephrine has also been noted (914). These two findings have been interpreted as indicating a deficiency of catecholamines and a reduced sympathetic nervous system activity. In addition, patients with dysautonomia appear to be hyperresponsive to methacholine, which suggests some disturbance in the parasympathetic nervous system (204).

ACRODYNIA ("PINK DISEASE")

Acrodynia, a disease of infants and young children which usually results from mercury poisoning, is frequently accompanied by abdominal pain, hypertension, tachycardia, profuse sweating, muscular weakness, paresthesias, psychic instability, and hyperglycemia (211, 450). However, typically these patients develop erythema of their fingers, toes, nose, and buttocks, and there may be desquamation of the palms and soles, photophobia, irritability, insomnia, stomatitis, and loss of teeth (318). Prolonged exposure to mercury may result in a characteristic brown reflex from the anterior lens capsule as seen by the slit-lamp; with a history of mercury exposure and the presence of increased levels of mercury in the urine, there should be no difficulty in differentiating acrodynia from pheochromocytoma. Nonetheless, the similarity between the manifestations of this tumor and acrodynia has been stressed, and a patient with pheochromocytoma may, though rarely, develop a bright pink color of the face, hands, and feet during a paroxysmal attack (464). It is particularly noteworthy that some patients with acrodynia have slight elevations of urinary catecholamines and VMA (450, 795). The finding of hyperplasia of the chromaffin system in acrodynia (Stolz, cited in 450) is particularly intriguing.

NEUROBLASTOMA, GANGLIONEUROBLASTOMA, AND GANGLIONEUROMA

Neuroblastoma (sympathoblastoma), which arises from immature and undifferentiated neuroblasts of neural crest ectoderm, is one of the commonest malignancies of infancy and early childhood, usually occurring in patients less than 5 years of age. Occasionally the diagnosis is made in the second decade of life. Most commonly the adrenal gland is the site of origin of this tumor and, rarely, it may occur bilaterally. It may arise elsewhere in the abdomen and pelvis, and in the chest, neck, or head (759, p. 3). It may occur in the adrenal glands or wherever sympathetic nervous tissue is located. Frequently these are functioning tumors which elaborate dopa, dopamine, and norepinephrine and, rarely, produce paroxysmal attacks with tachycardia, palpitations, diaphoresis, pallor, flushing, hypertension, irritability, polyuria, and polydipsia (759, p. 8; 998). In one series of patients with neuroblastoma, hypertension was found in about half of the cases examined (998). As mentioned earlier (see Chapter 4, under Pregnancy in Pheochromocytoma), neuroblastoma may occur in the fetus and, rarely, cause manifestations of excess circulating catecholamines in the mother (759, p. 5; 1000). In addition, there may be abdominal discomfort, distention, and a mass (sometimes with gastrointestinal and genitourinary symptoms due to compression of adjacent structures), anorexia, weight loss, metastatic subcutaneous nodules [sometimes with blanching in and around these lesions, due probably to the presence of vasoconstricting catecholamines (759, p. 6)], periorbital ecchymoses, unilateral proptosis, periorbital swelling, fever, bone or joint pain, weakness or paralysis of the lower extremities (if the tumor invades the extradural space and exerts pressure around the spinal cord), paresthesias, sensory loss, and opsoclonus (due to acute cerebellar encephalopathy) (759, p. 61; 998). Chronic diarrhea is seldom seen in neuroblastoma (998); however, a child may occasionally present with the "celiac triad": diarrhea, weight loss, and enlargement of the abdomen (759, p. 81). Anemia and x-ray evidence of metastases are sometimes present. Rarely,

cases of neuroblastoma (or ganglioneuroma) have been reported to coexist with neurofibromatosis (759, pp. 227–228). Cushing's syndrome also, on rare occasions, becomes manifest (759, p. 80).

In most cases, increased urinary excretion of dopa, dopamine, norepinephrine, normetanephrine, VMA, and HVA is found (998, 999). Increased concentrations of 3-methyl-4-hydroxyphenylalanine (365) and dihydroxyphenylacetic acid have also been reported in the urine of patients with neuroblastoma (926, 950). One patient was reported who was thought to have an epinephrine-secreting neuroblastoma (634); however, since epinephrine excretion is almost always normal in patients with neuroblastoma, an increased excretion of this catecholamine should be of value in differentiating neuroblastoma from pheochromocytoma.

In contrast, patients with pheochromocytoma usually excrete only increased quantities of norepinephrine and/or epinephrine, normetanephrine and/or metanephrine, and VMA. Only rarely are excessive amounts of dopa and dopamine excreted by patients with pheochromocytoma (16, 91, 586, 644, 888, 926, 1014); therefore, the presence of these substances and HVA in the urine of an infant or child strongly suggests and is almost diagnostic for the presence of a tumor originating from neuroblasts or sympathetic ganglia. Of 113 patients with untreated neuroblastoma, Gitlow and coworkers found significant elevations in the urine of MHPG, VMA, HVA, and total metanephrines, respectively, in 97, 96, 93, and 86 percent of patients. Ninety-seven percent of the patients excreted abnormal quantities of at least three of these catabolites, whereas less than 2 percent failed to excrete abnormal quantities of at least one of these catabolites (759, p. 133).

More recently, Goldstein and coworkers have shown that dopamine β-hydroxylase is significantly increased in the serum of patients with neuroblastoma (383). In contrast DBH in the serum of patients with pheochromocytoma is either not elevated (342) or only modestly elevated in some patients with this tumor (587). Granules associated with catecholamine production are present in neuroblastoma but are generally smaller and less numerous than in pheochromocytoma (90,

669). Why neuroblastomas frequently elaborate dopa and dopamine in addition to norepinephrine remains unexplained.

Although urinary cystathionine has been reported to be elevated in 81 percent of patients with progressive neuroblastoma (433), the significance of this finding and its diagnostic value are uncertain and remain to be clarified. Elevation of cystathionine may occur with a variety of neoplasms and is therefore not specific for neuroblastoma. Bone marrow aspiration and examination for neuroblastoma cells is positive in about 50 percent of cases at the time of diagnosis. Tumor biopsy can, of course, establish the diagnosis.

Ganglioneuroblastoma is a malignant tumor composed of immature neuroblasts and mature ganglion cells in varying proportions. This tumor is capable of producing catecholamines; however, symptomatology related to the pressor amines is rarely evident (998), although hypertension and profuse sweating have been reported (808). Chronic diarrhea with accompanying hypokalemia, failure to thrive, abdominal distention, flushing, and skin rash occur in some patients. The cause of the diarrhea remains unexplained but may be related to the elaboration of prostaglandin

by these tumors (844). Patients with ganglioneuroblastoma may excrete increased quantities of dopa, dopamine, norepinephrine, and their metabolites, as in neuroblastoma (808, 998, 999). Cushing's syndrome, or, rarely, virilization, has been observed in patients with ganglioneuroblastoma (759, p. 80).

Ganglioneuroma usually occurs in older children and adults and arises from the thoracic and lumbar sympathetic trunks. Composed of mature ganglion cells, it is a benign tumor which occasionally is accompanied by the chronic diarrhea syndrome noted in patients with ganglioneuroblastoma (998). Occasionally hypertension, diaphoresis, polyuria, and polydipsia occur (808), and increased excretion of dopamine, norepinephrine, VMA, and HVA have been found in patients with ganglioneuroma (365, 396, 808, 926). A patient with ganglioneuroma and Cushing's syndrome has also been reported (808). Voorhess was unable to demonstrate any abnormality of catecholamine metabolism in patients with ganglioneuroma unless associated with chronic diarrhea (998). It is noteworthy that one tumor has been described which was a mixed pheochromocytoma-ganglioneuroma (178). The content of catecholamines, dopa,

Table 5.2 *Content of Catecholamines and Related Compounds in Tissue of Neuroblastomas and Ganglioneuromas (µg/g tissue)[a,b]*

Authors	No. of cases	NE	E	Dopa	Dopamine	VMA	HVA
Neuroblastoma							
Page and Jacoby (729)	1	<1	0	—	1	0.56	—
Gjessing (365)	3	6–25	10–78	—	6–40	—	—
Greer et al. (399)	5	0.01–2.4	0.01–1.1	0.05–0.6	0.02–2.2	—	—
Käser (497)	5	0.2–4	0 (3) –0.07	—	0.04–1	—	—
Anton et al. (16)	1	2.0	1.1	0.05	0.3	—	—
Cameron et al. (127)	1	557	151	—	10.5	—	—
Bohuon and Guerinot (87)	11	0.01–10	0 (1) –11	0 (3) –3	0 (6) –0.5	—	—
Voorhees (998)	10	0.13–276	0 (2) –3.3	—	0 (7) –1.3	0 (2) –0.5	0 (3) –2.0
Silverman et al. (896)	5	[<0.1–6.5]		—	0.2–16.0	—	—
Hintersberger et al. (449)	4	[0.34–11.6]		—	0 (1) –6.4	2.9–3.6	0.8 (1)
Ganglioneuroma							
Greenberg and Gardner (396)	1	8.6	0.07	—	2.1	—	—
Rosenstein and Engelman (808)	1	10.4	—	0.72	1.83	—	—
Hintersberger et al. (449)	2	[6.3–30.0]		—	0.8–12.4	—	0.1
Rosenthal et al. (810)	1	95.0	0	—	3.0	—	—

[a] Adapted from Winkler, H. and Smith, A. D. Chap. 20. Pheochromocytomas and other catecholamine producing tumors. *In: Catecholamines.* Courtesy of Springer-Verlag, 1972, p. 918.

[b] Abbreviations: E = epinephrine; NE = norepinephrine; dopa = dihydroxyphenylalanine; VMA = vanilmandelic acid; HVA = homovanillic acid. Parentheses adjacent to concentrations () = number of observations. Brackets [ ] = range of total concentration of NE plus E.

Table 5.3 *Urinary Excretion of Catecholamines and Metabolites in Children with Neuroblastoma and Ganglioneuroma*[a,b]

Reference	No. of cases	No. in which determination was abnormal/No. in which determination was performed					
		Dopa	Dopamine	HVA	NE	NMN	VMA
Williams et al. (1042)	79	2/2	16/22	32/43	18/23	12/19	58/75
Studnitz et al. (950)	21	18/21	20/21	9/17	19/21	20/21	21/21
	100	20/23 (87%)	36/43 (84%)	41/60 (68%)	37/44 (84%)	32/40 (80%)	79/96 (82%)

[a] From Crout, J. R. Chap. I. Catecholamine metabolism in pheochromocytoma and essential hypertension. *In: Hormones and Hypertension.* Springfield. Courtesy of C. C. Thomas, 1966, p. 31.

[b] Abbreviations: Dopa = dihydroxyphenylalanine; HVA = homovanillic acid; NE = norepinephrine; NMN = normetanephrine; VMA = vanillylmandelic acid.

and their metabolites in neuroblastomas and ganglioneuromas as reported by a number of investigators is recorded in Table 5.2. The urinary excretion of these substances has also been quantitated by Williams and coworkers, and Studnitz and associates in 100 children (see Table 5.3). In contrast to the typical excretion patterns (namely, norepinephrine and epinephrine and their metabolites) of patients with pheochromocytoma, it is evident that a high percentage of patients harboring a neuroblastoma or ganglioneuroma excrete significant concentrations of dopa, dopamine, and homovanillic acid.

Differentiating tumors arising from neuroblasts and sympathetic ganglion cells from pheochromocytoma is primarily dependent on demonstrating the differences in excretion patterns of catecholamines and their metabolites mentioned previously. The history of chronic diarrhea in addition to the abnormal catecholamine metabolism suggests a neural crest tumor other than pheochromocytoma. Rarely, however, the diagnosis may be made only on laparotomy and biopsy. It is noteworthy that two patients with pheochromocytoma and associated ganglioneuroma have been reported (1070).

ACUTE INFECTIOUS DISEASE

Rarely, manifestations in a patient with pheochromocytoma may suggest an infectious process, particularly when fever, tachycardia, and leukocytosis are prominent manifestations. In one patient seen at Columbia Medical Center the presence of rheumatic fever was considered a possibility before the correct diagnosis of pheochromocytoma was established.

An example of pheochromocytoma masquerading as an overwhelming infection was reported by Fred and associates (326). They described a 62-year-old woman who experienced abdominal pains, vomiting, fever (up to 106.6°F on one occasion), a nonproductive cough, tachypnea, tachycardia, and hypotension followed by paroxysmal hypertension. The patient also developed a prominent systolic murmur, a marked leukocytosis (ranging between 14,500 and 23,600), and azotemia. The diagnostic possibilities considered were gram-negative bacteremia, pneumonia, multiple pulmonary emboli, and bacterial endocarditis. An unusual complication during the patient's hospital course was the development of a markedly distended cecum which required decompression. The patient died several days later and an epinephrine-secreting pheochromocytoma of the right adrenal gland was found at necropsy.

Fred and coworkers pointed out the striking similarity of the findings in their patient to those in the patient described by Hamrin (417). The patient of Hamrin had epigastric cramps, vomiting, fever (up to 104.9°F), tachycardia, leukocytosis, and azotemia. The blood pressure was initially normotensive, but she developed profound shock which responded to norepinephrine infusion, hydrocortisone, antibiotics, and fluid replacement. Subsequently, a tender mass, thought to be a perinephric abscess at the upper pole of the right kidney, was removed and found to be a pheochromocytoma which contained predominantly epinephrine.

RARE CAUSES OF PAROXYSMAL HYPERTENSION

In reviewing the literature on paroxysmal hypertension up to 1946 (including two monographs on the subject) Bauer and Belt reported that crises of hypertension had been observed in the following conditions: eclampsia, lead poisoning, essential hypertension, nephritis, aortitis, various diseases of the nervous system (e.g., epilepsy, tabes, traumatic or vascular damage to the brain, meningitis, vagus nerve compression, sciatic neuritis, disease of the gasserian ganglion), typhoid fever, and other acute infections and some allergic reactions (47). It has also been reported that periarteritis nodosa and thyroid crisis may cause paroxysmal hypertension (466). One patient with meningococcic meningitis had paroxysmal elevations of systolic blood pressure from 130 mmHg to 240 mmHg. Demole and Rutishauser described an unusual case of paroxysmal hypertension accompanied by hyperglycemia in a patient suffering from tuberculous destruction of the left adrenal gland. Transfusion of blood taken from this patient during a hypertensive crisis markedly raised a recipient's blood pressure and blood sugar; transfusion of blood obtained in the absence of a hypertensive crisis failed to cause this pressor rise (222). Burak and coworkers reported a patient with an adrenocortical adenoma which caused clinical manifestations simulating pheochromocytoma (112). Another patient was reported by Bauer and Belt to have had repeated elevations of blood pressure (160/90 to 280/140 mmHg) following consumption of a glass of Madeira wine. This response was considered an allergic reaction. Whether a pressor agent such as tyramine may have been implicated in this hypersensitive reaction to Madeira wine is uncertain.

Several unusual conditions which may mimic manifestations found in patients with pheochromocytoma are worth discussing since these could conceivably mislead the physician. Therefore, for completeness, the following causes of paroxysmal hypertension have been included in the differential diagnosis; however, only rarely should any of these conditions be confused with pheochromocytoma.

ACUTE INTERMITTENT PORPHYRIA

Acute intermittent porphyria is frequently accompanied by recurrent attacks of moderate or severe abdominal pain, gastrointestinal disturbances, and neurologic dysfunction. Frequently transient hypertension (sometimes with spasm of retinal arteries) (867), sinus tachycardia (with nonspecific ECG abnormalities), postural hypotension, nervousness, vomiting, fever, constipation, and epileptic seizures may occur and suggest the diagnosis of pheochromocytoma. However, manifestations of peripheral (primarily motor) and/or central nervous system involvement, personality changes, psychoses, and reversible pigmentation of exposed parts of the body support the diagnosis of acute porphyria.

Of some value in the diagnosis of acute porphyria is that it rarely occurs before puberty, is very rarely seen in blacks, and the attack rarely lasts less than 48 hr. In addition, attacks may be correlated with the menstrual cycle or may sometimes be precipitated by barbiturates, sulfonamides, contraceptive pills, and griseofulvin (867). Diagnosis of acute porphyria is also suggested if urine darkens when it is left standing, due to conversion of porphobilinogen and other precursors to porphyrin and porphobilin, a dark brown pigment (867). Diagnosis can be confirmed by excess quantities of porphobilinogen and aminolevulinic acid in the urine; however, lead intoxication also frequently causes increased excretion of aminolevulinic acid (867).

It is noteworthy that markedly increased concentrations of urinary catecholamines have been reported in some patients with attacks of acute intermittent porphyria accompanied by hypertension and tachycardia (25). Since increased excretion of catecholamines appears to result from increased sympathoadrenal activity, which may account for some of the clinical manifestations, it has been suggested that treatment of this disorder include adrenergic blocking drugs (25).

Conceivably, the differential diagnosis between acute intermittent porphyria and pheochromocytoma with paroxysmal hypertension might be confusing, and the importance of examining the urine for excess concentrations of porphobilinogen and aminolevulinic acid must be recalled.

ACUTE OR CHRONIC LEAD POISONING

Acute or chronic lead poisoning may cause paroxysmal hypertension in addition to gastrointestinal disturbances (colicky abdominal pains, nausea, vomiting, constipation), neuromuscular manifestations (muscular soreness, weakness, hypertonus, paralysis, wrist drop, etc., without sensory deficits), and symptoms and signs of encephalopathy (headache, insomnia, irritability, mania, delirium, confusion, projectile vomiting, lethargy, neurologic manifestations of cerebral and cerebellar dysfunction, blindness, deafness, convulsions, coma, and sometimes death) (318). The presence of a characteristic blue-black lead line along the gingival margin of the teeth and stippling of the retina adjacent to the optic disc are of diagnostic value when present. Increased intracranial pressure may occur and accounts for some of the manifestations of encephalopathy; however, it has been pointed out that when the onset is very acute (318) the optic discs may not reveal papilledema.

The presence of lead poisoning is confirmed by elevated lead content in blood and urine; however, the diagnosis of tetraethyl lead intoxication is based on a history of exposure and an increased lead content in the urine, since blood levels are usually normal (318). With a careful history, physical examination, and appropriate laboratory tests, differentiation of lead intoxication from pheochromocytoma should not be difficult. It is interesting that Bernal demonstrated a pressor effect in the recipient when, during a paroxysm of hypertension, 300 ml of blood were taken from a patient with chronic lead poisoning and transfused into a normal subject; no pressor effect occurred when the blood transfused was obtained from normal subjects or from the patient with lead poisoning during a normotensive period (65). Furthermore, it has recently been found that significantly increased urinary excretion of HVA and VMA may occur with increased lead absorption—even in asymptomatic or mildly symptomatic persons. Apparently, increased concentrations of lead in non-osseous tissues are associated with an altered catecholamine metabolism (895).

TABETIC CRISIS IN TABES DORSALIS

Paroxysmal elevations of blood pressure in patients with tabes dorsalis may be marked. One patient had a systolic pressure which rose from 90 mmHg to 235 mmHg during a crisis (828), and another patient's blood pressure rose from normotensive levels to as high as 300/190 mmHg (58). It has been reported that some patients with tabes dorsalis may have paroxysmal hypertension (apparently a disturbance of the autonomic nervous system) and symptoms so suggestive of pheochromocytoma that they have been subjected to surgical exploration (58, 828); tumors were not found in three such patients.

The differentiation of paroxysmal hypertension occurring during a tabetic crisis from that due to pheochromocytoma should be no problem today with the availability of biochemical tests to measure the catecholamines or their metabolites. A tabetic crisis is usually characterized by lightning pains which vary from mild to excruciating, and involve the extremities, especially the legs; however, visceral (gastric) crises are also relatively common and are frequently associated with retching and vomiting. Occasionally palpitations, weakness, pallor, and profuse sweating occur, and one patient had four episodes of convulsions, each followed by unconsciousness (58).

In two cases, hypertension accompanied by typical symptoms of a gastric crisis has been precipitated by the injection of epinephrine; in one patient the attack lasted 6 days and in the other patient it subsided after 48 hr (58). Use of a laxative containing cascara was thought to precipitate crises of hypertension, pallor, palpitations, diaphoresis, nausea, and vomiting. Patients with tabes dorsalis may have hypertensive episodes without any associated symptoms. One patient had both paroxysmal hypertension and postural hypotension.

It is noteworthy that the blood glucose, which was determined during a hypertensive crisis, was normal; furthermore, the histamine provocative test for pheochromocytoma has been uniformly negative in patients with tabes.

Loss or diminution of position and vibratory sensation occur in almost every case, and pupillary abnormalities, including miosis with poor or absent responsiveness to light but retained accommodation (Argyll-Robertson pupils), are usually present. One pupil may be larger and sluggishly reactive to light, whereas the other pupil may be miotic and unreactive to light. During a hypertensive crisis in one patient, the Argyll-Robertson pupils became widely dilated but were still unreactive to light (58). Ataxia, impaired gait with a broad base and slapping quality, areas of hypalgesia, diminution of deep pain sensation, impaired function of the urinary bladder (overflow incontinence) and bowel (constipation), paresthesias, and sexual impotence are present in many patients with tabes dorsalis. Occasionally Charcot's arthropathy occurs. The knee jerks are often hypoactive and the ankle jerks are nearly always absent.

Strongly positive serologic tests for syphilis are present in the early stages of tabes dorsalis, but late in this disease (especially if antisyphilitic treatment has been administered) serologic tests on both blood · and cerebrospinal fluid may be negative; not infrequently the serology is negative on blood and positive on cerebrospinal fluid.

ACUTE ENCEPHALITIS

Acute encephalitis may be accompanied by transient hypertension (sometimes paroxysmal), in addition to headache, nausea, vomiting, and seizures, such as may occur in patients with pheochromocytoma. However, high fever with meningeal signs, confusion, delirium, and signs of diffuse central nervous system dysfunction are typical findings in acute encephalitis but do not occur in patients with uncomplicated pheochromocytoma. If papilledema occurs, it is not accompanied by evidence of vasospastic and/or hypertensive retinopathy, which may occur in patients with pheochromocytoma. Focal or generalized slowing of EEG waves, increased uptake of radioactive isotopes by some areas of the brain, and displacement of the swollen brain on pneumographic or arteriographic studies may occur in acute encephalitis but are not found in patients with pheochromocytoma. Characteristic increases in white cells, and in proteins in the cerebrospinal fluid, aid in establishing the diagnosis of encephalitis.

CLONIDINE WITHDRAWAL

Marked elevations of blood pressure (e.g., 149/103 to 216/161 mmHg) have been noted in some patients with essential hypertension, usually on an average of 12 hr following *withdrawal from relatively large doses of clonidine (Catapres, Catapresan) medication* (418). Dr. Sibly Hoobler stated that in his experience and that of his colleagues the withdrawal reaction occurred only in patients receiving 1.2 mg (or more) of clonidine per day (personal communication from Dr. S. Hoobler, Emeritus Professor of Medicine, University of Michigan). Tremor, restlessness, insomnia, and nausea or anorexia developed in all those experiencing this blood pressure crisis. In addition, the patients frequently complained of severe headaches, and sometimes had vivid dreams, increased salivation, hiccups, and abdominal and muscle pains. We know of several patients who developed acute encephalopathy and expired following abrupt withdrawal of clonidine. Symptomatology and an elevation of urinary and plasma catecholamines indicated increased sympathetic discharge which could be controlled by combined α- and β-receptor blockade with phentolamine and propranolol, respectively (418).

HYPOVOLEMIA WITH INAPPROPRIATE REFLEX VASOCONSTRICTION

Paroxysmal hypertension with hypovolemia has been described by Cohn in three adult males (two black and one white) (163). When admitted to the hospital these patients had extreme blood pressure elevations with marked diaphoresis. In one patient the blood pressure was unobtainable and peripheral pulses were barely palpable, though femoral pulses were strong. Absence of Korotkoff sounds in this latter patient was thought to have resulted from intense peripheral vasoconstriction (164).

Clinical and laboratory manifestations such as apprehension, headache, nausea, vomiting, fever, marked skin vasoconstriction, tachycardia, seizures, shock, hemoconcentration, reduced plasma volume, and hyperglycemia in some of these patients suggested the diagnosis of pheochromocytoma. Also, pharmacologic testing with phentolamine was positive for the presence of this tumor, although this test may have been falsely positive in two of the patients because of interfering medication with Reserpine.

Repeated 24-hr urinary excretion of VMA and provocative tests with histamine and/or tyramine and x-ray studies were normal in the patients tested. Furthermore, the blood pressure returned to normal levels in two of these patients; only the remaining patient required chronic antihypertensive medication.

Vascular hyperresponsiveness to noxious stimuli and to infusions of norepinephrine was demonstrated in these three patients, and it was believed that, when hypertensive, they were in a state characterized by hypovolemia and inappropriately severe reflex vasoconstriction (163).

FIBROSARCOMA OF THE PULMONARY ARTERY

Fibrosarcoma of the pulmonary artery, which is itself an extreme rarity, has been reported masquerading as a pheochromocytoma (1056). A normotensive patient was reported who experienced episodic palpitations, dyspnea, and tachycardia associated with elevations of the blood pressure up to 180/130 mmHg, which could be promptly reduced to normal levels (120/70 mmHg) by administration of phentolamine. These clinical manifestations and response to phentolamine were strongly suggestive of pheochromocytoma.

A pressor substance was demonstrated in the urine of this patient but was not identified. Whether anoxia resulting from a compromised pulmonary circulation may have activated the sympathoadrenal system and released catecholamines into the circulation was not known. Conceivably the fibrosarcoma might have elaborated a pressor substance, or the tumor might have produced an insulin-like substance which induced hypoglycemia, thereby activating the sympathoadrenal system. Theoretically, any tumor capable of inducing hypoglycemia might cause manifestations suggesting catecholamine liberation.

PORK INGESTION

Very rarely, a most exotic form of hypertension is observed in patients ingesting pork (113). The substance in pork responsible for elevation of blood pressure, which may occur acutely, in combination with headaches of varying severity, giddiness, scotomatas, dyspepsia, palpitations and tinnitus, remains unknown. Burch points out that "some people are so sensitive to pork that mere traces of bacon grease or of pork seasoning in food are sufficient to increase arterial blood pressure to dangerous levels" (113). The history of members of one family as recorded by Burch is particularly instructive:

The history of Mrs. V. S., a 42-year-old Negro woman, illustrates the relation of pork intake to arterial hypertension. This patient develops a rather sudden elevation in arterial blood pressure when she eats pork chops (her favorite meat), develops a "splitting" and "unbearable" headache, blurring of vision, marked giddiness, pounding of her heart, tinnitus, and a feeling of being seriously ill and near collapse. Her blood pressure increases to 240/140 mmHg or more at rest on occasions after eating pork for a few successive days. These symptoms will last for hours and gradually subside if she abstains from pork. All clinical manifestations of illness disappear and her clinical state returns to normal, including her blood pressure, without medication.

This patient's 35-year-old brother, B. M., participated in a family feast in which a hog was killed and fresh pork was consumed in large quantities. He suddenly developed a malignant type of hypertension (220/170 mmHg) with hematemesis, hematuria, blood in his stools, palpitation, hyperhydrosis, markedly impaired vision, with the syndrome of hypertensive encephalopathy and coma, and then died quickly (113).

Similarities between the clinical manifestations of pork sensitivity and pheochromocytoma are worth underscoring.

HYPOTHALAMIC DYSREGULATION

Dysregulation of the hypothalamus was postulated as the cause of fever accompanied by hypertension which occurred precisely every 21 days and lasted for several hours in one patient. This syndrome appeared related to cyclical dysregulation of the hypothalamus, with both a derangement of thermoregulation and an excess stimulation of ACTH release. The latter caused a marked increase in the elaboration of 17-hydroxycorticosteroids, which in turn may have played a role in the development of hypertension. No abnormality of catecholamine metabolism was detected in the patient (personal communication from Dr. Sheldon Wolff, National Institutes of Health).

TETANUS

Severe tetanus can produce a syndrome consistent with continuous but fluctuating overactivity of the sympathetic nervous system. It may be accompanied by fluctuating tachycardia (up to 200–300 per min), irregularities of cardiac rhythm, peripheral vascular constriction, pallor, profuse sweating, pyrexia, and sustained but labile hypertension with elevations of blood pressure (to as high as 300 mmHg systolic and 166 mmHg diastolic) (773). Furthermore, the excretion of catecholamines in the urine may be markedly increased (172). The glycosuria and hyperglycemia noted in some patients with tetanus may be explained by activation of the sympathetic nervous system. Even gastrointestinal disturbances such as constipation and paralytic ileus may be attributed to sympathetic overactivity (508). Kerr and coworkers found that the hypertension observed in patients with tetanus was not necessarily related to hypercapnia or muscle spasm and did not appear the result of renal impairment. They postulated that the sympathetic nervous system may be continuously and variably overactive, similar to overactivity of somatic motor neurons in patients with tetanus. Usually there was a clear association between catecholamine excretion and the severity of this disease (508). Evidence has accumulated that tetanus toxin may be carried by motor axons by retrograde intraaxonal transport to the central nervous system; it may also reach the spinal ganglia via sensory axons (1023). It is possible that tetanus toxin also enters the adrenergic system, but we are not aware of any experimental studies on this point. It is interesting that the myocardial lesions occurring in some patients with pheochromocytoma, and in some patients dying from tetanus, appear identical and are probably catecholamine-induced (805).

There should never be any problem in identifying a typical case of tetanus. The history of an injury followed by an incubation period of usually 3 days to 4 weeks and by the development of the characteristic increased tone in various muscle groups, trismus, dysphagia, etc., is almost pathognomonic for tetanus. However, some physicians may be unaware that tetanus may be accompanied by sustained and fluctuating hypertension and other clinical manifestations of overactivity of the sympathetic nervous system. In addition, the presence of elevated urinary catecholamines may conceivably confuse the diagnosis, especially if the case is atypical and if a history of trauma or a portal of entry for *Clostridium tetani* is not evident.

Recently one of us (W.M.M.) saw an 18-year-old male who had developed a volvulus from adhesions resulting from a previous appendectomy. The patient had always been normotensive; however, shortly following the removal of about 3 feet of gangrenous distal ileum, he was found to have a blood pressure of about 170/110 mmHg, a pulse of 120/min and minimal fever, which persisted for several days. In consultation, Dr. Harold Neu (Department of Medicine, Columbia Medical Center, New York City) suggested that the hypertension might be related to toxemia from *Clostridium perfringens (welchii)*—one of the inhabitants of the gastrointestinal tract. Unfortunately, no catecholamine assays were performed on this patient's blood; yet it is intriguing to speculate that activation of the sympathetic nervous system may result from elaboration of toxins not only from *Clostridium tetani* but also from other bacteria of the Clostridia family.

GUILLAIN-BARRE SYNDROME

The Guillain-Barré syndrome may be accompanied by transient elevations of blood pressure; sustained hypertension and an elevation of urinary VMA have also been reported (899). Evidence of a polyneuropathy with bilateral muscle weakness and flaccid motor paralysis and sensory manifestations are characteristic of this syndrome. Occasional neck pain and muscle stiffness may occur, and papilledema may sometimes appear. Classic cerebrospinal fluid findings are a normal pressure and an elevated protein concentration, without an increased number of leukocytes; however, the protein concentration may be normal and, rarely, there may be a lymphocytosis in the cerebrospinal fluid (245).

FACTITIOUS PRODUCTION OF PAROXYSMAL HYPERTENSION

Factitious production of paroxysmal hypertension and symptomatology suggesting a catecholamine-secreting pheochromocytoma may, rarely, have to be considered.

Lurvey and associates reported the case of a 41-year-old female paramedical aide who gave a 15-month history of attacks of nausea, anxiety, headache, vertigo, palpitations, pallor, tachycardia, and hypertension, usually with a systolic pressure ranging from 210 to 220 mmHg and a diastolic pressure of about 110 mmHg (596). She had also experienced momentary loss of consciousness and anterior chest pain. ECGs revealed PVCs and elevated S–T segments. One attack was accompanied by cardiorespiratory arrest which was successfully treated. Physical examination revealed two café-au-lait spots on her chest but was otherwise unremarkable. Urinary catecholamines and VMA were elevated following attacks; however, attempts to provoke attacks by vigorous abdominal massage or the administration of glucagon or histamine were unsuccessful. Aortography and left adrenal venography (right adrenal venogram was unsuccessful) were unremarkable, and no hypertensive episodes were noted during these procedures. Plasma catecholamines in blood collected from various levels of the inferior vena cava were within normal limits. Treatment with phenoxybenzamine prevented attacks, and attacks, which recurred usually 4 days after discontinuing this medication, could be terminated with phentolamine administered intravenously.

Following an attack, selective adrenal arteriograms and venograms were performed but were again found to be negative. The pattern of catecholamine excretion was confusing and atypical in that the ratio of epinephrine to norepinephrine did not remain constant (e.g., following an attack, the urinary concentration of norepinephrine decreased, while that of epinephrine increased). Because of the confusing and atypical nature of the clinical and laboratory picture, in addition to her rather flat affect, occupational exposure to drugs,

and sophisticated knowledge of the manifestations of pheochromocytoma, her belongings were searched. Syringes with residual medications were found in her purse and an open ampule of isoproterenol and a vial of lidocaine were discovered in her suitcase.

When confronted with this evidence by a psychiatrist, she was found to be severely depressed and admitted self-administration of 500 μg isoproterenol and 100 mg lidocaine subcutaneously to induce attacks "so that people would believe she was really ill." Since she had learned to use lidocaine to control PVCs during her attacks, it seemed possible that the lidocaine had caused her cardiorespiratory arrest (596).

Lurvey and coworkers pointed out that side effects of isoproterenol could mimic many of the clinical manifestations of a patient with pheochromocytoma. They further indicated that isoproterenol was not separable from epinephrine in the routine clinical assay. They postulated that an initial hypotensive effect of isoproterenol could have reflexly activated the sympathetic nervous system and caused a release of norepinephrine; this latter sequence, coupled with a possible impairment of the norepinephrine uptake system by isoproterenol, might have accounted for the increased urinary excretion of norepinephrine in this patient (596).

The importance of surreptitious self-administration of pressor agents as a cause of pseudopheochromocytoma is underscored by the intriguing reports of two additional cases. One of these patients induced hypertension by self-administration of ephedrine and theo-ephedrine (912); the other was a 22-year-old female medical student who was employed as a nurse and induced hypertensive crises by self-administration of metaraminol and norepinephrine. In this latter woman, paroxysmal hypertension (up to as high as 260/140 mmHg) associated with headache, chest pain, nasal obstruction, nausea, and vomiting usually occurred in situations when she could be observed by physicians. Urinary catecholamines were frequently very elevated although normal on some occasions, but provocative tests with glucagon and histamine were negative. Since renal tomograms and left renal arteriography suggested a left adrenal tumor, laparotomy was performed but no intraabdominal neoplasm was discovered. The right adrenal gland was removed because it appeared somewhat enlarged; however, histologically it proved to be normal. Postoperative aggressive behavioral changes were interpreted as a "psychological reaction produced by prolonged hospitalization (four months) and rancor at not getting her medical problem settled" (912).

Ultimately, the possibility of self-induced crises was considered because of (a) the irregularity of catecholamine excretion (predominantly epinephrine on some occasions and norepinephrine on others); (b) negative responses to provocative tests; (c) negative surgical exploration; and (d) psychopathic behavior. An ampule of metaraminol and an ampule of levarterenol and several mandelic acid tablets were discovered hidden in her handbag. Sterile radioactive ^{131}I, was added to the metaraminol, and saline was substituted for the levarterenol in the same type of container. The patient was given iodine solution by mouth in an effort to block ^{131}I uptake. Following another crisis, blood and urine were found to be radioactive and a scan of the neck revealed a thyroid image. She refused to admit self-administration of pressor substances despite the fact that this had been established. It was apparent that she had a deep-seated psychiatric disorder, since she was willing to undergo laparotomy and to face the prospect of possibly having both her adrenal glands resected.

The reason for relating these cases in detail is to emphasize that, if one encounters clinical manifestations suggesting pheochromocytoma in a person having access to a variety of drugs, the remote possibility of factitious production of symptoms (i.e., pseudopheochromocytoma) should be considered. Conceivably, drug abuse with amphetamine, which has β- as well as α-receptor activity, may produce hypertension, tachycardia, cardiac arrhythmias, diaphoresis, and other sympathomimetic effects and may present some diagnostic confusion if self-administration of this drug is not evident. The presence of a psychiatric disturbance, variable and atypical catecholamine excretion patterns, negative provocative tests, and normal radiologic studies should raise a serious suspicion that crises may be due to surreptitious self-admin-

istration of pressor agents, especially in persons associated with the health care industry. Certainly, every effort should be made to exclude pseudopheochromocytoma before performing an exploratory laparotomy.

An additional point of interest is that one hypertensive patient, who secretly took methyldopa (Aldomet), was mistakenly diagnosed as having a pheochromocytoma on the basis of spuriously elevated catecholamines. (Interference by methyldopa with the fluorometric assay of catecholamines is discussed in Chapter 6.) Unfortunately, he was subjected to an unnecessary laparotomy (718).

FORTUITOUS CIRCUMSTANCES SIMULATING PHEOCHROMOCYTOMA

Finally, it should be mentioned that on rare occasions pheochromocytoma has been mimicked by a combination of coincidental circumstances. One such situation was that of coarctation of the abdominal aorta (at the level of the renal vessels) which simulated pheochromocytoma (384). Sometimes the patient, a 45-year-old woman, had recurrent attacks of nausea, vomiting, pressure in the neck, pounding headache, chest pain, flushing, and temporary unconsciousness; polyuria followed these attacks. Other attacks consisted of shaking chills, pallor, and cold sweats. Attacks were accompanied by increases in the systolic blood pressure from 115 to 160 or even to 230 mmHg. Tomograms revealed an indefinite shadow in the left adrenal region which proved to be due to distended collateral vessels. Both systolic and diastolic blood pressures were observed to increase about 40 mmHg when a syringe was brought to the bedside, and it is conceivable that some, if not most, of her blood pressure lability resulted from anxiety. However, another patient was cited in whom coarctation of the abdominal aorta was accompanied by sustained hypertension and wide fluctuations of pressure (384).

Another set of coincidental circumstances simulating pheochromocytoma was that of a renal cyst which occurred in a 48-year-old male who had recurrent attacks of severe palpitations, trembling, and marked weakness. Blood pressures ranged between 105/65 and 148/90 mmHg, and the patient had a marked pressor response to the intravenous administration of histamine, which was thought to suggest pheochromocytoma. Intravenous and retrograde pyelography were interpreted as demonstrating a mass in the left suprarenal area. At operation this lesion proved to be a cyst in the upper pole of the kidney and in retrospect it was concluded that his symptoms and signs simulating pheochromocytoma were due to recurrent states of acute anxiety (1011).

One very unusual case report was that of a woman with sustained hypertension who for many years had had innumerable attacks of palpitation, headache, dizziness, weakness, and angina. Urinary epinephrine was elevated to the pheochromocytoma range and a presacral pneumogram revealed a tumor above the kidney. Exploration was negative for pheochromocytoma; following the patient's death the tumor proved to be an adrenocortical adenoma (469). We are unaware of any other similar reports.

POTENTIAL SECONDARY DIAGNOSES

One must always be aware of the pathologic conditions which have been reported to occur more frequently in patients with pheochromocytoma than in the general population (particularly cholelithiasis, medullary thyroid carcinoma, hyperparathyroidism, Cushing's syndrome, neurofibromatosis, mucosal neuromas, thickened corneal nerves, alimentary-tract ganglioneuromatosis, marfanoid habitus, polycythemia, and von Hippel-Lindau disease). These secondary diagnoses, in addition to the various vascular and cardiac pathologic complications which sometimes occur in patients with this tumor (Table 3.11), may further obscure and confuse the diagnosis of pheochromocytoma unless their potential relationship to pheochromocytoma is appreciated.

It is recommended that in screening patients for the presence of medullary thyroid carcinoma, pentagastrin (Peptavlon) be initially injected, since it appears to be a more effective secretagogue for calcitonin than is calcium infusion (340); yet, since this is not uniformly so, a negative pentagastrin test should be followed by a calcium infusion test

in order to best eliminate the diagnosis of medullary thyroid carcinoma. It should be recalled that this type of thyroid carcinoma may elaborate not only calcitonin but also ACTH-like substances, prostaglandin, and serotonin and that these secretions can cause a variety of clinical manifestations which are not usually seen in patients with pheochromocytoma.

The detection of hypercalcemia in a patient with pheochromocytoma, in the absence of other conditions known to elevate serum calcium, suggests that hyperparathyroidism (due either to parathyroid adenomas or to chief cell hyperplasia) is present; however, it is important also to demonstrate an elevated parathormone. In rare instances, hypercalcemia may conceivably be due to production of a parathormone-like substance or some other calcium-affecting factor elaborated by the pheochromocytoma (891, 958). This latter point is worth remembering since it further underscores the importance of removing the pheochromocytoma before definitely concluding that hypercalcemia is the result of hyperparathyroidism.

In rare instances Cushing's syndrome with hyperadrenocorticism and hypokalemic alkalosis may become manifest in a patient with sporadic or familial pheochromocytoma. This appears almost always to result from elaboration of ACTH by the tumor, since it seems unlikely that a pheochromocytoma is capable of synthesizing cortisol. In patients with Cushing's syndrome there is a loss of the circadian rhythm of plasma cortisol levels observed in normal subjects, and the excretion of free cortisol in the urine is increased. When confronted with a patient with Cushing's syndrome, several tests as well as an ACTH assay can be used to decipher the etiology of this syndrome as follows:

1. Usually high levels of dexamethasone (8 mg/day) will suppress plasma cortisol in Cushing's disease but not if the syndrome is due to adrenal neoplasms or ectopically produced ACTH-like substance.
2. Administration of metyrapone will increase the urinary excretion of 17-hydroxy-corticosteroids in patients with Cushing's disease but not if the syndrome is due to adrenal neoplasms or ectopically produced

ACTH-like substances. Since metyrapone can cause a release of catecholamines from the adrenal medulla, it has been suggested that it should be administered cautiously to any patient who may have a pheochromocytoma (181).

3. The ACTH stimulation test will usually increase plasma cortisol and urinary 17-hydroxycorticosteroids in patients with Cushing's disease, but not when the syndrome is due to adrenal cortical carcinoma or ectopically produced ACTH-like substance.

4. Plasma ACTH levels are, of course, elevated in patients with Cushing's syndrome due to ectopically produced ACTH-like substance. The levels may also be elevated in Cushing's disease, whereas plasma ACTH is absent in patients with adrenal cortical neoplasms.

An additional point of diagnostic interest is that the excretion of very high levels of 17-ketosteroids (>50 mg/24 hr) is usually seen only in patients with adrenal cortical carcinoma or ectopic ACTH-producing tumors. Radiologic studies of the sella turcica and adrenals may also aid in the differential diagnosis, and sampling of adrenal vein blood can be of great value in differentiating a unilateral neoplasm from bilateral adrenal cortical disease.

On extremely rare occasions adrenal virilism or Addison's disease has been associated with pheochromocytoma, and one must be prepared to treat appropriately any patient with evidence of adrenal insufficiency. If there is ever any evidence suggestive of Addison's disease, the ACTH stimulation test may be decisive; failure of plasma cortisol levels to increase following ACTH administration is virtually pathognomonic of adrenal insufficiency. It must be reemphasized that ACTH infusion should be performed with extreme caution in patients with pheochromocytoma, and only if absolutely essential, since severe and even fatal attacks of hypertension and hypotension following ACTH administration have been reported (680, 730, 780).

Neurofibromatosis, as well as a pheochromocytoma, may, rarely, compromise the vascular supply to a kidney and thereby induce renal ischemia. Under the latter circumstances, a patient with neurofibromatosis and/or pheochromocytoma may develop hyperreninemia in the venous blood draining the affected kidney and this may be misinterpreted as the cause of the patient's hypertension.

Hyperglycemia is usually a manifestation of increased circulating catecholamines, yet the possibility that diabetes mellitus may coexist with a pheochromocytoma and require appropriate therapy must be considered.

Very rarely a patient may present with an acute abdomen or with chest pain suggesting myocardial infarction. These points should be kept in mind since it could be catastrophic to perform a laparotomy on a patient with pheochromocytoma without appropriate preoperative and intraoperative management. Because of the difficulties in recognizing and correctly diagnosing *hemorrhagic necrosis in a pheochromocytoma,* a detailed account of this entity is presented.

Although small areas of hemorrhage and necrosis are frequently evident in many pheochromocytomas, it is distinctly unusual to find a degree of *hemorrhagic necrosis* sufficient to cause clinical manifestations of an acute abdomen or a cardiovascular catastrophe.

Brody described an 18-year-old girl with severe sustained hypertension due to a pheochromocytoma who developed severe abdominal cramps and vomiting for which she was given 10 mg of prochlorperazine (Compazine) intramuscularly (102). Ten minutes later the blood pressure fell from 190/150 mmHg to 80/60 mmHg which required norepinephrine infusion for 5 hr to stabilize her blood pressure. Approximately 2.5 weeks later the blood pressure and urinary catecholamines had returned to normal levels. This patient's pheochromocytoma was removed and the entire central mass appeared necrotic and infarcted. It was speculated that the shock following prochlorperazine administration may have played a significant role in promoting the necrosis of this tumor.

Brody pointed out that others (574) had reported intramuscular administration of chlorpromazine (another phenothiazine derivative) to a patient with pheochromocytoma during a hypertensive crisis resulting in marked hypotension requiring a vasopressor agent. They suggested that patients with pheochromocytoma may be extraordinarily sensitive to phenothiazine drugs and that the occurrence of shock following their use should raise the suspicion that the patient may be harboring a pheochromocytoma. Subsequently, others have reported shock following administration of phenothiazines to patients with pheochromocytoma (140, 326, 594).

Following the intramuscular administration of meperidine (Demerol) and prochlorperazine (Compazine), one patient with pheochromocytoma developed shock, pulmonary edema, and pyrexia (103°F); the patient's history and clinical manifestations were considered to suggest dissecting aneurysms of the thoracic aorta, with rupture.

Autopsy revealed a partly cystic pheochromocytoma (with focal hemorrhage and necrosis), which contained approximately equal concentrations of epinephrine and norepinephrine. In addition, there were pulmonary edema, renal tubular necrosis, colonic mucosal necrosis (probably ischemic), and focal myocarditis (140).

Page and associates studied a group of patients with predominantly epinephrine-secreting pheochromocytomas (730); substantial secretion of epinephrine caused predominance of β-adrenergic effects, sometimes accompanied by bouts of profound hypotension. It is conceivable that prochlorperazine triggered a significant release of catecholamines from the pheochromocytoma of one patient who became hypotensive.

The mechanism whereby phenothiazines may induce shock or cause release of catecholamines in patients with pheochromocytoma remains obscure. Since phenothiazines [chlorpromazine (Thorazine); triflupromazine (Vesprin); prochlorperazine (Compazine); promazine (Sparine); promethazine (Phenergan); thiethylperazine (Torecon); etc.] are very commonly used to treat psychiatric patients or to control nausea and vomiting, it is important to observe some caution before prescribing these drugs to hypertensive patients if the cause of the hypertension is uncertain.

Hemorrhagic necrosis in pheochromocytomas has been reported in patients given anticoagulants (485, 638). In the patient reported by Jelliffe, anticoagulants had been given because severe substernal and epigastric pain had been considered the result of coronary thrombosis. A mobile mass the size of an orange was found to the left of the umbilicus; subsequently it moved to the right of the umbilicus and became more palpable. It was presumed that the paroxysms of the hypertension in addition to the anticoagulation contributed to the hemorrhage into the cystic, friable, necrotic tumor discovered at necropsy (485). A 36-year-old woman reported by McAlister and Koehler had labile hypertension and electrocardiographic evidence suggesting anterolateral myocardial ischemia (638). Numerous episodes of chest pain, palpitations, sweating, and occasionally vomiting were thought to be due to coronary insufficiency, and she was given anticoagulants. One week later she developed marked diaphoresis, pounding headache, tachycardia (120/min), and hypertension (170/130 mmHg). One hour later she complained of severe right upper quadrant pain and the blood pressure fell to zero, but was successfully supported with vasoconstrictors and hydrocortisone. In the next 2 days the hematocrit dropped from 38 to 17 percent and anticoagulants were discontinued. A right upper quadrant mass appeared and there was flank tenderness. Roentgenograms, which revealed obliteration of the right psoas shadow and a mass displacing the right kidney inferiorly and laterally, were considered consistent with a retroperitoneal hematoma. Cholecystography demonstrated a single large gallstone. Fortunately, the possibility of a hemorrhage in a pheochromocytoma was considered in this patient and the urinary catecholamines and VMA were found to be markedly elevated [7800 μg/24 hr (normal <100) and 250 mg/24 hr (normal up to 6), respectively]. A large hemorrhagic and necrotic pheochromocytoma and the gallbladder were successfully removed, and recovery was uneventful (638). Sobonya and coworkers reported the unusual case of a 20-year-old black woman who died in circulatory shock associated with hyperkalemia and hemorrhage into an extraadrenal (mainly epinephrine-producing) pheochromocytoma (923).

McAlister and Koehler stated that among tumors of the retroperitoneal space, pheochromocytoma is the most likely to undergo a spontaneous hemorrhage sufficient to cause an acute abdomen and shock. They emphasized the importance of being aware that retroperitoneal bleeding can cause an acute abdomen and shock. They also indicated that radiologic studies may be valuable in establishing the correct diagnosis of a hemorrhage into a pheochromocytoma (638); however, abdominal aortography may induce a fatal hemorrhage into the tumor and periadrenal region (520, 583).

Hemorrhagic necrosis in pheochromocytomas has followed the use of phentolamine (Regitine) (802, 990) and prochlorperazine (102), both of which drugs have α-adrenergic blocking effects. It is not clear whether the hemorrhagic necrosis was related in some way to these medications.

Rarely, retroperitoneal or intraperitoneal hemorrhage from a pheochromocytoma may result if hemorrhage within the tumor causes rupture of the capsule (220). Scott and associates have reported the cases of two patients with hemorrhagic infarction with spontaneous rupture of their pheochromocytomas which necessitated emergency operation (875a).

The extreme importance of recognizing the clinical picture of hemorrhagic necrosis in a pheochromocytoma cannot be overstated. Without prompt institution of appropriate therapy and extirpation of the tumor, the patient will almost certainly die. A high index of suspicion is, of course, fundamental in correctly diagnosing this unusual complication.

Diagnosis

CHAPTER SIX

GENERAL REMARKS

It is important to question very carefully any patients suspected of having a pheochromocytoma, since they may not spontaneously comment on certain symptoms and signs which, to the physician, are particularly valuable clues in suggesting that diagnosis. Patients may often have symptoms and signs caused by this tumor even for a number of years before the diagnosis is made. This has been our experience as well as that of others. Engelman has called this delay in diagnosis the "diagnosis gap," and suggests that it results from an insidious onset of symptoms which are not alarming to the patients (267). We have seen patients with pheochromocytoma whose clinical manifestations have been misinterpreted for a number of years as being due to anxiety, the menopause, paroxysmal tachycardia, etc.

Patients with pheochromocytoma and persistent hypertension are not infrequently misdiagnosed as having essential hypertension, especially when symptoms and signs are few or totally lacking. We have seen several patients who have carried the diagnosis of essential hypertension for more than a decade before the correct diagnosis was made.

As expounded in the section on differential diagnosis above (Chapter 5), the symptoms of patients with pheochromocytoma may closely simulate a large variety of disease entities. Furthermore, the complications which can occur in patients with this tumor may suggest a diagnosis of acute gastrointestinal disorder, primary renal disease, metastatic neoplasm, etc.

Despite the value of a detailed history in the differential diagnosis of pheochromocytoma, the preoperative diagnosis can be confirmed only by the demonstration of excess concentration of catecholamines or their metabolites in the plasma or urine.

Table 6.1 has been prepared to aid the clinician in selecting those patients who should be carefully screened for the presence of pheochromocytoma. The manifestations listed are based on vast experience, and if this table is used as a diagnostic guide, the chances of *not* recognizing a patient with this tumor should be minimized, if not eliminated. It has been stated that it is unrewarding and uneconomical to screen all hypertensives for this disorder (719); but the availability of fairly simple, quite reliable, and relatively inexpensive tests for detecting elevated catecholamine metabolites in the urine is a compelling argument to screen *all* patients with severe hypertension or with hypertension resistant to treatment in whom the cause of hypertension has not been established. The potential dangers and the lethal character of pheochromocytoma further underscore this argument.

As mentioned in Table 6.1, one must have a high index of suspicion when confronting any patient with hypertension, if the diagnosis is uncertain. Pheochromocytoma has been called "The Great Masquerader" and "The Great Mimic" because of its remarkably varied manifestations, which closely simulate a variety of diseases.

A GUIDE FOR SCREENING

Recorded in Table 6.1 is a list of manifestations and circumstances which should particularly alert the physician to screen a patient with sustained and/or paroxysmal hypertension most carefully for evidence of pheochromocytoma. Screening can be conveniently and adequately performed in the great majority of cases by appropriate chemical testing of the urine for evidence of excessive excretion of catecholamines and/or their metabolites. In some of these patients who are relatively normotensive, provocative tests and plasma catecholamine assays may be indicated. We have expressly emphasized the absolute need to screen all symptomatic patients with sustained or labile hypertension, and all patients with severe hypertension (Groups 2, 3, or 4) or with hypertension resistant to treatment in whom the cause of the hypertension has not been definitely established. Postoperative deaths continue to occur because the physician or surgeon did not consider the remote possibility of pheochromocytoma as the cause of hypertension. Today it is indefensible to perform a surgical procedure on a patient with sustained and/or labile hypertension without first making every attempt to exclude the presence of a pheochromocytoma. In addition, the family of any patient thought to have familial pheochromocytoma should also be screened for any evidence of this tumor. It is of utmost importance that the physician become acutely aware of the varied and bizarre manifestations that can occur in familial as well as sporadic pheochromocytoma. A point of extreme concern is the fact that manifestations of pheochromocytoma occasionally first appear during pregnancy and, if not lethal, may remit, only to return at a later date, sometimes in association with a subsequent pregnancy. As mentioned earlier, pregnancy and childbirth in the presence of undetected pheochromocytoma carry a high risk of maternal and fetal mortality.

Very rarely, patients with pheochromocytoma have been reported who have "attacks" of some of the classical symptoms and signs of pheochromocytoma, but without hypertension. The difficulty in detecting these somewhat "occult" pheochromocytomas is obvious and requires a meticulous history by an especially alert physician.

If the recommendations in Table 6.1 are diligently followed, practically all patients with pheochromocytoma can be detected. Therefore, we do not feel that routine screening of

Table 6.1 *Whom to Screen for Pheochromocytoma (the Physician Must Have High Index of Suspicion)*

SCREEN ALL SYMPTOMATIC HYPERTENSIVES (SUSTAINED AND/OR PAROXYSMAL) IF DIAGNOSIS IS UNCERTAIN. THIS WARNING IS ALL THE MORE IMPORTANT IF THE PATIENT IS ABOUT TO UNDERGO SURGERY!!!

SCREEN ALL PATIENTS WITH SEVERE HYPERTENSION (RETINOPATHY GROUPS 2, 3, AND 4) AND/OR HYPERTENSION RESISTANT TO THERAPY IF DIAGNOSIS UNCERTAIN!

PARTICULARLY PERFORM TESTS ON PATIENTS HAVING SUSTAINED AND/OR PAROXYSMAL HYPERTENSION WITH:

Recurrent "attacks" of symptoms and signs outlined in Tables 4.1 and 4.3, especially when precipitated by the following (even if "attacks" occur with normotension or paroxysmal hypotension):

Exertion or postural change (extending neck, straining, standing up quickly, bending over)
Palpation of area near pheochromocytoma
Emotion
Ingestion of some foods and/or liquids (cheese, wine or beer which contain tyramine; fruit juice rich in synephrine; hot or cold beverages)
Hyperventilation
Micturition

Injection of some drugs [histamine, glucagon, tyramine, tetraethylammonium, methacholine, ACTH, nicotine, anectine, diamorphine, nitroglycerine, saralasin (and other angiotensin analogues)]
Odor (cooking, perfume, ink)
Hot shower
Smoking

Weight loss (10% or more below standard weight)
Orthostatic hypotension
Hypermetabolism (BMR>20%) without hyperthyroidism
Hyperglycemia
Paradoxic response of BP to antihypertensive drugs (especially ganglionic blockers and guanethidine)
Severe pressor response during:

Anesthesia induction
Operation

Renal arteriography
Parturition

Unexplained circulatory shock

During anesthesia
During pregnancy; during delivery; in puerperium

During operation or postoperatively
Following administration of phenothiazine drugs

Miscellaneous

Short history of hypertension (2 years, or less)
< 35 years old

Hypertensive retinopathy (group 3, 4 or severe group 2)

Family history of pheochromocytoma (perform tests *even if no hypertension and asymptomatic*)
Evidence of certain other disease entities

Cholelithiasis
Medullary thyroid carcinoma
Hyperparathyroidism
Mucosal neuromas
Thickened corneal nerves
Marfanoid habitus
Alimentary-tract ganglioneuromatosis

Neurofibromatosis
Cushing's syndrome (rare)
von Hippel-Lindau disease (rare)
Polycythemia (rare)
Virilism (extremely rare)
Addison's disease (extremely rare)
Acromegaly (extremely rare)

"Toxemia" of pregnancy
Unexplained pyrexia
Transient ECG abnormalities during hypertensive episodes
X-ray evidence of a suprarenal mass

SCREEN FIRST DEGREE (PRIMARY) RELATIVES, I.E., SIBLINGS AND CHILDREN

SCREEN PATIENTS WITH "ATTACKS" OF SYMPTOMS AND SIGNS OUTLINED IN TABLES 4.1 AND 4.3 EVEN IN THE ABSENCE OF HYPERTENSION all asymptomatic hypertensives is mandatory. Recently it was pointed out that in the Royal Adelaide Hospital the cost of routinely screening patients with sustained hypertension in order to detect only one patient with pheochromocytoma was $28,784. This figure was based on the cost not only of VMA tests in Australia but also on the cost of hospitalization related to urine collection for the screening test (750). In the United States, even if only the $31.00 (the cost of the metaphrine test—see footnote c, Table 6.14) for each urinary screening test were considered, the cost estimate for detecting one patient with pheochromocytoma among patients with sus-

tained diastolic hypertension would be $31,000 (assuming an incidence of 0.1 percent and assuming that only one screening test was adequate in each patient).

PHEOCHROMOCYTOMA "PEARLS"

Table 6.2 contains several facts about pheochromocytoma which are worthwhile for the clinician and student to memorize. Because of their importance and, in some instances, their ease of recall, we have called them *Pheochromocytoma "Pearls."*

As noted, five major manifestations of pheochromocytoma begin with the letter "H"

Table 6.2 *Pheochromocytoma "Pearls" (Facts Worth Memorizing)*

5 H's[a]	Hypertension
	Headache
	Hyperhydrosis
	Hypermetabolism
	Hyperglycemia
95% will have	Headache or
	Hyperhydrosis or
	Palpitation
Rough rule of 10	10% familial
	10% bilateral (adrenal)[b]
	10% malignant
	10% multiple (other than bilateral adrenal)[b]
	10% extraadrenal[b]
	10% occur in children
MEN–type 2 triad	Medullary thyroid carcinoma
	Bilateral-familial pheochromocytoma (frequent)
	Hyperparathyroidism (~50%)
MEN–type 3 sextet	Medullary thyroid carcinoma
	Bilateral-familial pheochromocytoma (frequent)
	Mucosal neuromas
	Thickened corneal nerves
	Marfanoid habitus
	Alimentary-tract ganglioneuromatosis
	(Very rarely hyperparathyroidism)
4 C's	Cholelithiasis
	Cushing's syndrome (very rare)
	Cutaneous lesions
	Cerebellar hemangioblastoma (very rare)

Pheochromocytoma manifestations may appear during pregnancy!

[a] The term "Triad of H's" was used by Dr. John E. Howard and refers to hypertension, hyperglycemia, and hypermetabolism (without hyperthyroidism) occurring in patients with pheochromocytoma. We have extended this category to include 5 H's.

[b] Adults and children combined.

—hypertension, headache, hyperhydrosis, hypermetabolism, and hyperglycemia; and 95 percent of patients with this tumor will have one or more of the following: headaches, hyperhydrosis, or palpitations.

The "Rule of 10" immediately helps one recall that about 10 percent of pheochromocytomas are familial, 10 percent malignant, and 10 percent occur in children. Furthermore, if a statistical analysis combines the findings in adults and in children, 10 percent of these tumors are bilateral in the adrenals, 10 percent are multiple, and 10 percent are extraadrenal.

The two types of multiple endocrine neoplasia that may be associated with familial pheochromocytoma have been grouped separately according to their pathologic features and manifestations. Medullary thyroid carcinoma, pheochromocytoma, and hyperparathyroidism are grouped as a triad characteristic of the MEN–type 2 syndrome. Awareness of the occurrence of mucosal neuromas, skeletal anomalies, thickened corneal nerves (evident on slit-lamp examination), and symptoms and signs of alimentary-tract ganglioneuromatosis will aid in the early recognition of MEN–type 3 and will permit the differentiation of this syndrome from MEN–type 2.

Four conditions which occur more frequently in association with pheochromocytomas than in the general population begin with the letter "C," and are grouped together as a memory aid: cholelithiasis, Cushing's syndrome, cutaneous lesions, and cerebellar hemangioblastoma. In our experience, as mentioned earlier, the incidence of cholelithiasis has been 30 and 10 percent, respectively, in patients with paroxysmal and sustained hypertension due to pheochromocytoma, and, according to the literature, Cushing's syndrome has been reported in more than a dozen patients with this tumor. Cutaneous lesions—such as café-au-lait spots, axillary freckling, vascular nevi, hairy moles, and neurofibromatosis—may occur with increased frequency in patients with pheochromocytoma. Approximately 5 percent of patients with this tumor have neurofibromatosis, whereas perhaps 1 percent of persons with this latter disorder have pheochromocytoma. In addition, mucosal neuromas are a hall-

mark of MEN–type 3. Although the occurrence of cerebellar hemangioblastoma (Lindau's disease) is rare in patients with pheochromocytoma, yet there is an increased association of these tumors.

Finally, in Table 6.2, we have listed the fact that symptoms and signs may become manifest during pregnancy. This phenomenon is of signal importance, since an awareness of this fact may prevent the death of both mother and fetus!

A careful and detailed history and physical examination, concentrated especially on the symptoms and signs common to patients with pheochromocytoma, should, in the majority of cases, enable a physician with a high index of suspicion to suggest the correct diagnosis on clinical grounds alone. In addition, a number of laboratory and radiographic abnormalities may be demonstrated which may further suggest the diagnosis of pheochromocytoma.

LABORATORY FINDINGS

BLOOD GLUCOSE, GLYCOSURIA, AND GLUCOSE TOLERANCE

As mentioned earlier, about 65 percent of patients with pheochromocytoma and persistent hypertension have fasting hyperglycemia, whereas 56 percent of those with paroxysmal hypertension have this abnormality (see Table 6.3). However, it should be pointed out that samples for blood sugar analysis were usually obtained from patients with paroxysmal hypertension between attacks, when secretion of catecholamines from these tumors was probably minimal. A fasting blood glucose value as high as 400 mg/dl which was accompanied by a glycosuria of 60 to 80 g per day was reported in one patient with pheochromocytoma who became normoglycemic following removal of the tumor (229). Fasting hyperglycemia and any associated glycosuria are not usually pronounced.

In some, but not all, patients with paroxysmal hypertension, blood glucose concentrations may parallel changes in blood pressure. For example, in one patient the blood glucose rose quickly from a fasting level of 124 mg/dl to 224 mg/dl at the beginning of a hypertensive crisis; 25 min after the attack started the concentration was 218 mg/dl and

Table 6.3 *Fasting Blood Sugar, Basal Metabolic Rate, Proteinuria, and Blood Urea in 76 Patients with Pheochromocytoma with Paroxysmal or Persistent Hypertension[a]*

Parameter	Paroxysmal function		Persistent function	
	Patients	%[b]	Patients	%[b]
Fasting blood glucose (mg/dl)[c]				
<120 (Folin-Wu) or <90 (autoanalyzer)	15	44.1	10	34.5
120–149 (Folin-Wu) or 90–109 (autoanalyzer)	11	32.4	9	31.0
>149 (Folin-Wu) or >109 (autoanalyzer)	8	23.5	10	34.5
Not done	3	—	10	—
Basal metabolic rate				
(% <+10)[d]	18	56.3	3	9.1
+10 to +19	5	15.6	5	15.2
+20 to +49	9	28.1	17	51.5
+50 or more	0	—	8	24.2
Not done	5	—	6	—
Proteinuria, Grade 1 or more	13	35.1	25	64.1
Blood urea (mg/dl)[e]				
<40	26	81.3	28	75.7
40–59	5	15.6	7	18.9
60 or more	1	3.1	2	5.4
Not done	5	—	2	—

[a] Adapted from Gifford, R. W. Jr., Kvale, W. F., Mayer, F. T., Roth, G. M., and Priestley, J. T. *Mayo Clinic Proc. 39:* 287, 1964.

[b] Calculated on basis of number of patients who had tests.

[c] On December 1, 1958, the Mayo Clinic started to use the autoanalyzer for determination of blood glucose instead of the Folin-Wu method. Normal fasting blood glucose by the Folin-Wu and autoanalyzer methods are <120 mg and <90 mg/dl, respectively.

[d] Value considered unequivocal increase for BMR if >19 percent.

[e] Value considered increased for blood urea if >40 mg/dl.

0.5 hr after the attack ended it had fallen to 120 mg/dl. [It is interesting that in this same patient the total serum protein rose slightly during the crisis and fell promptly afterward, probably as the result of transient hemocontraction occurring during the hypertensive period. A slight concomitant rise in blood calcium may have been associated with the protein elevation (462).]

The impaired glucose tolerance noted in some patients with pheochromocytoma appears related, in part at least, to decreased peripheral sensitivity to insulin, perhaps due to elevated plasma free fatty acids (930), and the inhibitory effect on insulin release exerted by the catecholamines (930, 1035). Although hyperglycemia occurred more frequently in the patients with persistent (65.5 percent) than in those with paroxysmal (55.9 percent) hypertension, the difference was not striking.

Hermann and Mornex observed that the frequency of blood glucose disturbances increased proportionately to the increase of total epinephrine in the pheochromocytoma; however, tumors containing purely norepinephrine are capable of causing glucose disturbances (437, pp. 151–152).

Ketoacidosis almost never develops in patients with pheochromocytoma, probably because adequate endogenous insulin is present; furthermore, the hyperglycemia caused by excessive circulating catecholamines may oppose their lipolytic effect and thus reduce the ketogenic potential (930). It is noteworthy, however, that acetonuria has been produced in the experimental rat by injections of epinephrine (12).

Scott and associates reported that diabetic glucose tolerance tests which existed in nine of their patients reverted to normal in seven following pheochromocytoma extirpation. However, unless diabetes mellitus coexists, impaired glucose tolerance eventually disappears in practically all patients following removal of their pheochromocytoma. Reversion of glucose tolerance to normal is not always prompt and complete; sometimes gradual improvement may occur over a period of several years (930).

BASAL METABOLISM

The frequency with which certain laboratory abnormalities are encountered depends on whether the hypertension caused by pheochromocytoma is sustained or paroxysmal. For example, in Table 6.3, it is evident that about 76 percent of patients with persistent hypertension have elevated BMRs, whereas only about 28 percent of patients with paroxysmal hypertension have such an elevation. It is further apparent that BMR elevations >50 percent were observed only in the group with sustained blood pressure elevations. It should be appreciated that the above findings reflect values in patients with paroxysmal hypertension and pheochromocytoma during periods when hypertensive crises were absent and tumor function relatively quiescent. Marked elevations of blood glucose and BMR would be expected during hypertensive crises in the paroxysmal group similar to those occurring in patients with sustained hypertension and pheochromocytoma. Of the patients with pheochromocytoma reported by Gifford and coworkers, three with sustained hypertension had BMRs greater than 100 percent, and one had a rate of 261 percent (352).

PLASMA FREE FATTY ACIDS (FFA)

It has been demonstrated that intravenous administration of epinephrine (389) or norepinephrine (686) causes significant elevations of plasma FFA, an effect which may be due to the activation of lipase in adipose tissue (796) and the consequent mobilization of fat stores. Engelman and coworkers found that there was a correlation between the decrease in BMR and fall in plasma FFA caused by treatment. There was evidence also that administration of phenoxybenzamine or phentolamine can, at least in part, inhibit the action of catecholamines on the release of FFA. An increase in FFA concentration has been shown to increase oxygen consumption by skeletal muscle (248) as well as by leukocytes (304). Furthermore, β-adrenergic blockade (with pronethalol) of the norepinephrine-induced FFA rise abolished the increased oxygen consumption (270). Engelman and associates have attributed the increased BMRs in patients with pheochromocytoma to elevated plasma FFA (270).

The mean concentration for plasma FFA in eight untreated patients with pheochromocytoma reported by Engelman and coworkers (270) was 0.77 ± 0.21 mEq/liter (range: 0.44 to 1.09), whereas the mean value in normal subjects was 0.35 ± 0.12 mEq/liter (range: 0.11 to 0.70). These differences were highly significant ($p < 0.001$), despite the inclusion of one patient with paroxysmal hypertension who had normal FFA, BMR, and blood pressure. (In addition to the increased plasma FFA and glucose caused by excessive circulating catecholamines one would also anticipate an accompanying elevation of plasma glycerol (446a); however, to our knowledge glycerol concentrations have not been determined in patients with pheochromocytoma.)

While many who had an elevated BMR also had an elevated blood glucose, only about half of the patients with an increase in one of these parameters had an increase in the other.

SERUM CHOLESTEROL

Rare instances have been cited in the literature where serum cholesterol was significantly elevated preoperatively and then returned to normal levels after the pheochromocytoma was removed. This has been mentioned above in connection with the increased incidence of cholelithiasis in patients with pheochromocytoma; however, adequate data are not available to determine whether the hypercholesterolemia occasionally observed in patients with pheochromocytoma can be attributed to the catecholamines.

PERIPHERAL BLOOD COUNTS AND RED CELL VOLUME

Both *anemia* and *polycythemia* (96, 110, 909, 1002) have been described in patients with pheochromocytoma; usually, however, patients have relatively normal red blood cell counts. Bradley and coworkers first reported a patient (a 10-year-old white male) with pheochromocytoma and polycythemia as having the following: Hgb 21 g/dl; Hct 65 percent; RBC 3,300,000/mm^3; red cell mass 40 ml/kg; WBC 8000/mm^3; and platelets 745,000/mm^3 (96). They also demonstrated a marked decrease in plasma disappearance time of ^{59}Fe administered intravenously, and the presence of erythroid hyperplasia in the bone marrow. Inappropriate (i.e., where high red cell mass does not reflect tissue hypoxia) erythropoietic activity was demonstrated in the plasma and tumor extract. A remission with return to normal values occurred following removal of the tumor (96).

In a series of 15 patients with pheochromocytoma in whom red cell and plasma volumes were measured, the majority had red cell volumes within two standard deviations of normal; however, two male patients with widespread metastatic pheochromocytoma had severe anemia, with red cell volumes more than two standard deviations below the normal mean (909). Three patients had red cell volumes greater than two standard deviations above the mean normal value, and two of these had volumes of approximately 40 ml of red cells/kg of body weight (normal mean for men and women is about 30 and 26 ml/kg, respectively). The latter two patients had elevated hematocrits of 65 percent and 72 percent and hemoglobin concentrations over 20 g/dl. The peripheral white blood cell and platelet counts and the arterial oxygen saturation were normal, and there was no splenomegaly, suggesting that these two patients did not have a coincidental polycythemia vera. Furthermore, in one of these patients the pheochromocytoma was resected and the red cell volume, hematocrit, and hemoglobin returned to normal. Erythropoiesis-stimulating activity was demonstrated in the serum of both of these patients, and in an extract of the resected tumor.

Rosse and Waldmann, and others, have demonstrated an erythropoiesis-stimulating factor similar to, if not identical with, *erythropoietin*, which is elaborated by some cerebellar hemangioblastoma and renal tumors, known to cause polycythemia (233, 435, 816, 1003, 1004). It is now well-recognized that a variety of neoplastic tumors (e.g., renal carcinoma, adenoma or sarcoma, hepatoma, pulmonary carcinoma, cerebellar hemangioblastoma, adrenal adenoma, uterine fibroids, pheochromocytoma, and even renal cysts) can sometimes cause polycythemia (96, 233, 480).

It is noteworthy that two tumors (pheochromocytoma and cerebellar hemangioblastoma) which occasionally cause polycythemia sometimes occur in the same patient. Lindau emphasized the interesting observation that the two tumors (cerebellar hemangioblastoma and hypernephroma) most often associated with polycythemia are also occasionally found simultaneously (575). The association of these three tumors is intriguing, since it suggests that the cells from which these neoplasms originate have a similar background.

Halvorsen has presented strong support for the concept that the central nervous system is of fundamental importance in the regulation of erythropoiesis (411), and Fink and Fisher have shown that the adrenergic nervous system plays an important role in regulating kidney production of erythropoietin (314). Conceivably, vasoconstriction resulting from excessive circulating catecholamines may be severe enough in some patients with pheochromocytoma to cause renal hypoxia and contribute to an increased production of erythropoietin. It appears that the hypoxic kidney may produce a "renal erythropoietic factor" (erythrogenin) which may react with a serum protein to generate functionally active erythropoietin (387). Jacob has pointed out that this latter sequence is analogous to the blood pressure-elevating renin–angiotensinogen interaction which, interestingly, is also activated by hypoxia (480). However, it seems likely that the major (if not the only) reason for polycythemia is the elaboration of an erythropoiesis-stimulating factor by some of these tumors.

The *white blood cell* count is normal in almost all patients with uncomplicated pheochromocytoma and sustained hypertension; however, it is uncertain whether paroxysmal hypertensive crises are frequently associated with leukocytosis since this has not been adequately studied. French and Compagna reported a patient with pheochromocytoma whose blood pressure varied between hypertensive and hypotensive levels (329). The patient had a persistent polymorphonuclear leukocytosis (reaching 41,500 cells/mm³ on one occasion and without evidence of infection, hemorrhage, or necrosis) which subsided after the tumor was removed. They reviewed the literature and found that although most studies revealed a normal hemogram, six reports indicated varying degrees of leukocytosis in patients with pheochromocytoma. Richmond and coworkers reported a patient with bouts of paroxysmal hypotension, due to an epinephrine-secreting tumor, which were accompanied by marked leukocytosis (up to 33,000 per mm³); differential white blood counts usually revealed the leukocytosis to be due to an increase in neutrophils (86 percent), but on one occasion the increase was primarily in lymphocytes (69 percent) (791).

It has been shown that injection of epinephrine causes a leukocytosis in two phases: the first, which occurs about 17 min after injection, is accompanied by an increase in neutrophils, lymphocytes, and eosinophils, whereas the second is accompanied by an increase in polymorphonuclear leukocytes only (842, 1055). In the first phase, the degree of change in lymphocytes was greater than that observed in other white cell elements. The increase of leukocytes in the secondary phase was maximal at about 4 hr following epinephrine injection and was less pronounced than the primary phase (842). This latter rise was entirely due to mobilization of neutrophils since there was a concomitant decrease in lymphocytes and eosinophils. The mechanism for this rise in neutrophils remains unclear, but the lymphopenia and eosinopenia appear best explained by an increased adrenal cortical secretion resulting from ACTH release (842). Explanation for the increased WBC in the primary phase remains obscure, although studies by Lucia and coworkers suggest that the leukocytosis is not the result of splenic contraction or bone marrow stimulation (588). It is noteworthy that one patient with pheochromocytoma had an eosinophilia of 25 percent which disappeared after the tumor was removed (856). Infusions of norepinephrine apparently do not significantly alter the total or differential white blood cell count (791).

The *erythrocyte sedimentation rate* was only very rarely elevated in patients with pheochromocytoma unaccompanied by complications.

PLASMA AND TOTAL BLOOD VOLUME

Schnelle and associates have pointed out that both the plasma volume and the red cell mass may be markedly contracted in some patients with pheochromocytoma. They have emphasized the importance of determining both fractions (by means of chromate-51-tagged red cells and chromate-51-tagged protein) for accurate assessment of a patient's blood volume (869).

Brunjes and coworkers have suggested that many patients with pheochromocytoma have a decreased plasma and total blood volume, which accounts for the frequent occurrence of postoperative shock following resection of the tumor (110). On the other hand, Waldmann reported that only four of 18 patients with pheochromocytoma had plasma volumes more than two standard deviations below the mean of normal subjects (normal mean = about 41 ml/kg body weight); three of 15 patients with pheochromocytoma had total blood volumes more than 2 standard deviations below the normal mean. Furthermore, three of the four patients with low plasma volumes, and two of the three with low total blood volumes, had metastatic pheochromocytoma; hence, the majority of patients studied by Waldmann and associates had normal plasma and normal total blood volumes (909).

During treatment with α-methyl-*p*-tyrosine (an inhibitor of tyrosine hydroxylase and catecholamine synthesis) or phenoxybenzamine (an α-adrenergic blocking agent), Waldmann reported an 11 percent increase in the mean plasma volume, whereas he reported a mean increase of 6 percent following surgical resection. He felt that these changes were relatively unimportant biologically (909).

Johns and Brunjes in 1962 (489), Tarazi and coworkers in 1970 (966), and, more recently, Deoreo and coworkers (223) demonstrated hypovolemia in the majority of their patients with pheochromocytoma. In fact,

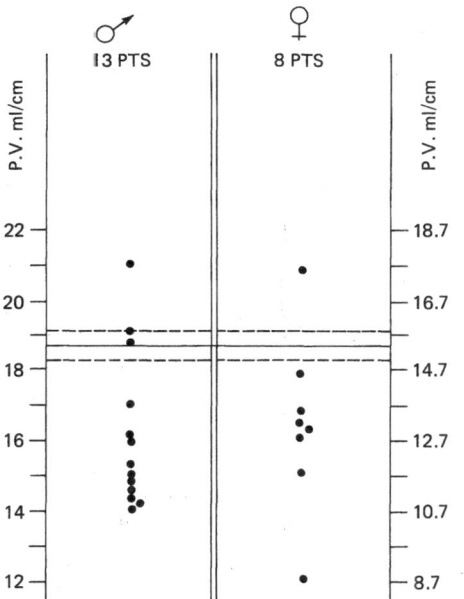

Fig. 6.1 Plasma volume in pheochromocytoma. Average plasma volume is 85.5 percent of normal for height (standard deviation: ±13.7; standard error: ±2.99). Normal values for male patients are 18.7 ml/cm body height ±0.33 S.E.M. and for female patients 15.3 ml/cm body height ±0.25 S.E.M. Plasma volume is expressed in relation to height instead of weight to avoid differences owing to age or obesity. Horizontal lines = mean and standard error of mean. From Deoreo, G. A., Jr., Stewart, B. H., Tarazi, R. C., and Gifford, R. W., Jr., *J. Urol. 111:* 719, 1974. By permission of Williams & Wilkins Co.

Tarazi observed a predictable inverse relationship between plasma volume and the diastolic blood pressure (223). The plasma volume in 21 patients with pheochromocytoma studied by Deoreo and coworkers is depicted in Figure 6.1. The average plasma volume for these patients was 85.5 percent of normal.

BLOOD UREA

The blood urea, blood urea nitrogen, and creatinine are within normal limits in the great majority of patients with pheochromocytoma; however, slight elevations of blood urea were occasionally noted. As seen in Table 6.3 above (results on 69 patients), approximately 81 and 76 percent of patients, respectively, with paroxysmally or persistently functioning tumors had normal blood urea values (<40 mg/dl). Only one out of 32 patients with paroxysmal hypertension, and two out of 37 patients with persistent hyperten-

sion, had blood urea values of 60 mg/dl or greater. Even an increase in blood urea clearance may occur in some patients (640).

Marked elevations of blood urea are distinctly unusual in patients with pheochromocytoma, but may occur if renal blood flow and glomerular filtration are seriously compromised by the effect of circulating catecholamines (556) or by some complication such as circulatory collapse and shock; very rarely, blood creatinine may also become elevated under the same circumstances.

PROTEINURIA

As mentioned previously, proteinuria of Grade 1 or more was a frequent finding, occurring in about 64 and 35 percent, respectively, of patients with tumors causing persistent or paroxysmal hypertension. Proteinuria may occur during a paroxysm or increase after an attack (462). Heavy proteinuria (>3 g daily) is practically never seen in patients with pheochromocytoma. It is noteworthy, however, that a 29-year-old man who had experienced frequent paroxysmal attacks for 10 to 11 years developed mild sustained hypertension (160/110 mmHg) and moderate renal insufficiency with a persistent proteinuria of 1 or 2 g per liter of urine (462). A more detailed discussion of the urinary findings and renal function in patients with pheochromocytoma appears in the section on differential diagnosis (Chapter 5) under "Renal Disease."

PLASMA RENIN AND ALDOSTERONE

Maebashi and coworkers found plasma renin elevated in five of seven patients with pheochromocytoma (601). They observed that elevated plasma renin levels were consistently found when the urinary excretion of norepinephrine was greater than epinephrine. On the other hand, plasma renin levels were normal in patients in whom the excretion of epinephrine was higher than that of norepinephrine. However, they stated that two of their patients were thought to have hypertension on the basis of renal artery stenosis (which could have accounted for hyperreninemia) due to compression of the renal artery by an extraadrenal pheochromocytoma located at the hilum of the kidney. Similarly, Van Way and associates have reported elevated renin in blood from the renal vein in a patient with a pheochromocytoma in the renal hilum which caused renal artery stenosis (989). The latter investigators reviewed the literature and discovered eight patients (ages 18 to 47 years) who had coexisting renal artery stenosis and pheochromocytoma. They concluded that arterial lesions resulted from direct pressure by an adjacent pheochromocytoma in some cases but that in others it seemed possible that catecholamines might have caused prolonged renal artery vasoconstriction which ultimately became a fibrous stenosis (989).

One report of renal artery stenosis due to compression by a pheochromocytoma in the renal hilum was particularly interesting since it occurred in an identical male twin. The other twin did not develop the tumor (509). In another patient, renal artery stenosis due to myointimal proliferation was believed to have resulted from a norepinephrine-secreting extraadrenal pheochromocytoma located adjacent to the renal artery. In this patient renal vein renins were elevated bilaterally without lateralization (328). It should be kept in mind that when pheochromocytoma and neurofibromatosis coexist, it is possible that renal arterial lesions can be caused by neurofibromas and may contribute to the hypertension (see Chapter 4).

Since renal artery stenosis may result in hyperreninemia, it was impossible to be certain in patients with coexisting lesions whether the stenosis or the effect of excessive circulating catecholamines from the pheochromocytoma was responsible for the elevated plasma renin levels. Meyer and associates reported increased plasma renin in five of seven patients with sustained hypertension and pheochromocytoma (658). They also found hyperaldosteronism in one of these patients. Similarly, Vetter and coworkers found elevated plasma renin activity ($>$20 ng/ml/3 hr) in seven of eight patients with pheochromocytoma, and four of these seven patients had abnormally high plasma aldosterone levels ($>$120 pg/ml) (992a). Hyperaldosteronism, a persistently low serum potassium, and a significantly reduced blood volume in a patient with pheochromocytoma was described by LeQuisne; however, renin or angiotensin levels were not mentioned (784). Mann-

hart and associates reported a patient with a pheochromocytoma in the neck who had secondary hyperaldosteronism which disappeared after extirpation of the pheochromocytoma (626). Several patients with pheochromocytoma were considered to have secondary aldosteronism as a result of hyperreninemia (515, 626, 1049). Other investigators have failed to demonstrate elevated plasma renin levels in patients with this tumor (103, 388); however, in some of these studies it was not indicated whether the patients had hypertension when the blood was sampled for renin. Werning and coworkers found plasma renin elevated in only two of six patients with pheochromocytoma (1027), but they were unable to explain why only two patients had renin elevations, since all patients had significantly increased urine catecholamines and VMA in addition to hypovolemia. All their patients were maintained on identical sodium intakes (1027). Others have found inconstant elevations of plasma renin in patients with pheochromocytoma (1027); occasionally the elevation may be extraordinarily high and return to normal following removal of the tumor (422). In one unusual case, plasma renin levels did not decline toward normal until 9 months following removal of an adrenal pheochromocytoma, despite the disappearance of renal artery stenosis caused by pressure from the tumor (474).

In reviewing the literature, Hiner and coworkers noted that an elevated plasma renin activity had been observed in more than 70 percent of patients with pheochromocytoma in whom renin had been quantitated (446b). These investigators reported an interesting study on an 11-year-old hypertensive (180/120 mmHg) boy who was originally thought to have renal artery stenosis because of an elevated plasma renin activity and an abnormal response to sodium deprivation. (Plasma renin activity on an unrestricted sodium diet was 7.3 ng/ml/hr whereas salt restriction caused a marked increase to 38 ng/ml/hr.) Urinary excretion of epinephrine, norepinephrine, VMA, and metanephrines was markedly increased, and angiography revealed a vascular mass in the right suprarenal area and no evidence of renal artery stenosis. Measurement of intrarenal blood distribution demonstrated that the outer cortical renal blood flow and percent flow to the outer cortex were 211 ml/min/100 g tissue and 73.9 percent in the left and 272 ml/min/100 g tissue and 72.4 percent in the right kidney. (Normal values in childhood for the outer cortical renal blood flow and percent flow to the outer cortex are 374 ± 16 ml/min/100 g tissue and 83 ± 1.9 percent.) Hiner and coworkers pointed out that the reduced renal cortical blood flow and reduced fractional flow to the outer cortex are consistent with the effects of catecholamines or with those of angiotensin on intrarenal hemodynamics. Subsequently a pheochromocytoma was removed with the right adrenal gland and the plasma renin activity returned to normal. Although renal hemodynamics were not measured postoperatively, these investigators concluded that the return of plasma renin activity to normal levels suggested that the initial abnormality was related to the effects of the pheochromocytoma. They further pointed out that elevation of plasma renin activity in patients with pheochromocytoma can result from a complex interplay of "volume- and catecholamine-induced effects" (446b). Increased circulating catecholamines may cause: (a) direct stimulation of the juxtaglomerular cells, (b) vasoconstriction of renal afferent and renal cortical arterioles, (c) direct stimulation of proximal tubular cells (with enhancement of sodium reabsorption), and (d) blood volume contraction. Experimental results indicate that any alteration in intrarenal hemodynamics which results in a decreased transmural tension in afferent arterioles and/or a decreased rate of sodium delivery to the macula densa may result in an increased secretion of renin (206b).

In conclusion, it appears from a review of the literature that plasma renin may be elevated in some. but not all, patients with pheochromocytoma. The sodium intake has not been rigidly controlled in most of the patients with pheochromocytoma thus far reported. Dietary control of salt intake is, of course, mandatory for an accurate comparative analysis of renin levels. Occasionally, increased plasma renin levels may be due to associated renal arterial disease or to renal artery compression by the pheochromocytoma; however, in most instances elevation of plasma renin results from the effects of increased circulat-

ing catecholamines on both kidneys. By determining the concentrations of plasma renin in blood collected from both renal veins, it may be possible to differentiate whether the increased renin secretion is due to the effects of increased circulating catecholamines (which would affect both kidneys) or to unilateral renal artery narrowing (992a). As suggested by Maebashi and coworkers, it is possible that intense renal vasoconstriction caused by excessive concentrations of circulating norepinephrine will increase plasma renin levels. Epinephrine also causes renal vasoconstriction, yet they noted elevations in plasma renin of dogs during infusions of epinephrine only when these animals had been premedicated with propranolol. Medication with this β-adrenergic blocker may have augmented renal vasoconstriction caused by epinephrine and may have modified renal hemodynamics to a degree similar to that caused by norepinephrine (601).

Despite the above conclusions, it is worth mentioning that experimental studies in animals regarding the role of the renal sympathetic nerves and catecholamines in renin release strongly suggest that a β-receptor in the kidney mediates an increase in renin secretion (206b, 207).

It is particularly noteworthy that in one patient with pheochromocytoma and widespread neurofibromatosis, infusion of saralasin (1-sar, 8-ala, angiotensin II; P113) caused a precipitous rise in the blood pressure from a relatively normotensive level to 230/170 mmHg (241). This hypertensive crisis was accompanied by severe headache, back pains, and profuse sweating. The initial plasma renin activity was 7.7 ng/ml/hr and it increased to 38 ng/ml/hr following the hypertensive crisis and the administration of phentolamine. It seems likely that saralasin triggered a release of catecholamines from the pheochromocytoma and that the hyperreninemia resulted from the effect of excessive circulating catecholamines on the kidneys. Because of this untoward experience and since angiotensin II and several angiotensin analogues (including saralasin) can cause release of catecholamines from the adrenal medulla, Dunn and coworkers have recommended caution whenever saralasin is administered, especially if pheochromocytoma is suspected (241).

Recently Dr. Koshiro Fukiyama stated that he has had two patients with pheochromocytoma who experienced hypertensive crises during infusion of 1-sarcosine-8-isoleucine angiotensin II. Phentolamine promptly returned the blood pressures to normal levels and, subsequently, the administration of phenoxybenzamine prevented recurrence of the hypertensive crises when this angiotensin analogue was reinfused (personal communication from Dr. Koshiro Fukiyama, Kyushu University, Japan).

It should be mentioned that "rebound hypertension" (sometimes accompanied by headache, nausea, vomiting, diaphoresis, seizures, and coma) may occur following an infusion of saralasin in some patients with renal hypertension. Unlike the hypertensive crises which have been observed *during* infusion of saralasin (or other angiotensin analogues) in patients with pheochromocytoma, the alarming "rebound hypertension" reported in patients with renal hypertension occurred *1 to 3 hr after saralasin infusion was stopped* (502a).

CHEMICAL ABNORMALITIES DUE TO ASSOCIATED CONDITIONS

Occasionally other chemical abnormalities may occur which do not result from secretion of the pheochromocytoma but are due to the elaboration of hormones by associated conditions (e.g., Cushing's disease, hyperparathyroidism, and medullary thyroid carcinoma). Diagnosis of these associated conditions may be made from the chemical abnormalities they produce. Of particular importance is the fact that, by finding a normal serum thyrocalcitonin level under basal conditions and also a normal thyrocalcitonin response to intravenous pentagastrin and calcium infusion tests, one can almost eliminate the presence of a medullary thyroid carcinoma or C-cell hyperplasia in a patient suspected of having Sipple's syndrome.

Normally, the serum thyrocalcitonin level does not increase above 0.55 ng/ml during a 4-hr calcium gluconate infusion (15 mg of calcium per kilogram of body weight). The upper limit of normal for the basal level of calcitonin is 0.35 ng/ml and in most normal subjects it is less than 0.10 ng/ml (83a). [The normal basal plasma immunoreactive calcitonin concentration in subjects studied at

the Mayo Clinic is ≤ 0.39 ng/ml (135).] Dr. C. E. Jackson has pointed out that sometimes patients with the Zollinger-Ellison syndrome, hypoparathyroidism, or pseudohypoparathyroidism have abnormal elevations of serum calcitonin. These patients may have normal or elevated levels under basal conditions or the levels may become elevated only following administration of pentagastrin or during a calcium infusion (personal communication from Dr. Charles E. Jackson, Henry Ford Hospital, Detroit). We are unaware of any hypertensive or hypotensive reactions to the administration of pentagastrin or calcium.

Recently Sizemore and Heath have demonstrated that pentagastrin injection (0.5 μg/kg of body weight, given as a bolus in 5 sec) is superior to calcium infusion (15 mg/kg of body weight given over a 4-hr period) for the diagnosis of medullary thyroid carcinoma or its precursor, parafollicular C-cell hyperplasia (903a). In their experience 20 percent of patients with familial thyroid carcinoma or C-cell hyperplasia had normal or indeterminate (nondiagnostic) immunoreactive basal calcitonin concentrations. In patients with medullary thyroid carcinoma or C-cell hyperplasia, the pentagastrin-provocative test invariably caused a diagnostic elevation of calcitonin whereas 18 percent of the calcium infusion results were falsely negative. In five kindreds the pentagastrin test correctly predicted medullary thyroid carcinoma or C-cell hyperplasia in 47 percent of the estimated 50 percent of members at risk (903a). As mentioned earlier, Gagel and associates indicated that the use of both the pentagastrin and calcium provocative tests may be more reliable than either test alone (340).

The laboratory abnormalities that may be observed in patients with pheochromocytoma and some associated conditions are enumerated in Table 6.4.

ELECTROCARDIOGRAPHIC CHANGES
CLINICAL

Electrocardiographic changes, particularly sinus tachycardia, may be frequently observed in patients with pheochromocytoma. Atrial or ventricular premature contractions or tachycardia are not infrequent during hyper-

Table 6.4 *Laboratory Findings Sometimes Present in Pheochromocytoma*

1. Fasting hyperglycemia (⅔ of sustained hypertensives)
2. Glucosuria
3. Impaired glucose tolerance
4. ↑ BMR (>20%) (¾ of sustained hypertensives)
5. ↑ Plasma FFA (mainly sustained hypertensives) (? ↑ glycerol)
6. ↑ Serum cholesterol
7. Anemia or polycythemia (WBC normal or ↑) (ESR normal or ↑)
8. ↓ Plasma and/or total blood volume
9. ↑ Blood urea < 60 mg% in 95%; with or without proteinuria (rarely slight serum creatinine ↑)
10. ↑ Plasma renin ± aldosteronism (? when NE > E, or when associated renal artery stenosis)
11. If associated with
    Cushing's syndrome
      ↑ Serum ACTH (elaborated by pheochromocytoma)
      ↑ Plasma cortisol
      ↑ Urinary steroids
    Hyperparathyroidism
      ↑ Serum calcium
      ↑ Serum parathyroid hormone
      ↓ Serum phosphate
    Medullary thyroid carcinoma
      ↑ Serum thyrocalcitonin
      ↑ Serum prostaglandin
      ↑ Serum serotonin
      ↑ Urinary 5-HIAA
      ↑ Serum histaminase

tensive crises. Supraventricular tachycardia up to 200/min in two patients and 160/min in a third patient has been recorded (836). Ectopic beats may result from stimulation of the myocardium by increased circulating catecholamines (242). Furthermore, myocardial "irritability" is increased if its concentration of catecholamines is excessive. In their review of alterations in the electrocardiogram of patients with pheochromocytoma, Sayer and associates have categorized these as abnormalities of rhythm or abnormalities suggesting myocardial ischemia, damage, or strain (856). Disorders of rhythm consisted of the following:

1. Wandering pacemaker
2. Sinoauricular dissociation
3. Auricular tachycardia
4. Auricular premature contractions
5. Auricular flutter
6. Auricular fibrillation
7. Nodal tachycardia
8. Ventricular premature contractions
9. Ventricular tachycardia

They found that arrhythmias occurred most frequently during paroxysms of hypertension and sometimes persisted after the blood pressure had returned to normal levels. All reported arrhythmias disappeared after the tumors were removed (856). Following administration of benzodioxane or phenoxybenzamine to one of their patients with pheochromocytoma and sustained hypertension, Sayer and coworkers observed a reversion toward normal of T waves, prolongation of the Q–T interval, and a clockwise rotation of the heart, with a shift to a more vertical position.

ECG abnormalities suggesting myocardial damage included the following:

1. Left axis deviation
2. Right axis deviation (occasionally with patterns similar to those seen in acute cor pulmonale and related to a marked increase in pulmonary artery pressure and a disproportionate increase in right ventricular work, which can be produced by catecholamine infusions (1055b).
3. Abnormally high or peaked P waves

4. Low or inverted T waves (often diffusely distributed)
5. S–T segment deviations and prolongation of Q–T interval

Sayer and coworkers reported that these changes occurred transiently during or between paroxysms of hypertension, and continuously in some patients with sustained hypertension (856). They stated that disappearance of these abnormalities sometimes occurred spontaneously, during hypertensive paroxysms or during a low-sodium regimen. Partial or complete reversal of these abnormalities to normal was noted in patients after tumor removal. It must be kept in mind, however, that evidence of irreversible myocardial damage [e.g., that associated with catecholamine cardiomyopathy as described by Kline (517) and van Vliet and coworkers (988) or with coronary atherosclerosis and/or myocardial infarction] may persist after a hypertensive crisis caused by pheochromocytoma or after tumor removal.

Sayer and coworkers emphasized that in the absence of any demonstrable etiologic factors the ECG abnormalities described above should alert the clinician to consider the possibility of pheochromocytoma. They appropriately stated that "the pathogenesis of the abnormal electrocardiogram produced by a pheochromocytoma is a complex interplay of the relative amounts of epinephrine and norepinephrine secreted by the tumor, the duration of the secretion, whether intermittent or sustained, and the net effects of these pressor amines upon the cardiac rate, rhythm, output, oxygen demand and supply, as well as the coronary circulation, pulmonary and peripheral arterial resistance, and perhaps the body electrolyte distribution" (856). It is well to remember, as indicated by Futterweit and associates (338) and noted by others, that a singularly striking feature of the ECG of some patients with pheochromocytoma is a diffuse distribution of T and S–T changes (124, 473, 856, 880); these changes are in contrast to those observed in patients with other forms of hypertension exhibiting a "strain pattern."

More recently, Saint-Pierre and coworkers have reviewed the electrocardiographic findings in patients with pheochromocytoma reported in the literature and have also presented the findings in 21 of their own patients. They noted that ventricular extrasystoles were particularly common and were recorded in about 50 percent of the reports in the literature (836). Auricular extrasystoles occurred less frequently.

Of the patients recently reported by Saint-Pierre and colleagues (835), the following ECG abnormalities were noted:

1. Left ventricular hypertrophy patterns
2. Arrhythmias (occurring sometimes without hypertension and liable to be induced by effort)
3. Coronary insufficiency patterns
4. Variable and transient repolarization disturbances (probably related to functional or autonomic disturbances caused by high concentrations of blood catecholamines)
5. Disturbances of repolarization accompanying clinical, roentgenologic, and hemodynamic manifestations of myocardial involvement (catecholamine cardiomyopathy)

None of the changes in the ECG described above can be considered specific; but, when they occur in association with the onset of palpitations, hypertension, and other symptoms and signs of increased circulating catecholamines, they take on greater diagnostic significance. The extent to which an associated coronary atherosclerosis might have contributed to some of the ECG abnormalities encountered is difficult to assess, especially since the effects of pheochromocytoma may possibly facilitate coronary atherogenesis (746).

A particularly fascinating electrocardiographic pattern, consistent with that observed in acute anterior myocardial infarction (note S–T elevations in precordial leads and Q wave in aVL), was observed in one of the patients with pheochromocytoma studied at the Mayo Clinic (Fig. 6.2). These ECG changes apparently were not the result of myocardial infarction but were probably related to the effects of excessive circulating catecholamines.

Electrocardiographic changes consistent with acute anteroseptal myocardial infarction have recently been reported in another patient with an adrenal pheochromocytoma studied at the Mayo Clinic (Fig. 6.3). This 59-year-old woman never experienced chest pains, and because of rapid reversal of the

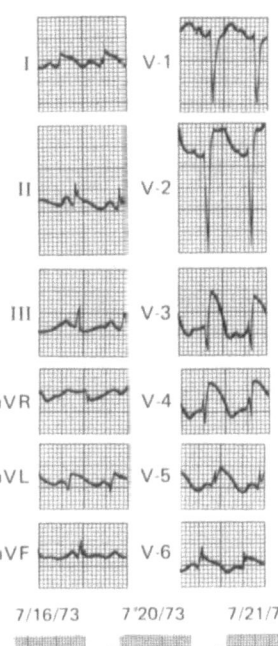

Fig. 6.2 This ECG was recorded about 24 hr before death in a 45-year-old man with a right adrenal pheochromocytoma who was in circulatory shock. He had not been recognized as having a pheochromocytoma and, following a left nephrectomy for transitional cell carcinoma of the kidney pelvis, was found to be in circulatory collapse. Postmortem examination revealed no evidence of acute myocardial infarction, no mural thrombus, and no significant coronary artherosclerosis; an incidental finding was an atrial septal defect. However, scattered throughout the myocardium were focal areas of necrosis associated with myocardial fiber degenerative changes and inflammatory cell infiltrations. It was felt by Dr. A. L. Brown (pathologist at the Mayo Clinic) that these pathologic lesions could best be explained on the basis of excessive circulating catecholamines from his pheochromocytoma. Note: This patient's myocardial pathology is shown in Figure 3.38A. Courtesy of Dr. H. B. Burchell, Senior Consultant in Cardiology, University of Minnesota.

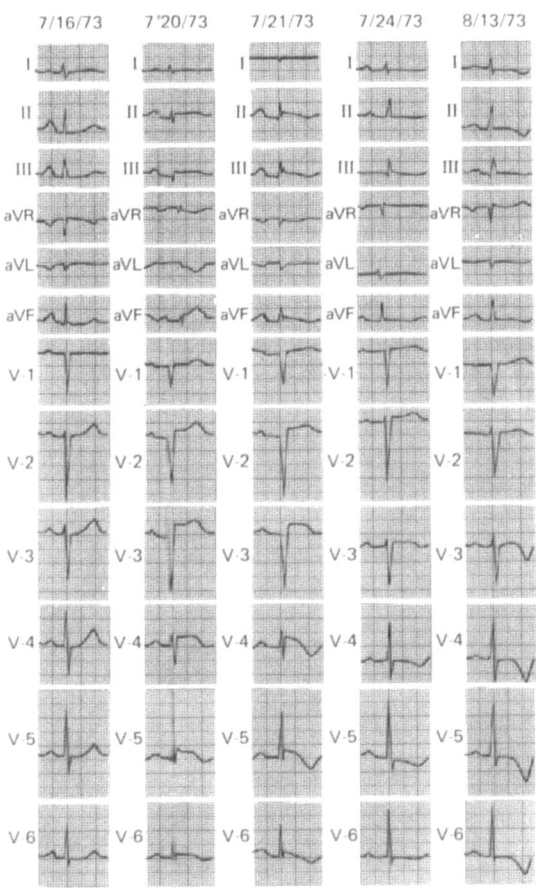

Fig. 6.3 Serial electrocardiograms. The S–T segment elevation and loss of R-wave voltage over anterior precordial leads on July 20, 1973 suggested acute anteroseptal infarction. There is S–T segment elevation in leads II, III, and aVF. Note also the rapid resolution of these changes: by July 24, 1973 R-wave voltage was returning to normal and by August 13, 1973 it was normal and only widespread T-wave inversion was evident. The ECG was that of a 59-year-old white woman who developed a paroxysm of hypertension (250/105 mmHg) and became apathetic, disoriented, and transiently blind. A left hemisensory deficit, dysesthesia of the left leg, and a left Babinski were noted and shortly thereafter she became unresponsive, diaphoretic, and showed signs of peripheral vasoconstriction. The ECG became abnormal at this time and thereafter sequential changes were observed as shown in the figure. She regained her sight in a few hours but peripheral vasoconstriction persisted and the sensory deficits improved only gradually. She was treated with α- and β-adrenergic blocking agents, and subsequently a pheochromocytoma was successfully removed from the region of the left adrenal gland. From Radtke, W. E., Kazmier, F. J., Rutherford, B. D., and Sheps, S. G., *Am. J. Cardiol 35:* 702, 1975.

changes were attributed to a toxic myocarditis due to catecholamines, rather than to a transmural infarction (778). Others have reported a similar case (742).

Cheng and Bashour have recently reported the case of a 51-year-old black woman with pheochromocytoma who presented with striking cardiographic changes mimicking ischemic heart disease at one time and acute pulmonary embolism at other times. Paroxysmal episodes were accompanied by abnormalities of repolarization of the Q–T interval and deep and wide symmetrically inverted T waves without changes in the QRS complex. Prominent P waves in Leads II, III, and aVF were frequently observed with no significant change in the QRS axis. The Q–T interval remained prolonged even when T waves were upright. Normal ECGs were recorded during several attacks of paroxysmal hypertension. These investigators pointed out that symmetric T-wave inversion with or without a prolonged Q–T interval is not specific for coronary artery disease; similar ECG changes have been seen in acute pancreatitis, gallbladder disease, acute cerebrovascular accidents, during administration of quinidine, atypical angina with normal coronary arteriograms, and diencephalic discharges. Although the mechanism whereby these changes induce repolarization abnormalities is not well understood, a diencephalic discharge of catecholamines has been implicated in some of these conditions. Finally, Cheng and Bashour cite evidence for the toxic effects of excessive levels of catecholamines on the myocardium. It was also noted that reversible T-wave inversions have been induced in normal man by intravenous infusion of norepinephrine (149a).

It is interesting that electrocardiographic changes similar to those which occurred in the patient of Cheng and Bashour were observed in a patient who inadvertently received an overdose of norepinephrine and developed circulatory shock (personal communication from Dr. Howard B. Burchell, Senior Consultant in Cardiology, University of Minnesota).

Occasionally bradycardia instead of tachycardia occurs in patients with pheochromocytoma (322, 416, 431, 924). Vagal response to elevated blood pressure during hypertensive crises in some of these patients evidently causes sinus slowing instead of the usual sinus tachycardia, premature beats, and ectopic tachycardias which result from β-adrenergic stimulation of the myocardium (322). Rarely, reflex bradycardia with depression of the sinus node and escape of lower pacemakers have been recorded in patients with pheochromocytoma during a severe hypertensive crisis (116, 280, 322). Nodal escape and A-V

dissociation have been observed during hypertensive crises in association with both bradycardia (116, 280, 322) and tachycardia (338).

Forde and coworkers have reported two patients with intermittent chest pain and arrhythmia who were initially suspected of having acute myocardial infarction (322). Constant ECG and blood pressure monitoring revealed that episodically severe hypertension (associated with anterior chest pressure or pain, palpitations, and other clinical manifestations) occurred coincidentally with reflex bradycardia and nodal espace rhythm and A-V dissociation (Figs. 6.4 and 6.5). With

Fig. 6.4 Sequential changes in cardiac rhythm during an episode of hypertension in Case 1, demonstrating slowing of the sinus pacemaker and nodal escape rhythm with A-V dissociation as the blood pressure rises, and restoration of sinus rhythm, culminating in sinus tachycardia, as the blood pressure falls toward normal (paper speed 25 mm/sec). Note the initial drop in blood pressure (shown in Table 6.5) at the onset of this attack when epinephrine becomes elevated. On one occasion the blood pressure rose from 120/80 to 250/100 mmHg during the development of A-V dissociation and then fell to 80/60 mmHg. This is particularly interesting since, as mentioned earlier, hypotensive periods have occasionally been reported in patients harboring a pheochromocytoma which secretes predominantly epinephrine. This is patient No. 30 described in Chapter 7. Numbers on the left hand margin indicate time in minutes. From Forde, T. P., Yormak, S. S., and Killip, T., *Am. Heart J. 76:* 389, 1968.

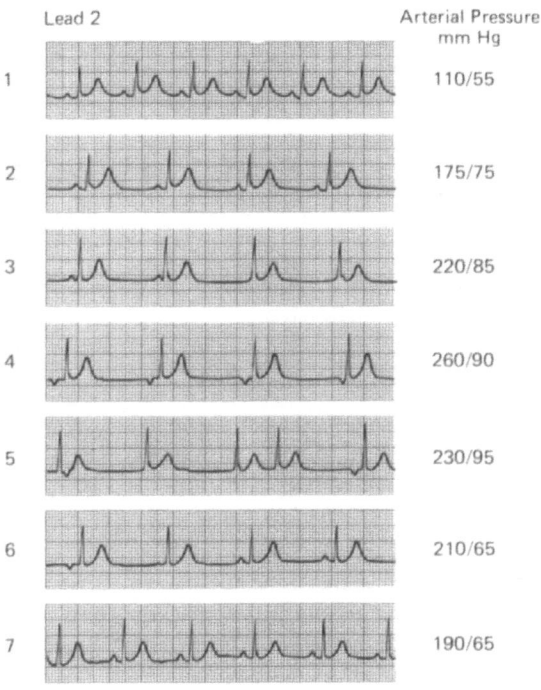

Lead 2	Arterial Pressure mm Hg
1	110/55
2	175/75
3	220/85
4	260/90
5	230/95
6	210/65
7	190/65

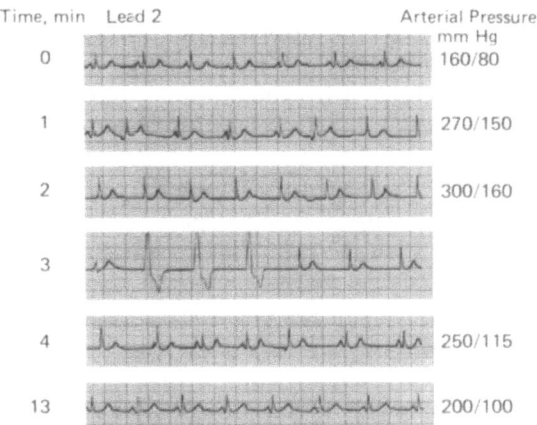

Time, min   Lead 2   Arterial Pressure
                                            mm Hg
0   160/80
1   270/150
2   300/160
3
4   250/115
13   200/100

Fig. 6.5 Sequential changes in cardiac rhythm during an episode of hypertension precipitated by massage of right upper abdominal quadrant in Case 2. Note depression of sinus pacemaker and appearance of lower foci as blood pressure rises. When blood pressure declines, sinus mechanism is restored (paper speed 25 mm/sec). This is patient No. 32 described in Chapter 7. From Forde, T. P., Yormak, S. S., and Killip, T., *Am. Heart J. 76:* 391, 1968.

(Fig. 6.5), both epinephrine and norepinephrine plasma concentrations reached very high levels when hypertension was induced by massage of the right upper abdomen (Table 6.5). It is noteworthy that sinus bradycardia and occasionally complete A-V dissociation have been produced by intravenous infusion of norepinephrine into human subjects (42).

As emphasized by Forde, Yormak, and Killip, the diagnosis of pheochromocytoma should be considered in any patient with periodic bradycardia and escape of lower pacemakers (322). Careful documentation of the blood pressure before and during such arrhythmias is mandatory, and if it is disclosed that these electrocardiographic abnormalities are induced by hypertensive crises, a pheochromocytoma must be strongly suspected. To date, reflex bradycardia with nodal escape rhythm in patients with pheochromocytoma has almost invariably been described in those who have paroxysmal and not persistent hypertension. One 44-year-old woman with slight hypertension (160/108 mmHg recumbent) had isoelectric T waves in Leads I and aVL, diphasic T waves in Leads V3–4, and inverted T waves in Leads II, III, and V5–6. Slight S–T depression in Leads V5–6 and a prominent P wave in Lead II were also present (338). She developed a blood pressure rise of

subsidence of the hypertensive crises, the ECG reverted to normal sinus rhythm. The rise in blood pressure always preceded the onset of the arrhythmia. In case 1 (Fig. 6.4), we found that only the plasma epinephrine became markedly elevated during a spontaneous hypertensive crisis, whereas in case 2

Table 6.5 *Plasma Levels of Epinephrine and Norepinephrine in Two Cases of Pheochromocytoma with Reflex Bradycardia and Nodal Escape Rhythm[a]*

	Blood pressure (mmHg)	Plasma epinephrine[b] (μg/liter plasma)	Plasma norepinephrine[b] (μg/liter plasma)
Normal concentrations (upper limit)		<1.5	<6.6
Case 1			
Control	154/80	1.3[e]	3.8[e]
During spontaneous hypertensive attack			
Onset	80/50	2.6	3.5
Rising	205/68	26.7	3.6
Peak	240/130		
Falling	198/73	2.9	3.4
Case 2			
Control	158/80	3.1[e]	8.2[e]
During hypertensive attack induced by pressure in right upper quadrant			
Peak	300/160	28.5[e]	27.3[e]

[a] Modified from Forde, T. P., Yormak, S. S., and Killip, T.III. *Am. Heart J. 76:* 391, 1968.
[b] Performed by Dr. W. M. Manger, New York University Medical Center, New York City.
[e] Average of two rapid sequence samples.

80/46 mmHg above the basal level following a histamine (0.025 mg I.V.) provocative test, and simultaneously the ECG revealed further peaking of the P waves, A-V dissociation, and supraventricular and ventricular extrasystoles. The ECG returned to the prestimulation state 20 min after histamine administration. Three days following pheochromocytoma extirpation no ECG abnormalities were evident.

An electrocardiographic finding which has been noted (116, 329, 755) in patients with pheochromocytoma, but not previously emphasized, was observed in case 2 mentioned above (W. M. Manger and S. S. Yormak, unpublished data). Figure 6.6 reveals a continuous recording from Lead II in this patient during a paroxysmal attack of hypertension. During the periods of bradycardia and nodal escape, the T waves became exceptionally high and decreased toward normal when the blood pressure returned to normal and the bradycardia subsided. Also, there was a slight and transient depression of the S–T segment. The finding of a huge T wave is in no way specific for pheochromocytoma. Enlarged T

waves may be seen in myocardial infarction or hyperkalemia; however, one would usually expect other typical ECG changes to occur concomitantly with these latter conditions.

The ECG of a patient with pheochromocytoma reported by French and Campagna, revealed a prolonged Q–T interval, prominent U waves, depressed S–T segments, and high, peaked T waves (329)—abnormalities that were clearly reversible.

A summary of the electrocardiographic abnormalities which may be seen in patients with pheochromocytomas which are actively secreting catecholamines is given in Table 6.6.

EXPERIMENTAL

Tenzer stated that epinephrine injected into the normal man increases cardiac frequency and the amplitude of the P waves, shortens the P–R interval, increases myocardial excitability, and provokes alterations in rhythm (973). In addition, he mentions that therapeutic doses of epinephrine can cause elevation of T waves, whereas larger doses will cause T-wave inversion. When moderate doses of norepinephrine were injected, bradycardia and depression of the P wave occurred; in addition, nodal rhythm sometimes appeared, and frequently the T waves became elevated (973).

It is noteworthy that infusions of epinephrine or norepinephrine into the coronary artery of dogs produced high, upright, peaked T waves with depressed S–T segments (40). Large upright T waves, associated with prominent U waves, prolonged Q–T interval, and T–U fusion have not infrequently been observed as an electrocardiographic manifestation of intracranial disease (114).

Experimental animal studies on the effect of hypothalamic or stellate ganglion stimulation, and stellate ganglionectomy, suggest that sympathetic pathways are involved in some of these ECG alterations (651, 1066). Increased concentrations of circulating catecholamines may conceivably cause disturbances in the myocardium in a manner similar to those induced by activation of the sympathetic innervation of the heart. Intravenous administration of epinephrine or norepinephrine to healthy subjects leads to reversible ECG alterations. Sjöstrand found that epinephrine invariably caused the appearance of

Fig. 6.6 Continuous recording from Lead II (coronary care unit monitoring electrodes) in a 58-year-old white male with pheochromocytoma during paroxysmal attack of hypertension. This is the same patient whose ECG tracing appears in Figure 6.4 and is patient No. 32 described in Chapter 7. From Manger, W. M. and Yormak, S. S., unpublished.

A. Onset of attack (BP = > 300/115, normal BP = 130/65). Nodal escape rhythm—heart rate = 58/min.

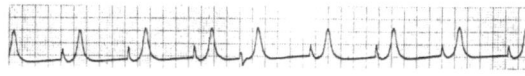

B. Symptoms subsiding. Nodal escape with some sinus rhythm—heart rate = 51-63/min.

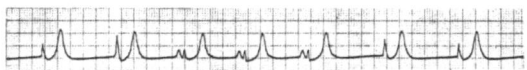

C. 3-5 minutes after onset, symptoms gone (BP = 135/60). Regular sinus rhythm—heart rate = 82/min.

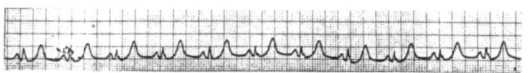

Table 6.6 *ECG Abnormalities Sometimes Seen in Patients with Pheochromocytoma*

Atrial, nodal, or ventricular tachycardia
Atrial or ventricular premature contractions (with or without bigeminy)
Bradycardia with or without complete A-V dissociation with or without
  T-wave peaking
Wandering pacemaker
Atrial flutter or fibrillation
Left or right axis deviation
Abnormally high or peaked P waves
Low or inverted T waves
S–T segment deviations
Prolonged Q–T interval

(Reversibility of ECG abnormalities + absence of etiologic explanation
suggests pheochromocytoma.)

a positive after-potential following the T wave which was coupled with an associated depression of the T wave and S–T segment (911). After vagal block, the ECG changes caused by epinephrine were augmented. On the other hand, administration of norepinephrine caused the reverse of the epinephrine effect; i.e., norepinephrine in the same dose produced a slight rise in the T wave, while the positive after-potential was either decreased or unchanged and the heart rate was slowed. ECG changes similar to those evoked by epinephrine were encountered in seven of eight patients with pheochromocytoma (131). Cannon and Sjöstrand emphasized that marked and variable reversible ECG changes occurring in a very short time should suggest the possibility of pheochromocytoma (131).

Watkins had commented that ECG alterations could be related to shifts in cellular potassium accompanying hyperglycemia caused by increased circulating catecholamines (1009). Consistent with this concept, French and Campagna (329) suggested that altered potassium metabolism, with consequent development of hypokalemia, could account for prolonged Q–T intervals, S–T depression, and prominent U waves, in addition to the positive after-potential (where the U or T wave descends and merges with the P wave before reaching the base line) noted in their patient and described by Cannon

and Sjöstrand. They further pointed out that although the upright, peaked T wave in their patient was not consistent with hypokalemia, catecholamines can secondarily cause a marked vagal effect, which could account for the T-wave peaking (130). Dr. Howard B. Burchell, who kindly reviewed this manuscript, suggested the possibility that a disparate flow of catecholamines into the myocardium might occur and result in local differences in sympathetic "drive" which could produce large T waves; he felt, however, that a transient ischemia of the subendocardial zone was a more likely explanation of the huge T waves (personal communication from Dr. Howard B. Burchell).

It should be pointed out that concentrations of serum potassium during paroxysms of hypertension in patients with pheochromocytoma have not been adequately studied. During a constant intravenous infusion of epinephrine (10–18 μg/min) in 12 normal young men, the mean serum potassium decreased very significantly by 17.3 percent without any remarkable change in serum sodium or chloride (481). Concomitantly, there was a decrease in urinary sodium, chloride, and potassium. The alteration in serum potassium was thought to reflect an intracellular shift. Keys noted a similar decrease in potassium in normal men following intravenous injection of 0.005 to 0.3 mg of epinephrine chloride but a return to levels slightly above preinjection values within 40 to 60 min (510). [These findings were in contrast to the immediate marked rise in plasma potassium caused by intravenous injections of epinephrine to dogs, cats, and rabbits (510).] A number of other investigators have found that administration of epinephrine causes a decrease in serum potassium (101, 143, 243, 801).

Graded intravenous infusions of norepinephrine in six normal young men caused a sharp fall in potassium clearance by the kidney without remarkably affecting clearance of sodium or chloride (774); also, there was a slight but statistically significant rise in serum potassium concentration (which averaged 5.2 percent) without any remarkable change in serum sodium or chloride. These results suggested that norepinephrine might cause a migration of potassium from intracellular to extracellular fluid. MacKeith, however, reported one patient with pheochromocytoma who had very elevated serum potassium between hypertensive attacks; he pointed out that intravenous epinephrine may produce an 86 percent rise in blood potassium (598). Only rarely has the serum potassium been reported elevated in patients with pheochromocytoma (640). Serum electrolytes are nearly always within normal limits in those patients with pheochromocytoma who have sustained hypertension; they are also normal between the hypertensive crises in those patients who have paroxysmal hypertension with pheochromocytoma.

CONCLUDING REMARKS

In the final analysis, we must recognize how totally imprecise are the contributions made by the electrocardiogram to the diagnosis of pheochromocytoma. After kindly reviewing this section on electrocardiography, Dr. Raymond Pruitt emphasized the desirability of pointing out the near total lack of specificity of the electrocardiographic changes occurring in patients with pheochromocytoma. He remarked that the origin of ECG changes may be more readily identified from clinical phenomena which suggest the presence of pheochromocytoma than from the ECG changes themselves (personal communication from Dr. Raymond D. Pruitt, Emeritus Dean, Mayo Medical School).

PHARMACOLOGIC TESTS IN THE DIAGNOSIS OF PHEOCHROMOCYTOMA

Prior to the advent of chemical methods for accurately detecting excess quantities of catecholamines or their metabolites in urine or blood, pharmacologic tests were heavily relied upon for making a preoperative diagnosis of pheochromocytoma. Two types of pharmacologic testing were employed: (1) the intravenous administration of an α-blocking agent which primarily blocked the vasoconstrictor effect of circulating catecholamines and thereby produced a pronounced decrease in the blood pressure of patients with hypertension caused by pheochromocytoma but produced no significant decrease in patients with other hypertensive conditions; and (2) the intravenous administration of an agent which caused a sudden release of catecholamines (from the tumor and/or possibly from excess stores in sympathetic nerves) into the circulation and thereby provoked a hypertensive crisis usually accompanied by symptoms and signs characteristically accompanying spontaneous paroxysmal attacks of hypertension (provocative test).

Today the preoperative diagnosis of pheochromocytoma can be made with confidence only when the concentration of catecholamines or their metabolites have been demonstrated by chemical determination to be significantly elevated in the urine or plasma.

Although the pharmacologic tests are now not frequently utilized, a provocative test, when combined with chemical quantitation of urine or plasma catecholamines or their metabolites, can prove indispensable in the diagnosis of a paroxysmally secreting pheochromocytoma. In 1954 we first demonstrated the diagnostic value of performing a provocative test combined with plasma catecholamine assay in certain patients with intermittently secreting tumors who had relatively normal blood pressures and normal plasma catecholamines (616). Diagnostic elevations of plasma catecholamines were induced in these patients by a provocative test (616, 623, 624). In evaluating patients suspected of having paroxysmal hypertension due to pheochromocytoma, we have found provocative tests to be especially valuable, since roughly 37.5 percent of such patients have normal plasma catecholamines when the blood pressure is normal or minimally elevated. A positive provocative test may also be helpful intraoperatively (223) and postoperatively after tumor extirpation in demonstrating the presence of additional pheochromocytomas.

METHODS OF PHARMACOLOGIC TESTING

A summary outline of the methods of pharmacologic testing and the criteria for judging results is indicated in Table 6.7. Provocative or α-adrenergic blocking tests may be performed on hospitalized or ambulatory patients.

Provocative Tests When the diagnosis of pheochromocytoma is suspected, a provocative test is indicated in those patients with relatively normal or minimally elevated blood pressures in association with normal or borderline elevations of catecholamines and/or their metabolites in plasma and/or urine.

A provocative test is now not performed if the blood pressure is greater than 170/110 mmHg, since we have invariably been able to establish the diagnosis of pheochromocytoma by chemical analysis of plasma or urine catecholamines and their metabolites in patients with sustained hypertension due to pheochromocytoma.

It is imperative that medications which may interfere with blood pressure responsiveness to provocative drugs or with determinations of catecholamines be avoided. No sedatives or narcotics should be taken for at least 48 hr, and all antihypertensive medication should be omitted for 1 week if this can be done without hazard to the patient. Furthermore, sympathomimetic medications as well as MAO and COMT inhibitors must be avoided, preferably for 1 week, since they may not only interfere with blood pressure responses to provocative drugs but may also result in erroneous quantitation of plasma and urine catecholamines and their metabolites when these determinations are performed in conjunction with the provocative tests.

Because of variability in vascular pressor responsiveness, it is mandatory that the blood pressure response to provocative drugs be compared with the pressor response to the standard cold pressor test. After the patient has remained recumbent and comfortable for

approximately 20 to 30 min and is in a relatively basal state, i.e., when the blood pressure has stabilized, as evidenced by repeated determinations, one hand is immersed in ice water up to the wrist for 1 min, during which time blood pressures are recorded every 15 to 20 sec in the other arm in order to determine the maximal blood pressure elevation resulting from this cold stimulus. Roth and associates reported that the average increase in the blood pressure during the cold pressor test was 40/29 mmHg, with a systolic range of 12 to 68 mmHg and a diastolic range from 10 to 78 mmHg. They never observed an attack induced by the cold pressor test in the large series of patients with pheochromocytoma which they investigated (820). After the cold pressor test, an indwelling needle (19 or

Table 6.7 *Pharmacologic Tests*

A. Provocative[a] (when BP relatively normal; not if BP > 170/110)
  1. Patient in basal state ─20 min (when BP stable)
  2. Avoid sympathomimetic medications and MAO and COMT inhibitors 1 week or more
   No sedatives or narcotics 48 hr
   No antihypertensive drugs 1 week or more
  3. Perform cold pressor test
  4. After blood pressure returns to basal state[a]
   Administer rapidly I.V. glucagon (1 mg) and then histamine (0.025–0.05 mg *base*) if glucagon test negative
   Histamine contraindicated in asthmatics (tyramine test unreliable)
Positive test: ↑BP 20/15 above peak cold pressor response and usually with accompanying symptoms and signs
False negative 20%; false positive very rare
Always have phentolamine to lower blood pressure!
B. Adrenergic blocking (when BP > 170/110)
  1. Patient in basal state
  2. Patient off drugs (see above)
   Phentolamine (Regitine) (5 mg I.V. rapidly)
   Positive test: ↓BP 35/25 but unreliable—many false positives from interfering drugs and nonspecific depressor response

---

[a] Plasma and/or urine should be collected before and following a provocative test and analyzed for catecholamines and/or their metabolites when possible.

Note: Medications to treat hypertensive crises, arrhythmias, or hypotension should *always* be available when provocative tests are performed.

20 gauge) or catheter is inserted into an antecubital vein. [The latter may be connected to a slow-infusion drip of normal saline or 5 percent dextrose in water and the provocative drugs injected directly into the tubing (near the vein) or via a 3-way stopcock interposed between the tubing and the needle or catheter.] We feel it is simpler and preferable to connect a syringe containing the provocative agent directly to the indwelling catheter or needle. The latter procedure will eliminate any "dead space" and the need for flushing to ensure that the provocative agent has been completely injected. Because of an occasional significant difference in the blood pressure between the right and left arms, recordings with a sphygmomanometer should always be made on the same arm. It is more convenient to take blood pressures on the arm used for ice water immersion; the other arm can then be kept stationary and used exclusively for intravenous injections and blood sampling as desired.

When the blood pressure has again stabilized, over a period of about 20 min, 1 mg of glucagon hydrochloride in about 1 ml of diluent is rapidly injected intravenously in one bolus and the blood pressure recorded every 15 to 20 sec for 5 min. If a pressure response occurs, the pressure is determined every minute until the pressor response subsides. The glucagon test is considered positive if an increase in blood pressure occurs which is at least 20 mmHg systolic and 15 mmHg diastolic above the peak blood pressure response induced by the cold pressor test. A positive test is usually accompanied by symptoms and signs characteristic of pheochromocytoma.

If the glucagon test is negative, the indwelling catheter or needle can be connected to an infusion of saline or dextrose in water to prevent blood clotting in the catheter or needle. Then in about 15 min, or later, when the blood pressure has stabilized, 0.05 mg (i.e., 0.05 ml volume) of histamine base (0.025 mg is adequate if the patient weighs less than 100 lb) is injected rapidly in one bolus and the blood pressure recorded as described after glucagon.

Histamine causes a transient vasodilation which is accompanied by an initial moderate to marked decrease in blood pressure, usually

observed about 30 sec after its intravenous injection. Absence of this initial characteristic blood pressure decrease suggests that the dose of histamine might not have been administered into the circulation, and in this event the test would be unreliable. Only rarely is a brief and slight decrease of 10 to

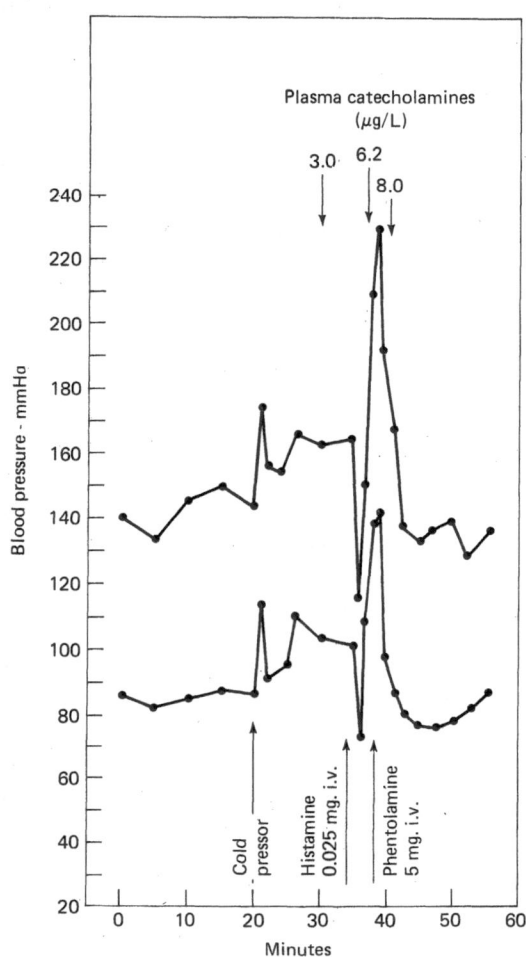

Fig. 6.7 Positive pressor response following intravenous administration of 0.025 mg of histamine base to a 57-year-old woman with metastatic pheochromocytoma. Note the immediate depressor response which is invariably present within 30 sec after injecting histamine intravenously. Failure to obtain this immediate depressor response indicates subcutaneous rather than intravenous injection. The pressor response follows the initial fall in blood pressure and is usually maximal within 2 min. To be significant, it should be at least 20/15 mmHg greater than the maximal pressor response to the cold pressor test. When it is obvious that a response has been obtained, phentolamine should be administered intravenously to terminate abruptly the pressor response and its potential hazards. From Gifford, R. W., Jr., Kvale, W. F., Mayer, F. T., Roth, G. M., and Priestley, J. T., *Mayo Clinic Proc.* 39: 293, 1964.

15 mmHg in systolic blood pressure noted within the first minutes after glucagon administration (555, 887). An example of a positive response to the histamine provocative test in a patient with pheochromocytoma is seen in Figure 6.7. The criteria for a positive test to histamine are identical to those for glucagon. In patients with pheochromocytoma and paroxysmal hypertension, Roth and coworkers found that in those having normal blood pressures between episodes the basal pressure averaged 117/78 mmHg, and this increased by 105/59 mmHg following the histamine test; in those having a more labile pressure the basal pressure averaged 151/105 mmHg and this increased by 75/46 mmHg (820). The maximal pressor response to glucagon or histamine usually occurs within 2 to 3 min after drug injection (352, 887), and all responses are seen within 5 min (887).

It is imperative that phentolamine be available (preferably 5 mg in each of several syringes) so that 5 mg may be immediately administered intravenously in an effort to promptly abort a positive response, shorten the induced attack, relieve any symptoms, and prevent possible vascular complications. Rarely, a second or third injection of 5 mg of phentolamine is required to terminate an attack. One patient reported by Roth and as-

sociates (820) had a 700 g pheochromocytoma, and required a total of 50 mg to reduce the blood pressure to basal levels in 10 min following a histamine test (Fig. 6.8). These investigators pointed out that this knowledge was important in the care of this patient since 50 mg of phentolamine was required during operation to keep the blood pressure at safe levels. A more typical response to histamine is also shown in this figure. Intravenous sodium nitroprusside is also an equally effective and safe antihypertensive agent; however, phentolamine is more conveniently prepared for use in counteracting an excessively severe hypertensive crisis and for alleviating some of the unpleasant symptomatology which may accompany the induced paroxysm.

Histamine was first used by Mayo in 1927 in an attempt to abort paroxysmal crises in a patient with pheochromocytoma (636). Subsequently, in 1943, Hyman and Mencher demonstrated that histamine was able to induce paroxysmal hypertension in patients with pheochromocytoma (470). Since the introduction of the histamine test by Roth and Kvale in 1945 (822), this drug has proved most reliable in causing a liberation of catecholamines into the circulation and inducing a paroxysmal attack of hypertension in pa-

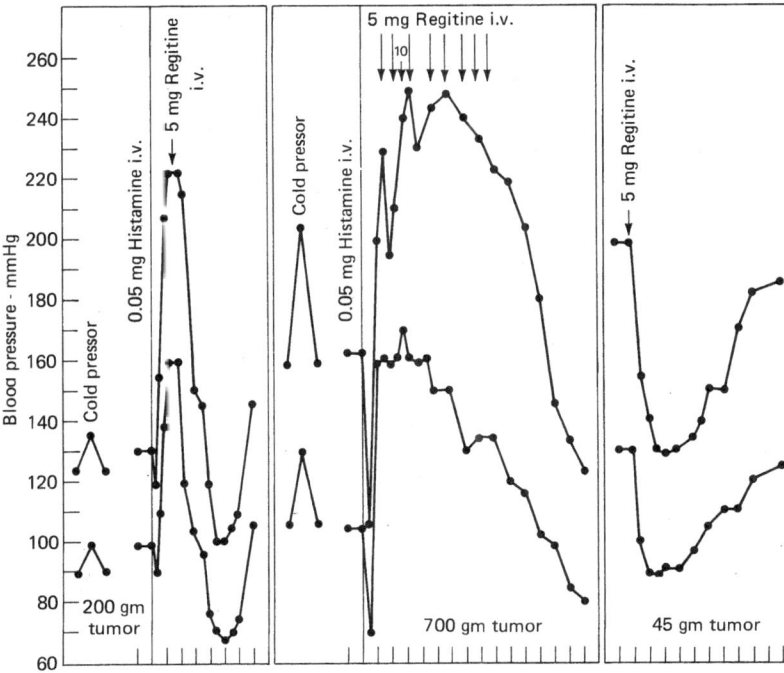

Fig. 6.8 Changes in blood pressure during the cold pressor, histamine, and Regitine tests. Left and center: patient had paroxysmal hypertension. Right: patient had sustained hypertension. From Roth, G. M., Flock, E. V., Kvale, W. F., Waugh, J. M., and Ogg, J., *Circulation 21:* 770, 1960. By permission of the American Heart Association, Inc.

tients with pheochromocytoma. Shortly following histamine injection, many patients transiently experience dryness of the mouth, a warm sensation, flushing, and mild headache; those with pheochromocytoma often experience an intense throbbing headache, marked anxiety, severe palpitations, and a pronounced sensation of warmth. Patients without this tumor may also occasionally experience an intense histamine cephalgia and pronounced flushing and sensation of warmth. Our experience and that of some other investigators indicate that the histamine test is positive in roughly 70 to 75 percent of patients with paroxysmal hypertension due to pheochromocytoma (218, 223); however, Sheps and Maher reported the histamine test was positive in only about 42 percent of the patients with pheochromocytoma whom they evaluated (887). The explanation for the smaller number of positive responses to histamine which they obtained is not clear, but conceivably it was related to the relatively small series studied and/or to the fact that the dose of histamine base administered intravenously was never more than 0.025 mg.

In our experience falsely positive responses to histamine occur only very rarely, although some have observed false positive responses in up to 11 percent of tests (888). Roth and coworkers pointed out that in patients with paroxysmal hypertension, sedatives inhibit the blood pressure rise evoked by the cold pressor test without remarkably influencing the pressure response to histamine; consequently a falsely positive histamine test could result (820). Falsely positive tests to histamine occurred in one patient who had taken phentolamine by mouth for 2 months and in another patient in whom a migraine headache was induced by histamine (820). Falsely negative responses may occur in approximately 25 percent of patients with pheochromocytoma and paroxysmal hypertension. A falsely negative response can result from antihypertensive medication, which can prevent a positive blood pressure rise following the histamine test in patients with pheochromocytoma (820, 824). Falsely negative responses to histamine occur more commonly when the test is performed in patients having sustained hypertension caused by this tumor (352). However, as mentioned previously, there is today no need to perform provocative tests on patients with sustained hypertension, since the diagnosis can almost invariably be made by chemical determination of plasma or urinary catecholamines and their metabolites.

In 1965 Lawrence proposed the use of glucagon as a provocative test for pheochromocytoma (553). Shortly thereafter, additional studies demonstrated the usefulness of this provocative agent. Sheps and Maher performed a comparative study on the accuracy and merits of glucagon versus histamine as a provocative test for pheochromocytoma (887). They found that the glucagon test was well tolerated and that only occasionally did patients experience "slight headaches, mild flushed feeling, vague nausea, and mild palpitations, all of momentary duration" (887). Lawrence also reported that side effects from glucagon testing were minimal; occasionally, others have observed nausea, pallor, tachycardia, excessive diaphoresis, and epigastric discomfort (183, 841).

In some instances Sheps and Maher observed a greater pressor response after glucagon than after histamine, but invariably subjective sensations were more marked after histamine. A change in pulse rate did not occur after glucagon in the absence of a pressor response. Patients without pheochromocytoma who were tested with 0.5 mg of glucagon had distinctly lower pressor responses than those given 1 mg, the dose used in almost all cases. These investigators felt that larger doses were contraindicated for screening patients, since the pressor responses to 1 mg of glucagon in some patients with pheochromocytoma were so pronounced (887). (Probably 0.5 mg of glucagon is adequate in patients weighing less than 100 lb.) Poutasse and Gifford have found that larger doses are no more desirable, and that a 1 mg glucagon dose appears to be optimal (769).

In a small series studied by Sheps and Maher, six of eleven patients with pheochromocytoma had positive pressor responses to glucagon, whereas five of twelve patients with this tumor had positive responses to histamine (887). There were no false positive responses to 1 mg of glucagon in their series, and they did not find any reports of false positives to this test in the literature.

Sheps and Maher concluded that since 1 mg of glucagon produces (1) no false positive responses, (2) fewer unpleasant side effects, and (3) a higher percentage of positive pressor responses in patients with pheochromocytoma, it is preferable to the test employing 0.025 mg of histamine as the provocative agent (887). Others have also reported on the advantages and superior reliability of the glucagon test compared to other provocative tests in detecting patients with pheochromocytoma (488, 554, 562).

On the other hand, our experience indicates that histamine (at least when given in a dosage of 0.05 mg) results in more positive tests in patients with pheochromocytoma than does glucagon, and only rarely causes a false positive response. A false positive response to glucagon has been reported (1034), but the investigators did not employ a cold pressor test for proper interpretation of the pressor response to glucagon. We and others (887) have occasionally seen patients with pheochromocytoma who have a positive pressor response to one provocative agent and not the other. Because of this finding, and because it causes fewer unpleasant side effects, we recommend that a glucagon test be performed first, and then, if negative, be followed by a histamine test. This approach of following up a negative glucagon response with a histamine test seems particularly justifiable in the light of a recent report by Siqueira-Filho and coworkers in which the glucagon test was negative in a series of six patients with pheochromocytoma (898). Two of the patients had nonfamilial pheochromocytomas and four had familial tumors (MEN–type 2, with the triad of bilateral pheochromocytoma, medullary thyroid carcinoma, and parathyroid hyperplasia). In addition, the glucagon test did not increase the plasma catecholamine concentrations of those with normal levels (one patient with a nonfamilial tumor and three with familial tumors) into a range diagnostic for pheochromocytoma. All of these patients were normotensive except for one patient with a nonfamilial tumor who was very mildly hypertensive. These investigators also reported that the blood pressure and plasma catecholamine response to glucagon were negative in every instance in 19 subjects who were relatives of patients with

MEN–type 2 (898). Urinary catecholamines, metanephrines, and VMA, and also plasma catecholamines (before and after the glucagon test) were within normal limits in one of the patients with nonfamilial pheochromocytoma and two of the patients with MEN–type 2. From their findings they concluded that the early diagnosis of pheochromocytoma in MEN–type 2 may be especially difficult and may require multiple biochemical and roentgenographic investigations (898). Certainly, appropriate plasma catecholamine assay, combined with both a glucagon test and then a histamine test (if the former is negative), is indicated in patients with paroxysmal hypertension or normotension suspected of having pheochromocytoma. This approach may be especially important in screening patients with MEN–type 2 or 3, particularly since positive responses to glucagon or histamine may occur less frequently in these conditions (139, 799a, 883, 947).

Provocative tests should not be performed on precariously ill patients, particularly those with recent cardiovascular complications such as cerebrovascular accidents or myocardial infarction. As always, one must weigh the potential risks of any test against the value of the information derived from the test. Histamine should, of course, not be administered to asthmatics, since it may produce severe bronchospasm in sensitive persons.

Levey and coworkers characterized the glucagon receptors in a pheochromocytoma. It appears that release of catecholamines secondary to glucagon stimulation may be mediated by activation of tumor adenyl cyclase and the subsequent increase in intracellular cyclic AMP. They cited the findings of others that glucagon (as well as ACTH and TSH) can stimulate adenyl cyclase in tissue homogenates from pheochromocytoma. On the other hand, histamine did not activate adenyl cyclase, and it is postulated that the histamine-mediated release of catecholamines is indirect (569).

A variety of other drugs has been used as provocative agents (e.g., methacholine, tetraethyl ammonium chloride or bromide, and tyramine hydrochloride), but none has proved as reliable as histamine and glucagon. Administration of nitroglycerine was reported to cause positive pressor responses in each of three patients with pheochromocytoma (218), but the reliability of this drug has not been adequately evaluated.

In 1964, Engelman and Sjoerdsma reported that tyramine appeared to be a suitable substitute for histamine in the pharmacologic diagnosis of pheochromocytoma (274). Furthermore, they emphasized that there is a morbidity associated with the intravenous injection of histamine. These views are contrary to our experience and those of our colleagues. We have observed the tyramine test to be positive in only about 39 percent of patients with pheochromocytoma and positive also in 30 to 50 percent of patients with essential hypertension. When Sheps and coworkers compared the histamine and tyramine tests in the diagnosis of pheochromocytoma, they found tyramine to be an unreliable provocative agent (886). With regard to the safety of the histamine test, Roth performed 14,235 tests and did not have any untoward reactions (personal communication from Dr. Grace M. Roth, Emeritus Professor of Physiology at the Mayo Clinic). However, it is noteworthy that a nearly fatal complication was reported in a 22-year-old man in whom myocardial infarction developed at the height of the pressor response induced by histamine (400). Also, in rare instances the acute rise in blood pressure precipitated by a provocative agent may cause a serious arrhythmia [e.g., multifocal ventricular extrasystoles (391)]. The importance of performing any provocative test properly, with meticulous attention to the dosage of the drug employed, and with appropriate precautions, cannot, of course, be overstated! Phentolamine or nitroprusside should be available for administration to promptly abort an extreme blood pressure increase. (Although other serious reactions are

Table 6.8 *Pharmacologic Testing in Pheochromocytoma[a]*

Agent used	No. patients tested	Patients with 1 or more positive responses	
		No.	%
Histamine	34	24	71
Glucagon	19	12	63
Tyramine	18	7	39

[a] From Deoreo, G. A. Jr., Stewart, B. H., Tarazi, R. C., and Gifford, R. W. Jr. *J. Urol. 111:* 716, 1974.

extremely unlikely, lidocaine and propranolol should be available to control hazardous ventricular arrhythmias which might possibly occur and persist; furthermore, norepinephrine and volume expanders should be available to combat hypotension which might conceivably complicate an untoward reaction.)

A more recent assessment of the positive pressor responses induced by various provocative agents in patients with pheochromocytoma is indicated in Table 6.8.

α-Adrenergic Blocking Test In previous years, when the resting blood pressure of a patient suspected of having a pheochromocytoma was greater than 170/110 mmHg, an α-adrenergic blocking drug was administered. With the advent of chemical assays for catecholamines and their metabolites, the use of α-adrenergic blocking drugs to screen patients suspected of having pheochromocytoma has become obsolete.

The term "adrenergic" was introduced by Dale to designate agents which induce a response in effector cells innervated by the sympathetic nerves (202). Accordingly, an adrenergic blocking drug is one that inhibits certain responses of effector cells to catecholamines and related compounds, and to sympathetic nerve impulses. It has been correctly pointed out that the terms "adrenolytic" and "sympatholytic," which also have been used interchangeably with "adrenergic" blocking agents, are misnomers, since no lytic process occurs in the adrenergic agents, the sympathetic nerves, or the effector cells (707). The agent which appears most satisfactory for neutralizing the pressor effect of circulating catecholamines is Regitine (phentolamine mesylate). Piperoxane (Benzodioxane), another agent which blocks the pressor action of circulating catecholamines, has also been used (376, 381), but it has proved less reliable in screening patients with pheochromocytoma than phentolamine, and undesirable reactions may accompany its administration (237, 395).

Grimson first reported the successful use of phentolamine (Regitine; imidazoline) to control blood pressure before and during operation and removal of a pheochromocytoma (404). Iseri and associates also used phentolamine to treat a patient with pheochromocytoma, and suggested that parenteral administration of phentolamine could prove valuable in the detection of these tumors (473).

Nasal congestion, lacrimation, pupillary constriction, nausea, sweating, abdominal cramps, and diarrhea have been reported as side effects of phentolamine (430); however, with intravenous administration of only 5 mg, which is the optimal test dose for screening patients suspected of having pheochromocytoma, only rarely are a warm sensation and flushing of the skin noted (261, 353). Although our experience and that at the Mayo Clinic has indicated that phentolamine is an extremely safe drug with essentially no serious side effects, it is noteworthy that Roland reported the death of a 21-year-old pregnant patient with pheochromocytoma following the injection of phentolamine (802). He also cited vasomotor collapse with death following the use of phentolamine in a 65-year-old woman with a pheochromocytoma and in a 35-year-old nonpregnant woman without pheochromocytoma (802). Because of these latter reports some do not perform this test on ambulatory patients (400).

The medications withheld before the provocative test must be similarly avoided before the α-adrenergic blocking (phentolamine) test. The protocol for the test is essentially the same as that for the provocative test except that the preliminary cold pressor test is omitted. With the patient in a relatively basal state, 5 mg of phentolamine (dissolved in about 1 ml of sterile water) is rapidly injected intravenously in one bolus, and blood pressures are taken every 15 to 20 sec for 2 min, and every 30 sec for 10 min thereafter, if there is a positive response. A prompt depressor response of 35 mmHg systolic and 25 mmHg diastolic or more is considered positive for the presence of pheochromocytoma. Usually the pressure remains depressed for 10 min or more before returning to the pre-test levels (Fig. 6.9). The average blood pressure in a series of patients with pheochromocytoma and sustained hypertension studied at the Mayo Clinic was 215/146 mmHg. The average fall in blood pressure following the phentolamine test in these patients was 78/53 mmHg (820).

Many falsely positive responses have resulted from interfering drugs [e.g., sedatives, narcotics, antihypertensive and vasoconstrictor drugs (820, 824)], and nonspecific depres-

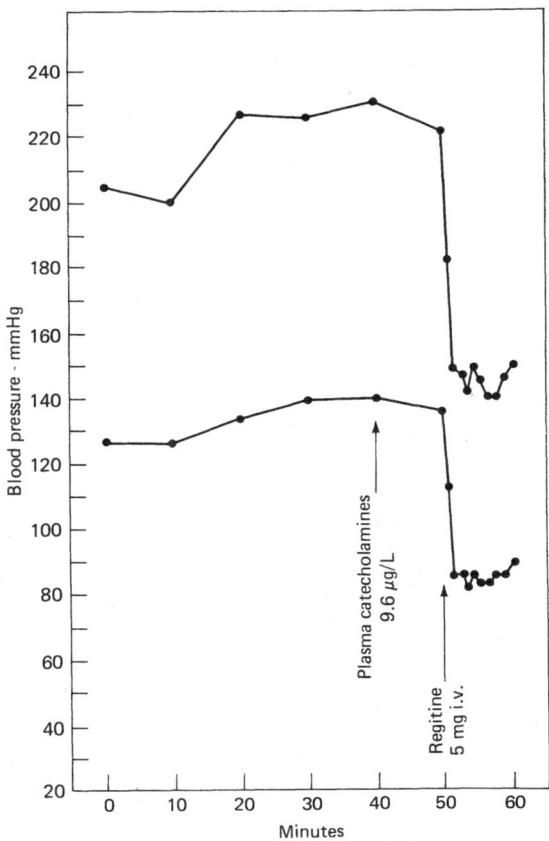

Fig. 6.9 Positive depressor response following intravenous administration of 5 mg of phentolamine (Regitine) to a 29-year-old man with metastatic pheochromocytoma. The depressor response is characteristically prompt and profound (usually greater than 35/25 mmHg) when positive. From Gifford, R. W., Jr., Kvale, W. F., Maher, F. T., Roth, G. M., and Priestley, J. T., *Mayo Clin. Proc.* **39:** 292, 1964.

sor responses occasionally occur; positive responses may occur in the presence of azotemia, or cerebrovascular accidents, and in patients treated with reserpine (261, 353, 469, 815, 848). Falsely negative tests are most common in patients with paroxysmal hypertension and pheochromocytoma, since, if the test is made when the plasma catecholamines are not significantly elevated, no depressor response will follow the injection of phentolamine (352). The results at the Mayo Clinic of testing patients harboring pheochromocytoma with phentolamine or piperoxane are indicated in Table 6.9. Since vasomotor collapse following phentolamine testing has been reported (802), it is well to have a pressor agent (e.g., norepinephrine) and volume expander available for immediate use if necessary.

Table 6.9 *Results of Testing Patients Harboring Pheochromocytomas with α-Adrenergic Blocking Agents*[a]

| | No. of tests | | | | | |
| | Paroxysmal function[b] | | | Persistent function[b] | | |
	Positive	Negative	Equivocal	Positive	Negative	Equivocal
Phentolamine	8	5	0	44	6	1
Piperoxane	0	2	0	13	7	2

[a] From Gifford, R. W., Jr., Kvale, W. T., Maher, F. T., Roth, G. M., and Priestley, J. T. *Mayo Clin. Proc. 39:* 296, 1964.
[b] Tumors causing paroxysmal or persistent hypertension.

A modified phentolamine test for the diagnosis of pheochromocytoma has been proposed by Spergel and coworkers (930, 931). In this test, blood samples for insulin and glucose determinations are collected 20 min after the start of an infusion of 10 percent glucose in water (2 ml/min). Administration of 5 mg phentolamine to patients with pheochromocytoma results in the characteristic blood pressure decrease mentioned above; in addition, however, the inhibitory effect of catecholamines on insulin release from the pancreas (764) is blocked by phentolamine. As a result, plasma insulin levels increase and plasma glucose levels decrease significantly in patients with pheochromocytoma and excessive circulating catecholamines. On the other hand, patients without pheochromocytoma show very little change in their plasma insulin and glucose (Fig. 6.10) (931).

Fig. 6.10 A. Changes in blood pressure and plasma glucose and insulin levels after injection of saline and 5 mg phentolamine mesylate in patient with pheochromocytoma. Abscissa is marked in 1-min intervals. B. Sample study in patient with false-positive response to phentolamine. Note lack of change in plasma glucose and insulin values despite significant change in blood pressure. Abscissa is marked in 1-min intervals. From Spergel, G., Levy, L. J., Chowdhury, F. R., Rodman, H. M., Ertel, N. H., and Bleicher, S. J., *J. Am. Med. Assoc. 211:* 267, 1970. Copyright 1970, American Medical Association.

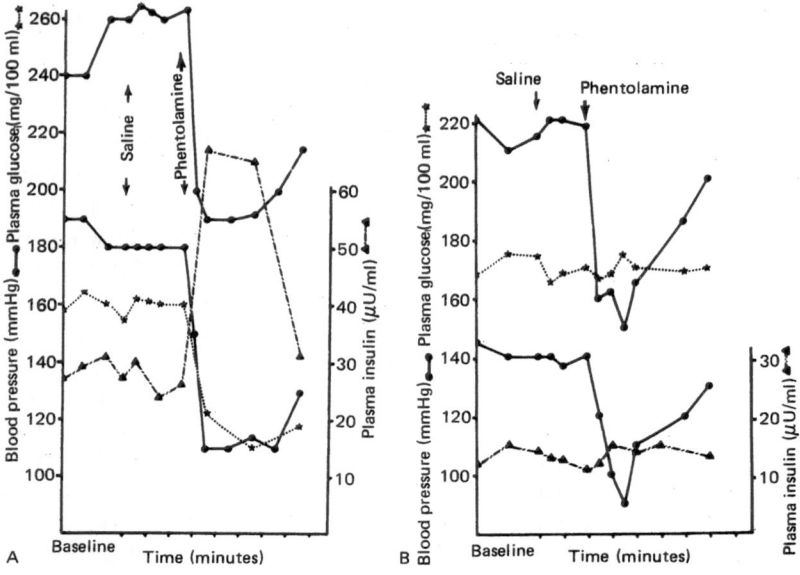

Based on the data accumulated by Spergel and coworkers, "a fall in plasma glucose concentration greater than 18 mg/dl (mean + 2 S.D.) and a rise in plasma insulin values greater than 13 microunits/ml (mean + 2 S.D.) appears to separate false-positive and negative results from those associated with active pheochromocytoma" (931). Since measurement of plasma insulin is not universally available, they suggested that at least plasma glucose determinations be made when the modified phentolamine test is performed on pheochromocytoma suspects (931). This observation is interesting but usually of limited clinical value.

Phentolamine is now rarely used diagnostically, since the diagnosis of pheochromocytoma today rests on the chemical demonstration of elevated catecholamines and/or their metabolites. However, on the rare occasion when a patient presents in a hypertensive crisis or in a sustained malignant hypertensive state, the blood pressure response to the intravenous administration of phentolamine may be of great value in a preliminary differential diagnosis and a guide to the type of therapy to institute initially. It should be remembered, of course, that falsely positive phentolamine tests may be observed in some patients with uremia. Ertel has made the interesting suggestion that plasma glucose determinations during the *modified phentolamine test* (discussed above) may be especially valuable in the occasional situation (e.g., acute hypertensive encephalopathy or extremely severe hypertension) when the diagnosis of pheochromocytoma must be established or excluded very promptly, i.e., before catecholamines or their metabolites can be determined (personal communication from Dr. Norman H. Ertel, Professor of Medicine, New Jersey Medical School).

Although phentolamine has proved to be an extremely safe drug to administer intravenously, a convulsive seizure and four fatal terminations following phentolamine testing have been reported (262, 437, p. 92). Despite the fact that we and our colleagues at the Mayo Clinic have never encountered a serious reaction to phentolamine or any of the provocative tests, we recommend that every safety precaution be taken when using these drugs in any patient with pheochromo-

cytoma. Therefore, whenever phentolamine is to be used, it is recommended that an intravenous needle or catheter be inserted and kept in place for at least a short time after administration of the drug. A solution of norepinephrine containing about 8 μg/ml should be available to infuse and counteract a prolonged hypotensive episode.

When the provocative drugs are to be used, one should not only have adequate phentolamine available to combat a hypertensive crisis but it is also a worthwhile precaution to have sodium nitroprusside ready for immediate infusion, since at least one patient with pheochromocytoma has been reported who was resistant to phentolamine but did respond to nitroprusside (712). As mentioned above, lidocaine, propranolol, norepinephrine, and volume expanders should also be available.

In conclusion, it should be particularly stressed that any procedure which may lower the blood pressure significantly or precipitate a hypertensive crisis (whether the administration of drugs or some physical maneuver) must be performed with considerable caution and repeated blood pressure measurements. One must always be fully prepared to control blood pressure and arrhythmias, since a rare patient with pheochromocytoma may be sensitive to various drugs or be especially brittle under mildly stressful circumstances.

BIOCHEMICAL TESTS

The *sine qua non* for the preoperative diagnosis of pheochromocytoma is the demonstration of elevated concentrations of catecholamines or their metabolites in the urine or plasma. Operation in search of a catecholamine-secreting tumor without chemical confirmation is virtually indefensible, except for the rare situation where the pheochromocytoma appears to be nonfunctioning despite the use of provocative tests.

Between 1950 and 1954, Engel and von Euler (263), Goldenberg and Rapport (379, 380), Lund (590), Burn (117), von Euler and associates (298), Pekkarinen (740) and Manger and associates (616) demonstrated the great value of quantitating urine and plasma catecholamines to detect patients with pheochromocytoma. Subsequently, a number of chemical tests have been developed which permit quantitation of catecholamines and their metabolites. The virtue of measuring these metabolites is emphasized by the fact that no more than 1 percent of normally synthesized norepinephrine or 10 percent of that formed by a pheochromocytoma is eliminated unchanged (359). Occasionally, in the past, bioassays have been used to demonstrate excess pressor substances in blood or urine; however, because these require test animal preparations and are not very sensitive, they have been abandoned and replaced by the chemical assays. A bioassay, of course, has the distinct advantage of establishing whether biologic activity (e.g., a pressor response) is present—a virtue not shared by chemical tests.

URINE ASSAYS

A major problem encountered with chemical analysis has been one of specificity. Also, some methods have been inadequately sensitive and not sufficiently reproducible. Most of the reliable quantitative methods are relatively difficult and require rigidly controlled conditions. Some assays are particularly time consuming and present formidable technical problems which may interfere with their accuracy. Various chemical tests used for demonstrating increased excretion of catecholamines, metanephrine, and normetanephrine (together termed "metanephrines"), VMA (vanillylmandelic or vanilmandelic acid, or 3-methoxy-4-hydroxymandelic acid), and MHPG (3-methoxy-4-hydroxyphenylglycol) have proved invaluable in detecting patients with pheochromocytoma (11, 185, 186, 191, 263, 358–360, 362, 363, 380, 590, 784, 820, 846, 888, 909, 948, 1037). Pitfalls encountered with chemical assays on urine have been presented and appraised adequately (354, 357, 358, 361, 362, 748, 846). A specific isotope dilution method for quantitating VMA has been reported by Weise and coworkers (1021), but it has not been used extensively.

Most investigators and commercial laboratories have quantitated concentrations of catecholamines, VMA, and total metanephrines in 24-hr collections of urine (185, 186, 191, 784, 888, 909). Alternatively, Gitlow and associates have quantitated VMA and total metanephrine concentrations in random urines.

They expressed concentrations in terms of creatinine content, since the excretion of these catecholamine metabolites and creatinine varied only slightly from hour to hour and assays appeared reliable and reproducible (358, 359, 361). While the technique of random urine sampling has proved highly reliable in detecting patients with pheochromocytoma, it should be appreciated that occasionally a patient may be encountered whose tumor is quiescent for a prolonged period of time during which the pheochromocytoma appears to release little or no catecholamines into the circulation. Consequently, if a random urine sample is obtained on such a patient during such a quiescent interval, the urine concentration of catecholamines or metabolites can fall within the normal range. Under such circumstances, 24-hr collections of urine would give a greater chance of detecting these tumors which only intermittently release their catecholamines. Completeness of the 24-hr urine collection is mandatory for accurate interpretation of the results. Unfortunately, 24-hr urinary excretion of creatinine (even if corrected for body weight and surface area) cannot be used as a precise index for the completeness of the urine collection (398). Recently it has been suggested that measurement of catecholamine metabolites in overnight urine collections is adequate for separating patients with pheochromocytoma from those with essential hypertension, provided the laboratory has determined the upper limit of normal for overnight excretion (954).

Rarely, we have encountered patients with pheochromocytoma who repeatedly had normal concentrations of catecholamines and metabolites in both random *and* 24-hr collections of urine when they were normotensive. With these patients it is imperative that plasma and/or urine be obtained for catecholamine and/or metabolite determinations during a hypertensive period (either occurring spontaneously or induced by a provocative agent or by some physical maneuver), since there are occasions when a definite preoperative diagnosis can be made only through this approach. Gitlow has stated that no more than 1 to 2 percent of patients with pheochromocytoma should require diagnostic procedures, other than and in addition to analysis of urine for VMA and total metanephrines (358). In keeping with this statement, Sato and coworkers have reported that in 29 patients with pheochromocytoma (19 with sustained and 10 with paroxysmal hypertension) measurement of catecholamines in 24-hr urines never failed to establish the correct diagnosis (853). Catecholamine excretion was apparently lower in patients with paroxysmal than in those with sustained hypertension; however, urinary catecholamine levels were significantly elevated in all their patients, even during periods of normotension. They suggested that the paradox of normotension despite increased excretion of catecholamines might be explained by the fact that patients with pheochromocytoma are relatively insensitive to exogenous catecholamines (853).

Although one can almost invariably demonstrate elevated catecholamines or their metabolites in the urine or plasma of patients with sustained hypertension due to pheochromocytoma, we believe that patients with paroxysmal hypertension present a more difficult diagnostic problem when they are normotensive. The late Marcel Goldenberg said that, in the series of patients with pheochromocytoma studied at Columbia Medical Center, he found normal concentrations of catecholamines in the urine of four patients during periods of normal blood pressure (personal conversation). It should be appreciated that estimates of the percentage of falsely positive or negative tests for pheochromocytomas are always open to question, since proof of the presence or absence of these tumors can only be established by surgical exploration.

Experience at National Institute of Health

Crout, Pisano, Sjoerdsma, Engelman, and coworkers have had considerable experience in quantitating the urine catecholamines as well as their metabolites in patients with pheochromocytoma (185, 191, 193, 267, 909).

METHODS EMPLOYED

For determination of free (unconjugated) epinephrine and norepinephrine in urine, Crout, Pisano, and Sjoerdsma employed a modification (189) of the method of von Euler and Floding (290). Spectrophotometric methods were used to quantitate urinary VMA (758) and total metanephrines (i.e., normetanephrine plus metanephrine) (757). Twenty-four-hour urine specimens collected in 10 to 15 ml of 6 N hydrochloric acid could be stored at $0°C$ for many months without any deterioration of the catecholamines or their metabolites. Free catecholamines of unhydrolyzed urine are determined since hydrolysis may cause some destruction of these amines. However, since a high proportion of metanephrine and normetanephrine is excreted in the conjugated form, hydrolysis is performed before their measurement. VMA exists in the free form and hydrolysis is unnecessary.

RESULTS

Crout, and coworkers reported (191) that in 114 hypertensive patients who were not acutely ill the excretion of total free catecholamines (epinephrine plus norepinephrine) was 32 ± 18 μg per day (mean $\pm$ S.D.). The upper limit of "normal" was considered 100 μg per day, and only two patients without pheochromocytoma excreted slightly more than this amount.

In 91 patients with essential hypertension and 30 normotensive subjects, excretion of total metanephrine was 0.62 ± 0.28 mg per day (mean $\pm$ S.D.). No difference was observed between these hypertensives and normotensives. The upper limit of "normal" was considered 1.3 mg per day. Modest elevations above this limit encountered in three patients were found to result from interfering substances. No drugs appeared to interfere directly with the assay. However, MAO inhibitors were observed to increase excretion values to as high as 2.2 mg per day. Elevations may persist for even 2 weeks after discontinuing these enzyme inhibitors.

In 20 patients with essential hypertension, VMA excretion was 3.7 ± 1.1 mg per day (mean $\pm$ S.D.) and the upper limit of normal was considered 6.0 mg per day. Only one patient had a value slightly above this limit.

Crout and coworkers found that the major substance excreted in the urine of 23 patients with pheochromocytoma was VMA; the metanephrines were less prominent. The catecholamines comprised only a small fraction of the substances excreted. In order to represent the relative increase in excretion of these substances they displayed the results as multiples

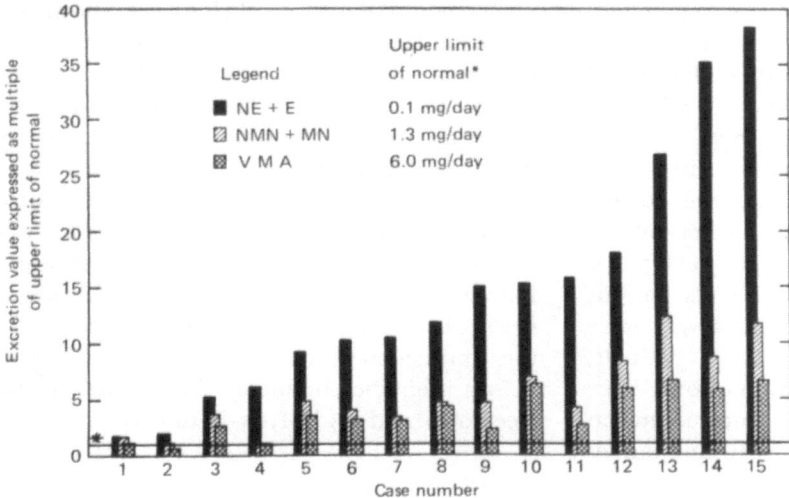

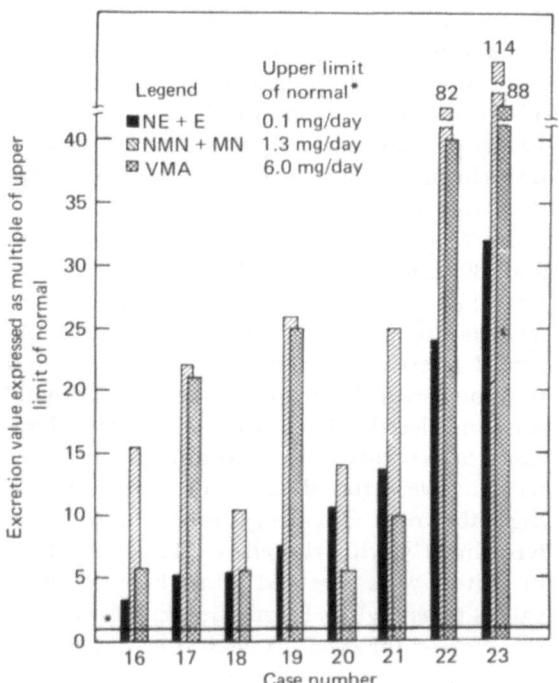

Fig. 6.11 Pattern of excretion of urinary catecholamines and metabolites in 15 patients with pheochromocytomas who excreted a relative excess of free catecholamines over metabolites. Note that all values are expressed as multiples of the upper limit of normal. Most of these patients had tumors weighing less than 50 g and containing less than 100 mg total content of catecholamines ("low" group). These tumors have a rapid rate of catecholamine turnover. From Crout, J. R. Chap. 1. Catecholamine metabolism in pheochromocytoma and essential hypertension. In: *Hormones and Hypertension.* Courtesy of C. C. Thomas, 1966, p. 22.

Fig. 6.12 Pattern of urinary excretion in eight patients with pheochromocytoma in whom 0-methylated metabolites showed the greatest relative increase above normal. These patients had tumors weighing more than 50 g and containing more than 100 mg total content of catecholamines ("high" group). These tumors have a slow rate of catecholamine turnover. From Crout, J. R. Chap. 1. Catecholamine metabolism in pheochromocytoma and essential hypertension. In: *Hormones and Hypertension.* Courtesy of C. C. Thomas, 1966, p. 23.

of the upper limit of normal (Figs. 6.11 and 6.12). Two patterns of excretion were observed. In Figure 6.11 it is evident that in these 15 cases there was a relatively greater increase in the excretion of catecholamines than in the excretion of metabolites. Most of these tumors weighed less than 50 g, contained less than 100 mg total catecholamine content, and had a rapid rate of catecholamine turnover. On the other hand, Figure 6.12 shows that in these eight cases there was a relatively greater increase in the excretion

of metabolites than in the excretion of catecholamines; most of these tumors weighed more than 50 g, contained more than 100 mg total catecholamine content, and had a slow rate of catecholamine turnover. In almost all patients with pheochromocytoma the relative increase of the metanephrines was greater than that of VMA.

A diagnostic elevation of urinary catecholamines, as well as of VMA and metanephrines, was found in 20 of the 23 patients; however, in three patients (cases 1, 2, and 4) only the catecholamines were elevated and diagnostic of pheochromocytoma. Crout and coworkers pointed out that quantitation of catecholamines may be particularly valuable in patients with minimally secreting tumors (cases 1–4, Fig. 6.11). However, they cited two case reports in the literature which showed increased excretion of VMA at a time when catecholamine values were normal; they suggested that these patients were, possibly, similar to those depicted in Figure 6.12, and had pheochromocytomas in which a large proportion of the catecholamine was metabolized within the tumor.

SCREENING AND DIAGNOSTIC CRITERIA

Crout and associates concluded that, since determination of metanephrines is highly reliable and comparatively easy to perform, and since it is at least as helpful diagnostically as VMA excretion, quantitation of total metanephrines is favored for screening patients suspected of having pheochromocytoma. They stated that a metanephrine value of 1.0 mg or less per day in a patient with sustained hypertension rules out pheochromocytoma, whereas a value of 2.5 mg or more per day (in the absence of other conditions known to elevate the metanephrines) is diagnostic for

Table 6.10 *Urinary Catecholamine Excretion in Patients with and without Pheochromocytoma during Spontaneous and Histamine-Induced Attacks[a]*

Patient	Type of test or attack	When urine sampled[b]	Catecholamine excretion (μg/hour)[c] NE	E
No pheochromocytoma				
1	Histamine test negative	During test	1.5	1.2
		Control	1.9	1.0
2	Histamine test negative	During test	1.0	0.3
		Control	0.6	0.1
3	Histamine test negative	During test	3.5	0.2
		Control	4.9	0.0
4[d]	Histamine test false positive	During test	2.0	—
		Control	2.0	—
5[d]	Histamine test false positive	During test	3.1	—
		Control	2.0	—
6[d]	Histamine test false positive	During test	0.9	—
		Control	1.1	—
7	Spontaneous attack with increase in blood pressure	During attack	2.0	0.2
		Control	1.7	0.2
With pheochromocytoma				
8	Histamine test positive	During test	39.0	0.0
		Control	25.0	0.0
9	Spontaneous attack	During attack	41.0	16.0
		Control	21.0	7.2
10	Spontaneous attack	During attack	6.1	7.3
		Control	2.2	1.4

[a] From Crout, J. R. Chap. 1. Catecholamine metabolism in pheochromocytoma and essential hypertension. *In: Hormones and Hypertension.* Courtesy of C. C. Thomas, 1966, p. 29.

[b] Control period is either the hour prior to the histamine test or, in the case of attacks, a comparable period on another day when the blood pressure was stable.

[c] Normal urinary excretion of catecholamines in micrograms per hour is almost invariably ≤ 4.8.

[d] Data from Engelman, K. and Sjoerdsma, A. *JAMA, 189:* 107–112, 1964.

this tumor. If values are equivocal (i.e., values between 1.0 and 2.5 mg per day, which occurred in 6 percent of their patients with pheochromocytoma), and if no interfering substances are present, then they recommend that urine catecholamines be determined. In the event that the patient has paroxysmal hypertension but is normotensive with a normal excretion of metanephrines during the period of urine collection, then urine is collected again, this time during and following a paroxysm of hypertension, either one spontaneously induced, or one induced by a provocative test or a physical maneuver. A twofold increase of epinephrine or norepinephrine excretion during the hypertensive period supports the diagnosis of pheochromocytoma, whereas no catecholamine elevation suggests that a tumor is not present (191). Table 6.10 reveals the effect of a histamine test or a spontaneous attack on urinary catecholamine excretion in patients with and without pheochromocytoma. It is noteworthy that, despite falsely positive pharmacologic tests in three of the patients without pheochromocytoma, no significant elevation in urinary catecholamines followed the hypertensive episode.

Crout has stated that, although most patients with pheochromocytoma and paroxysmal hypertension excrete increased amounts of catecholamines and/or their metabolites "even between attacks," some do not (185). He has emphasized that "the demonstration of normal excretion of norepinephrine and epinephrine during a period of hypertension excludes pheochromocytoma as the cause of the hypertension" (185).

In the experience of Crout and associates very few patients will be misdiagnosed if 24-hr urines are assayed with accurate methodology, since elevations of catecholamines or metabolites can be demonstrated in 90 to 95 percent of patients with pheochromocytoma. Despite the collection of urine during a carefully timed period which "bracketed" the attack (either spontaneous or provoked), in only one case (patient 10, Table 6.10) of Crout and coworkers did this approach aid in establishing the diagnosis. Crout has pointed out that urine samples "bracketing attacks" should be analyzed for the catecholamines in preference to their metabolites, since catecholamines appear in the urine at the same time their circulating levels are increased,

whereas their metabolites appear only slowly over a period of hours.

Finally, Crout has recommended that if the diagnosis of pheochromocytoma remains doubtful after adequate urinary assays, then it is best to wait 6 to 12 months and reevaluate the patient. Although pharmacologic tests are rarely used today for diagnostic purposes, except as mentioned above, Crout suggested that phentolamine could be of value in detecting a pheochromocytoma in that rare circumstance when an episode of hypertension occurs during operation on a patient not previously suspected of harboring this tumor.

In 1966 Sjoerdsma and associates reported a summary of results of assaying 24-hr urine specimens for catecholamines, VMA, and metanephrines in 64 patients with pheochromocytoma (Fig. 6.13) (909). As is evident in Figure 6.13 there was a very high degree of accuracy in detecting the presence of a pheochromocytoma with any of these tests. Except in very rare instances, when tumor secretion was truly intermittent (about 1 percent of cases), the measurement of any of these compounds established the diagnosis of pheochromocytoma (267).

It has been recognized that a number of tests used for the measurement of VMA are quite nonspecific and are, in fact, screening tests for phenolic acids; interference by the ingestion of a variety of substances (e.g., raw fruits, vanilla, coffee, and tea) can cause spurious elevations of VMA. It is strongly recommended that test "kits" which accept VMA values up to 10 to 14 mg per 24 hr be avoided because of their lack of specificity. Engelman has emphasized that patients have been needlessly subjected to operation based on the erroneous results of these nonspecific tests and he makes the plea that such tests be eliminated (267).

Experience at Mount Sinai Medical Center, New York City Gitlow and associates have reviewed their 10 years of experience in the use of a variety of biochemical techniques for detecting and establishing the presence of a pheochromocytoma (358). They found that estimation of the urinary catecholamines in patients suspected of harboring pheochromocytoma was less desirable than assay of the metabolites. They found urinary concentrations of catecholamines were lower and more

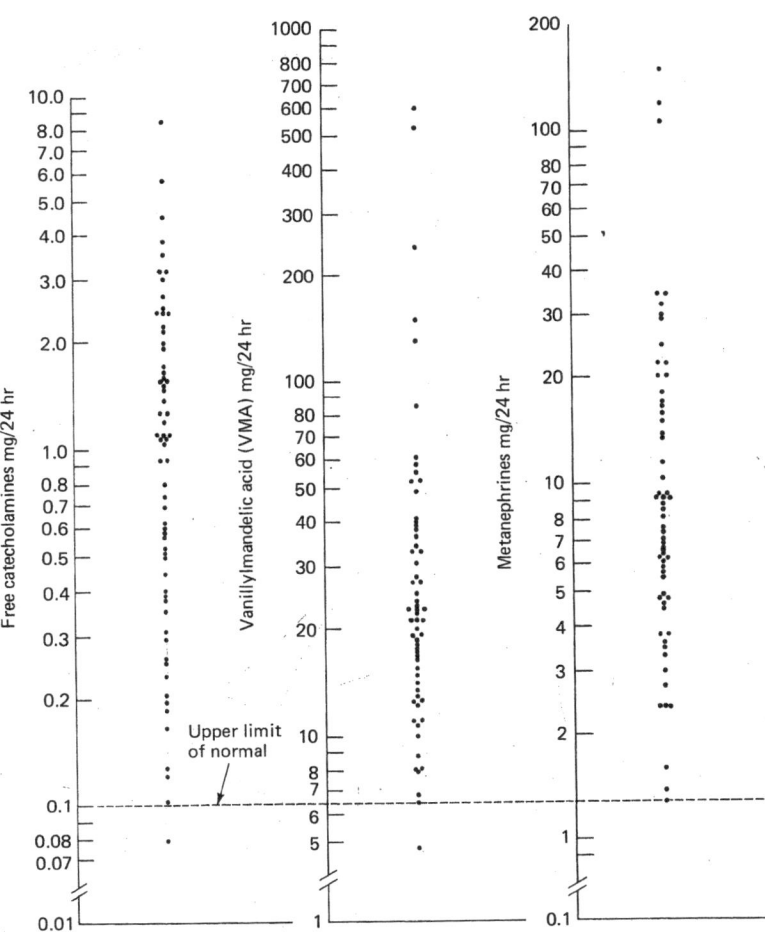

Fig. 6.13 Urinary excretion of catecholamines and metabolites in pheochromocytoma. Summary of results of urinary assays on 64 patients with proved pheochromocytoma, representing the experience of the Experimental Therapeutics Branch of the National Institute of Health up to 1966. The range of values was so great that it required use of differing logarithmic scales. The horizontal broken line designates the upper limits of normal, these being catecholamines = 0.1 mg, vanillylmandelic acid (VMA) = 6.5 mg, and metanephrines = 1.3 mg/24 hr. From Sjoerdsma, A., Engelman, K., Waldman, T. A., Cooperman, L. H., and Hammond, W. G., *Ann. Intern. Med. 65:* 1306, 1966.

variable than their metabolites; moreover, the techniques of the catecholamine assay and the interference from medication presented more problems than those experienced with quantitation of VMA and the metanephrines (358). In addition, they observed high levels of VMA in several patients with pheochromocytoma who excreted normal amounts of catecholamines (360). They also cited the report by Kraupp and coworkers (527) of a patient with a pheochromocytoma who excreted large quantities of VMA and catecholamines during paroxysmal hypertension but only an elevated VMA between paroxysms. Consequently, when investigating patients suspected of having neural crest neoplasms, they elected to assay catecholamine metabolites.

METHODS EMPLOYED

Colorimetric (360, 363) and chromatoelectrophoretic (1057) techniques were used to screen for elevated excretions of VMA and total metanephrines, respectively. VMA was

quantitated with a bidirectional paper chromatographic procedure (23, 359) or a gas-liquid chromatographic procedure (1038). Spectrophotometric methods were used to determine the concentrations of the metanephrines (361, 757, 1036). Urinary MHPG and dopamine were quantitated by gas-liquid chromatography (1037), whereas bidirectional paper chromatography was used to determine HVA (359).

In general, the methods for quantitating urinary catecholamines and MHPG are more complex and difficult to perform than those for the analysis of VMA and metanephrines. Consequently, methods for accurately determining urinary catecholamines are used less frequently for evaluating patients suspected of having pheochromocytoma. Gitlow and associates found that the determination of catecholamines in urine was less reliable diagnostically than assay of the metabolites, a view in keeping with the results of others (185, 223, 784). Since catecholamine concentrations were relatively less elevated and more variable than their metabolites, interference from drugs was a greater problem with catecholamine measurements than it was with metabolite assays (359, 360). In their experience the assay of epinephrine or metanephrine to aid in localization of tumors in the adrenal gland was of little value in the management of their patients (358). They pointed out that VMA and MHPG have a common precursor (3-methoxy-4-hydroxymandelic aldehyde), which probably explains a parallel increase in the urinary excretion of these metabolites. They therefore concluded that assay of MHPG did not offer any additional advantage over that gained from quantitating only VMA and the metanephrines (358).

The clinical indications used by Gitlow and associates (358) for chemically testing urine in order to establish or exclude a diagnosis of pheochromocytoma were very similar to our own criteria presented in Table 6.1. Positive chemical screening tests were always followed by quantitative assays for VMA and total metanephrines (358).

RESULTS

Gitlow and coworkers analyzed their series, which consisted of 92 patients with proved pheochromocytoma and 9,500 control subjects, and found:

1. Total metanephrines were increased in 100 percent of patients with pheochromocytoma, but occasionally they were increased in its absence.
2. VMA and MHPG were increased in about 97 percent of patients with pheochromocytoma, but rarely increased in its absence.
3. Dopamine and its metabolite HVA were increased in only one patient with pheochromocytoma, and in this case the tumor was malignant.

They found that hemorrhagic shock, overwhelming sepsis, or pulmonary insufficiency were sometimes accompanied by a slightly increased excretion of catecholamines and their metabolites. One of their patients with accelerated hypertension accompanied by severe hypertensive encephalopathy had an elevated excretion of VMA following intravenous administration of phentolamine (360). They also encountered three semicomatose patients with increased intracranial pressure resulting from intracranial hemorrhage who excreted increased amounts of VMA and total metanephrines in the absence of pheochromocytoma; excretion of these metabolites returned to normal with clinical recovery (358). Patients with metastatic carcinoid were observed to excrete slightly elevated amounts of VMA, but none excreted more than 5 μg/mg creatinine. Each of these patients with carcinoid excreted excessive quantities of 5-hydroxyindoleacetic acid (5-HIAA), which was identifiable on the chromatographic assays used to detect VMA and the metanephines (748).

VMA and total metanephrine levels expressed in micrograms per milligram of creatinine in the urine were higher and more variable in normal children up to 15 years of age than in adults (361). Table 6.11 reveals

Table 6.11 *Excretion of Catecholamine Catabolites by Normal Children[a,b]*

No. subjects	Age (years)	VMA			HVA			M + NM		
		Mean	S.D.	Range	Mean	S.D.	Range	Mean	S.D.	Range
43	1–12 months	6.9	3.2	1.40–15	12.9	9.58	1.2–35	1.64	1.32	0.001–4.60
15	1–2	4.6	2.22	1.25–8	12.6	6.26	4–23	1.68	1.13	0.27–5.38
21	2–5	3.95	1.72	1.5–7.5	7.58	3.56	0.5–13.5	1.25	0.77	0.35–2.99
23	5–10	3.3	1.40	0.5–6.0	4.7	2.66	0.5–9.0	1.13	0.78	0.43–2.70
24	10–15	1.91	0.77	0.25–3.25	2.5	2.42	0.25–12.0	0.60	0.48	0.001–1.87
14	15–18	1.34	0.61	0.1–2.75	1.0	0.65	0.5–2.0	0.24	0.23	0.001–0.67

[a] From Gitlow, S. E., Mendlowitz, M., Wilk, E. K., Wilk, S., Wolf, R. L., and Bertani, L. M. *J. Lab. Clin. Med.* 72: 614, 1968.

[b] Excretion in urine expressed as micrograms per milligram of creatinine. VMA = vanillylmandelic acid; HVA = homovanillic acid; M = metanephrine; NM = normetanephrine; S.D. = standard deviation.

the mean, standard deviation, and range of VMA, HVA, and the metanephrines in subjects varying in age from 1 month to 18 years. Obviously, if an accurate interpretation of the result is to be made, the age of the patient tested for these substances must be considered. Gitlow has stated that if the concentration of any of these catecholamine metabolites is above the mean concentration plus three standard deviations corresponding to the age of the patient, then the presence of a neural crest tumor must be strongly considered (S. E. Gitlow, personal communication). It is noteworthy that Sandler and Ruthven (845), using a spectrophotometric method, found that, for various age groups, the mean excretion of VMA in mg/24 hr was as follows: 0.3 (neonates); 1.5 (1 to 5 years); 2.5 (5 to 10 years); 3.5 (10 to 15 years); 4.0 (adults). Mean excretion of catecholamines and their metabolites would, of course, be expected to be higher in adults than in children because of the larger size of the adrenergic system in the older subjects. A point worth reemphasizing is the importance of a complete 24-hr collection for proper interpretation of results. In a child it may be extremely difficult if not impossible to collect the entire 24-hr specimen. In such instances random urine sampling, and the expression of concentrations of catecholamines or their metabolites per milligram of urinary creatinine, would seem a more reasonable and reliable diagnostic procedure—especially since perhaps 90 percent of children with pheochromocytoma have sustained hypertension and a continuously functioning tumor.

Gitlow and coworkers cautioned that, in over 30 percent of patients with pheochromocytoma, nonspecific techniques for colorimetric assay of VMA had little diagnostic value (358). A rapid, inexpensive, simple, sensitive, and specific chromatoelectrophoretic test for the assay of the metanephrines and 3-methoxy-4-hydroxyphenylglycol developed by Wolf and associates (1057) has been found to be extremely accurate in detecting patients with pheochromocytoma; the test requires no dietary restrictions. Currently in use at Columbia Presbyterian Medical Center, this test has proved very reliable in screening patients suspected of harboring a pheochromocytoma, since the band representing the metanephrines in the chromatogram is highly specific.

On the other hand, the band for MHPG occurs in the same region as that for HVA and is increased by use of methyldopa. Furthermore, VMA determined by this screening assay can be altered by diet (personal communication, Dr. Ray Gambino, Chief of Clinical Chemistry, Columbia Medical Center, New York). Nevertheless, the quantitative urine metanephrine assay is more reliable in detecting pheochromocytomas.

Since Gitlow and coworkers (358) found that all 92 patients with pheochromocytoma excreted increased amounts of metanephrines in random urinary samples, they suggested that the 13 percent incidence of normal total metanephrine excretion observed in patients with pheochromocytoma by Crout and coworkers (191) might have resulted from incomplete collection of the 24-hr urine sample in the latter study. Gitlow has strongly suggested that all patients having elevated total metanephrines should have the diagnosis of pheochromocytoma further substantiated by a VMA determination (Dr. S. E. Gitlow, personal communication).

Experience at the Mayo Clinic In 1974 Remine and associates reviewed the experience at the Mayo Clinic in the biochemical evaluation of patients with pheochromocytoma (784). The precise concentrations of catecholamines and the metabolites were not recorded since the report was concerned only with whether the substance measured was elevated or within the normal range. Procedures for the quantitation of 24-hr urinary catecholamines, VMA, and metanephrines have been described elsewhere (91, 487, 888).

RESULTS
Measurement of urinary catecholamines and VMA in 51 patients with pheochromocytoma revealed that in 10 patients (20 percent), both substances were normal, whereas in 31 (60 percent), both were elevated. In four (8 percent), VMA was increased whereas catecholamines were normal; and in six (12 percent), VMA was normal, whereas the catecholamines were elevated. [It is conceivable that the normal values for VMA obtained in some of these patients may have been due to the sensitivity of the assay employed, since Gitlow has recently claimed that, in his experience, at least 95 percent of patients with pheo-

chromocytoma have elevated urinary VMA concentrations (Dr. S. E. Gitlow, personal communication).]

Determination of metanephrines and VMA in 47 patients revealed that only two (4 percent) had normal levels of both substances, whereas 33 (70 percent) had elevations of both metabolites. In 12 (25 percent), metanephrines were elevated, whereas VMA was normal.

Quantitation of metanephrines and catecholamines in 47 patients revealed both substances were normal in two patients (4 percent), and both substances were elevated in 34 (75 percent). In 11 (21 percent), metanephrines were elevated whereas catecholamines were normal. These results are recorded in Table 6.12.

Since 1960, with improved biochemical methods for measuring urinary catecholamines and their metabolites, the preoperative diagnosis of pheochromocytoma has been correctly made in almost all patients studied at the Mayo Clinic (784). In keeping with the views of Crout and coworkers (191), Gitlow and associates (358), and Deoreo and associates (223), the experience at the Mayo Clinic demonstrates that the determination of urinary metanephrines is the most reliable single test for screening and identifying patients with pheochromocytoma (784). When the metanephrines were determined, falsely negative tests occurred in only two out of 52 patients (4 percent) with pheochromocytoma. Negative tests for catecholamines occurred in 13 out of 60 patients (21 percent), and normal test results occurred in 15 out of 52 patients (29 percent) in whom VMA was determined.

As further support in establishing a preoperative diagnosis of pheochromocytoma in the presence of elevated metanephrines, additional urine collections are indicated for confirmation of the elevated metanephrines and for quantitation of VMA and catecholamines. Sheps and coworkers found that when assays were performed on multiple urine specimens from the same patient harboring a pheochromocytoma, there were often considerable variations in catecholamine output, but less so in the excretion of VMA and the total metanephrines (888).

More recently, Siqueira-Filho and associates (898) have noted an increased frequency of patients with multiple endocrine neoplasia type 2 (MEN–type 2—medullary thyroid carcinoma, pheochromocytoma, and parathyroid hyperplasia) studied at the Mayo Clinic. It was particularly noteworthy that of four normotensive patients with MEN–type 2, only two had an increased excretion of VMA and only one had an elevated concentration of the metanephrines. Urinary catecholamines were normal in all four, and plasma catecholamines were elevated in only one. A slight increase in urinary HVA was also noted in one of these patients as mentioned earlier in this chapter. It was of some concern that none of these patients had a positive response to the glucagon provocative test. Siqueira-Filho and coworkers have stressed the importance of extensive biochemical studies and carefully

Table 6.12 *Results of Biochemical Assays on 24-hr Urine Samples Collected from Patients with Pheochromocytoma (Studied at the Mayo Clinic)[a,b]*

No. of patients	Assays performed	Patients with both assays normal[c]	Patients with assays elevated[c]			
			Both	CA only	VMA only	MN only
51	CA and VMA	20	60	12	8	—
47	MN and VMA	4	70	—	0	25
47	MN and CA	4	75	0	—	21

[a] This table is based on data reported by Remine, W. H., Chong, GC., van Heerden, J. A., Sheps, S. G., and Harrison, E. G., Jr. *Ann. Surg. 179:* 740–748, 1974.

[b] CA = catecholamines; VMA = vanillylmandelic acid; MN = total metanephrines.

[c] Figures indicate percent of total number of patients.

performed nephrotomography in this unique familial endocrinopathy (898). Hamilton and coworkers have recommended that urinary epinephrine be determined in patients with MEN–type 2 since their pheochromocytomas are almost always located in the adrenal glands and often secrete a significant amount of epinephrine. In four of seven patients in one family with Sipple's syndrome epinephrine was the main catecholamine abnormality (414). Weiss reported a patient with Sipple's syndrome who had a hypertensive response to a glucagon test which was followed by a threefold rise in urinary epinephrine concentration (1022).

Experience at the Cleveland Clinic   A report in 1974 by Deoreo and associates (223) at the Cleveland Clinic reviewed their experience of assaying 24-hr urines for catecholamines, the metanephrines, and VMA in patients with hypertension. In the event hypertension was paroxysmal they performed a provocative test with histamine or glucagon. Urine collection was begun immediately after the test and continued for 24 hr and then, with conventional methodology, assayed for catecholamines, the metanephrines, and VMA. Urinary concentrations of the catecholamines and metabolites were not recorded; however, the report indicated whether or not the substance assayed was elevated on one or more occasions.

RESULTS
Of 25 patients with pheochromocytoma in

whom urinary metanephrines were determined, 25 (100 percent) had elevated values; 27 out of 33 patients (82 percent) had elevated VMA levels; and 18 out of 27 patients (67 percent) had elevated urinary catecholamines. The results of Deoreo and associates once again confirm the superior accuracy and reliability of the assay of metanephrines for screening and identifying patients with pheochromocytoma.

Remarks Concerning the Excretion of Dopamine   The normal excretion of dopamine in urine is approximately 100 to 200 μg/day, up to 5 times that of norepinephrine (285, 905). In 1951 von Euler found dopamine excretion was about 2000 μg/day in a patient with pheochromocytoma (285). Shortly thereafter, Manger and associates (616), and then Weil-Malherbe (1014) and McMillan (644) demonstrated the presence of dopamine in some pheochromocytomas. In addition, Weil-Malherbe demonstrated for the first time the presence of dopa in two pheochromocytomas. He also noted that despite a significantly greater concentration of norepinephrine than dopamine in one of these tumors, the excretion of dopamine in the urine was far greater than the excretion of epinephrine and norepinephrine (Table 6.13). It is interesting that despite the much higher concentration of dopamine than norepinephrine in the tumor of the patient reported by McMillan, greater concentrations of norepinephrine than of dopamine were excreted. This tumor was thought to be malignant (Table 6.13).

Table 6.13   *Concentrations of Catecholamines and Dopa in Pheochromocytomas and Urine of Patients Studied by Weil-Malherbe and McMillan[a]*

Patient[b]	Tumor (μg/g)				Urine (μg/24 hr)		
	E	NE	Dopamine	Dopa	E	NE	Dopamine
1	124	770	494	147	37	257	3420
2	107	764	49.8	⌐8	—	—	—
3	0	150	1970	0	0	124	50
					0	1045	450

[a] This table is based on data reported by Weil-Malherbe, H. *Lancet* 2: 282–284, 1956, and by McMillan, M. *Lancet* 2: 284, 1956.
[b] Patients 1 and 2 were reported by Weil-Malherbe; patient 3 was reported by McMillan.

Subsequently, dopamine (91) and dopa have, rarely, been detected in pheochromocytomas (586) (Table 2.4). As mentioned earlier, the presence of dopamine and its precursor does not always indicate, as previously postulated (16), that the tumor is malignant (91, 586, 888). We believe, however, that the incidence of malignancy is significantly greater in pheochromocytomas containing dopamine than in those containing only epinephrine and norepinephrine. Bollman and associates reported that analysis of a metastatic pheochromocytoma which occurred 2 years after the primary tumor was removed revealed that it contained 0.1 mg of dopamine per gram of tissue but no epinephrine or norepinephrine (91). Sheps and coworkers reported one patient who excreted large amounts of HVA (a metabolite of dopamine) and whose pheochromocytoma revealed the intriguing finding of neuroid features (i.e., no sharp division between pheochromocytes and ganglion-like cells); it was felt that this tumor represented a pheochromocytoma with associated elements of a ganglioneuroblastoma (888). There is no need to quantitate urinary dopamine or its metabolite HVA (homovanillic acid) or dopa for purposes of detecting a patient with pheochromocytoma, since these substances are only very rarely elevated, whereas the excretion of the catecholamines and/or their metabolites are almost always increased. Urine assay for dopamine, HVA, and dopa should be reserved as an aid in differentiating pheochromocytoma from other neural crest tumors (ganglioneuroma, neuroblastoma, ganglioneuroblastoma), since the latter tend to elaborate these substances in preference to epinephrine and norepinephrine. However, differentiation of pheochromocytoma from other neural crest tumors on a biochemical basis alone is not totally reliable since occasionally a pheochromocytoma will also secrete these substances (see Chapter 5 under Neuroblastoma).

The excretion of atypical urinary compounds (e.g., tyramine, 3-methoxytyramine, *p*-sympathol, *n*-methylmetanephrine, *m*-hydroxyhippuric, and *p*-hydroxyhippuric acid) has been reported on rare occasions in patients with pheochromocytoma (437, pp. 105 and 106).

Effect of Diet and Drugs   Certain drugs may alter or interfere with even the best assays, but few create problems in the diagnosis of pheochromocytoma.

The drugs which interfere with the biosynthesis and/or metabolism of the catecholamines are as follows:

1. The antihypertensive drugs which depress the activity of the sympathetic nervous system (57, 358).
2. MAO inhibitors [e.g., iproniazid (Marsilid), pargyline, tranylcypromine] (358, 946).
3. Dehydrogenase inhibitors [e.g., disulfiram (direct inhibitor) and ethanol (competitive inhibitor via acetaldehyde)] (358, 915). [There is evidence that ethanol can increase catecholamine synthesis and may thereby elevate blood pressure when large amounts of ethanol are consumed (personal communication from Dr. Stanley E. Gitlow).]

Although these drugs usually will not alter the excretion of the catecholamines and their metabolites to a degree which will confuse the diagnosis of pheochromocytoma, this possibility must always be kept in mind. The drugs which cause actual or spurious elevations in the values of catecholamine excretion (e.g., methyldopa and L-dopa) and their metabolites (e.g., MAO inhibitors) must, of course, be avoided for proper interpretation.

According to Gitlow, methyldopa (Aldomet) failed to significantly alter the levels of VMA or the metanephrines (358). On the other hand, some investigators have reported that methyldopa increases values for the total metanephrines in the urine (941). Other investigators have noted that methyldopa causes a decrease in urinary VMA in patients with essential hypertension (981); but the decrease of VMA in patients with pheochromocytoma has been minimal (344) or transient (885). Methyldopa (354) and L-dopa will markedly and spuriously elevate the catecholamine values when the fluorometric method is being used for measuring these amines in the urine or plasma. Other drugs which may cause significant interference with the fluorometric methods and spuriously augment the values obtained for catecholamines are: tetracycline, chlortetracycline, oxytetracycline, erythromycin (701), quinine, quinidine (354), and chlorpromazine (820). Excess biliary pigment in the urine has been reported to interfere with chromatographic determination of urine catecholamines (11).

It is also important to emphasize that interference with Pisano's urinary metanephrine assay by certain x-ray contrast media has been reported (490). It appears that radiopaque media which contain methylglucamine [e.g., Renovist, Renografin, Hypaque-M (75 or 90 percent), Cardiografin, Urografin, or Conray] can prevent oxidation of metanephrines to vanillin and lead to falsely negative results. Hypaque sodium, which does not contain methylglucamine, does not cause any interference with the measurement of metanephrines. It is recommended that urines be collected before or at least 3 days after the administration of substances containing methylglucamine. Interference with the metanephrine assay by radiopaque material has also been noted by one of us (R.W.G.).

Since MAO inhibitors will inhibit the conversion of the metanephrines to VMA, therapy with MAO inhibitors may cause an increase of metanephrine into a range diagnostic of pheochromocytoma. Although MAO inhibitors can result in a decrease in VMA, they would very rarely reduce VMA to a normal range in a patient with pheochromocytoma (267). A transient increase in VMA excretion has been noted in some patients at the start of treatment with MAO inhibitors (946).

Neg-gram (the antibacterial, nalidixic acid) has been noted to spuriously increase VMA levels, whereas Atromid-S (the cholesterol-lowering agent, clofibrate) has been reported to spuriously lower VMA (267).

Assays for urinary catecholamines, metanephrines, and VMA employed by Crout and coworkers (135) were not significantly influenced by the following drugs: barbiturates, thiazides, reserpine, hydralazine, cardiac glycosides, guanethidine, ganglionic blocking agents, and phentolamine. Crout and Sjoerdsma reported that the ingestion of even three bananas (which contain norepinephrine) could cause an increased excretion of hydrolyzable conjugates of catecholamines in the urine into a range seen in some patients with pheochromocytoma (192, 194); however, others have noted that after ingestion of three or four bananas the urinary excretion of catecholamines, VMA, or metanephrines did not exceed the normal range (881, 1055a).

Gitlow and associates found that diet did not appear to influence the accuracy of their assays or the excretion of VMA or total metanephrines (358). However, techniques which depend on measurement of VMA by its conversion to vanillin may be distorted significantly by the ingestion of citrus fruits (phenoxy acids), coffee, tea, chocolate, bananas, or vanilla and result in abnormally elevated VMA concentrations. Also, the ingestion of small doses of a large variety of drugs, including the antihypertensives and diuretics, did not remarkably alter the excretion of VMA and the metanephrines. Large doses of reserpine or guanethidine increased HVA excretion and slightly lowered the urine concentrations of VMA, the metanephrines, and MHPG; however, VMA excretions were never depressed to the normal range by these two antihypertensive drugs. Ethanol or disulfiram (Antabuse), inhibitors of aldehyde dehydrogenase, increased MHPG and decreased VMA excretion. Methocarbamol (Robaxin) and trihexyphenidyl hydrochloride (Artane) obscured the chromatographic measurement of MHPG but not that of VMA. Large doses of L-dopa caused elevations in the excretion of all the catecholamine metabolites (358). Less specific screening methods employing the diazo reagent to measure VMA give spuriously high values for urinary VMA in patients receiving methocarbamol (129) or *p*-aminosalicylic acid and in patients being tested with bromsulphothalein (BSP) and phenolsulfonphthalein (PSP) (11). Aspirin, sulfa drugs, mephenesin, and glyceryl guaiacolate may also interfere with colorimetric methods used to measure VMA.

Gitlow and coworkers have evaluated the effect of a large number of drugs and foods on the accuracy of various assays they employ. Specifically, they have found that administration of the following drugs does not appear to seriously alter the determination of VMA by the paper chromatographic or the double extraction screening tests which they employ (360): tetracycline, novobiocin, acetylsalicylic acid, digoxin, meperidine, chlorothiazide, phenylephrine, naphazoline, ephedrine, isopropyl-arterenol, phenobarbital, secobarbital, atropine, coffee, tea, fruit, or vanilla-containing substances. Even ingestion of as much as 8 mg of epinephrine did not elevate VMA to the pheochromocytoma range.

The screening accuracy of the rapid chromatoelectrophoretic test employed by Wolf and coworkers (1057) to assay urinary metanephrines and 3-methoxy-4-hydroxyphenylglycol was not disturbed by the following drugs: spironolactone, benzothiadiazine, phthalimidine, guanethidine sulfate, meprobamate, Rauwolfia serpentina derivatives, digitalis, diphenylhydantoin sodium, ephedrine, and barbiturates.

Furthermore, ingestion of small doses of reserpine, guanethidine, α-methyldopa, common antihistamines, acetylsalicylic acid, phenobarbital, meprobamate, digitalis, chlorothiazine, spironolactone, epinephrine, amphetamines, neosynephrine, and isoproterenol did not significantly enough modify the excretion of VMA or metanephrines to impair the value of the chromatoelectrophoretic test in screening patients suspected of harboring a pheochromocytoma (358).

Authors' Views Regarding Diagnosis of Pheochromocytoma by Urine Assay We subscribe to the view that determination of urine metanephrines is the best test available for screening patients suspected of having a pheochromocytoma. This view seems to be shared by most investigators who have had the largest amount of experience in studying patients with pheochromocytoma. Determination of

Table 6.14 *Chemical Tests[a]*

		Normal adult levels in urine		
		Upper limit of normal (mg/24 hr)	Range (μg/mg of creatinine)	Effect of drugs, diet, certain radiopaque media, and fluorescent substances[b]
Catecholamines				↑ Catecholamines
Epinephrine		0.02		↑ Drugs containing catecholamines
Norepinephrine		0.08		↑ Amphetamine
	Total	0.10		↑ Ethanol
Dopamine		0.20	0.08–0.23	↑ Isoproterenol[c]
				↑ L-Dopa
				↑ Methyldopa
				↑ Tetracyclines[c]
				↑ Erythromycin[c]
				↑ Chlorpromazine[c]
				↑ Other fluorescent substances[c] (e.g., quinine, quinidine, bile in urine)
				↑ MAO inhibitors ?
				↑ Rapid clonidine withdrawal?
				↑ Excess ingestion of bananas
				↓ Large doses: reserpine;[d] guanethidine;[d] ganglionic blockers; fenfluramine?
Metanephrines				↑ Catecholamines
Metanephrine		0.4		↑ Drugs containing catecholamines
Normetanephrine		0.9		↑ MAO inhibitors
	Total	1.3	0.001–2.2	↑ L-Dopa
				↑ Rapid clonidine withdrawal
				↑ Ethanol
				↑ Excess ingestion of bananas
				↑ Aldomet (Methyldopa)[c]
				↓ Renovist, Renografin (sodium diatrizoate)
				↓ Large doses: reserpine;[d] guanethidine;[d] ganglionic blockers; fenfluramine?

Table 6.14 *Continued*

VMA	6.5	0.2 –3.5	↑ **Catecholamines** (slight increase)
			↑ **Drugs containing catecholamines** (slight increase)
			↑ L-**Dopa**
			↑ **NegGram**[c] (nalidixic acid)
			↑ **Rapid clonidine withdrawal**
			↑ **Excess ingestion of bananas**
			↑ **Robaxin** (methocarbamol)[e]
			↑ Mepheresin[e]
			↑ BSP or PSP[c,e]
			↑ Excess ingestion of chocolate, tea, **coffee**, citrus fruit, or vanilla[e]
			↑ p-Aminosalicylic acid[d]
			↑ Aspirin[e]
			↑ Sulfa drugs[e]
			↑ **Glycerol guaiacolate**[e]
			↓ Aldomet (Methyldopa)[c,e]
			↓ Clofibrate (Atromid-S)
			↓ Large doses: reserpine;[d] guanethidine;[d] ganglionic blockers; fenfluramine?
			↓ **Disulfiram** (Antabuse)
			↓ **Ethanol**
			↓ **MAO inhibitors**
			↓ Chlorpromazine
MHPG	1.8	0.25–2.0	↑ **Catecholamines**
			↑ **Drugs containing catecholamines**
			↑ **Disulfiram** (Antabuse)
			↑ **Ethanol**
			↑ **Artane** (trihexyphenidyl)[e]
			↑ **Robaxin**[e]
			↑ **Rapid clonidine withdrawal**
			↑ Excess ingestion of bananas
			↓ Large doses: reserpine;[d] guanethidine;[d] ganglionic blockers; fenfluramine?
			↓ **MAO inhibitors**
HVA	8.0	0.2–3.5	↑ **Catecholamines**
			↑ **Drugs containing dopamine**
			↑ Large doses: reserpine, guanethidine, ganglionic blockers
			↑ L-**Dopa**

[a] The charge for some of these tests at one of the large and representative medical centers in New York City in 1976 was as follows:

Assay of 24-hr urine for catecholamines	$31.00
Assay of 24-hr urine for total metanephrines	$31.00
Assay of 24-hr urine for VMA	$34.00
chromatoelectrophoresis for metanephrines	$31.00

Abbreviations: VMA = vanillylmandelic acid; 3-methoxy-4-hydroxymandelic acid; MHPG = 3-methoxy-4-hydroxyphenylglycol; HVA = homovanillic acid; MAO = monoamine oxidase; BSP = bromsulphthalein; PSP = phenolsulfonphthalein.

[b] Substances in bold type may cause significant alteration of even most specific assays.

[c] Probably spurious interference.

[d] When chronically administered. (Acute administration of reserpine and guanethidine may cause an initial increase of the catecholamines and their metabolites.)

[e] Cause interference with only less specific assays.

the total metanephrines is relatively easy to perform, accurate, inexpensive, and less subject to falsely positive or negative results. Furthermore, the concentrations of metanephrine and normetanephrine or total metanephrines more accurately reflect the amounts of epinephrine and norepinephrine that have reached the circulation as free amines than does the measurement of VMA (187). The precaution, as with other tests, must be taken to avoid carefully (preferably for 1 week) any drugs which significantly alter catecholamine metabolism and change the actual concentration of metanephrines (Table 6.14). Fortunately, the number of drugs significantly influencing the concentration of metanephrines, or possibly interfering with the assay, appears to be very small. One must be aware of conditions other than pheochromocytoma which may elevate excretion of catecholamines and their metabolites, in order to avoid misinterpretation which might result in an erroneous diagnosis.

Measurement of urinary VMA is also a highly reliable assay for detecting patients with pheochromocytoma, but it must be performed accurately by a reliable laboratory and with the proper precautions to have discontinued any interfering drugs, preferably for 1 week (Table 6.14). Urinary catecholamines are more difficult to measure accurately than their metabolites, and the expertise for quantitation of the catecholamines is therefore not as readily available. "There is safety in numbers," so when feasible, and when pheochromocytoma is strongly suspected, assays of all three substances (i.e., metanephrines, VMA, and catecholamines) would be ideal. The fact that many interfering substances alter only one of the biochemical assays is another argument against depending on the quantitation of only one of these substances in the urine. The biochemical vagaries of pheochromocytomas, as clearly demonstrated by Crout and coworkers (191), account for a relatively greater secretion of catecholamines than metabolites by some pheochromocytomas, whereas the reverse is true in other pheochromocytomas. If results are equivocal, tests should, of course, be repeated.

When a patient has sustained hypertension, an assay either on random samples of urine or on a 24-hr specimen should be equally reliable if performed properly. If a random sample is used, it is, of course, necessary to determine the concentration of catecholamines or their metabolites per milligram of creatinine in order to interpret whether any excess of catecholamine, VMA, or metanephrine is present. If a 24-hr urine is assayed no creatinine determination is required. Yet it is, of course, essential that the entire 24-hr specimen be collected to permit an accurate interpretation. Completeness of collection can be assessed fairly accurately by creatinine estimations if there is no significant impairment of renal function. Because of the inconvenience of collecting all the urinary output for 24 hr, the reliability of the collection may be suspect—a point worth remembering. In many children, and occasionally in adults, it may be difficult if not impossible to collect a 24-hr urine specimen. In this situation we recommend that measurement of urine catecholamines and their metabolites be expressed in concentration per milligram of creatinine.

In the presence of polyuria or oliguria quantitation of the catecholamines and their metabolites in terms of creatinine is also more reliable than their estimation in 24-hr urines, since relating results to creatinine will correct for variations in urine volume. Excretion of creatinine appears to be quite well correlated with the excretion of norepinephrine, VMA, HVA, and the total metanephrines (361, 454a); hence, in renal insufficiency one may sometimes find a marked decrease in the 24-hr urine excretion of both creatinine and the catecholamines and/or their metabolites. If the clearance of both creatinine and the catecholamines (and their metabolites) is markedly impaired, it is essential to express results in terms of creatinine in order to make a valid interpretation. We are aware of one patient (see the case in Chapter 7 of the 29-year-old woman described under "Special Case Report—Pheochromocytoma Masquerading as Eclampsia") who, despite a 24-hr urine volume of 2050 ml and severe sustained hypertension due to pheochromocytoma, had a creatinine clearance of only 2.2 ml/min, and also unelevated 24-hr excretions of catecholamines and total metanephrines.

If the urine of a patient with paroxysmal hypertension has not been collected during, and several hrs following, a hypertensive period, then the presence of a pheochromocytoma cannot be excluded with absolute certainty, despite normal urinary catecholamines and/or their metabolites. As mentioned earlier, we believe that a 24-hr urine collection from all patients with intermittent hypertension is preferable to random urine sampling, since there is a better chance of detecting an occasional increase in excretion of catecholamines and their metabolites in the urine specimen which surveys a 24-hr period. When analysis of a 24-hr urine sample reveals normal excretion of catecholamines and/or metabolites in a patient with minimal hypertension or paroxysmal hypertension who is strongly suspected of having a pheochromocytoma, then we consider it mandatory to attempt to induce a paroxysm of hypertension by a physical maneuver (e.g., flank massage, bending, rolling onto the side, or some maneuver noted by the patient to cause an attack), or by a provocative drug. As stated previously, we administer glucagon initially and, if this pharmacologic test proves negative (i.e., the blood pressure rise is not significant), we follow up shortly thereafter with a histamine test. Urine and blood (if plasma analysis is feasible) should be collected for catecholamine assay shortly before and immediately following each provocative procedure. Urine should also be collected for several hours following the provocative procedure for assay of catecholamines, VMA, and the metanephrines. Normal concentrations of catecholamines and their metabolites in urine collected during and following hypertension exclude pheochromocytoma as the cause of the hypertension. However, it must be appreciated that, rarely, a patient with pheochromocytoma and normotension may be encountered in whom every effort to provoke an elevation of blood pressure accompanied by a diagnostic increase in urinary and plasma catecholamines and/or metabolites may fail. Under these circumstances, and if radiologic studies are negative, it seems reasonable and prudent to avoid exploratory laparotomy and to retest the patient every few months for any evidence of a pheochromocytoma—despite a strong clinical impression that a tumor may be present.

The upper limit for the quantity of catecholamines and their metabolites excreted in 24 hr by normal subjects is recorded in Table 6.14. The range of the urine concentration of these amines and metabolites per milligram of creatinine is also included, as are the drugs, diet, certain radiopaque media, and fluorescent substances which *may significantly influence* either their actual or "apparent" concentrations by, respectively, altering catecholamine metabolism or interfering with various assays. There are obviously a large number of drugs which may depress or excite the central and peripheral adrenergic systems. Since many of them have not been evaluated, it is impossible to prepare an all-inclusive list of these agents. The drugs and foods which interfere only with the less specific methods are those not listed in bold type. In human subjects administration of ACTH, ACTH peptides, and large doses of cortisone has been reported to cause a marked decrease in norepinephrine; epinephrine excretion remained the same during ACTH administration but tended to increase during cortisone therapy (286, p. 295). To our knowledge, ACTH or cortisone therapy has almost never altered catecholamine metabolism to a degree which could interfere with the diagnostic assays in patients with pheochromocytoma. However, as mentioned earlier, ACTH (and perhaps cortisone) may precipitate a severe hypertensive crisis and even death in a patient harboring a pheochromocytoma.

In general, it is probably preferable but not always practical to avoid the use of all substances which may interfere with the accurate determination of catecholamines and their metabolites for approximately 1 week before collection of urine for biochemical assay. Iproniazid, for example, may result in a depression of VMA excretion for as much as 5 days after withdrawal (946); an elevation in the metanephrines for the same length of time may also occur. In addition to the drugs and radiopaque media mentioned earlier which were found to interfere with the quantitation of urine catecholamines and their metabolites (Table 6.14), various conditions other than pheochromocytoma may also cause an increase or decrease in the excretion of the urinary catecholamines and their metabolites. Many of these conditions, which are indicated in Table 6.15, have been mentioned and briefly reviewed by some investigators (11,

358, 956); however, it seems worthwhile to include all of these conditions in one comprehensive table for convenient reference.

Although a number of circumstances or disease states which are associated with in-creased excretion of catecholamines and their metabolites have been discussed earlier, certain general comments regarding increased activity of the adrenergic nervous system seem warranted. A variety of stressful circum-

Table 6.15 *Important Points Regarding Catecholamine Excretion When Evaluating Patients*

I. Conditions (other than pheochromocytoma) which may be accompanied by
   A. Significantly increased excretion of catecholamines and metabolites
      1. Some types of stress: congestive heart failure; circulatory shock; electroshock; marked hypotension; myocardial infarction; pulmonary infarction; hypoxia; mesenteric thrombosis; sepsis; acidosis (diabetic, respiratory, circulatory shock, uremic, lactic, etc.); acute spinal cord injury; ↑ intracranial pressure; terminal state; hypoglycemia; strenuous exercise; trauma; severe cold; surgery; burns; parturition; gravitational or hypobaric stress; emotional upset; iron deficiency anemia; oxygen toxicity (especially with convulsions); hypovolemia; delirium tremens.
      2. Other neural crest tumors [e.g., ganglioneuroma, neuroblastoma, ganglioneuroblastoma; retinoblastoma (1 case); melanotic progonoma (1 case)]
      3. Certain diseases in addition to those associated with stress: acute porphyria; lead poisoning; tetanus; Guillain-Barré syndrome; acrodynia; carcinoid; quadriplegics (hyperreflexic state); toxemia of pregnancy with convulsions; some intracranial lesions; amyotrophic lateral sclerosis with chronic muscle fasciculation (1 case); leukemia (1 case)
      4. Certain drugs, foods, and fluorescent substances (Table 6.14). (Some of these cause spurious increases.)
   B. Significantly decreased excretion of catecholamines and metabolites
      1. Certain drugs and radiopaque media (Table 6.14). (Some of these cause spurious decreases.)
      2. Certain diseases [familial dysautonomia; quadriplegia (quiescent state); orthostatic hypotension (due to a deficient sympathetic nervous system); malnutrition].
      3. In some patients with renal insufficiency and/or oliguria (if 24-hr urine sample quantitated and results not expressed in terms of milligrams creatinine).

II. Noteworthy points regarding analysis of urinary catecholamines and metabolites
   A. Avoid screening "Kits" for VMA measurement!
   B. Avoid drugs and stressful conditions which may alter excretion of catecholamines and their metabolites or interfere with their assay.
   C. If normotensive with equivocal results, collect urine shortly after paroxysm of hypertension (either spontaneously occurring or induced by provocative procedure) and analyze for catecholamines and their metabolites.
   D. The ratio of urinary catecholamines to metabolites depends on tumor metabolism. Hence may, rarely, have only catecholamine *or* metabolite elevated.
   E. If significant amount of urinary catecholamines is epinephrine or its metabolite (metanephrine) the tumor is in the adrenal, organ of Zuckerkandl, or rarely, thorax or bladder.

stances can activate the sympathoadrenal system and result in significant increases in the excretion of catecholamines and their metabolites. Many of the conditions, which have been shown experimentally or clinically to be associated with an increased secretion of catecholamines, were reviewed in 1956 by von Euler (286) and are listed here:

1. splanchnic nerve stimulation;
2. reflex liberation caused by hypotension (via carotid sinus reflex), afferent nerve stimulation, tilting to 70° from recumbent position;
3. stimulation of hypothalamic secretory centers;
4. asphyxia, oxygen lack, hypercarbia;
5. hypoglycemia;
6. muscular work (especially strenuous and fatiguing exercise);
7. immersion in cold water;
8. administration of certain drugs (e.g., acetylcholine, nicotine, histamine, serotonin, potassium salts, ether, phosphonates, possibly bile salts or ferrous salts, thallium poisoning);
9. electroshock therapy;
10. surgical and traumatic stress (surgery complicated by pain, fever, and slow healing; cerebral trauma; pneumoencephalogram); and
11. emotional stress (e.g., flying in transport planes as well as piloting).

In general, one would expect some correlation between the severity of the stimulus and the degree of activation of the sympathoadrenal system (as reflected by the amount of catecholamines released into the circulation and the concentrations of catecholamines and their metabolites excreted into the urine). Some forms of stress may cause a liberation of epinephrine and norepinephrine simultaneously. On the other hand, a variety of stresses result in an increased secretion of epinephrine without changing the secretion rate of norepinephrine; the reverse may also occur (286). The finding that preferential secretion of epinephrine or norepinephrine is a common phenomenon implies that an increased secretion of adrenal medullary cells may occur independently (i.e., without a simultaneous increased secretion from the sympathetic nerves, and vice versa).

More recently, Hingerty and O'Boyle (448) have reviewed some of the reports on sympathoadrenal response to stress. In addition to the conditions enumerated by von Euler, anxiety, aggressiveness, and anticipation of competition appeared to cause increased secretion of catecholamines under a large variety of circumstances (e.g., competitive sports; final examinations; hospital admission; military training; exciting, amusing, sexually arousing films; performance of tasks under disagreeable or distracting conditions; sleep deprivation; flights at supersonic speeds; parachute jumping; exposure to 12 g in a centrifuge; routine automobile driving). It is interesting that racing drivers sometimes had a 20-fold increase in norepinephrine excretion after a 20 min race, with a pulse rate reading 180 to 210 at the start and persisting throughout the race. [Weil-Malherbe found marked increases in the urinary excretion of epinephrine, norepinephrine, and dopamine in racing car drivers; however, there was no comparable effect on the excretion of VMA or the metanephrines (1013).] Patients with severe head injuries were at times observed to have urinary norepinephrine and epinephrine elevated, respectively, to 7 and 30 times normal values. High catecholamine excretion rates (14 to 17 times normal) may occur and persist for several hours after exhausting competitive exercises (e.g., skiing, marathon running, woodcutting). Observations on the effect of exercise suggest that untrained individuals exhibit a greater catecholamine response to exercise than trained athletes. Drinking coffee or smoking tobacco caused increases in catecholamine excretion, but these elevations were relatively small. Consumption of alcohol and amphetamines can also increase catecholamine excretion (448).

Hingerty and O'Boyle also reviewed studies on the effect of myocardial infarction on catecholamine secretion which, they pointed out, could be influenced by multiple stresses (e.g., pain, tissue damage, circulatory disturbances, and emotion). Significantly, elevated catecholamine secretion may be observed within the first 24 hr post myocardial infarction, and may not return to normal for 5 days in the uncomplicated case. Acute coronary insufficiency without myocardial infarction can also result in significantly elevated secretion of catecholamines. Two patients studied at the Cleveland Clinic had recurrent angina due to the Prinzmetal syndrome; their urinary metanephrines were significantly elevated and the presence of a pheochromocytoma had to be excluded (personal communication from Dr. Frederick Heupler, cardiologist, Cleveland Clinic).

It is essential that the diagnostician be fully aware of conditions (Table 6.15) other than pheochromocytoma which may significantly alter the excretion of catecholamines and their metabolites. It is only with such knowledge that the diagnostician can properly evaluate the results of urinary assays of these substances in order to establish or exclude the presence of a functioning pheochromocytoma. Although mild physical stress, or most types of emotional crises, even with pronounced anxiety, will not remarkably influence the excretion rate of the catecholamines or their metabolites, many types of severe physical stress can elevate their excretion into the range seen in some patients with pheochromocytoma. Because of the fact that concentrations of urinary and plasma catecholamines are only transiently elevated in some patients critically ill with conditions such as myocardial infarction, hypotension, acidosis, etc., it may be of value to perform serial determinations of catecholamines (985).

Undoubtedly there are other forms of stress or disease states (not recorded in Table 6.15) which may cause increased excretion of catecholamines and their metabolites. One particularly unusual circumstance in which increased catecholamine excretion occurred was reported by von Euler and associates (293). These investigators found that bilaterally adrenalectomized patients, receiving maintenance doses of cortisone, not infrequently excreted increased quantities of norepinephrine; excretion of epinephrine was markedly reduced. No explanation was offered for the increased excretion of norepinephrine which occurred in some of these patients. One of us (W.M.M.) has recently seen a 39-year-old woman with Addison's disease who was receiving fludrocortisone and cortisone replacement therapy. She periodically excreted slightly increased concentrations of total catecholamines, total metanephrines, and VMA. Although

purely speculative, it is conceivable that elevations of her urinary catecholamines and metabolites may have resulted from periods of hypovolemia—perhaps accompanying inadequate steroid replacement therapy.

It is extremely important for one to keep in mind the host of drugs, foods, radiopaque media, and fluorescent substances which may alter the excretion of the catecholamines and their metabolites or interfere with their measurement. For example, even the use of "cold" tablets, bronchodilators for asthma, cough medicines, or nose drops containing catecholamines may result in elevations of these amines and some metabolites into the range diagnostic of pheochromocytoma.

The occurrence of increased catecholamine excretion in neural crest tumors and in some diseases has been discussed earlier. In regard to these conditions it should be stated that a "true" chemodectoma is considered by some to be almost invariably a nonfunctioning paraganglioma. Hence, the inclusion of this neural crest tumor with the functioning tumors in Table 6.15 must be questioned.

Although the presence of increased excretion of dopa, dopamine, and/or homovanillic acid points strongly to a diagnosis of a neural crest tumor other than pheochromocytoma, yet it must be reemphasized that on rare occasions pheochromocytomas may also excrete excessive amounts of these substances. It should be mentioned that increased quantities of dopa and homovanillic acid may also be excreted in the urine of some patients with metastatic malignant melanoma (personal communication from Dr. A. W. Kopf, Professor of Dermatology, New York University Medical Center). We are unaware of any studies on the excretion of the catecholamines, VMA, or the metanephrines in patients with metastatic melanoma.

It is particularly important to emphasize the fact that increased intracranial pressure can significantly activate the adrenergic system and result in increased excretion of the catecholamines and their metabolites. We observed increased plasma catecholamines in a patient with increased intracranial pressure and hypertension resulting from a brain tumor (624). In addition, excess excretion of urinary catecholamines (606) and their metabolites (358) has been found in patients with intracranial hemorrhage and hypertension without pheochromocytoma. Since severe hypertension, encephalopathy, increased intracranial pressure, and intracranial hemorrhage can occur in patients without pheochromocytoma as well as in those with this tumor, the differential diagnosis may at times be challenging.

Crout reported the intriguing situation in which a patient with amyotrophic lateral sclerosis and chronic muscle fasiculation excreted increased quantities of norepinephrine —an increase which was attributed to excessive muscular activity (185). As mentioned earlier, some quadriplegic patients may experience hypertensive crises during a hyperreflexic state and this may be accompanied by a significantly increased excretion of catecholamine metabolites. On the other hand, during a quiescent period (in the absence of a hyperreflexic state) quadriplegics usually excrete decreased amounts of catecholamines and their metabolites.

Recently, Voorhess and associates have reported the interesting observation that iron deficiency anemia may be accompanied by increased excretion of urinary norepinephrine and VMA. The norepinephrine concentrations may at times reach levels sometimes seen in patients with pheochromocytoma. Excretions of dopamine, epinephrine, and the total metanephrines remained normal (999). This exotic relationship between iron deficiency and increased excretion of norepinephrine and one of its metabolites may be related to a decreased tissue MAO activity, which has been demonstrated in experimentally induced iron deficiency; however, since MAO inhibitors increase metanephrine excretion and decrease VMA excretion, one would have anticipated this pattern of excretion in iron deficiency anemia if the defect in this condition is related to a decrease of tissue MAO.

Several investigators have reported that polyuria has been accompanied by increased excretion of epinephrine and/or norepinephrine (109, 210, 859). Sunderman studied the relation between urine volume and the excretion of VMA during a 24-hr period in 558 hypertensive patients (956). Although he found no significant differences in the mean excretion of VMA in urine volumes varying from 800 to 3600 ml per day, there was a significantly lower value with urine volumes of 400 to 800 ml per day. It was therefore recommended that adults should excrete more than 800 ml daily if VMA is to be measured. Despite these reports indicating that urine volume may influence the excretion of catecholamines and VMA, other investigators have found that in normal volunteers on regimens of different fluid intakes, the urinary excretion of free and conjugated fractions of epinephrine, norepinephrine, and dopamine remained remarkably constant despite the fact that the daily fluid output varied from less than 1000 to almost 4000 ml (451). We are not aware of any cases of pheochromocytoma in which the correct diagnosis was obscured because of polyuria or oliguria. The fact that some adults and many children with pheochromocytoma experience polyuria should not influence the diagnostic accuracy of the urinary assays.

It should also be mentioned that the urinary excretion of epinephrine and possibly norepinephrine has been reported to be negatively correlated with the urine pH, more catecholamines being excreted in acid urine (454a); however, to our knowledge this has not presented any problem in evaluating patients suspected of having a pheochromocytoma.

With regard to random sampling of urine for assay of the catecholamines or their metabolites, it is noteworthy that a patient with a pheochromocytoma may have a diurnal variation in the rate of excretion of these substances, as do normal adults. For example, in normal subjects and in one patient with a pheochromocytoma the lowest excretion rate for VMA was between 11 p.m. and 7 a.m. (956), i.e., during a period of minimal physical activity. The urinary excretion of catecholamines and their metabolites in patients with sustained hypertension and pheochromocytoma appears to be quite variable, but the levels remain above normal when determined over a period of many days (505).

In Table 6.15 are also listed the conditions associated with decreased excretion of catecholamines and their metabolites. Certain drugs may decrease the excretion of catecholamines and their metabolites (Table 6.14). Chronic administration of large doses of fenfluramine, an anorectic drug with moderate antihypertensive action, has been shown to reduce markedly the plasma concentration of norepinephrine (991a); it is likely that significant reductions in the concentrations of the catecholamines and their metabolites in the urine would also occur. Possibly diazepam (Valium) should be included in this group of drugs which decrease catecholamine concentrations; however, the effect of this drug on catecholamine metabolism has not been adequately studied. It must be appreciated that certain drugs and radiopaque media can interfere with the measurement of the catecholamines or their metabolites. Although Renovist or Renografin may spuriously normalize levels of metanephrines in patients with pheochromocytoma, we are not aware of any patient with a pheochromocytoma in whom drug therapy lowered the excretion rate of the catecholamines and/or all their metabolites to a normal range.

Finally, the following noteworthy points regarding analysis of urinary catecholamines and their metabolites in patients with pheochromocytoma are also made in Table 6.15:

1. Simple screening "kits" for VMA measurements should be avoided because of the lack of specificity and unreliability. Sunderman reported studies indicating that the "Pheoset" technique for measuring VMA is an unsatisfactory screening procedure for pheochromocytoma. Also, the qualitative screening test developed by Hingerty (448) for detecting excessive amounts of urinary catecholamines has proved valuable in detecting patients with pheochromocytoma (91, 448, 505). However, Kelleher and coworkers have stressed that in order to eliminate false negatives, the upper limit of normal by this assay should be considered 90 μg/24 hr. These investigators considered the determination of total metanephrines the best confirmatory test for pheochromocytoma (505). Salicylates, tetracyclines, and methyldopa can give falsely positive results with the Hingerty method even 1 week after administration of these drugs has been discontinued (448).

2. The drugs listed in Table 6.14 (which interfere with even the most specific assays) should be avoided for at least 1 week. Also, any drug which has not been evaluated for its effect on the excretion of the catecholamines and their metabolites or on their chemical assay must be considered suspect if results are equivocal or positive. Under such circumstances these unevaluated drugs should be eliminated and the urinary catecholamines or their metabolites reassayed 1 week later.

   A point which has not been adequately emphasized or considered is the possibility that some borderline results or slight elevations in the excretion of the catecholamines or their metabolites could result from excessive stress occurring during the 24-hr period when the urine was collected. For example, strenuous physical exertion, severe cold stress, etc., could conceivably result in a higher than normal excretion of catecholamines and their metabolites. This fact can be explained to patients so that they will understand the importance of avoiding severe stress during the period of urine collection.

3. In normotensive subjects where the result of biochemical assay has been negative or only borderline elevated, urine must be collected during or shortly after a spontaneous or induced paroxysm of hypertension in order to establish whether or not a patient has a pheochromocytoma.

4. The relative amount of catecholamines and metabolites excreted by patients with pheochromocytoma depends on the tumor metabolism.

5. If a significant fraction of the urinary catecholamines is epinephrine or its metabolite (metanephrine), then the chances are excellent that the tumor will be in the adrenal gland, although occasionally such tumors occur in the organ of Zuckerkandl, or, very rarely, in the thorax or bladder.

If accurate biochemical assays are used, and if the conditons which may cause elevated urinary values of catecholamines and their metabolites have been eliminated, a significantly elevated excretion of the catecholamines or their metabolites can be considered pathognomonic for pheochromocytoma.

PLASMA ASSAYS

Introduction Estimation of the plasma catecholamines has proved invaluable in assessing sympathoadrenal activity under a variety of stressful circumstances. It has also been found to be highly reliable not only in detecting patients with pheochromocytoma but also in localizing these tumors. [Methods are available for estimating VMA in the serum (716, 955), but these methods have been used only very rarely for diagnosis and localization of a pheochromocytoma (955). To our knowledge, quantitation of the metanephrines in the blood has not been used to detect patients harboring this tumor.]

A pressor substance in the blood of patients with pheochromocytoma was first demonstrated by means of a bioassay technique in 1937 by Beer, King, and Prinzmetal (53), and in 1943 by Hyman and Mencher (470). However, it was not until 1951 that Lund and Møller, employing the trihydroxyindole fluorometric method of analysis, accurately quantitated the concentration of plasma catecholamines in a patient with pheochromocytoma (593). A year later, Lund reported five patients in whom the plasma catecholamines were elevated to between 14 and 98 μg per liter (normal value being <1 μg per liter) during episodes of paroxysmal hypertension (590). Four of these patients were found to have pheochromocytoma, but no tumor was discovered in the fifth. In 1953, von Euler, Lund, Olson, and Sandblom used the same chemical assay to determine both the plasma and urine catecholamines in another patient with pheochromocytoma (298). The following year Manger and coworkers, using the ethylenediamine fluorometric assay, reported studies on 13 patients with pheochromocytoma, and further established the diagnostic value of quantitating plasma catecholamines in patients suspected of having pheochromocytoma (616). The latter investigators also demonstrated the diagnostic importance of combining the histamine provocative test with analysis of plasma catecholamines in some patients with pheochromocytoma who have normal plasma catecholamine levels during normotensive periods. The dramatic way in which anesthesia and/or operative manipulation can some-

times trigger an abrupt release of catecholamines into the circulation and cause a striking increase in plasma catecholamines and the blood pressure was also reported (616). Subsequently, more detailed studies on plasma catecholamines in a series of 23 patients with pheochromocytoma (16 with sustained and seven with paroxysmal hypertension) were presented by Manger and coworkers (611a, 622–624). We have now completed plasma catecholamine determinations on 40 patients with pheochromocytoma, and we have correlated the plasma concentrations of epinephrine and norepinephrine with the tumor concentrations of these amines. The findings in 38 of these patients are presented in detail in Chapter 7.

During the past few years the diagnostic accuracy of determining plasma catecholamines to identify patients with pheochromocytoma has been further substantiated by Louis and coworkers (266, 342, 584). These investigators used the double-isotope technique of Engelman and Portnoy (271).

Since the hypertension in patients with pheochromocytoma is due to increased circulating catecholamines, the plasma catecholamines should invariably be elevated in those patients with an actively secreting tumor which is causing sustained hypertension. Undoubtedly, however, a patient will eventually be found who has a paroxysmally functioning pheochromocytoma in addition to essential hypertension. An elevated blood pressure in the presence of normal plasma catecholamines might conceivably result in the erroneous belief that the patient is not harboring a pheochromocytoma when, in fact, an intermittently secreting tumor is present.

The unique advantage of performing plasma catecholamine assays is that blood can be conveniently collected immediately before and after a provocative test and correlated with blood pressure responses. Such a correlation can be diagnostic in patients with pheochromocytoma and paroxysmal hypertension who have normal concentrations of catecholamines and their metabolites in the urine and plasma. The determination of both epinephrine and norepinephrine in plasma may be very helpful in localizing a pheochromocytoma since, if epinephrine is significantly increased, the tumor nearly always proves to be one arising from the adrenal area; however, as mentioned earlier, such tumors may occasionally arise from the organ of Zuckerkandl; and, very rarely, a tumor of the chest or the urinary bladder may secrete epinephrine as well as norepinephrine. Also, as stated above, the determination of both metanephrine and normetanephrine may similarly provide information which strongly suggests an adrenal location of a pheochromocytoma; however, usually only the total metanephrines (i.e., metanephrine plus normetanephrine) are measured since this is a simpler analytical procedure.

Because of the relative simplicity and availability of methods for estimating total urinary metanephrines and VMA (especially the screening procedures), and because of the reliability of measuring these substances in order to detect patients with pheochromocytoma, quantitation of plasma catecholamines has remained largely an experimental tool and had, until recently, rarely been used for diagnostic purposes except by us and our colleagues at the Mayo Clinic. On the other hand, since quantitation of catecholamines in plasma samples obtained from various sites in the vena cava has proved extremely valuable in localizing pheochromocytomas, it has been utilized by a number of investigators. Central venous blood sampling can be particularly valuable in localizing an actively secreting tumor which has defied localization by other means. The subject of preoperative tumor localization is considered in detail later in this chapter.

Finally, one virtue of quantitating plasma catecholamines instead of urinary concentration of these amines or their metabolites is the fact that with blood collection one feels secure that samples were properly collected, preserved, and not contaminated during collection. A distinct *dis*advantage of collecting a blood sample for a screening assay is evident in *some* patients with paroxysmal hypertension due to pheochromocytoma, since in about 37.5 percent of these subjects the plasma catecholamines may be normal during normotensive periods (see Chapter 7). Obviously, urine collection over a period of 24 hr would be more likely to detect a periodically secreting tumor.

Results Using the Ethylenediamine Method Employed by Manger and Coworkers Initially, a modification (624) of the ethylenediamine fluorometric method of Weil-Malherbe and Bone (1018, 1019) was used to quantitate the plasma catecholamines in experimental and clinical studies. The method is comparatively simple and, when employed by most investigators, has given reproducible results (624). Concentrations were initially expressed in micrograms per liter (μg/liter) of plasma of "epinephrine-like substance." The estimate of "epinephrine-like substance" is based on a calculation that assumes that all the fluorescence is due to epinephrine; however, the fluorescence of extracts of plasma is usually due to both epinephrine and norepinephrine. Since norepinephrine exhibits only about one-third of the fluorescence that epinephrine does, the concentration of "epinephrine-like substance" is less than the arithmetic sum of the concentrations of epinephrine and norepinephrine when both are present. The term "epinephrine-like" was introduced by Weil-Malherbe and has been retained since some of our initial determinations were performed before a method of estimating the individual concentrations of epinephrine and norepinephrine had been devised.

Our original procedure to quantitate epinephrine and norepinephrine necessitated utilization of two aliquots which had to be analyzed separately by different chemical techniques requiring considerable manipulation. Our mean recovery for epinephrine added to plasma was about 100 percent, whereas that for norepinephrine was approximately 82 percent, which is in good agreement with the results of other investigators using the method (624).

Since 1958, we have employed a modification similar to our initial method except that two interchangeable secondary filters are used to permit the quantitation of epinephrine and norepinephrine in a single aliquot. This modification has yielded results quite similar to those obtained by the original method and has an accuracy of $\pm$10 percent. It has simplified our analytical procedure and has improved our accuracy in differentiating and quantitating epinephrine and norepinephrine. Evaluation of the method we have employed for quantitating the catecholamines has indicated that it is highly sensitive and fairly specific, although less so than the trihydroxyindole procedure. Furthermore, the reproducibility of results, the simplicity of the method, and the relatively stable fluorescent substances produced by the condensation of the ethylenediamine with the catecholamines are all virtues not equalled by other fluorometric chemical methods (624, 1015). A comparative study of our modification of the ethylenediamine method with an improved trihydroxyindole method as modified by Steinsland revealed fairly good agreement between the results obtained by these two methods during infusions of catecholamines or during periods of hemorrhagic shock and acidosis. Under these latter circumstances the ethylenediamine procedure appeared superior to the trihydroxyindole method in differentiating epinephrine and norepinephrine (620). Certainly, both methods are admirably suited for detecting an increase in circulating catecholamines which occurs in patients with pheochromocytoma or in many stressful situations which cause sympathoadrenal activation (624). Over the past 24 years, we have used the fluorometric ethylenediamine method to perform approximately 9000 plasma catecholamine determinations in a large variety of clinical and experimental conditions. Our results conclusively indicate that

elevations of the concentrations of plasma catecholamines correlate extremely well with the activation of the adrenergic nervous system. On the other hand, absence of a significant increase in the concentrations of plasma catecholamines does not necessarily exclude the possibility that some degree of adrenergic stimulation occurred.

CLINICAL STUDIES

We have also demonstrated the excellent capability of the ethylenediamine method to detect and accurately differentiate epinephrine from norepinephrine during infusions of norepinephrine in normotensive and hypertensive subjects (617).

Table 6.16 reveals the concentrations of epinephrine-like substance in peripheral venous plasma of 37 healthy men and women, 45 men and women with essential hypertension, and 21 patients with pheochromocytoma who were not exhibiting a paroxysmal attack of hypertension at the time blood samples were collected. Without exception, the concentration of epinephrine-like substance was less than 3.5 μg/liter in all subjects without pheochromocytoma. Very rarely, a patient without pheochromocytoma was found to have a single elevation above this value; however, when several determinations were performed on such a patient, the mean value was invariably below 3.5 μg/liter. Values above this

Table 6.16 *Concentration (μg/liter) of Epinephrine-like Substance (ELS) in Peripheral Venous Plasma of 37 Healthy Men and Women, 45 Men and Women with Essential Hypertension, and 21 Patients with Pheochromocytoma[a,b]*

| | Healthy | | Hypertensive | | | | Patients with pheochromocytoma and hypertension | | | |
| | Men | Women | Men | | Women | | Sustained hypertension | | Paroxysmal hypertension | |
	ELS	ELS	BP	ELS	BP	ELS	BP	ELS	BP	ELS
No. of subjects	28	9	20	20	25	25	16	15	5	6
Mean	1.6 ± 0.12	1.3 ± 0.19	$\frac{197}{120}$	1.6 ± 0.18	$\frac{200}{118}$	2.0 ± 0.13	$\frac{188}{122}$	6.9 ± 0.93	$\frac{133}{86}$	5.0 ± 1.3
S.D.	0.66	0.57	—	0.82	—	0.67	—	3.61	—	3.22
Range	0.4–3.0	0.3–2.3	$\frac{160–292}{90–190}$	0.1–3.1	$\frac{154–240}{92–156}$	0.7–3.2	$\frac{148–250}{89–170}$	3.6–16.6	$\frac{120–144}{80–92}$	1.0–9.4

[a] Data taken from Manger, W. M., Wakim, K. G., and Bollman, J. L. *Chemical Quantitation of Epinephrine and Norepinephrine in Plasma.* Courtesy of C. C. Thomas, 1959, from Tables 1,II; 2,II; and 7,II; pp. 79, 80, and 92.

[b] In patients with paroxysmal hypertension, only values of ELS in blood obtained in the absence of a paroxysm were included in this table. BP = blood pressure; figures after ± = standard error of the mean; S.D. = standard deviation; all patients were Caucasian.

level were invariably found in patients with pheochromocytomas which were actively secreting (i.e., in those patients with tumors causing sustained hypertension or during a paroxysm of hypertension). However, as mentioned earlier, some patients with pheochromocytoma and normotension between attacks may also have normal plasma catecholamine concentrations.

Figure 6.14 graphically depicts the results of our studies up until 1958, during which period we expressed the plasma catecholamine content in terms of "epinephrine-like substance," as defined above. The figure represents the percentage distribution of concentration of epinephrine-like substance in the plasma of the 37 normotensive subjects, the 45 patients with essential hypertension, and 21 patients with pheochromocytoma. The average concentration of epinephrine-like substance for each patient was used to construct this graph. Regarding patients with pheochromocytoma and paroxysmal hypertension, only the elevated preoperative values occurring in the course of a spontaneous or induced paroxysm of hypertension were used. Although the mean concentration of epinephrine-like substance for the hypertensive group (1.8 µg/liter) was slightly greater than that for the normotensive group (1.5 µg/liter), the overlapping of concentrations of epinephrine-like substance in these two groups is striking. The mean concentration of epinephrine-like

substance in the 21 patients with pheochromocytoma was 6.8 µg/liter of plasma.

On the one hand, Figure 6.14 graphically demonstrates that the concentrations of epinephrine-like substance in the plasma of normotensive and essential hypertensive subjects overlap; on the other hand, it demonstrates that the concentrations of epinephrine-like substance in the plasma of patients who have actively secreting pheochromocytomas are invariably greater than those in subjects with normotension or essential hypertension.

Our original studies on 23 patients with pheochromocytoma have been reported in detail previously (623, 624); however, some of our findings on these patients will be recapitulated in Chapter 7 to permit comparison with some of our subsequent studies of other patients with pheochromocytoma.

Since 1958 we have employed the improved and simplified fluorometric technique which permits the determination of both epinephrine and norepinephrine; therefore, the concentrations of both these catecholamines have been reported and the term "epinephrine-like" substance has subsequently been discarded.

Quantitation of epinephrine and norepinephrine was performed on normal subjects and patients with essential hypertension as follows:

Used in this study were 20 normal subjects (13 men and seven women) ages 19 to 65

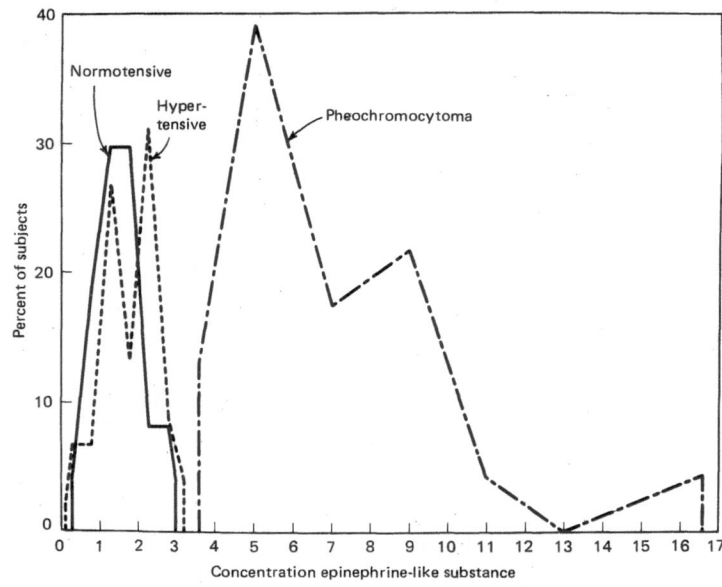

Fig. 6.14 Percentage distribution of 37 normal subjects, 45 patients with essential hypertension, and 21 patients with actively secreting pheochromocytomas, according to concentration of epinephrine-like substance in plasma. From Manger, W. M., Wakim, K. G., and Bollman, J. L. *Chemical Quantitation of Epinephrine and Norepinephrine in Plasma.* Courtesy of C. C. Thomas, 1959, p. 93.

years, and 31 patients with uncomplicated essential hypertension (18 men and 13 women) ages 18 to 60 years. In most instances, the diagnosis of essential hypertension was established by the exclusion of secondary causes, including the absence of renal arterial lesions by radiographic studies. Eighty-five percent of normotensives and 71 percent of hypertensives were Caucasian. After obtaining the patient's informed consent, we took samples of venous and sometimes arterial blood simultaneously from indwelling catheters in the antecubital vein and brachial artery or via venepuncture. All persons were recumbent for at least 15 min, in a relatively basal state, having been on no medication for approximately 1 month and almost always on a regular diet. All patients were hospitalized. Blood pressure was measured by the auscultatory method or by means of the arterial catheter connected to a Statham p23 Db

strain gauge; direct pressures were recorded on an oscillograph.

Table 6.17 reveals the mean ages, blood pressures, and concentrations of epinephrine and norepinephrine in venous and arterial plasma of normotensive and hypertensive men and women. The percentage of total plasma catecholamines that was norepinephrine is also indicated. Ages were quite similar in the groups compared except that the hypertensive women whose venous plasma was analyzed were significantly ($p<0.01$) older (50 $\pm$ 2.5 years) than the normotensive women (37 $\pm$ 3.5 years) in the same group. Mean arterial blood pressures (MABP) between normotensive men and women were not remarkably different, and this was also true of the hypertensives, although the hypertensive women had moderately higher systolic pressures than did the men.

Figure 6.15 reveals the venous plasma con-

Table 6.17 *Age, Blood Pressure, and Concentration of Plasma Catecholamines (μg/liter) in Normal Subjects and Patients with Essential Hypertension*[a]

	Normotensive			Hypertensive			p values for differences between normotensive and hypertensive subjects		
	Total	Men	Women	Total	Men	Women	Total	Men	Women
A. Groups in which venous plasma analyzed									
No.	20	13	7	31	18	13			
Age	36 ± 2.6	36 ± 3.7	37 ± 3.5	43 ± 2.0	38 ± 2.2	50 ± 2.5	<0.05	NS	<0.01
BP	123 ± 3	126 ± 3	117 ± 4	174 ± 6	164 ± 4	189 ± 12	<0.001	<0.001	<0.001
	77 ± 1	79 ± 1	74 ± 3	108 ± 3	110 ± 4	105 ± 3	<0.001	<0.001	<0.001
MABP	92 ± 1	94 ± 1	88 ± 3	130 ± 3	128 ± 4	133 ± 5	<0.001	<0.001	<0.001
E	0.6 ± 0.08	0.5 ± 0.10	0.7 ± 0.10	0.6 ± 0.06	0.5 ± 0.07	0.6 ± 0.10	NS	NS	NS
NE	2.4 ± 0.23	2.7 ± 0.27	2.1 ± 0.42	3.2 ± 0.24	3.0 ± 0.33	3.3 ± 0.35	<0.05	NS	<0.05
Total CA	3.0 ± 0.24	3.1 ± 0.31	2.8 ± 0.40	3.7 ± 0.24	3.6 ± 0.34	3.9 ± 0.37	<0.05	NS	NS
% NE	81	85	74	85	85	85			
B. Groups in which arterial plasma analyzed									
No.	7	5	2	8	4	4			
Age	37 ± 4.2	32 ± 3.9	50	45 ± 3.2	40 ± 5.0	49 ± 2.5	NS	NS	NS
BP	130 ± 4	131 ± 6	129	217 ± 17	194 ± 16	240 ± 28	<0.001	<0.025	<0.05
	78 ± 6	79 ± 1	77	103 ± 4	106 ± 8	100 ± 4	<0.001	<0.015	<0.05
MABP	96 ± 2	96 ± 2	95	141 ± 7	136 ± 8	147 ± 12	<0.001	<0.005	<0.025
E	0.5 ± 0.11	0.5 ± 0.16	0.6	0.4 ± 0.06	0.3 ± 0.10	0.5 ± 0.03	NS	NS	NS
NE	2.8 ± 0.36	2.9 ± 0.52	2.7	2.3 ± 0.45	2.9 ± 0.84	2.0 ± 0.61	NS	NS	NS
Total CA	3.3 ± 0.42	3.4 ± 0.61	3.3	2.7 ± 0.47	3.2 ± 0.92	2.4 ± 0.59	NS	NS	NS
% NE	85	85	83	86	90	81			

[a] All values represent mean ± standard error of the mean. BP = blood pressure; CA = catecholamines; E = epinephrine; MABP = mean arterial blood pressure; NE = norepinephrine; NS = not significant.

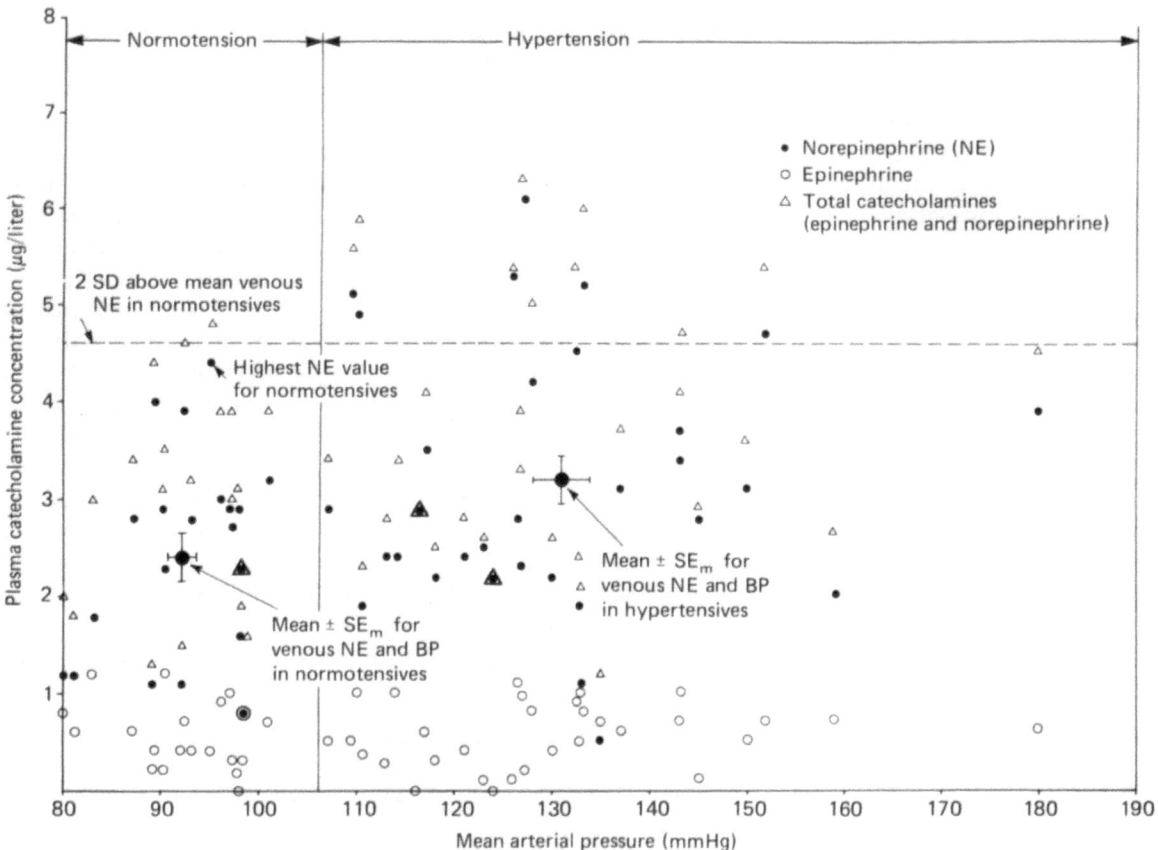

Fig. 6.15 Venous plasma catecholamines and mean arterial blood pressure in healthy normotensive subjects and patients with essential hypertension.

centrations of norepinephrine, epinephrine, and total catecholamines plotted against the mean arterial pressure of 20 subjects with normotension and 31 patients with essential hypertension. The mean $\pm$ SE$_m$ for norepinephrine and that for blood pressure for normotensives and hypertensives are also recorded.

We observed that seven of the hypertensives [four men (two black and two white) and three women (two black and one white)] had venous norepinephrine values which were slightly higher than the highest value (4.4 μg/liter) of the normotensives. All four men and two of these women had norepinephrine values greater than two standard deviations above the mean concentration for norepinephrine in the normotensives. Epinephrine concentrations were similar in both groups (Table 6.17 and Fig. 6.15). In these seven patients, representing about 23 percent of the hypertensives, some of those having the highest mean pressures also had the highest plasma norepinephrine; however,

a correlation between level of norepinephrine and pressure was not apparent. In the remaining 77 percent of patients, there was no appreciable correlation of norepinephrine concentration with the height of the systolic, diastolic, or mean arterial pressure, and absolutely no correlation between the concentration of epinephrine and blood pressure. Actually, some norepinephrine concentrations in this remaining 77 percent were lower than the mean norepinephrine value of the normotensives. As a result, the 28 percent greater mean venous concentration of norepinephrine in the hypertensive group (3.2 $\pm$ 0.24 μg/liter) than in the normotensives (2.4 $\pm$ 0.23 μg/liter) was barely statistically significant ($p < 0.05$) (Table 6.17). The percentage distribution of venous norepinephrine in these 20 normal subjects and 31 patients with essential hypertension is displayed in Figure 6.16. Although there is considerable overlapping of the values of the normotensives and hypertensives, it is evident that a proportion (perhaps one-fourth) of the hyper-

Table 6.18 *Age, Blood Pressure and Venous Plasma Catecholamines in Black and White Patients with Essential Hypertension*[a]

Subjects (n)	Age (years)	BP (mmHg)	E (μg/liter)	NE (μg/liter)
Black ♀ (5)	53 ± 2	$\dfrac{188 \pm 7}{108 \pm 4}$	0.7 ± 0.17	3.5 ± 0.71
White ♀ (8)	49 ± 4	$\dfrac{189 \pm 19}{103 \pm 4}$	0.5 ± 0.13	3.2 ± 0.40
p	NS	NS	NS	NS
Black ♂ (4)	45 ± 2	$\dfrac{171 \pm 11}{116 \pm 9}$	0.5 ± 0.21	4.0 ± 0.86
White ♂ (14)	36 ± 2	$\dfrac{162 \pm 5}{108 \pm 5}$	0.6 ± 0.75	2.8 ± 0.32
p	<0.05	NS	NS	NS

[a] No significant differences in catecholamine concentrations between sexes. BP = blood pressure; E = epinephrine; NE = norepinephrine; NS = not significant.

tensives have values above the highest value of the normotensives.

The correlation coefficients relating venous norepinephrine to mean arterial pressure in the 20 normotensives (0.31) and 31 hypertensives (0.035) were not statistically significant. Even when the values for all 51 subjects were combined, the correlation coefficient (0.27) was of only borderline significance ($p<0.05$). Also, the correlation coefficients relating venous norepinephrine to diastolic pressure for normals (0.17), hypertensives (−0.076), and for the combined subjects (0.20) were not significant.

There was no remarkable difference in arterial catecholamine concentrations between those with normotension and those with essential hypertension. Concentrations of catecholamines in normotensive men and women were not significantly different; this was also the case in the hypertensive patients, although the hypertensives had higher mean norepinephrine values (Table 6.17). The percentage of the total venous catecholamines that was norepinephrine in the normotensives and hypertensives was, respectively, 81 percent and 85 percent (Table 6.17); however, this percentage increased to a mean of approximately 90 percent (range 83 to 98 percent) for the seven hypertensives having norepinephrine values exceeding the highest value for normotensives. Although the concentrations of venous epinephrine and norepinephrine for the nine black hypertensives (0.6 ± 0.13, and 3.7 ± 0.52) were higher than those for the

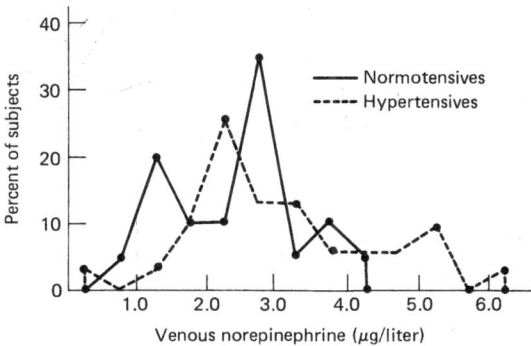

Fig. 6.16 Percentage distribution of venous norepinephrine in 20 normal subjects and 31 patients with essential hypertension.

22 white hypertensives (0.5 ± 0.06, and 2.9 ± 0.25), the differences were not statistically significant. No significant differences in plasma catecholamine concentrations were noted between black and Caucasian males or females (Table 6.18).

As can readily be seen in Figure 6.15, the highest plasma norepinephrine concentration occurred in a patient with essential hypertension, whereas the highest concentrations of epinephrine were not remarkably different between the normotensives and hypertensives. It is, of course, important to select the highest values for plasma norepinephrine (or total plasma catecholamines) obtained in subjects without pheochromocytoma (under relatively basal conditions) for use as a guide for detecting patients harboring this tumor.

We invariably found patients having plasma epinephrine concentrations greater than 1.3 μg/liter and/or norepinephrine concentrations greater than 6.3 μg/liter to be harboring a pheochromocytoma. It is implicit in the preceding statement that the blood samples for assay are collected from these patients under relatively basal circumstances, and that no conditions which may cause significant sympathoadrenal activation are present (Table 6.15). Interference by drugs which contain catecholamines or which spuriously elevate the catecholamine levels because of their fluorescent characteristics must, of course, be excluded.

As will be discussed later in Chapter 7, all of our patients with sustained hypertension due to pheochromocytoma had elevated plasma catecholamines in at least one of several samples assayed; however, as already stated, the concentrations of plasma catecholamines were within normal limits in about 37.5 percent of those patients harboring pheochromocytomas who were relatively normotensive when blood was sampled for assay.

CONDITIONS CAUSING ELEVATION
OF PLASMA CATECHOLAMINES

We and our colleagues have previously reported that the following conditions may result in significant elevations of the plasma catecholamines into the range seen in some patients with pheochromocytoma:

1. Hypotension (moderate or marked; e.g., as caused by hemorrhagic or anaphylactic shock or a large I.V. dose of histamine) (614, 624).
2. Increased intracranial pressure (624, 625).
3. Exercise (624).
4. Electroshock therapy (619, 624).
5. Electric stimulation of the splanchnic nerve (624).
6. Anoxia and asphyxia (624).
7. Acute severance of the spinal cord (624).
8. Pricking the medulla oblongata (624).
9. Some anesthetic agents (e.g., ether and chloroform) (624).
10. Palpation and manipulation of the adrenal gland during surgical exploration (624).
11. Possibly lymphoma (624).
12. Administration of certain drugs (e.g., mescaline) and drugs containing catecholamines (619, 624).
13. Hypoglycemia (132).
14. Acidosis (133, 607, 696, 697).

We have also demonstrated that renal insufficiency (616, 624), hemolysis or hyperbilirubinemia, or administration of some drugs [e.g., tetracycline, chlorpromazine (624), methyldopa (354), or L-dopa (620)] will cause spurious elevations of the plasma catecholamines. Some drugs (e.g., acetylcholine, tyramine) release catecholamines from the adrenal gland when they are perfused through the isolated gland (697); Woods and associates found that certain drugs (nicotine, potassium chloride, lactic acid, sodium carbonate, ammonium chloride, procaine, decaborane, or barium chloride injected intra-aortically greatly increase the concentration of circulating catecholamines (624, p. 184). Relatively large amounts of histamine or glucagon given intravenously may very significantly increase the concentration of circulating catecholamines, whereas small doses (as used in the provocative test) will never increase the plasma catecholamines to levels seen in patients harboring an actively secreting pheochromocytoma. From studies on shock induced by hemorrhage, anaphylaxis, or the administration of a large dose of histamine I.V., it seems reasonable to conclude that any drug which causes pronounced hypotension may result in a reflex secretion of catecholamines with an increase in plasma catecholamines, unless, of course, the hypotension is brought about by blocking the action of the sympathoadrenal system (624).

There are undoubtedly many untested drugs which may cause a liberation of catecholamines on administration in small and/or large dosage. Occasionally some drugs (e.g., clonidine) may even cause an increased release of catecholamines upon withdrawal. There are, of course, a number of drugs which may interfere with the biochemical assays in such a way as to cause spurious results. These possibilities must alway be considered if erroneous interpretations resulting in diagnostic errors are to be avoided. Table 6.19 reveals mean values and the upper limits obtained with three different biochemical assays for determining concentrations of plasma catecholamines in normal subjects and in patients with essential hypertension. The drugs which may alter the plasma catecholamine concentrations or interfere with the assays are listed. Dietary restrictions do not appear to be necessary; we are unaware of any foods which remarkably alter the results obtained by any of the assays used for determining plasma catecholamines. Furthermore, we found that rapid ingestion of four bananas [previously reported to increase catecholamine conjugates in the urine (192, 194)] caused no significant change in the concentration of catecholamines in plasma obtained at 20-min intervals for 1 hr after ingestion (T. W. Rock and W. M. Manger, unpublished data).

Several pertinent facts regarding some of the conditions listed above are worth mentioning.

We previously reported one patient with persistent hypertension who, for many years, had been using Asthma-Nefrin (a solution of epinephrine hydrochloride) in a nebulizer for treatment of recurrent attacks of asthma. There was also mild azotemia. Despite the fact that Asthma-Nefrin had not been used for a period of about 40 hr, the concentration of epinephrine-like substance was 5.1 μg/liter of plasma, and the phentolamine test gave equivocal results. The patient subsequently used nebulized Asthma-Nefrin during an acute attack of asthma, and approximately 41 hr later the concentration of epinephrine-like substance averaged 12.2 μg/liter of plasma, and the phentolamine test again gave equivocal results. Because a diagnosis of pheochromocytoma could not be excluded, an exploratory laparotomy was performed but no tumor was found. Following operation, the concentration of epinephrine-like substance was 2.6 and 1.9 μg/liter of plasma, 5 and 7

Table 6.19 *Comparison of Methods Used to Assay Venous Plasma Catecholamines*[a]

	Methods					
	Fluorometric EDA[b]		Fluorometric THI[c]		Double isotope[d]	
Patients	E μg/liter	NE μg/liter	E μg/liter	NE μg/liter	E μg/liter	NE μg/liter
Normotensives						
Ref. 17			0.48	0.97		
Ref. 162			0.06	0.3		
Ref. 1072	0.7 (1.3)	2.7 (3.8)	0.2 (0.7)	2.2 (3.2)		
Fig. 6.15 and Table 6.17	0.6 (1.3)	2.4 (4.4)				
Essential hypertensives						
Ref. 584; 585					0.07 (0.12)	0.24 (1.0)
Fig. 6.14 and Table 6.17	0.6 (1.3)	3.2 (6.3)	CA μg/liter			
Normotensives						
Ref. 487			0.17 (0.45)[e]			
Mostly essential hypertensives						
Ref. 487			0.21 (1.5)[e]			

[a] All values except those in parentheses are mean concentrations. Values in parentheses are upper limits. E = epinephrine; NE = norepinephrine; CA = total catecholamines.

[b] EDA = Modifications of ethylenediamine fluorometric method (620, 1072). Note: large amounts of dopac, catechol, phenol, pyrogallol, hemolysis, hyperbilirubinemia, and certain substances which accumulate in the presence of uremia can cause spurious elevations of plasma catecholamine values. Dopamine, if present, will also be detected.

[c] THI = Trihydroxyindole fluorometric method (modified by several investigators). Mean concentrations of epinephrine and norepinephrine in normal subjects found by three different groups of investigators (17, 162, 1072) indicate the variability of results obtained with this method. Total catecholamine concentrations have been reported by others (487). Note: Dopamine causes minimal fluorescence with this method.

[d] Modification of Engelman-Portnoy double isotope method by Louis and coworkers (584, 585). Note: Dopamine (or α-methyldopamine) and L-dopa are minimally detected (272).

[e] Values uncorrected for 65 percent recovery.

Note that food or drugs containing catecholamines or L-dopa can give increased values for plasma catecholamines. Chronic administration of large doses of fenfluramine and certain antihypertensive drugs (see Table 6.14) may significantly decrease plasma catecholamines. Fluorescent substances such as tetracycline, erythromycin, quinine, quinidine, and chlorpromazine can cause spurious elevations of catecholamine values with fluorometric methods but not with the double isotope procedure. Isoproterenol and methyldopa (or its synthetic product α-methyl-norepinephrine) can cause spurious elevations with any of these methods.

days, respectively, after the last use of nebulized epinephrine. Results of phentolamine tests were also normal. It was thought that absorption of epinephrine from the pulmonary parenchyma might have been slow and the excretion impaired (blood urea preoperatively was 70 mg/100 ml) sufficiently to result in these elevated concentrations of pressor amines for a considerable time after inhalation of Asthma-Nefrin (612, 624).

With regard to conditions which may increase plasma catecholamines, it is noteworthy that experimental induction of hypertension by increasing intracranial pressure in the dog causes activation of the sympathoadrenal system and is usually accompanied by a marked rise in the plasma catecholamines and an elevation of blood sugar. These findings have been confirmed by others (789). The mechanism of hypertension and hyperglycemia, and the occasional glycosuria seen in some patients with brain tumor and increased intracranial pressure, are perhaps analogous to our experimental model (624). The findings of Gitlow and associates that some patients with increased intracranial pressure excreted excessive amounts of catecholamine metabolites in the urine (358) is consistent with our results.

Mild exercise may cause minimal or no change in the concentration of plasma catecholamines; for a significant change to occur, the exercise must be moderately severe or strenuous (621, 624, p. 176). In one patient a strenuous 3-mile run caused an increase in plasma epinephrine concentration from 0 to 3.5 μg/liter and an increase in norepinephrine concentration from 2.9 to 8 μg/liter (382a).

With regard to the experimental finding that acidosis causes a marked liberation of catecholamines into the circulation, it is noteworthy that one of our patients with severe diabetic acidosis was found to have an elevated level of norepinephrine (9.3 μg/liter), i.e., in the range of concentrations seen in patients with pheochromocytoma (K. Steel and W. M. Manger—unpublished data); epinephrine was within normal limits (0.9 μg/liter). This patient was a 57-year-old white woman with profound diabetic ketoacidosis (blood glucose = 700 mg/dl; pH = 6.92; CO_2 content = 3.8 mEq/liter; K = 5.4 mEq/liter; BUN = 36 mg/dl; glucose, acetone, and

diacetic acid all 4+ in the urine). The blood pressure was 160/60 mmHg, pulse 70/min, respirations 40/min (Kussmaul in type), and the temperature was 103°F. Following appropriate treatment and recovery of this patient, the concentrations of norepinephrine and epinephrine were found to be respectively 3.0 and 0 μg/liter. It seems quite possible that acidosis may have stimulated the sympathetic nervous system and caused an increased liberation of norepinephrine; yet this latter speculation is not established, since we have had a 25-year-old woman with diabetic ketoacidosis (blood glucose = 350 mg/dl; pH = 7.11; CO_2 content = 4.9 mEq/liter; K = 3.6 mEq/liter; BUN = 11 mg/dl; glucose, acetone, and diacetic acid all 4+ in the urine) whose concentrations of plasma norepinephrine (4.6 μg/liter) and epinephrine (0 μg/liter) were within normal limits.

In 1954 and subsequently we suggested that patients with azotemia may have falsely elevated values for the concentrations of plasma catecholamines (616, 624). The explanation for this finding appeared to result from the retention in patients with azotemia of substances which caused fluorescence when condensed with ethylenediamine. The identity of these interfering substances remains undetermined. Although it seems unlikely that phenol is one of these substances (624), phenolic compounds which occur in large concentration in the plasma of patients with severe renal insufficiency may play a role (1072). Since only the ethylenediamine method is affected by these substances (1072), it is necessary to use the trihydroxyindole or the double-isotope method to measure plasma catecholamines in patients with renal insufficiency.

COMMENT ON
ETHYLENEDIAMINE METHOD

As noted in Table 6.19, dopamine, if present in significant amount, will also cause fluorescence in the ethylenediamine procedure which will result in falsely elevated levels for norepinephrine and epinephrine, especially the latter. Although such interference will, of course, vitiate the accuracy of quantitating epinephrine and norepinephrine, in one sense, the detection of fluorescence due to excessive quantities of circulating dopamine enhances the diagnostic accuracy of the ethylenediamine method in screening patients suspected of harboring a pheochromocytoma. This statement is based on the fact that, rarely, a pheochromotoma, like other neural crest tumors, may secrete dopamine. (We have felt fairly certain that dopamine was not secreted in significant amounts by the pheochromocytomas in almost all the patients we have studied, since identification of the catecholamines, by means of paper chromatography, in the removed tumors has revealed only epinephrine and norepinephrine.) Dopamine causes only minimal fluorescence in the trihydroxyindole method and is not detected by the double-isotope method of Engelman and Portnoy (271).

Fluorescence in the ethylenediamine procedure will also be augmented by large concentrations of dihydroxyphenylacetic acid (dopac, a metabolite of dopamine) in plasma. Consequently, a large increase of dopac in the plasma of patients with pheochromocytoma would also be detected by the ethylenediamine method, but not by the trihydroxyindole or double-isotope assays. Again, such interfering fluorescence, though vitiating the accuracy of quantitating epinephrine and norepinephrine by the ethylenediamine procedure, would further enhance the value of this method in screening patients suspected of having a pheochromocytoma or other neural crest tumor.

Von Euler and associates (283) found both dopamine and dopac in normal urine but only dopac in bovine plasma (291). Weil-Malherbe also found dopac in normal urine (1016). Anton and coworkers did not detect dopac in urine of normal subjects but found significant amounts in urine of several patients with neuroblastoma or malignant pheochromocytoma (16). Although Anton and coworkers detected negligible amounts of dopamine and dihydroxyphenylalanine (dopa) in plasma of normal subjects, they found considerable quantities of both dopamine and dopa in plasma of a patient with malignant pheochromocytoma (16). Dopa is not detected by the ethylenediamine or trihydroxyindole method except when present in huge concentration, as occurs in patients receiving large doses of L-dopa, or conceivably, as might rarely occur, in a patient whose pheochromo-

cytoma is elaborating huge amounts of this catecholamine precursor. Dopa is not detected by the double-isotope method.

From the foregoing it can be concluded that the ethylenediamine method is uniquely qualified as a highly sensitive procedure for screening patients suspected of harboring an actively secreting pheochromocytoma or some other neural crest tumor.

Our colleagues at the Mayo Clinic have also used the ethylenediamine method as modified by Manger (624) and they have determined the concentrations of epinephrine-like substance in a large series of patients with pheochromocytoma (91, 820, 888).

Bollman and coworkers found the mean concentration of epinephrine-like substance in 1127 patients (considered not to have a pheochromocytoma but whose symptoms suggested the possible presence of this tumor) to be 2.4 μg/liter $\pm$ 1.1 (S.D.); 95 percent of the values were less than 4.5 μg/liter. The concentrations in 15 of 18 patients with pheochromocytoma ranged from 6.0 to 86.5 μg/liter, significantly greater than those in the patients without pheochromocytoma. Concentrations were always high, but variable on different days in these 15 patients, whereas patients with paroxysmal hypertension due to pheochromocytoma usually had normal levels of plasma catecholamines when they were normotensive (91).

When Roth and associates quantitated epinephrine-like substance in 490 patients without pheochromocytoma, they found the mean value was 2.5 μg/liter (range 0.75 to 5.5 μg/liter). They found the concentrations in 36 patients with pheochromocytoma were significantly elevated, ranging from 6.9 to 360 μg/liter (820).

Sheps and coworkers reported that of 28 patients with pheochromocytoma, five with sustained hypertension had elevated basal plasma catecholamine levels. Of 23 patients with pheochromocytoma and paroxysmal hypertension, only 12 had elevated plasma catecholamines when the pressure was normotensive. A provocative test with histamine almost invariably caused an increase in plasma catecholamines to an abnormal level. Of 101 patients considered not to have a pheochromocytoma, only two had elevated plasma catecholamines; however, in one of these patients only one sample was slightly elevated whereas five were normal. The other patient had significantly elevated plasma catecholamines on four determinations, slightly elevated urinary catecholamines twice, slightly elevated total metanephrines once out of two determinations, normal VMA concentrations twice, and a negative histamine test. Also, a paraaortic mass was seen on nephrotomography, but since operation was refused, one cannot with certainty exclude the possibility that this mass was in fact a pheochromocytoma (888).

In general, the results of plasma catecholamine determinations performed by our colleagues at the Mayo Clinic are in agreement with our results. Our upper limit of normal for epinephrine-like substance was somewhat lower than that reported by some of our colleagues; however, they did not always find it possible to exclude the use of drugs which might have increased the concentration of plasma catecholamines or might have interfered with their measurement by the fluorometric assay. We have invariably questioned our subjects in detail regarding medications they are taking or have taken recently, and in addition, we have carefully recorded all drugs which are being administered to hospitalized patients. We strongly urge that a most detailed history regarding drugs and conditions known to alter the levels or measurement of plasma catecholamines be included for proper interpretation of the results of any assay.

Our colleagues at the Mayo Clinic reported only the concentrations of epinephrine-like substance in plasma; however, as mentioned previously, we and others have found the determination of both epinephrine and norepinephrine in plasma to be of some help in the localization of pheochromocytomas, since the presence of an increased concentration of epinephrine almost always signifies that the tumor is located in the adrenal gland.

Results Using the Double-Isotope Method of Engelman and Portnoy Although the double-isotope method of measuring plasma catecholamines has been claimed to be specific and highly sensitive (perhaps 20 times more sensitive than the trihydroxyindole fluorescence method), it is technically compli-

cated, difficult, and time-consuming, especially so if both epinephrine and norepinephrine are separated by thin-layer chromatography for quantitation. Some investigators have had problems of poor recoveries and reproducibility. Louis and coworkers reported recoveries for total catecholamines ranging from 14 to 24 percent, and for epinephrine and norepinephrine (when the differential assay is employed) ranging from 5 to 16 percent (584). As discussed below, various investigators have occasionally obtained different results in patients with essential hypertension. Modifications have been introduced in an attempt to improve and simplify the method; however, since the procedure requires special expertise, and currently is being used primarily as a research tool, it is not available or suitable in the routine diagnostic chemistry laboratory.

Even when the double-isotope assay is employed by highly competent investigators, results may sometimes be obtained which suggest significant methodologic problems. For example, one group reported that intravenous infusion of l-norepinephrine (0.07 to 0.15 $\mu g/kg/min$) to patients with quadriplegia resulted in elevations of norepinephrine and epinephrine from mean values of 0.05 and 0.004 $\mu g/liter$ to 3.28 and 0.08 $\mu g/liter$, respectively. The marked elevation in norepinephrine was, of course, anticipated; however, it is conceivable that the unexpected elevation in epinephrine may have resulted from methodologic problems. [We did not encounter a similar problem when the ethylenediamine method was used to quantitate plasma epinephrine and norepinephrine during infusions of epinephrine or norepinephrine in dogs, normotensive subjects, or hypertensive patients (617, 620).]

Using this enzymatic double-isotope assay for plasma catecholamines, Engelman and coworkers found that patients with essential hypertension had mean total plasma catecholamines which were about twice that of normotensives, the difference being highly significant ($p < 0.001$). Seventy-five percent of their hypertensive patients had catecholamine values more than two standard deviations above the mean for the normotensives (273). Eighty percent of the total catecholamines was norepinephrine (similar to that of normotensives), and concentrations of catecholamines were similar in both sexes (273). Plasma catecholamine concentrations in normotensive patients with psychiatric depression were reported to be equal to or greater than those in hypertensives (765).

Using a similar assay, De Quattro and Chan reported that plasma catecholamines were 30 percent higher in supine patients with sustained essential hypertension than in supine normotensive subjects ($p < 0.05$). In their patients with essential hypertension, total catecholamine values exceeded the mean for healthy normotensive subjects by more than two standard deviations in 26 and 33 percent of cases, respectively, for the supine and standing positions; also, total catecholamines were greater in women than in men (224). They also found a slight correlation of diastolic pressure and total catecholamines in hypertensives and normotensives.

Using the same double-isotope assay, Louis and coworkers found a close correlation in essential hypertensive patients between resting diastolic pressure and basal plasma norepinephrine but not epinephrine (585). Geffen and coworkers also reported that in patients with essential hypertension there was a positive correlation between diastolic pressure, plasma dopamine-β-hydroxylase (DBH), and norepinephrine concentrations which they felt suggested increased sympathetic activity rather than decreased norepinephrine inactivation (343).

On the other hand, Christensen and Christensen, using the double-isotope assay, found no significant difference between plasma catecholamine concentrations in normal subjects and in patients with essential or renal hypertension (152).

Other radioenzymatic methods which have been used more recently to quantitate plasma catecholamines in normotensive and in hypertensive patients have given divergent results. De Champlain and coworkers reported that more than 50 percent of patients with essential hypertension had circulating catecholamines greater than the highest value measured in normotensives (214). With their method they measured the total circulating catecholamines, and they were also able to differentiate dopamine from the other plasma catecholamines. It is interesting that dopa-

mine was detected only sporadically and in only a few normotensive and hypertensive subjects. When dopamine was detectable, the values were identical in the supine and erect posture, suggesting that the plasma concentration of this amine is independent of sympathetic nerve activity (214). Contrariwise, Lake and associates found no significant difference between plasma concentration of norepinephrine (and DBH) in age-controlled hypertensive and normotensive subjects (544). The method employed by Lake and coworkers permitted the determination of only norepinephrine.

The double-isotope procedure has been used successfully by several investigators to quantitate total plasma catecholamines in patients with pheochromocytoma (152, 266, 343, 584). Figure 6.17 reveals that in 47 normal subjects the concentrations for total plasma catecholamines, under basal resting conditions, ranged from 0.09 to 0.44 μg/liter (mean $= 0.26 \pm 0.08$); in 22 essential hypertensives, from 0.2 to 0.79 μg/liter (mean $= 0.47 \pm 0.19$); and in 13 patients with pheochromocytoma, from about 0.6 to 20.0 μg/liter (mean $= 6.2 \pm 5.6$). This again establishes the diagnostic value of quantitating total plasma catecholamines in patients with pheochromocytoma; however, Engelman pointed out that the values in three patients with this tumor were only slightly elevated, "indicating significant limitation on the use of isolated plasma catecholamine content for the diagnosis of pheochromocytoma" (266).

The double-isotope assay has been used successfully in the diagnosis of pheochromocytoma by Louis and Doyle (584) and Geffen and coworkers (342). Vena caval catheterization with blood sampling at various levels for catecholamine assay enabled precise localization in patients with pheochromocytoma [e.g., one patient with a pheochromocytoma of the pericardium which drained into the superior vena cava and azygous veins had the highest concentrations of catecholamines (entirely norepinephrine) in the superior vena cava]. In addition, central venous blood sampling permitted exclusion of tumors in some of their patients with borderline elevations of plasma or urine catecholamines (584). The presence of an elevated concentration of plasma epinephrine proved of value in sug-

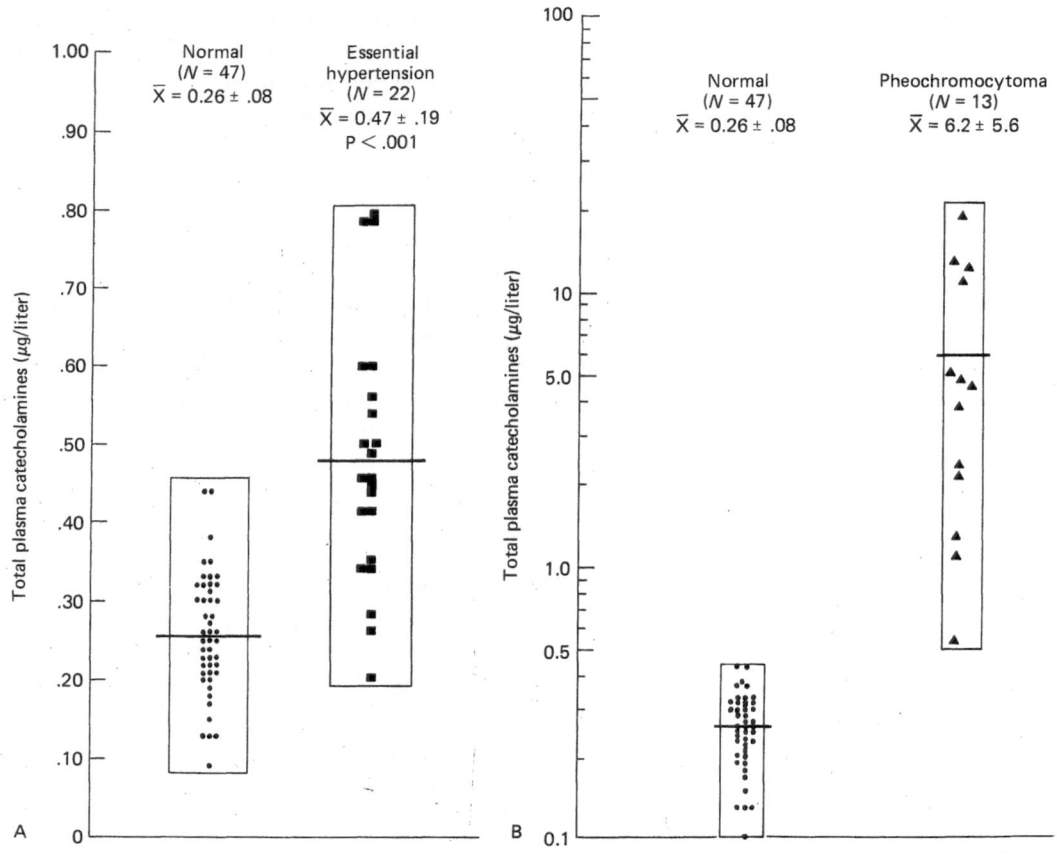

Fig. 6.17 A. Individual values of plasma catecholamine content under resting conditions in 47 normal adults and 22 patients with essential hypertension. The statistical data indicate the mean value ± standard deviation. There was no difference between the concentrations of epinephrine and norepinephrine in males or females in either group and the epinephrine content was consistently in the range of 20 percent of the total. B. Total plasma catecholamine content in 13 patients with pheochromocytoma during basal conditions compared to the values in 47 normal subjects. The statistical data represent the mean ± standard deviation. Note that the values on the ordinate are on a logarithmic scale. From Engelman, K. Assay of plasma catecholamines. In: Laragh, J. H., ed. *Hypertension Manual.* Courtesy of Dun-Donnelley, Yorke Medical Books, 1974, pp. 614, 615.

gesting that the tumor was located in the adrenal medulla (584). This finding was consistent with the observation of Crout and Sjoerdsma that patients who excreted elevated concentrations of epinephrine (with or without increased excretion of norepinephrine) almost always had a pheochromocytoma located in the adrenal gland. On the other hand, in patients excreting only increased concentrations of norepinephrine, about 35 percent of tumors were extraadrenal (193). Louis and Doyle have pointed out that a difficulty of the fluorometric measurement of the catecholamines in the urine lies in the fact that when the concentration of epinephrine is 5 to 10 percent of the total catecholamines,

accurate assay or even detection of epinephrine is impossible. The latter situation could prevail whenever the excretion of norepinephrine is sufficiently high to mask some elevation of epinephrine. With the double-isotope assay they did not encounter this problem of accurately identifying and quantitating norepinephrine and epinephrine (584).

Geffen and coworkers have also used the double-isotope method to quantitate total plasma catecholamines in 11 patients with pheochromocytoma. They also measured DBH in the plasma of eight of these patients (342). All but one of the total catecholamine values in the patients with pheochromocytoma were greater than the highest value in

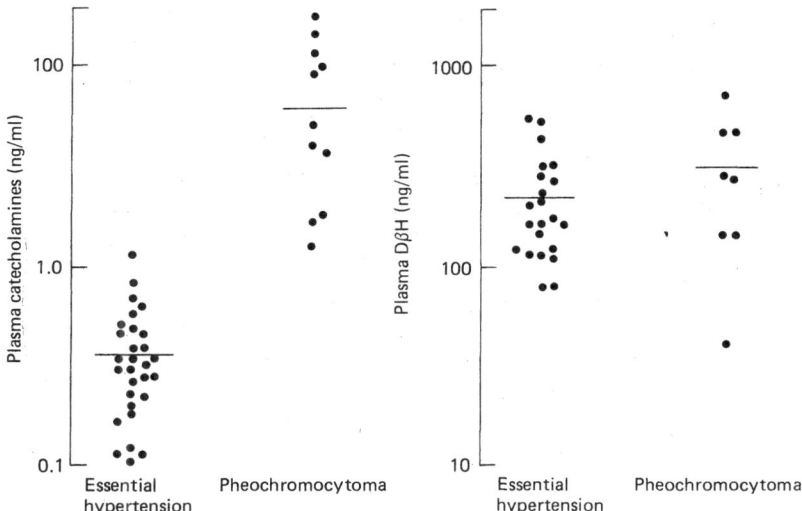

Fig. 6.18 Individual values for circulating plasma catecholamines and dopamine-β-hydroxylase in patients with pheochromocytoma or essential hypertension. From Geffen, L. B., Rush, R. A., Louis, W. J., and Doyle, A. E., *Clin. Sci. 44:* 422, 1973. By permission of Blackwell Scientific Publications.

patients with essential hypertension (Fig. 6.18). The mean concentration of catecholamines in the patients with essential hypertension was 0.34 ± 0.04 ng/ml (equivalent to μg/liter), whereas in patients with pheochromocytoma the mean was 5.75 ± 1.39 ng/ml, the difference being highly significant ($p < 0.001$). The mean concentrations of DBH in the patients with pheochromocytoma and essential hypertension were 329 ± 81 ng/ml and 226 ± 29 ng/ml, respectively, and these differences were not significant.

As pointed out by Geffen and coworkers, these results support the hypothesis proposed by Winkler and Smith (1052) that secretion of catecholamines from a pheochromocytoma does not occur via the process of neurally induced exocytosis, since release of catecholamines was not associated with a concomitant extrusion of DBH into the circulation (342). The findings are therefore in keeping with the concept discussed in Chapter 2 that there is excessive catecholamine synthesis in pheochromocytomas and that these amines bypass the normal storage and secretion mechanism and simply diffuse into the circulation; however, the fact that DBH decreased slightly in three patients with pheochromocytoma studied postoperatively indicated that a small amount of DBH is released from some of these tumors.

COMMENT ON DOUBLE-ISOTOPE METHOD

Despite the demanding technical aspects of the double-isotope method, it can be of great value in the diagnosis and localization of a pheochromocytoma. It is difficult to judge the limitations of this procedure from the above studies, since the blood pressures in the patients with pheochromocytoma were not reported. The possibility must be considered that the patients with normal plasma catecholamine concentrations reported by Engelman and by Geffen and associates might have had tumors which were not secreting catecholamines when blood was sampled. As mentioned earlier, in our experience (using the ethylenediamine fluorometric method) all patients with sustained hypertension (or during a paroxysm of hypertension) due to pheochromocytoma had diagnostically elevated plasma catecholamines. Again, we should like to stress the importance of performing a provocative test combined with appropriate blood sampling for catecholamine assay in those patients who are suspected of harboring a pheochromocytoma but who are relatively normotensive and have normal plasma catecholamines.

A final point worth noting is a report by Christensen that patients with myxedema may have elevated concentrations of plasma norepinephrine (153a). In previous studies employing the ethylenediamine method we found no remarkable or consistent difference between the concentrations of epinephrine and norepinephrine in normal subjects and those in a few patients with hyperthyroidism or myxedema (624, pp. 108 and 120). Furthermore, we did not detect any changes in plasma catecholamines in dogs administered large doses of thyroxine or triiodothyronine, (624, p. 282) or following hypophysectomy (624, p. 177). On the other hand, Goldfien and coworkers found significantly higher concentrations of epinephrine in hyperthyroid patients than in euthyroid subjects. The mean concentration in their patients with hyperthyroidism was only about twice that in normal subjects, i.e., well below the concentrations of epinephrine found in patients with pheochromocytomas which are actively secreting epinephrine (382a).

Using a modification of the double-isotope assay, Christensen more recently reported that the average plasma norepinephrine concentration was increased approximately threefold in patients with myxedema whereas the concentration was significantly decreased in patients with thyrotoxicosis; plasma epinephrine concentration in both these conditions was similar to that in euthyroid subjects (153a). Therefore, if the double-isotope assay is used, Christensen's finding of an increased level of plasma norepinephrine in patients with myxedema (many of whom are hypertensive) should be kept in mind when evaluating a patient suspected of having a pheochromocytoma.

We are unaware of any patients with myxedema who were erroneously thought to have pheochromocytoma because of abnormal levels of plasma catecholamines. Furthermore, although a slight increase of urinary norepinephrine excretion in patients with myxedema was reported by one group of investigators, no gross abnormalities in the excretion of catecholamines and their metabolites in patients with hypothyroidism or hyperthyroidism was evident (1055a).

Results Using Modifications of the Trihydroxyindole Fluorometric Method for Assay of Plasma Catecholamines Devised in 1949 by Lund and modified in 1950 to permit determination of the concentration of plasma catecholamines, the trihydroxyindole method was the first reasonably accurate fluorometric assay (591). Many modifications have since been made by different groups of investigators (17, 162, 289, 297, 350, 486, 487, 785, 992). In most instances the recovery of epinephrine or norepinephrine or both, added to plasma, varied from 65 to 90 percent, depending on which modification was employed. Considerable technical difficulties (e.g., in the preparation of blanks, in the timing, and in the technical precision mandatory for producing fluorescent products, and in the relative instability of these products) have sometimes resulted in erratic results. Since many of the modifications lacked the sensitivity to measure the small concentrations of catecholamines in plasma, no very precise comparisons of basal plasma catecholamine levels in normal subjects and in patients with essential hypertension were possible. As a result, some have questioned the sensitivity and specificity of the method (188, 982).

Recognition of the importance of stabilizing ascorbic acid [emphasized by von Euler and Lishajko (297)] and of rigidly controlling temperature [advocated by Gerst and coworkers (350)] and attention to critical timing, have considerably improved the trihydroxyindole method, and have minimized some of the previously encountered difficulties. More recently, Renzini and associates have introduced a two-column method for chromatographic purification of plasma samples, and have purportedly increased the specificity and sensitivity of the trihydroxyindole method (785). This method has recently been evaluated by Jiang and coworkers at the Mayo Clinic (486, 487). They measured only total plasma catecholamines. Five out of seven of their patients with pheochromocytoma had diagnostically elevated plasma catecholamines, whereas two had values within normal limits. There was a 15 percent incidence of abnormally elevated values in the hypertensives without pheochromocytoma despite the fact that all hypertensive patients without pheochromocytoma had urinary metanephrines within normal limits. (Unfortunately, they were unable to absolutely exclude the possibility that some patients were using medications that might interfere with the assay.)

Jiang and coworkers stated that "determination of urinary metanephrine is superior to the plasma catecholamine determination as a routine screening test for pheochromocytoma in hypertensive patients" (486). They felt, however, that plasma catecholamine determination was a valuable ancillary test, since the plasma catecholamine was considerably elevated in two patients with pheochromocytoma when their urine metanephrine was within normal limits. Finally, they reported that plasma catecholamine determinations enhanced the usefulness of the provocative test, since the latter strikingly increased plasma catecholamines in one patient without causing a positive pressor response (486).

On the other hand, the trihydroxyindole method has been the method of choice in quantitating urinary catecholamines; it has also been used successfully by a number of investigators in measuring plasma catecholamines, and as an aid not only in diagnosing pheochromocytomas but also in localizing them (2, 76, 162, 193, 239, 294, 298, 299, 316, 424, 590, 593, 603, 642, 741, 905, 992).

COMMENT ON TRIHYDROXYINDOLE METHOD (VALUE OF PLASMA VS. URINE ASSAY)

The small quantities of plasma catecholamines in plasma at basal conditions make it impossible to be certain that the fluorescent substances detected by any fluorometric method are entirely catecholamines. However, there is no question that knowledge of the plasma catecholamine concentration determined by the fluorometric methods can be exceedingly valuable in the diagnosis and localization of pheochromocytoma.

We question the conclusion of Jiang and coworkers in their report on seven patients with pheochromocytoma, studied at the Mayo Clinic, that determination of urine metanephrine is superior to determination of plasma catecholamines for detecting patients who might have a pheochromocytoma (487). Two of their patients with pheochromocytoma had normal concentrations of urinary metanephrine but high concentrations of plasma catecholamines. In one of the patients with pheochromocytoma who had normal plasma catecholamines in the presence of an elevated urine metanephrine, a provocative test with histamine caused a marked increase of the plasma catecholamines into a range diagnostic of pheochromocytoma. As stated

earlier, the accuracy of a plasma assay in the diagnosis of pheochromocytoma appears, then, to depend on whether the tumor is functioning and secreting catecholamines at the time a blood sample is collected. Jiang and coworkers did not mention the blood pressures of their patients with pheochromocytoma. It is conceivable that the tumors of the two patients with normal plasma catecholamines were quiescent when blood was sampled.

Recently, Remine and associates reported that 26 out of 56 patients with pheochromocytoma had elevated basal plasma catecholamine levels; i.e., 47 percent had falsely negative tests (784). Again, there was no mention of blood pressures in this series, and very likely there were many patients whose tumors were not secreting when blood samples were collected. On the other hand, if many of their patients with plasma catecholamines within normal limits had significant hypertension, presumably secondary to a pheochromocytoma which was actively secreting catecholamines into the circulation, then one would have to question the reliability of the method used to measure the plasma catecholamines.

In conclusion, the fact must be accepted that all plasma catecholamine assays have methodologic problems which make it difficult to accurately quantitate plasma catecholamines under relatively basal conditions in normal subjects. However, the fluorometric and radioenzymatic methods which detect both epinephrine and norepinephrine should consistently permit diagnosis of patients who have increased circulating catecholamines due to an actively secreting pheochromocytoma. We are convinced that in patients with sustained hypertension (or during a paroxysm) due to pheochromocytoma, the plasma catecholamines are almost invariably elevated above the highest value occurring in patients with essential hypertension. It is implicit in this latter statement that other conditions which alter plasma catecholamine concentrations or alter their assay be excluded.

Effects of Pharmacologic Tests and Hypertensive Episodes on Blood Pressure and Plasma Catecholamines In 1954 we demonstrated, for the first time, the value of quantitating plasma catecholamines in association with a provocative histamine test (616). As stated earlier, a significant percentage (perhaps 37.5 percent) of patients who have paroxysmal hypertension due to pheochromocytoma but are relatively normotensive when blood is sampled have normal plasma catecholamine concentrations. In such patients it is essential that a sample of blood be obtained at the time of a paroxysmal attack of hypertension, either one occurring spontaneously or one induced by physical maneuvers or provocative tests. In this manner, the diagnosis of pheochromocytoma may be established by a diagnostic elevation of plasma catecholamines, which almost always accompanies a positive provocative test.

It is evident from Table 6.20 that the rapid intravenous administration of 5 mg of phentolamine [followed in one instance by 10 mg of piperoxane (Benodaine)] to three patients with both pheochromocytoma and severe sustained hypertension resulted in a positive pharmacologic test (i.e., a decrease of at least 35/25 mmHg); however, when phentolamine was administered on another date in one of these patients (No. 6), this pharmacologic test was negative. In three patients with

Table 6.20　*Effect of Pharmacologic Tests and Hypertensive Episodes on Catecholamines in Peripheral Venous Plasma of Patients with and without Pheochromocytoma[a,b]*

Patients	Drug used or condition	Concentration (μg/liter of plasma)							
		Before administration of drug				After administration of drug			
		Approximate BP (mmHg)	ELS	E	NE	Approximate BP (mmHg)	ELS	E	NE
With pheochromocytoma									
6,s	Phentolamine then piperoxane I.V.	180/150	7.8	—	—	144/110[c]	7.1	—	—
6,s	Phentolamine I.V.	168/136	11.4	—	—	146/120	9.9	—	—
7,s	Phentolamine I.V.	224/134	10.6	—	—	128/68	12.8	—	—
8,s[d]	Phentolamine I.V.	238/164	4.4	0.9	12.8	158/90[e]	4.2	0.8	12.5
11,s	Histamine I.V.	190/100	4.8	2.8	7.4	240/138	6.6	5.3	4.9
12,s	Histamine I.V.	182/100	2.2	1.2	3.7	264/164	15.8	15.8	0
12,s	Histamine I.V.	194/120	4.5	—	—	228/150	18.1	—	—
13,s	Histamine I.V.	156/106	4.2	—	—	290/190	246.9	—	—
14,s	Histamine I.V.	188/102		—	—	274/180	28.6	20.4	30.1
15,s	Histamine I.V.	170/88	8.5			194/114	8.4	—	—
16,s	Histamine then phentolamine I.V.	148/98	—	—	—	194/124	4.7	—	—
						144/98[f]	6.0[f]	—	—
22,p	Histamine then phentolamine I.V.	134/94	8.1	3.5	16.7	244/164	15.7	4.9	39.5
24,p	Histamine I.V.	128/90	1.9 (2.1)	—	—	250/160	9.5	—	—
27,p	Histamine I.V.	158/100	6.0	—	—	194/114	7.2	—	—
30,p	Spontaneous paroxysm	154/80	—	1.1	3.6	205/68	—	26.7	3.6
32,p	Paroxysm induced by palpation	148/80	—	3.1	8.2	300/160	—	28.5	27.3
33,p	Paroxysm induced by exercise	135/90	—	4.4	11.6	190/120	—	6.5	15.5
34,p	Histamine I.V.	120/65	—	0.6 [0.7 (0.8	4.5 4.6] 3.7)	215/105		1.8 [7.3 (3.8	4.1 7.4] 3.3)
35,p	Paroxysm induced by exercise	110/78	—	6.7	9.0	225/?	—	7.7	10.4

Table 6.20 *Continued*

Patients	Drug used or condition	Before administration of drug				After administration of drug			
		Approximate BP (mmHg)	ELS	E	NE	Approximate BP (mmHg)	ELS	E	NE
38,p	Spontaneous paroxysm	156/80	—	—	—	230/110	6.6	0	24.2
After removal of pheochromocytoma									
8 mo after 10,s	Histamine I.V.	124/90	1.6	—	—	140/94	2.0	—	—
4 mo after 11,s	Histamine I.V.	164/108	3.3	0.5	10.2	180/120	2.6	0.0	9.5
5 mo after 11,s[g]	Histamine I.V.	158/120	6.6	—	—	218/138	7.0	—	—
14 mo after, 16,s	Histamine I.V.	130/90	0.7	—	—	148/110	1.3	—	—
20 mo after, 16,s	Histamine I.V.	140/90	1.9	—	—	146/100	1.8	—	—
Without pheochromocytoma, but with									
Hyperdynamic β-adrenergic state	Glucagon I.V.	132/100	—	0.0	2.2	140/110	—	0.0	2.2
Hyperlabile BP	Glucagon then	120/80	—	[0.4	2.0]	120/85	—	[0.5	2.8]
				(0.4	1.6)			(1.0	2.7)
	histamine I.V.	122/84	—	[0.5	1.7]	165/105	—	[0.0	1.8]
				(0.6	2.2)			(0.1	1.6)
Essential hypertension	Histamine I.V.	178/106	—	0.5	4.2	200/122	—	0.7	4.5
Essential hypertension	Glucagon then	140/110	—	0.7	1.0	160/130	—	0.6	1.0
				(0.4	1.1)			(0.5	1.1)
	histamine I.V.	145/108	—	0.6	1.2	155/120	—	0.8	1.6
17 controls[h]									
Mean	Histamine I.V.	168/102	1.7	—	—	186/113	1.6	—	—
Range		114–204 / 74–120	0.3–3.4	—	—	110–226 / 70–142	0.5–3.3	—	—
3 Controls[i]									
Mean	Phentolamine I.V.	235/155	2.2	—	—	189/139	2.5	—	—
Range		184–298 / 128–180	1.0–3.5	—	—	144–266 / 108–186	1.1–3.5	—	—

Concentration (μg/liter of plasma)

[a] In part from Manger, W. M., Wakim, K. G., and Bollman, J. L. *Chemical Quantitation of Epinephrine and Norepinephrine in Plasma.* Courtesy of C. C. Thomas, 1959, p. 96.

[b] BP = blood pressure; ELS = epinephrine-like substance; E = epinephrine; NE = norepinephrine; s = sustained hypertension; p = paroxysmal hypertension; I.V. = intravenous; ( ) = arterial plasma; [ ] = plasma from inferior vena cava above adrenal drainage.

Dose of drugs used: phentolamine, 5 mg; piperoxane, 20 mg; histamine base, 0.05 mg; glucagon, 1 mg. Note: None of these drugs in the dosage used appears to interfere with the catecholamine assay. However, in very high concentrations phentolamine will produce fluorescence by the ethylenediamine method.

[c] Response of blood pressure to drugs; actually blood pressure was 170/136 mmHg when blood sample was obtained.

[d] Recurrence of tumor.

[e] Response of blood pressure to phentolamine test; actually blood pressure was 182/108 mmHg when blood sample was obtained.

[f] Estimated 30 min after preceding value.

[g] Found to have a recurrent tumor 13½ months after operation.

[h] Group of 13 patients with essential hypertension, 3 hyperreactors, and 1 patient with subsiding toxemia of pregnancy (postpartum).

[i] One patient with essential hypertension, 1 with periarteritis nodosa and 1 with toxemia of pregnancy.

hypertension due to causes other than pheochromocytoma, this pharmacologic test was negative. No remarkable change in the concentration of plasma catecholamines resulted from the administration of phentolamine to patients with or without pheochromocytoma. The finding that phentolamine alone, or phentolamine followed by piperoxane, caused no appreciable change in the concentration of catecholamines in the patients with pheochromocytoma supports the view that neither of these drugs destroys the catecholamines or inhibits their release.

The rapid intravenous administration of 0.05 mg of histamine base to 10 patients with pheochromocytomas, and with blood pressures varying from moderate hypertension to normotension, resulted in moderate to marked pressor responses which were almost invariably positive pharmacologic provocative tests (i.e., an increase of at least 20/15 mmHg above the standard cold pressor test). An increase in epinephrine-like substance occurred in six out of seven patients on whom this measurement was made before and after administration of histamine. The patient who had no change in epinephrine-like substance (patient No. 15) was also the only patient who apparently had a negative histamine provocative test (i.e., a blood pressure response to histamine not significantly greater than the cold pressor response). It is noteworthy that patients with pheochromocytomas who respond positively to a provocative test on one occasion will almost always respond positively if the same test drug is administered subsequently. This was evident in patient No. 12; a provocative test with histamine was performed on two different occasions and each time the test caused an elevation of blood pressure and plasma catecholamines which was diagnostic for the presence of pheochromocytoma.

A particularly instructive observation was the response to histamine in patient No. 34 (described subsequently in detail under "Case Reports" in Chapter 7). Despite a positive provocative blood pressure response to histamine, the total catecholamines were minimally elevated; however, a point of importance is that, following the histamine test, the concentration of venous epinephrine became significantly elevated into the range seen in

patients with functioning pheochromocytoma. This latter observation indicates the value of quantitating both epinephrine and norepinephrine in patients suspected of harboring a pheochromocytoma, particularly when the concentration of total plasma catecholamines is not elevated. In this particular patient it was also helpful to quantitate the catecholamines in arterial blood and especially in blood sampled from the inferior vena cava above the point of venous drainage from the adrenal glands, since considerably greater increments in the concentrations of catecholamines were noted in these sites than in peripheral venous plasma. A pheochromocytoma was removed from this patient's left adrenal gland, an adrenal location having been suggested by the significant elevations of plasma epinephrine.

The value of quantitating both epinephrine and norepinephrine as a guide to tumor location, which has been mentioned earlier, is another compelling reason to determine both of these catecholamines when possible. In our series of patients with pheochromocytoma, a significantly elevated concentration of plasma epinephrine has correctly pointed to a location of the tumor in the adrenal area in all but patient No. 11, who was found to have a pheochromocytoma in the hilus of the liver. This latter tumor is the first pheochromocytoma we are aware of in this area to secrete significant amounts of epinephrine.

Histamine tests combined with plasma catecholamine determinations were performed on three patients following pheochromocytoma removal. In two of these patients no remarkable increase in their normotensive blood pressures occurred, and their plasma catecholamines remained within normal limits; however, the third patient remained hypertensive and had an elevated concentration of plasma norepinephrine when measured 4 months postoperatively. Again, the importance of quantitating both epinephrine and norepinephrine is indicated, since the concentration of epinephrine-like substance was within normal limits at that time and no increase in plasma catecholamines was caused by a provocative histamine test. The blood pressure response to the latter pharmacologic test was also negative. The findings in this third patient are pertinent, since 5 months postoperatively, the concentration of epinephrine-like substance was abnormally elevated. The blood pressure response to histamine was more pronounced than in the month preceding, but the epinephrine-like substance was not significantly increased by the histamine test (Table 6.20). This patient was found to have a recurrent pheochromocytoma 13.5 months postoperatively.

Histamine administered to patients with essential hypertension, hyperlabile blood pressures (hyperreactors), periarteritis nodosa, or toxemia of pregnancy was invariably accompanied by negative provocative tests and insignificant changes in the concentrations of epinephrine-like substance, epinephrine, and norepinephrine.

As mentioned earlier, rapid administration of 1 mg of glucagon intravenously has also been shown to be a useful provocative test in patients suspected of having pheochromocytoma, especially when combined with plasma catecholamine determinations (887, 947). We have found the blood pressure response to glucagon in patients with pheochromocytoma to be almost as reliable as the histamine provocative test. However, we have only recently supplemented the glucagon test with measurement of plasma catecholamines. In patients with essential hypertension, the hyperdynamic-β-adrenergic state, or hyperlabile blood pressure who did not harbor a pheochromocytoma, the pharmacologic provocative test with glucagon was negative. Furthermore, following administration of glucagon, only slight increases in the concentrations of epinephrine and norepinephrine were found in the patient with hyperlabile blood pressure, and these occurred in plasma sampled from an artery and the inferior vena cava (Table 6.20). We have not yet measured plasma catecholamines in a patient with pheochromocytoma before and after the glucagon test.

Also included in Table 6.20 are the pronounced changes in blood pressure and plasma concentrations of epinephrine and norepinephrine in patients with pheochromocytoma during a spontaneous paroxysmal attack or a paroxysm induced by palpation of the tumor or induced by exercise. It is noteworthy that patient No. 30, who had a marked increase in the liberation of epineph-

rine without any change in norepinephrine, had an increase in systolic blood pressure but a reduction in diastolic pressure, which is consistent with hemodynamic changes accompanying an increase in circulating epinephrine.

One of us (W. M. M.) has recently studied two patients with pheochromocytoma who were being treated with dibenzyline (phenoxybenzamine) to control their paroxysmal blood pressure attacks. Cold pressor tests alone were performed, and, although in both patients the blood pressures changed minimally on exposure to cold, the plasma catecholamines became significantly elevated in both. In one patient, a white male 27 years old, blood pressure was 122/90 before and 130/90 mmHg immediately after the cold pressor test, and this stress was accompanied by a rise of epinephrine from 0.9 to 4.2 μg/liter and of norepinephrine from 2.9 to 3.4 μg/liter. The other patient, a white male 22 years old, had a blood pressure of 140/95 before and 140/100 mmHg after the cold pressor test, and this stress was accompanied by a rise in epinephrine from 0.7 to 1.9 μg/liter and in norepinephrine from 3.8 to 7.6 μg/liter. The mechanism for this increase of catecholamines following the cold pressor test in these patients on phenoxybenzamine is unclear, but it suggests the possibility that in these two patients excessive stores in the sympathetic nerve granules may have been reflexly released; furthermore, the uptake mechanisms for released catecholamines might have been significantly blocked by phenoxybenzamine. [Iversen and coworkers have found that phenoxybenzamine and many congeners inhibit the uptake of catecholamines into adrenergic nerve terminals (uptake$_1$) and into extraneuronal tissue (uptake$_2$) (477a).]

It seems probable that in patients receiving equivalent blocking doses of phenoxybenzamine, the cold pressor test, which stimulates the adrenergic system, should induce a relatively greater elevation of plasma catecholamines in patients with pheochromocytoma (i.e., if they have excessive stores of catecholamines in their sympathetic nerves) than in subjects without this tumor. If this finding proves to be consistently true, it is conceivable that the effect of the cold pressor test on plasma catecholamines in patients receiving phenoxybenzamine may prove valuable in detecting patients with pheochromocytoma. Such a test would be particularly desirable since it would not be accompanied by any of the hazards or undesirable side effects of the provocative tests; however, since a positive result appears to depend on the presence of excessive catecholamine stores in the sympathetic nerves, it is probable that some patients with relatively quiescent pheochromocytomas and essentially normal catecholamine stores would not be detected in this way. The possible diagnostic value of utilizing the cold pressor test in some patients with pheochromocytoma who are receiving phenoxybenzamine is purely speculative at the present time, but the hypothesis deserves evaluation.

Thus far we have not found that sedatives, narcotics, or antihypertensive drugs reduce the concentration of plasma catecholamines to normal ranges in patients with pheochromocytoma. Paroxysmal hypertension may occur in a variety of conditions other than pheochromocytoma, which are listed with an asterisk in Table 1.1B. Of paramount importance is the recognition that some of the conditions which produce paroxysmal hypertension (e.g., intracranial lesions with or without increased intracranial pressure, hypoglycemia, autonomic hyperreflexia in a patient with a spinal cord lesion, certain neural crest tumors, lead poisoning, acute intermittent porphyria, acrodynia, carcinoid, clonidine withdrawal, tetanus, the Guillain-Barré syndrome, and factitious administration of some pressor agents) may be accompanied by increased excretion of catecholamines and their metabolites.

Roth and associates at the Mayo Clinic (820) reported the interesting case of a 21-year-old normotensive paraplegic patient who periodically had hypertensive episodes accompanied by severe headaches and excessive sweating in response to a full urinary bladder. A pheochromocytoma of the bladder was suspected. Figure 6.19 reveals that when the

Fig. 6.19 Pressor responses in paraplegic patient with full bladder and empty bladder. From Roth, G. M., Flock, E. V., Kvale, W. F., Waugh, J. M., and Ogg, J., *Circulation 21:* 775, 1960. By permission of the American Heart Association, Inc.

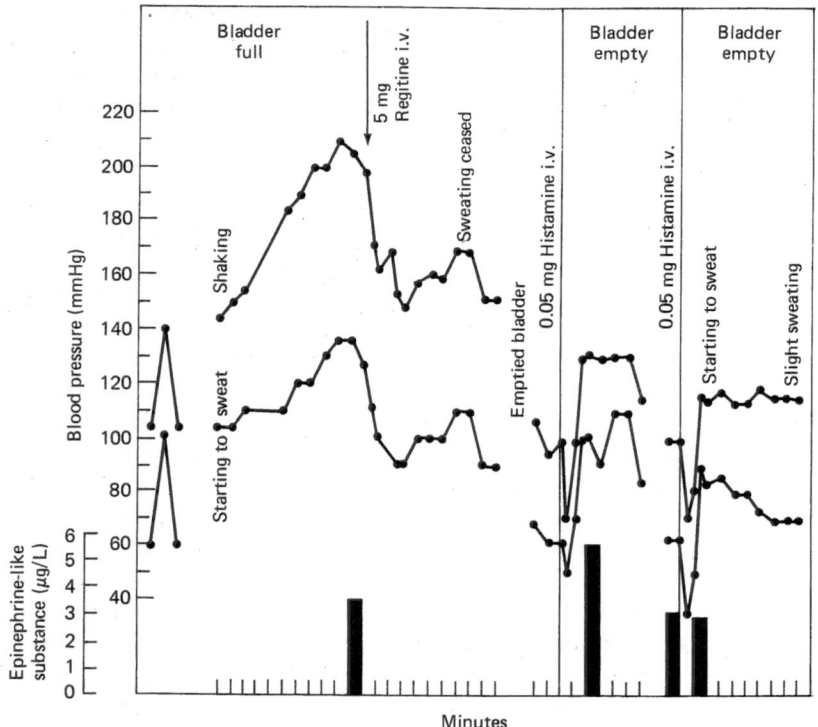

bladder was full the initial blood pressure was normotensive, and a slightly hyperreactive response to the cold pressor test was observed. During the next 40 min the pressure rose to 210/132 mmHg and the patient experienced sweating, shaking, and a severe headache. The concentration of epinephrine-like substance at this time was slightly elevated above normal, and the blood pressure response to the I.V. administration of 5 mg of phentolamine resulted in a positive pharmacologic test compatible with the presence of a functioning pheochromocytoma. Sweating ceased about 10 min later, when the pressure was lower. When the bladder was emptied, the blood pressure returned to normal, and a histamine test resulted in a negative provocative blood pressure response; however, the plasma epinephrine-like substance remained significantly elevated. The following day a repeat histamine test, after the bladder had been emptied, was again negative, and at that time the plasma concentrations of epinephrine-like substance (before and at the peak blood pressure response following histamine administration) were normal. If the bladder was distended with air in increments of 20 to 30 ml, the blood pressure could be elevated to 210/132 mmHg, and was accompanied by sweating and headache. As we have discussed earlier, autonomic hyperreflexia with hypertensive crises, accompanied by sweating and flushing of the face and neck but with pallor and vasoconstriction elsewhere, occurs frequently in quadriplegic patients, especially with a noxious stimulus such as bladder distention. Although a similar massive reflex response is unusual in paraplegics, it is observed in some patients with transverse spinal cord lesions as low as the level of the 10th thoracic dorsal segment.

The differential diagnosis of the conditions causing paroxysms of hypertension has been discussed in some detail in Chapter 5. A detailed history and careful physical examination plus appropriate laboratory studies, including histamine and glucagon' provocative tests combined with quantitation of the plasma catecholamines, will minimize, if not eliminate, errors in the differential diagnosis.

By using the ethylenediamine method as modified by Manger (624), our colleagues at the Mayo Clinic have further confirmed the value of combining a provocative test with the measurement of plasma catecholamines in patients suspected of having a pheochromocytoma (91, 820, 888).

Some patients with pheochromocytoma had a profound increase of epinephrine-like substance (from 86.5 to 360 µg/liter) following a histamine test on 1 day but a smaller increase (from 47 to 58 µg/liter) following a repeat test 2 days later (91). Subsequent experience at the Mayo Clinic confirmed our previous finding (624) that some patients with elevated basal plasma catecholamine concentrations had no further increases after histamine administration (91, 818).

One patient with a pheochromocytoma had frequently experienced attacks with hyperventilation. Histamine and phentolamine tests were repeatedly negative, and determinations of plasma and urinary catecholamines on 5 different days over a period of 21 months were normal. However, several minutes of hyperventilation and mild exercise caused the blood pressure to rise from 150/116 to 194/120 mmHg, and concomitantly the plasma epinephrine-like substance increased from 3.0 to 9.8 µg/liter; 0.5 hr later the urine catecholamines were abnormally increased to 40 µg/dl. Subsequently, a 32 g tumor was removed (91, 820). This patient is of particular interest, since occasionally precipitation of a typical hypertensive attack can be induced by some physical maneuver or manipulation when a provocative test fails to do so. Furthermore, precipitation of an attack by some physical means, combined with determination of plasma and/or urinary catecholamines or their metabolites, may permit a diagnosis to be made without the use of provocative drugs. Palpation and massage in the area where a pheochromocytoma is situated has been used by many as an aid to diagnosis and tumor localization; however, instances have occurred where palpation in one flank precipitated a hypertensive attack when, in fact, the tumor was located on the opposite side. One of our patients (see patient No. 33 under "Case Reports" in Chapter 7) developed a typical hypertensive crisis with elevations of his plasma catecholamines after he simulated shoveling (a maneuver which he claimed frequently resulted in attacks).

Sheps and coworkers reported one patient

with a pheochromocytoma in whom urinary concentrations of catecholamines and their metabolites were repeatedly normal; one of these urines was collected during a period when a histamine test produced a positive pressor response which was accompanied by high plasma catecholamines (888).

Figure 6.20 reveals the experience with the histamine test in patients with pheochromocytoma reported by Sheps and coworkers in 1966 (888). Their patients were divided into positive and negative pressor responses, and these are correlated in the figure with the con-

centrations of plasma epinephrine-like substance before and after histamine administration. A positive histamine response was associated with an increase (often marked) in plasma catecholamines to abnormal levels in all but one instance. Those patients having a negative histamine response had little or no increase in their catecholamine levels, indicating that the pressor response to the histamine test is due to the increase in circulating catecholamines released by these tumors. The catecholamine level prior to the administration of histamine appeared to have no bearing on the degree of pressor response provoked by the histamine test (888). The upper limit of normal, for epinephrine-like substance (5.7 µg/liter) selected by Sheps is considerably higher than our upper limit (3.5 µg/liter). Sheps and associates also found the tyramine test to be a less reliable provocative agent than histamine; furthermore, plasma catecholamines were not increased by the administration of tyramine (886, 888).

Finally, Sheps and coworkers reported that a positive phentolamine test was invariably associated with abnormally elevated basal plasma catecholamines in patients with pheochromocytoma. However, some of their patients with elevated plasma catecholamines had negative phentolamine tests. No direct relationship between the concentration of epinephrine-like substance and the degree of the hypotensive response to phentolamine was noted.

In some patients with pheochromocytoma we have found only slight or no elevation of plasma catecholamines following a positive histamine test, but in these instances the concentrations before the administration of histamine were abnormally elevated. In those patients with normal levels of plasma catecholamines before histamine administration we have found the catecholamines invariably increased if the histamine pressor response was positive. As mentioned earlier, we feel it is important to measure both epinephrine and norepinephrine since only one amine may increase and this increase may be only slightly into an abnormal range. Also, it is likely that the time when blood is sampled following a positive provocative test may not be optimal for detecting the maximal increase in circulating catecholamines in every patient.

Fig. 6.20 Plasma catecholamine (CA) concentrations before and after injection of histamine in 34 tests in 24 patients with pheochromocytoma. The left column illustrates 26 positive responses in 18 patients. In 15 of these tests, the plasma CA increased from a normal value to an abnormal one; in one instance, it remained normal; in 10, the resting value was abnormal and it increased further in the test. The right column illustrates eight tests in six patients in whom no pressor response was observed; very little change in plasma CA was seen. From Sheps, S. G., Tyce, G. M., Flock, E. V., and Maher, F. T., *Circulation 34:* 475, 1966. By permission of the American Heart Association, Inc.

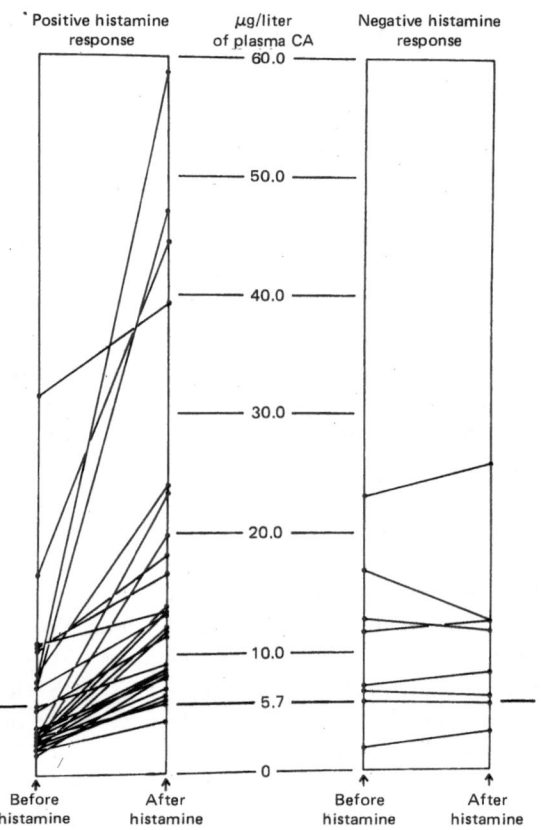

Sequential sampling might possibly detect significant increases in the concentration of plasma catecholamines following a positive provocative test which would otherwise be missed. It is noteworthy that one patient studied by Litchfield and Peart did not appear to have elevated urinary catecholamines following a paroxysmal attack; however, a bioassay technique was used to study this latter patient's urine (579).

In summary, Bollman, Roth, and Sheps and their coworkers [using Manger's modification of the ethylenediamine method (624)] confirmed the remarkable reliability of the determination of plasma catecholamines in detecting patients with pheochromocytoma—with the proviso that provocative tests be performed in conjunction with catecholamine determinations in patients with paroxysmally functioning tumors who have normal basal plasma catecholamine concentrations. This latter view is in complete agreement with our original observations in 1954 (616) and also our subsequent experience (623, 624).

PREOPERATIVE LOCALIZATION OF PHEOCHROMOCYTOMA

RADIOGRAPHIC TECHNIQUES

Since about 93 percent of pheochromocytomas occur in the abdomen, it is especially important for the radiologist to establish a protocol which will permit the most accurate and safe preoperative localization of these tumors. In adults, almost 90 percent of these tumors occur in the adrenal glands and, of these, roughly 7 percent are bilateral. Ten percent are extraadrenal. It must be constantly recalled that in children only about 78 percent of patients have intraadrenal pheochromocytomas, and of these, *roughly 24 percent are bilateral; 30 percent have extraadrenal tumors* (8 percent of these also have intraadrenal tumors).

Intravenous Pyelography and Survey Films
Survey films of the abdomen may occasionally localize a pheochromocytoma, especially if it is relatively large and not obscured by an adjacent organ. Our experience at the Mayo

Clinic has indicated that when scout films are combined with the intravenous pyelogram (IVP), evidence of an abdominal pheochromocytoma can be detected in about 23 percent of cases. This is true for tumors that produce paroxysmal as well as for those that produce sustained hypertension (352). The IVP provides additional valuable information in establishing the presence of both kidneys and evidence of their functional integrity.

Nephrotomography Nephrotomograms can increase the contrast between normal renal parenchyma and an adjacent mass, thereby sometimes better defining a lesion. This technique is similar to the IVP except that the dose of contrast material is doubled and a series of tomograms is obtained in rapid sequence. Urography and tomography (laminography) should be combined routinely, since together they may be very helpful in identifying and outlining a lesion in the vicinity of the kidney. In some instances, nephrotomograms may suggest the presence of a cyst rather than a solid tumor. The cystic nature of the lesion may further be supported by typical echographic findings; however, since pheochromocytomas may be solid or cystic, this differential point is of no great value.

Zelch and associates found that intravenous urography and adrenal laminography gave a clue suggesting the location of pheochromocytomas in less than one-third of their patients (1070). In their series of 37 tumors, only 10 (27 percent) were discovered by intravenous urography and an additional two by adrenal laminography (32 percent when the diagnostic accuracy of both techniques was combined). The usual urographic abnormality consists in displacement of the upper pole of the kidney; laminography may aid in defining a mass. Many tumors which were located anterior or posterior to the kidney, or those retrocaval in location, or those overlying the liver were rarely seen by laminography; however, the suprarenal mass was best seen with laminography. Being mainly a screening test, urography does not define the extent and precise location of a tumor (1070).

Experience at the Mayo Clinic has indicated that nephrotomography has accurately localized pheochromocytoma in 67.4 percent of their patients; however, 90 percent of the tumors were intraadrenal; no pheochromocytoma less than 2.5 cm in diameter was demonstrated in their series (784). Infusion and bolus nephrotomography have proved exceptionally accurate in identifying tumors of the adrenal gland (753).

According to Greer and associates, the average weight of pheochromocytomas causing pyelographic abnormalities (71 percent of cases) as compared with those causing no pyelographic changes was, respectively, 186 g (range: 25 to 615 g) and 48 g (range: 8 to 150 g) (400).

Computerized Axial Tomography Very recently, an additional tomographic technique has been introduced which may be of value in locating pheochromocytomas. This new procedure, also known as CT or CAT (computerized axial tomography) scan, which was originally designed to study the brain, has now been adapted for body scanning as well. Initial experience has demonstrated its usefulness in delineating retroperitoneal tumors, including pheochromocytomas (Fig. 6.21). It is premature to predict its ultimate role in localizing pheochromocytomas, especially in ectopic locations, but preliminary results are promising (personal communication from Dr. R. J. Alfidi, Radiologist at the Cleveland Clinic).

Retroperitoneal Pneumography Perirenal insufflation was introduced by Mencher in 1937 as a radiologic technique for identifying lesions in the region of the kidney and the adrenal gland (655). Subsequently, this technique of retroperitoneal pneumography was frequently employed to localize pheochromocytomas. Meyers described an "apical sign" which may sometimes be seen with retroperitoneal pneumography (or in the capillary phase of angiography of the adrenal gland) (659). Clear visualization of a normal adrenal apex (entirely cortex) in the presence of tumefaction in the remaining gland (mostly medulla) was said to be pathognomonic of an adrenal pheochromocytoma. On the other hand, an egg- or wedge-shaped outline ("wedge sign") was claimed to be pathognomonic of cortical adenoma (659). Significant morbidity and even occasional mortality associated with pneumography have virtually

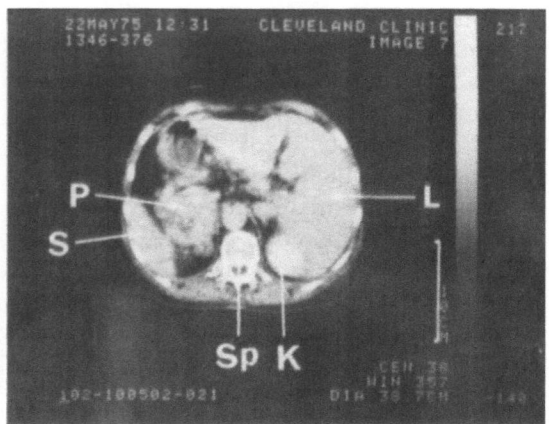

Fig. 6.21 Computerized axial tomographic scan demonstrating a pheochromocytoma (P) in left adrenal gland, medial to spleen (S). Also shown are the spine (Sp), liver (L), and upper pole of right kidney (K). Courtesy of Dr. R. J. Alfidi, Cleveland Clinic Foundation.

condemned its use, and the procedure is only rarely employed today to localize a pheochromocytoma.

Hermann and Mornex have found pneumography very valuable in localizing tumors (437). Apparently they have not experienced the serious reactions reported by others. Examples of the radiologic information that pneumography can give is illustrated in Figures 6.22 and 6.23. Occasionally this technique may demonstrate lesions less than 2 cm in size (493). Retroperitoneal insufflation, however, may be misleading in the case of extraadrenal tumors (817). Despite the excellent experience with this procedure in the hands of Meyers (659) and of Hermann and Mornex (437), we strongly urge that it should not be used in patients with pheochromocytoma, since angiography (arteriography and venography) is not only more accurate in localizing a pheochromocytoma but is also less hazardous. With the availability of other modalities, insufflation is rarely used to localize a pheochromocytoma or other abdominal lesions. In the patient who is sensitive to iodinated contrast media, insufflation may be of some value in detecting retroperitoneal tumors.

Angiography (Arteriography and Venography) Anyone involved with arteriography and venography of the adrenal gland must

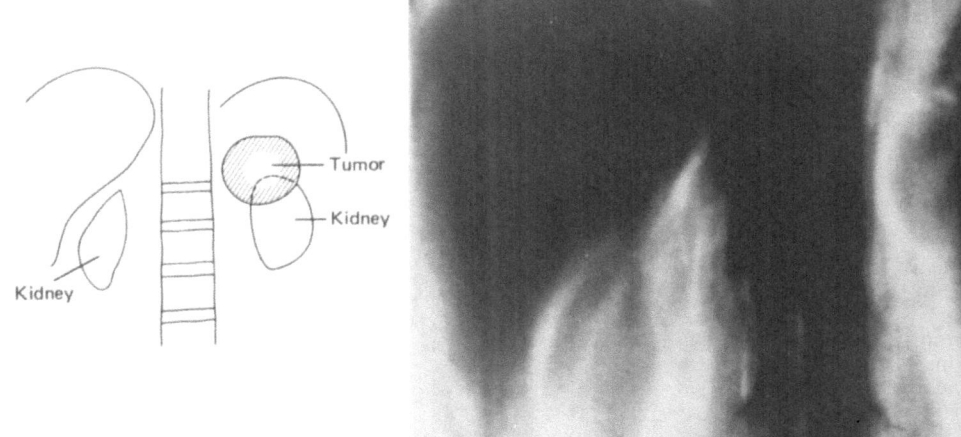

Fig. 6.22 Frontal tomography after pneumoretroperitoneum. From Hermann, H. and Mornex, R. *Human Tumors Secreting Catecholamines.* Courtesy of Pergamon Press. Oxford, England, 1964, p. 138.

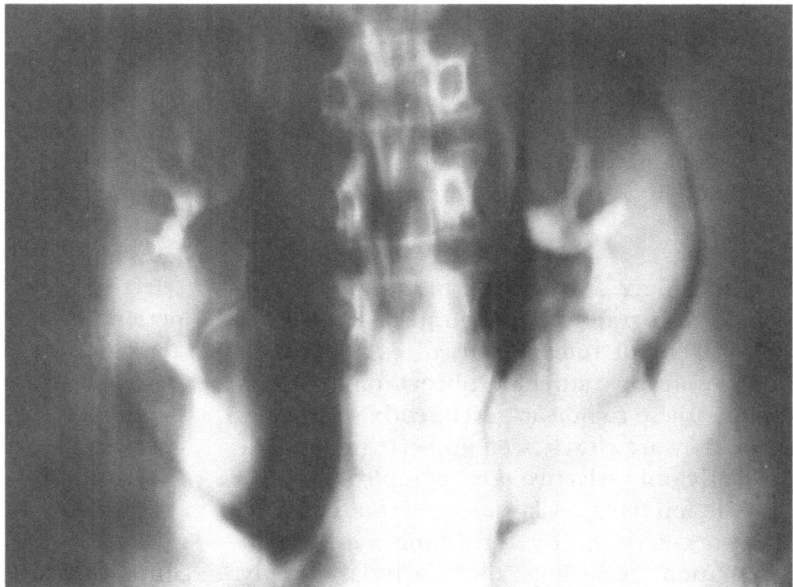

Fig. 6.23 Retroperitoneal air insufflation and nephrotomogram. This 46-year-old woman with hypertension had an intravenous urogram which revealed no abnormalities except for a minimal change in the axis of the right kidney and a duplicated collecting system on the left. Air introduced into the retrorectal space dispersed up the right flank and surrounded the right kidney and adrenal. A mass 8 cm in diameter is evident in the right adrenal area and is well outlined by the radiolucent air. It proved to be a pheochromocytoma. From Bosniak, M. A., Siegelman, S. S., and Evans, J. A. *The Adrenal, Retroperitoneum and Lower Urinary Tract (An Atlas of Tumor Radiology).* Courtesy of Year Book Medical Publishers, Chicago, 1976, Figure 28.

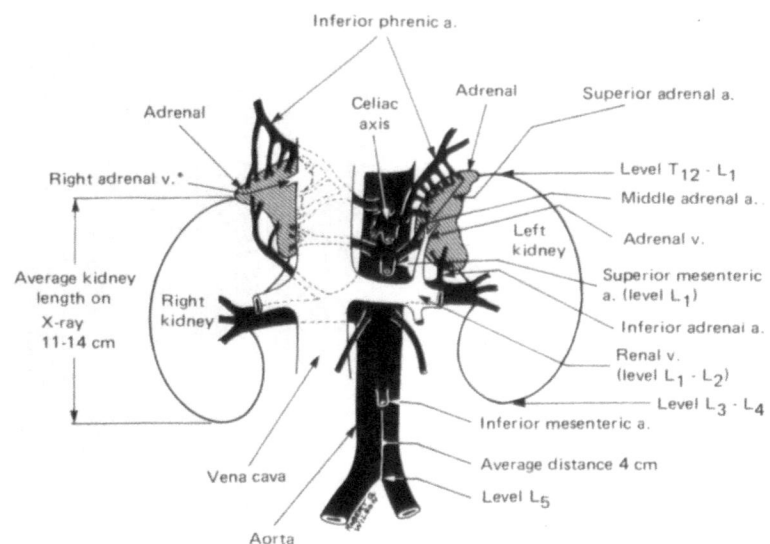

Fig. 6.24 Vasculature of the adrenal glands and important anatomic landmarks. This figure, created by W. M. Manger, is a composite of the anatomy and anatomic landmarks obtained from various sources, but in particular from Hollinshead, W. H., *Surg. Clin. North Am. 32:* 1136, 1952.

*May rarely drain into angle of inferior vena cava and renal v. or directly into renal v.

NOTE (according to Merklin, R.J. and Michels, N.A., J. Internat. Coll. Surgeons 29:41-76, 1958:

Superior adrenal a. usually derives from inferior phrenic a. (rarely from aorta)
Middle adrenal a. derives from aorta or inferior phrenic a. (rarely from renal or celiac a.)
Inferior adrenal a. derives from renal or aorta (2 to 3 times more often from renal a.)

have an understanding of its vasculature. This is equally true for those employing central venous blood sampling for catecholamine assay as a means of diagnosing and localizing a pheochromocytoma. Figure 6.24 reveals the arteries and veins of the adrenal glands in addition to their origins and pertinent landmarks.

AORTOGRAPHY AND SELECTIVE ARTERIOGRAPHY
Since aortography can accurately detect 80 to 85 percent of tumors, it is of extreme value in localizing adrenal pheochromocytomas. While these tumors are frequently so vascular that they are clearly seen on aortograms, occasionally only selective arteriography will show the lesion (493). Classically, a fine vascular network is seen. By furnishing valuable information regarding their arterial supply, arteriography can contribute to the efficient and safe extirpation of these tumors. Selective arteriography of the feeding vessels to these tumors (e.g., renal, celiac, superior and inferior mesenteric, inferior phrenic, middle adrenal, and pelvic arteries) can be of great value in localization. Thoracic aortography is only rarely performed to locate a possible pheochromocytoma in the chest, since tumors are rare in this location and since routine

chest x-rays with oblique views practically exclude a mediastinal lesion.

Since the early use of aortography for demonstrating adrenal tumors in 1934 (827), the procedure has become increasingly more popular and accurate as a diagnostic tool in detecting pheochromocytomas. Boijsen and colleagues reported localization of pheochromocytoma in five patients by aortography or selective nephroangiography (89). As more experience has been gained, the diagnostic angiographic approach has been modified for greater accuracy and safety. By 1973 angiographic diagnosis of more than 150 pheochromocytomas had been reported in the literature (2).

ADRENAL VENOGRAPHY
Since a small number of chromaffin tumors may be relatively avascular (336), adrenal venography may sometimes be of great value in localizing and establishing the presence of an adrenal pheochromocytoma. In one of our patients, selective arteriography only suggested the presence of a tumor, whereas an adrenal phlebogram delineated the lesion clearly (Fig. 6.27). Adrenal phlebography may be superior to arteriography in detecting small tumors (698) and those which are hypo-

vascular ("arteriographically avascular"). Displacement of vessels is characteristically evident. Significant necrosis may occasionally occur and account for the hypovascularity of some pheochromocytomas (38).

In 1968 Rossi and associates reviewed the techniques, usefulness, and hazards of arteriography in localizing and diagnosing pheochromocytoma (817). They concluded that the main usefulness of arteriography is in the localization of the tumor, since the diagnosis can be made without radiologic demonstration. They emphasized that preoperative location may be important in a poor-risk patient; however, more important is the demonstration of extraadrenal pheochromocytomas. In addition, they felt that arteriography was more informative than determination of catecholamines in blood samples from the vena cava. They suggested that the inability to detect some tumors reported in the literature could be attributed to one or more of the following: (1) An amount of contrast medium insufficient to visualize small arteries; (2) placement of the catheter tip below the renal arteries (with inadequate filling of the vessels above); and (3) omission of selective catheterization.

In a very thorough study by Agee and associates, 10 hypertensive patients (three of whom had Sipple's syndrome) were investigated for the presence of pheochromocytoma by a combination of arteriography, venography, and plasma catecholamine analysis of samples of central venous blood recovered from various sites. The success of their approach merits a detailed review of their protocol and methodology, which consisted of the following:

1. *Aortography and selective angiography*

In 10 patients, 40 to 50 ml of 76 percent contrast medium was injected into the aorta with the catheter tip at the level of T12; in three of them a supplemental injection was made, near the bifurcation of the aorta, to establish the presence of a tumor in the lower abdomen. In addition, selective angiography of the adrenal, renal, celiac, inferior phrenic, or lumbar arteries was performed on seven of the 10. Finally, an intraarterial injection of 6 to 8 μg of epinephrine was administered into the renal arteries of three

patients immediately before arteriograms were performed. Epinephrine has been reported to constrict most visceral arteries markedly without appreciably affecting the adrenal arteries. Consequently, since epinephrine can cause a shift of blood and contrast material to the adrenal arterial supply, sometimes injection of this catecholamine can materially improve selective adrenal arteriography and tumor visualization (493, 499). Thus far, no untoward reactions have been reported following the injection of these quantities of epinephrine.

2. *Adrenal phlebography*

In three patients, 4 to 8 ml of 60 percent contrast medium was injected into the adrenal veins and serial radiography performed.

3. *Venous Catheterization*

Blood was obtained (via venous catheterization) from various levels of the inferior vena cava in seven patients, from the renal veins in six, and from the left adrenal veins in two.

Of the 10 patients studied by Agee and colleagues, two had bilateral tumors in the adrenal areas and one had bilateral tumors medial to the inferior renal hila. Except for one patient who had a tumor to the left of the aortic bifurcation, all tumors occurred in the adrenal areas. The locations of the pheochromocytomas and the results of combining radiographic techniques and chemical assay to localize these tumors preoperatively are depicted in Figure 6.25 and Table 6.21.

Their results can be summarized as follows:

1. Eleven of 13 tumors were definitely demonstrated by aortography. (One tumor was missed and another was uncertain.)
2. Selective arteriography demonstrated five out of six tumors studied. This technique better defined the tumors and their blood supply than did aortography. One tumor, which was missed on aortography, was discovered on celiac arteriography performed after intraarterial injection of 6 μg of epinephrine. (One tumor listed as uncertain by aortography was also considered uncertain by selective arteriography.)
3. Adrenal phlebography easily demonstrated three out of four tumors; however, one, the

Fig. 6.25 Depiction of site and size of pheochromocytoma in all cases. The values of catecholamine determinations obtained at specific sites appear on the individual diagrams. Numerical values are in µg/liter. NE = norepinephrine; E = epinephrine; NE E = a combination of the two. Case 1 (A), precise measurement not available; measurements from both renal veins and superior portion of inferior vena cava significantly lower. Case 7 (G), left adrenal vein assay during hypertensive crisis following adrenal phlebography. Control sample unsuitable for analysis. Other samples obtained before hypertensive crisis, all 6½ months after removal of right adrenal pheochromocytoma.
From Agee, O. F., Kaude, J., and Lepasoon, J., Preoperative localization of pheochromocytoma. *Acta Radiol. (Diagn.) 14:* 548, 549, 1973.

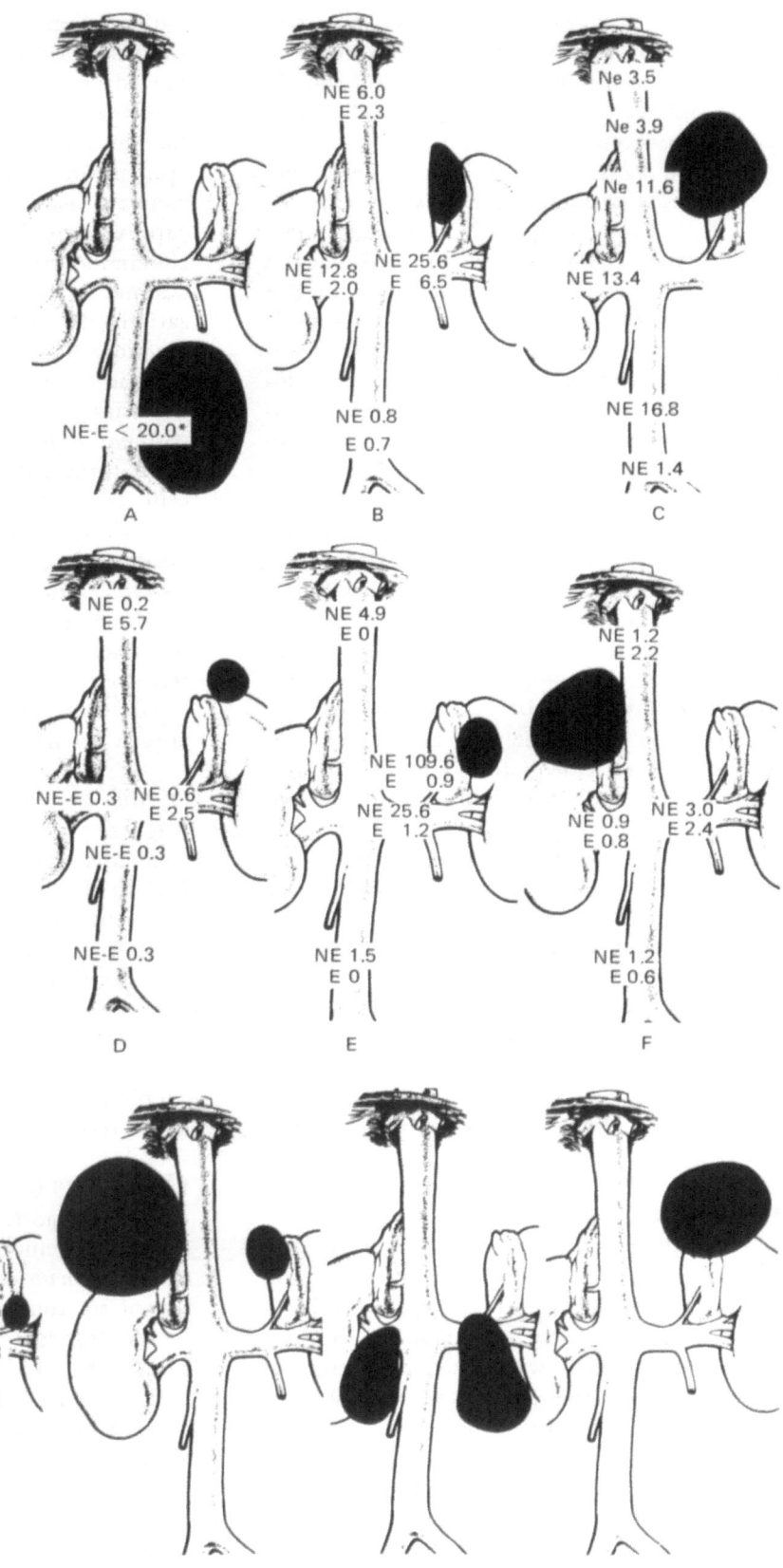

Table 6.21 Results of Biochemical Assays and Radiographic Examination on 10 Patients with 13 Histologically Proved Benign Pheochromocytomas[a,b]

Case	Age, sex, and maximum blood pressure	Highest 24-hr urine excretion of VMA or catecholamines[c]	Peripheral venous catecholamine[c] (μg/liter)	Site and amount highest central venous catecholamine (μg/liter)	Aortographic tumor localization	Selective angiographic tumor localization	Adrenal phlebographic tumor localization	Angiographic tumor size (cm)
1	37 F 200/135	VMA—42 mg		Low inferior caval vein NE-E 20	Left of aortic bifurcation			7 × 10
2	28 F 200/110	VMA—20 mg NME—90 μg NE—5 μg		L renal NE—26	L adrenal			2 × 4
3	54 M 170/120	VMA—40 mg		Low inferior caval vein NE—17	L adrenal	L adrenal		6
4	37 F 250/140	VMA—normal	NE 4 E 2	L renal E—2.5 High inf. caval vein E—5.0	Not found	L adrenal		2
5	44 F 200/120	VMA—18 mg NE—226 μg		L adrenal NE—110	L adrenal	L adrenal	L adrenal	3
6	42 F normal	VMA—17 mg		L renal NE—3	R adrenal	R adrenal		6
7	43 F 250/110	VMA—24 mg		L adrenal[d] NE-E—61	? L adrenal	? L adrenal[e]	? L adrenal	R 10 L 1
8	36 F 150/100	VMA—39 mg	NE 48 E 4	Sample unsuitable for analysis	Bilateral adrenal	Bilateral, medial to inferior renal hila	Bilateral adrenal	R 12 L 3
9	50 M 220/100	VMA—67 mg			Bilateral, medial to inferior renal hila	Bilateral, medial to inferior renal hila		R 6 L 6
10	53 F 200/120	VMA—67 mg			L adrenal			8

[a] From Agee, O. F., Kaude, J., and Lepasoon, J. *Acta Radiol. (Diagn.) (Stockh.) 14: 546, 1973.* VMA = vanillylmandelic acid; E = epinephrine; NE = norepinephrine; NME = normetanephrine.

[b] Catecholamines in cases 1 to 4 were determined by Dr. A. H. Anton, Gainesville, Fla.; catecholamines in cases 5 to 7 determined in Malmo, Sweden; and catecholamines in case 8 determined by Dr. M. S. Christensen, Aarhus, Denmark.

[c] Normal 24-hr excretion: VMA < 6.0 mg; NE < 150 μg; NME < 240 μg. Normal plasma values: E < 0.5 μg/liter and NE < 6.0 μg/liter.

[d] Sampling performed after extirpation of right adrenal tumor.

[e] Right adrenal not examined selectively.

smallest tumor in the series (about 1 cm in diameter), was not definitely identified by phlebography until a correlation was made with the findings on arteriography and the results of catecholamine assay.

4. Catecholamine elevations in plasma from the inferior vena cava, renal, or adrenal veins indicated pheochromocytoma in all seven cases where an assay was performed; however, the site of the tumor predicted from these elevations was correct in only four of the seven. The highest catecholamine concentrations occurred in the adrenal veins draining the tumors. The smallest tumor in the series, which could not be demonstrated with certainty on either arteriography or phlebography, was definitely localized by chemical assay.

5. By the combined use of radiographic techniques and determination of plasma catecholamines in blood sampled from various points in the central venous system, Agee and coworkers preoperatively correctly located all 13 pheochromocytomas in their series on 10 patients (2).

Aortography will almost invariably demonstrate tumors which are large and well-vascularized; however, Lanner and Rosencrantz have pointed out that angiographic studies in some pheochromocytomas which are not richly vascularized may lack pathologic vasculature in the arterial phase; only accumulation of contrast medium in the late capillary and venous phase may be evident (548).

Agee and associates emphasized that adrenal phlebography can provide valuable preoperative information since arteriography usually will not demonstrate the venous system draining the tumor. It must be appreciated, however, that phlebography has its limitations in evaluating adrenal tumors on the right because of variations in the normal anatomy of the veins draining the adrenal. Phlebography is successful in almost 100 percent of attempts on the left, but only in perhaps 70 percent on the right (2).

Agee and coworkers stated that, ideally, venous catheterization, with blood sampling for catecholamines, followed by phlebography, should be performed before arteriography. Catheterization and phlebographic studies may provide information which sug-

gests that arteriographic studies be focused on a particularly suspicious area. By following such a protocol, the arteriographic search for pheochromocytoma may be less extensive, less time-consuming, and less of a risk to the patient (2).

At the Cleveland Clinic, Zelch and co-workers have had extensive radiologic experience in evaluating 34 patients with a total of 37 pheochromocytomas (31 in the adrenal areas and six ectopic) (1070). In addition, two of their patients had medullary thyroid carcinoma and two had ganglioneuroma. They found that utilizing arteriography as a localizing and provocative test will give high diagnostic accuracy.

Zelch and associates have stated that "the angiographic sequence is the key to a safe and accurate study," and they recommend the following investigational procedure:

1. If localization is suggested by initial radiographic studies (survey films, urography, or laminography), selective renal arteriography is first performed on the suspected side.

2. If no localization is suggested by initial studies, then a selective right renal arteriogram is obtained because of the more constant arterial anatomy and the higher incidence of right-sided adrenal pheochromocytoma.

3. In the event that the right renal arteriogram is negative, a left renal arteriogram is next performed.

4. Following the above procedures, a high (with the catheter tip placed above the celiac axis) and then a low (with the catheter tip placed above the inferior mesenteric artery to visualize this vessel and the iliac arteries) aortographic study are carried out. (The aortogram is considered an integral part of all examinations because of its value in visualizing ectopic tumors and adrenal tumors whose blood supply is not from a branch of the renal artery.)

The above sequence is preferred since injection of contrast media into the aorta may initiate a hypertensive crisis before tumor localization. Injection into a renal artery not feeding a tumor will not significantly elevate blood pressure. On the other hand, regardless of the angiographic findings, a hypertensive response to selective angiography is considered a positive sign for pheochromocytoma (1070).

5. When the arteriographic findings are normal or questionable, adrenal venography is then employed. The importance of phlebography is emphasized, since 30 percent of the pheochromocytomas studied by Zelch and his associates were hypovascular and extremely difficult to locate by arteriography. Frequently these hypovascular tumors had only a "faint 'tumor stain' or draped vessels" (1070).

Let us summarize the experience of Zelch and associates, which was reported in 1974:

1. Aortograms were positive or suggestive in about 83 percent of 35 tumors studied. (Twenty out of 22 right adrenal tumors were detected, but because of hypovascularity only four out of seven lesions on the left were detected. Five out of six ectopic pheochromocytomas were also visualized.) That the aortogram was negative in six cases and only suggestive in four others emphasizes the need for selective arteriography and, sometimes, phlebography.

2. Adrenal venograms established the diagnosis in four tumors.

3. Fifty-three percent of patients had blood pressure elevations with intraarterial injection of contrast material, and two patients had elevations during injection into the adrenal vein.

Zelch and coworkers also observed that the degree of vascularity of pheochromocytomas did not appear related to their clinical or pathological presentation. The mechanism whereby contrast material may provoke a release of catecholamines from a pheochromocytoma is uncertain, but it seems likely that, at least in some instances, a mechanical effect may flush amine-rich blood from the tumor into the circulation; however, since hypertensive crises sometimes follow injections of only 0.5 ml of contrast material (646), it is possible that release of catecholamines may be caused by other mechanisms.

Usually, the vascular pattern noted with adrenal arteriography is rather characteristic, an early phase showing hypertrophic adrenal arteries and a network of small arteries with a reticular pattern, and, subsequently, a homogeneous density with discrete margins in the capillary phase. Occasionally, arteriography may demonstrate a "tumor blush" with a central radiolucent area which may represent relative avascularity with or without central necrosis or cyst formation (817). Angiographic findings in pheochromocytoma of the organs of Zuckerkandl have been described previously (609).

Fig. 6.26 Radiographic findings in a 42-year-old woman with classical paroxysmal hypertension. A. IVP reveals right suprarenal mass. B and C. Arteriograms confirm diagnosis and no ectopic tumors are suggested. From Deoreo, G. A., Jr., Stewart, B. H., Tarazi, R. C., and Gifford, R. W., Jr., *J. Urol. 111:* 716, 1974. By permission of Williams & Wilkins Co.

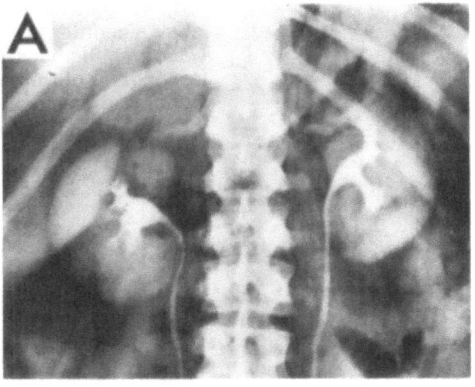

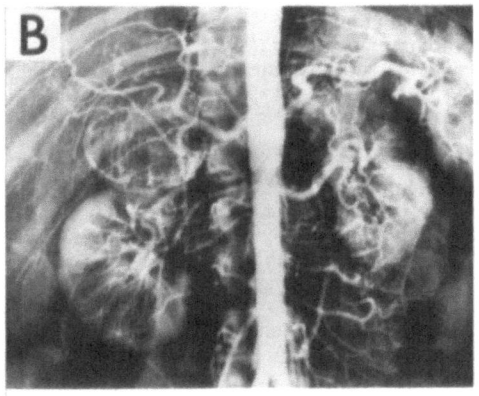

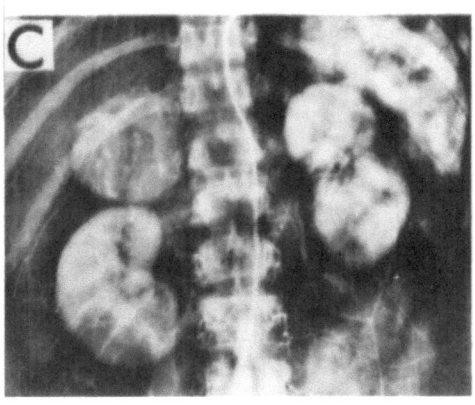

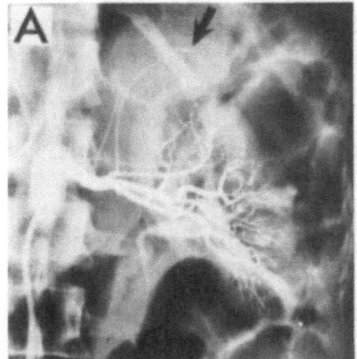 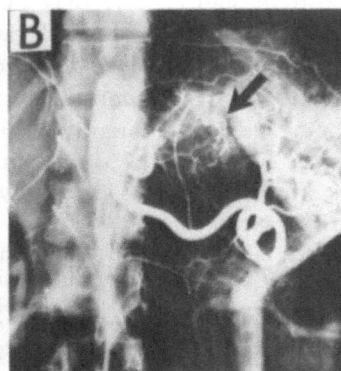 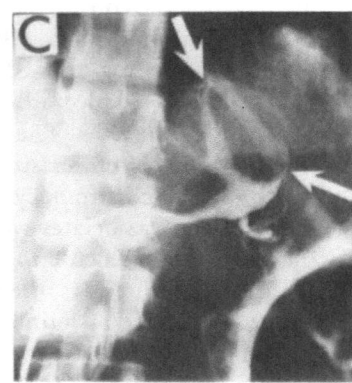

Fig. 6.27 Radiographic findings in a 35-year-old woman with a 5-year history of paroxysmal symptoms and hypertension. IVP was not diagnostic. A. Selective renal arteriogram demonstrates small irregular vessels (arrow) originating from left inferior adrenal artery. B. Selective celiac injection shows additional arterial supply (arrow) going to left adrenal. C. Left adrenal venogram demonstrates 5-cm mass (arrows) within adrenal gland. Compare vascularity of this tumor with the one in Figure 6.26. In this case venogram confirmed diagnosis only suggested on arteriograms. From Deoreo, G. A., Jr., Stewart, B. H., Tarazi, R. C., and Gifford, R. W., Jr., *J. Urol. 111:* 717, 1974. By permission of Williams & Wilkins Co.

Fig. 6.28 Radiographic findings and exposure of a pheochromocytoma in a 16-year-old boy with abdominal pain and hypertension. Palpation of lower abdomen suggested mass and produced flushing and hypertension. Arterial study of inferior mesenteric artery in early (A) and late (B) injection shows tumor blush lateral to aorta (arrows). C. Intraoperative exposure shows tumor of organ of Zuckerkandl being removed. Arteries supplying tumor (inferior mesenteric and left lumbar) have been ligated. From Deoreo, G. A., Jr., Stewart, B. H., Tarazi, R. C., and Gifford, R. W., Jr., *J. Urol. 111:* 718, 1974. By permission of Williams & Wilkins Co.

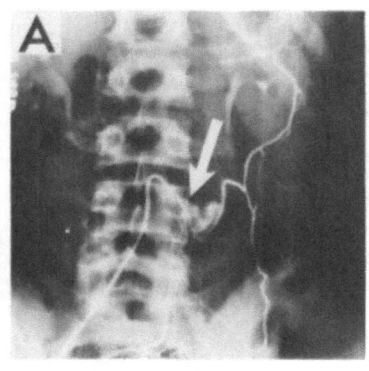 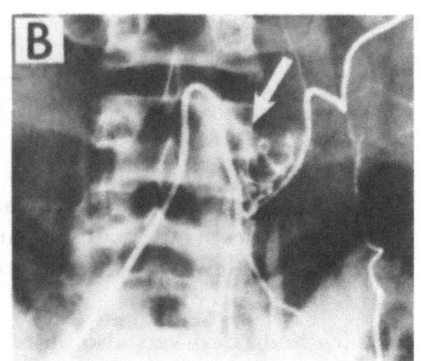

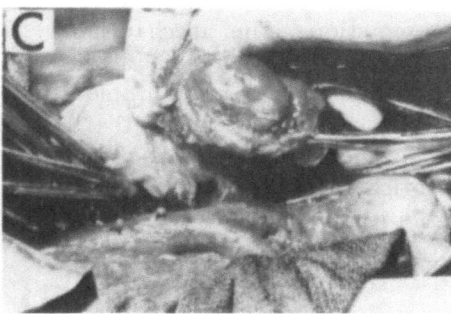

Some of the radiographic experience with arteriography and adrenal phlebography at the Cleveland Clinic is shown in Figures 6.26–6.29.

Extraadrenal pheochromocytomas, which account for about 10 percent of these tumors, present an arteriographic appearance similar to their adrenal counterpart. Frequently, a hypertensive crisis is induced by the injection of contrast medium (512, 646). Displacement of adjacent structures and even erosion of a vertebra may occur; however, differentiation

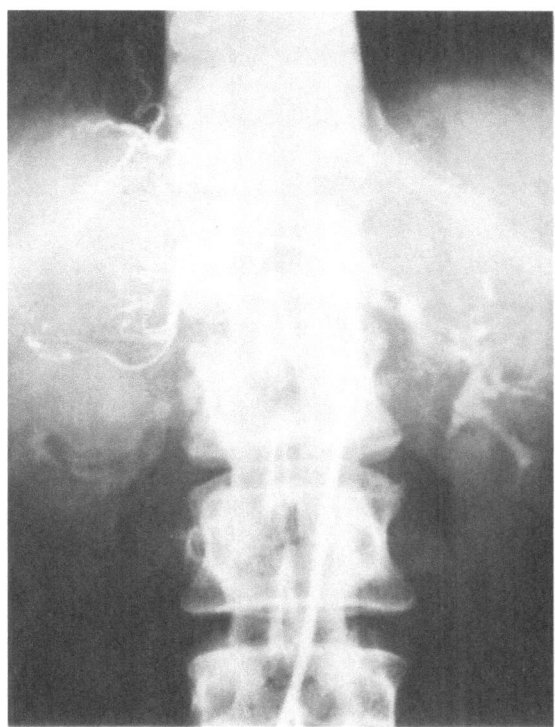 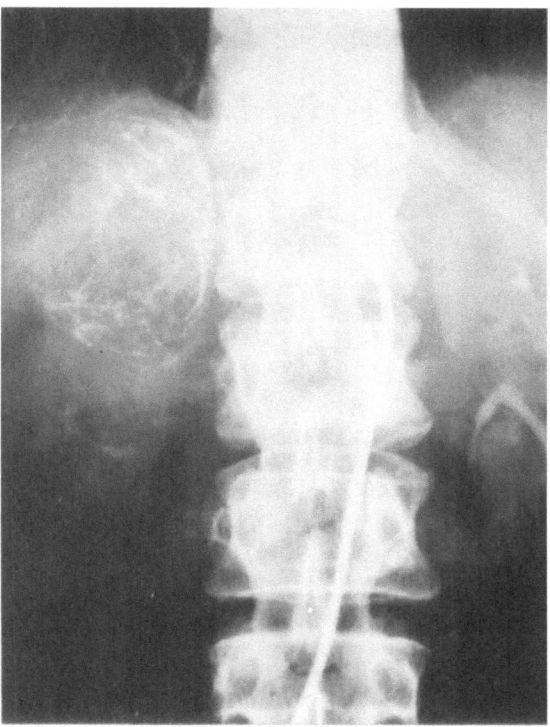

Fig. 6.29 Early (A) and late (B) phase of arteriogram demonstrating a large (40 g) right adrenal pheochromocytoma in a 58-year-old woman whose hypertension was discovered only several weeks before extirpation. She gave an 18-month history of episodes of nausea, dyspnea, weakness, headaches, light headedness, and tingling in the extremities. Urinary VMA and catecholamines were elevated. One month postoperative blood pressure was 170/90 mmHg. Dr. R. W. Gifford, Jr. Cleveland Clinic, unpublished.

between benign and malignant lesions by angiography appears impossible (512, 646).

Recently, Bosniak, Siegelman, and Evans have presented an extensive atlas of the radiographic findings in tumors of the adrenal gland, in the retroperitoneum, and in the lower urinary tract (94). Studies on a large number of pheochromocytomas were reported, including the angiographic findings in a patient with pheochromocytoma of the urinary bladder (Fig. 6.30). This patient was a 27-year-old woman who had developed gross hematuria, which became massive and resulted in circulatory shock requiring multiple blood transfusions. Cystoscopy revealed blood clots in the bladder and a nipple-like protrusion on the lateral wall which was edematous and bleeding. Biopsy of the lesion caused profuse bleeding, which was difficult

to control, and histologic examination indicated that the lesion was a pheochromocytoma. Her blood pressure remained normal and there was no history of hypertension or attacks or symptoms and signs suggestive of excessive catecholamine release. Partial cystectomy was performed and a bright red tumor mass, 1.5 cm in diameter, which proved histologically to be a pheochromocytoma, was found in the submucosa specimen.

The history of this patient is recounted in detail since this is the only patient we know of in whom angiographic study of a pheochromocytoma of the bladder has thus far been reported. It is the opinion of Bosniak and coauthors that the angiographic appearance of these tumors would be similar to the vascular pattern seen in pheochromocytomas elsewhere in the body.

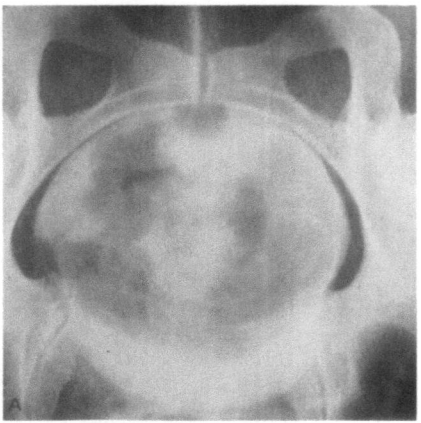

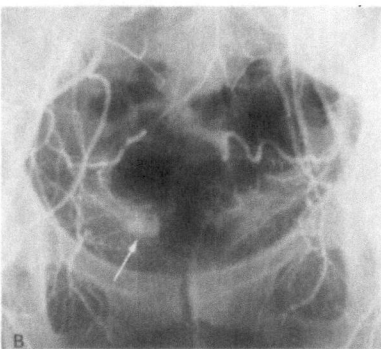 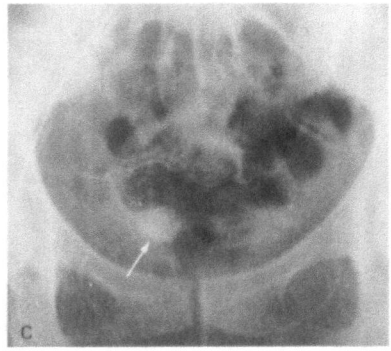

Fig. 6.30 A. Intravenous urogram (closeup of bladder). The bladder is filled with filling defects which represent blood clots. A specific tumor defect that represents the pheochromocytoma is not seen. B. Pelvic angiogram (anterior projection) in arterial phase. A vascular "tumor stain" is seen (arrow) in the right side of the pelvis supplied by vesicle arteries. C. Same study as B in the capillary phase. A "tumor stain" (arrow) is seen in the right side of the pelvis indicating a small vascular tumor in the right side of the bladder. From Bosniak, M. A., Siegelman, S. S., and Evans, J. A. *The Adrenal, Retroperitoneum and Lower Urinary Tract (An Atlas of Tumor Radiology)*. Chicago, Year Book Medical Publishers, 1976, Figure 171.

RISKS OF ANGIOGRAPHY

Rossi and associates employ the retrograde transfemoral technique for arteriographic studies. They point out that hemorrhage, shock, and death occurred in three of 18 patients with pheochromocytoma who were subjected to translumbar aortography. The three fatalities occurred in patients injected with iodopyracet (Diodrast) or acetrizoate (Urokon) sodium. Currently, less toxic media, such as diatrizoate (Hypaque), are used by almost all radiologists. Meaney and Buonocore have used 50 percent Hypaque and have emphasized the importance of controlling the amount of contrast material injected (646).

Rossi and associates routinely use an α-adrenergic blocking agent (phenoxybenzamine) to induce normotension for several days prior to angiography. They prefer not to employ angiography as a provocative test. Furthermore, they have observed wide variations in blood pressure during aortography in both normotensive and essential hypertensive patients (817).

Agee and associates carefully monitored blood pressure, with phentolamine available to counteract hypertensive crises. α-Receptor blockers were administered prophylactically in five patients. A hypertensive crisis occurred in one patient following aortography, in another during catheterization of the middle adrenal artery (without contrast injection), and in still another during adrenal phlebography. The first two patients had not received blocking agents and they responded promptly to phentolamine. The third patient, who had received an α-receptor blocking agent, was receiving an intravenous infusion of phenoxybenzamine when the blood pressure became transiently elevated with an injection of 6 ml of contrast medium into the left adrenal vein. Agee and associates also believe that premedication with α-adrenergic blocking drugs is desirable prior to phlebography or arteriography (2).

It is now well recognized that there is some hazard to any angiogram, and that the risk of inducing a hypertensive crisis in a patient with pheochromocytoma is significant, occurring in perhaps 50 percent of patients undergoing arteriography (1070). A hypertensive crisis may also, rarely, occur during renal venography (372). However, a hypertensive reaction may be viewed as additional evidence for the presence and location of a tumor, and crises can be easily controlled and aborted with phentolamine or sodium nitroprusside. It has been aptly stated that an angiogram provides a "vascular road-map for the surgeon" which is "more than adequate pay for the risk of the study" (499).

Deaths have resulted from angiography in patients with pheochromocytoma (520, 817, 839); however, with proper monitoring of blood pressure hypertensive crises can be readily recognized and controlled without serious risk to the patient. We concur with Zelch and colleagues regarding the value of angiography as a provocative test, and we agree with the concept that the benefits of detecting a small neoplasm or demonstrating multiple or ectopic tumors far outweigh the risk involved (1070). Since they use arteriography as a provocative test, in addition to a radiographic technique, for localizing pheochromocytomas, premedication with α-adrenergic blocking drugs is avoided. Blood pressure is carefully monitored throughout the examination, and, if the systolic pressure increases as much as 40 mmHg or the diastolic pressure as much as 20 mmHg, phentolamine is administered as needed through an indwelling venous catheter. In patients with essential hypertension or hypertension secondary to renal artery disease, contrast injection caused no change in pressure or only a transient rise not exceeding 10 mmHg (646). [However, it should be mentioned that in one patient without a pheochromocytoma, De-

Quattro and associates encountered both a rise in blood pressure and an elevation of plasma catecholamines induced by the injection of contrast medium via an adrenal vein catheter (225).] Test injections with 1 ml of contrast material prior to selective renal angiography and 5 ml prior to aortography are recommended.

VIEWS OF THE AUTHORS REGARDING RISKS OF ANGIOGRAPHY

Controversy exists as to whether all patients suspected of having a pheochromocytoma should be treated with phenoxybenzamine (dibenzyline, an α-adrenergic blocking agent), prior to angiography in order to prevent hypertensive crises which may be precipitated by the injection of contrast media. We believe that any patient who has been precariously ill or has been having a particularly stormy course with severe hypertensive crises, particularly if accompanied by arrhythmias, should be blocked with phenoxybenzamine prior to angiographic studies. Obviously, one must avoid stimulation of a tumor under such circumstances. In most instances we see no great advantage in having a patient *un*-blocked during angiographic studies, since the location of an abdominal tumor will be detected, in the vast majority of patients, by aortography and selective arteriography. Therefore, a hypertensive response during administration of contrast media is very rarely of crucial value in detecting the location of a tumor.

A previous negative surgical exploration of the abdomen and/or negative radiographic studies is an indication for avoiding adrenergic blockade in a patient suspected of harboring a pheochromocytoma. A hypertensive response during selective arteriography can sometimes be an important aid in confirming the diagnosis and in the localization of a pheochromocytoma. A patient with a history suggestive of paroxysmal hypertension due to pheochromocytoma in whom the chemical diagnosis remains equivocal, despite provocative tests, should not be given an α-adrenergic blocking agent prior to arteriography, since the drug can mask an informative hypertensive response. If the radiologist is alert to the potential hazards of arteriography in a patient with pheochromocytoma, and if he is *fully prepared to promptly combat any hypertensive crisis* with the administration of phentolamine or sodium nitroprusside, then there should actually be only minimal—if any—risk involved in the performance of any angiographic procedure. It is always wise to err on the side of caution and have available 5 mg of phentolamine in a syringe (in addition to five extra vials of 5 mg each) and/or a nitroprusside solution (250 ml of 0.9 percent saline or 5 percent dextrose in water containing 250 μg sodium nitroprusside per ml). Five mg of phentolamine or 250 μg (i.e., 0.25 mg) of sodium nitroprusside should be given as a bolus and repeated as necessary. An intravenous drip of nitroprusside can be started to control a prolonged hypertensive crisis. (The bottle containing this solution should be protected from light by some form of covering to prevent decomposition of the nitroprusside.) It is essential to have an indwelling venous catheter already in place and available for the prompt administration of these drugs. In addition, the blood pressure and also the ECG should be monitored by a competent assistant to the radiologist performing arteriographic studies. Lidocaine and propranolol should also be available to combat any persistent arrhythmia that does not respond to lowering of the blood pressure; volume expanders and norepinephrine should be available for infusion in the event that marked or prolonged hypotension should develop. It would be ideal to have a cardiologist in attendance, in the event that a serious cardiac complication were to develop. Our associates in radiology have never encountered any serious complication from a hypertensive reaction during angiography, yet it is wise to always be exceptionally cautious in performing these studies on patients with pheochromocytoma.

Finally, it is worthy of note that angiograms may occasionally be misleading. Gitlow cited four patients with hypertension and angiograms "diagnostic" of pheochromocytoma. Biochemical urine assays were within normal limits in each case; subsequently, tumors could not be found by exploration in two patients and by repeat angiography in the other two (358). Rarely, a pheochromocytoma overlying the kidney may simulate an intrarenal lesion on selective renal arteriog-

raphy; however, lack of distortion of intrarenal vasculature suggests that the location of the neoplasm is exterior to the kidney (894).

Some investigators believe that because of the "brittle" condition of patients with pheochromocytoma no further radiologic work-up is indicated after an excretory urogram has been obtained. Gitlow and associates perform an IVP, in an effort not only to localize the tumor but also to establish, prior to operation, that both kidneys are present and functioning adequately (personal communication from Dr. Stanley E. Gitlow). This point is well taken, since removal of a pheochromocytoma might conceivably require removal of an adjacent kidney. They reserve more extensive radiologic investigations and central venous blood sampling (for catecholamine assay) mainly for patients with recurrent tumors, or for patients with chemical evidence of pheochromocytoma in whom previous laparotomy has failed to reveal the tumor site.

It is our opinion that if a pheochromocytoma cannot be localized by IVP and nephrotomography, arteriography is indicated. If the latter fails to localize the tumor, then, when feasible, adrenal venography and central venous blood sampling are indicated. We feel that establishing the location of the tumor preoperatively will facilitate its quick and safe surgical removal. Preoperative localization should minimize that rare possibility of an unnecessary abdominal exploration when the tumor is, in fact, located in the thorax or neck—an error that could be disastrous; it may also avert an unwarranted adrenalectomy. In the final analysis, the radiologic investigation must also vary, and depends somewhat on the age, history, and clinical status of each patient.

Unusual Radiologic Features Certain unusual radiologic features of pheochromocytoma occurring in the abdomen should be kept in mind. Meyers and King have reemphasized that occasionally a tumor of the organ of Zuckerkandl may present on intravenous pyelography as a mass overlying the psoas muscle, which displaces the ureter laterally (407, 661). They have further noted that x-rays in the left posterior oblique position often best reveal a tumor of the organ of Zuckerkandl (661).

As mentioned earlier, calcification, which may occur in both intra- and extraadrenal pheochromocytomas, may be visualized on x-ray. In 1959 Meyers and King reported two cases of their own and reviewed 22 cases in the literature of patients who had detectable calcification in their tumors. The age of these patients ranged from 23 months to 74 years, one-half being in the fourth and fifth decades. Since the duration of symptoms was often 8 years or longer, it appears that a long course favors hemorrhage and necrosis and eventually secondary deposition of calcium. A curvilinear or egg-shell type of calcification of the tumor is not infrequently noted (94, 673). Usually, flecks and plaques of calcium have been described in pheochromocytoma (120, 661), whereas a "scattered flocculent type of calcification is most characteristic of adrenal carcinoma or neuroblastoma, in which a supra-adrenal mass is almost invariably demonstrable on intravenous urography" (660, 661). The radiologic differential diagnosis should include adrenal carcinoma and cyst, Addison's disease, neuroblastoma, and ganglioneuroma, since these are the commonest causes of calcification in the adrenal area (661). However, only neuroblastoma and ganglioneuroma might conceivably cause clinical and biochemical manifestations resembling somewhat those observed in patients with pheochromocytoma.

Occasionally, a peripheral ring of calcification may outline a moderate-sized pseudocyst resulting from hemorrhage and necrosis within the tumor (311). A small calcified ring may even resemble a gallstone (681), and a 1.5 cm calcific ring has been described in a pheochromocytoma of the urinary bladder (309). Apparently, calcium is deposited in the fibrous lining of these cysts (259).

It has been claimed that complete delineation of an adrenal tumor by retroperitoneal insufflation is a sign of benignity; however, Meyers and King have pointed out that metastases can occur without evidence of local tumor invasion. A malignant pheochromocytoma was entirely outlined by retroperitoneal pneumography in one of their patients. On the other hand, it has been said that irregular opacification and poor delinea-

tion by arteriography in an extraadrenal pheochromocytoma suggests a locally invasive rather than a benign tumor (455). Despite these claims and guides for differentiating benign from malignant pheochromocytomas, there is virtually no way to detect radiologically whether or not a pheochromocytoma is malignant except by evidence of tumor metastases. Any patient suspected of having a malignant pheochromocytoma, which occurs in about 10 percent of cases, should have, in addition to other radiologic studies, a skeletal survey and a liver scan, in an attempt to detect any evidence of metastatic disease.

Isotopic Localization of Adrenal Pheochromocytoma Lieberman and coworkers (573) and Sturman and associates (951) have had some success in diagnosis of adrenal disease by visualizing the human adrenal cortex with ^{131}I-19-iodocholesterol. Normal functioning adrenal glands may be visualized, but replacement of an adrenal gland by a tumor, such as a pheochromocytoma, can prevent visualization because of replacement, or compression and destruction of the involved gland.

Adrenal cortical imaging with ^{131}I-19-iodocholesterol may be of value in demonstrating adrenal cortical neoplasms or hyperplasia; this noninvasive radioisotope technique has been used successfully to localize adrenal pheochromocytomas. Since the cholesterol isotope will only concentrate in the adrenal cortex, a pheochromocytoma will not in itself appear radioactive but will be manifest by compression and/or displacement of radioactive cortical tissue. The usefulness of this technique has not yet been adequately explored; it cannot be used to detect extraadrenal pheochromocytomas.

Since the normal adrenal medulla accumulates radiolabeled catecholamines and their precursors, it is conceivable that in time a scanning technique will be developed which may be valuable in preoperatively localizing pheochromocytoma in an extraadrenal site as well as in an intraadrenal location. Anderson and coworkers have reported preliminary results which indicate that, following the intravenous injection of ^{14}C-labeled dopamine, radioactivity became considerably more concentrated in pheochromocytoma tissue than in liver, muscle, or fat (13).

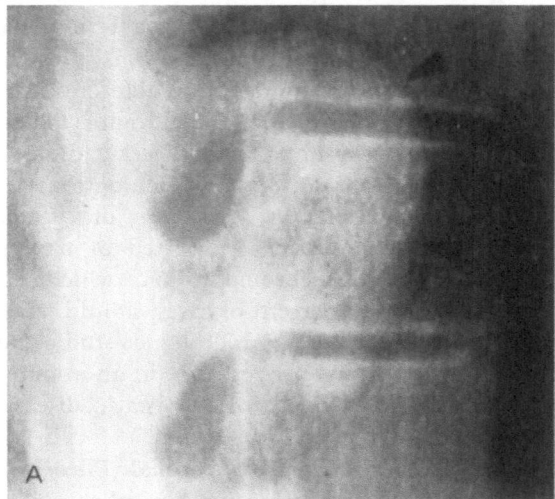
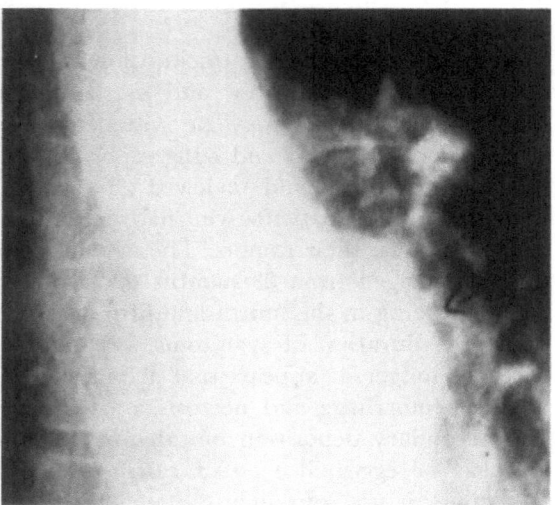
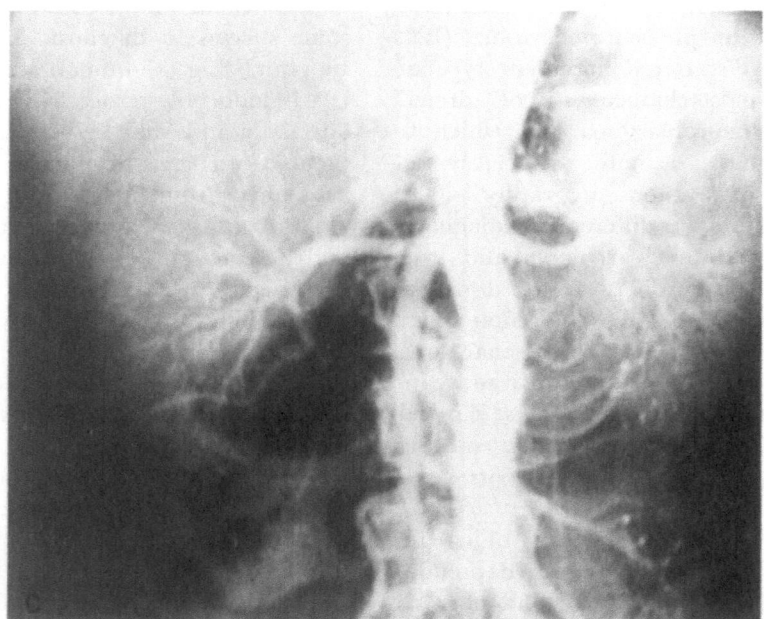

Fig. 6.31 A. Tomogram demonstrating a smooth extrapulmonary mediastinal tumor situated in the left costovertebral angle at the level of the eighth vertebral body. B. Aortography revealing the vascular nature of the mediastinal mass. C. Aortography showing the abnormal circulation at the left renal hilum.

The patient was a 52-year-old male who was asymptomatic and normotensive until he developed symptoms of gallstones. Cholecystectomy was accompanied by hypotension and profuse sweating. Postoperatively, sweating persisted and electrocardiographic changes were thought to represent anterolateral myocardial infarction although pathologic Q waves were not seen. Subsequently the patient was found to have vascular pheochromocytomas in the thorax and left renal hilum. These were removed successfully. T-wave inversion persisted in Leads I, AVL, V5, and V6. From McNeill, A. D., Groden, B. M., and Neville, A. M., *Br. J. Surg. 57:* 458, 1970.

Chest, Neck, and Head x-Rays   In any radiologic investigation of a patient suspected of having a pheochromocytoma, especially when no lesion can be demonstrated in the abdomen and pelvis, one must be aware that very rarely (probably <2 percent) tumors may occur in the chest or neck or even, possibly in the head. It is particularly important in searching for a chest lesion to obtain oblique films, since the tumor almost always has its origin in chromaffin tissue in the paravertebral gutter adjacent to the spine, and therefore a small

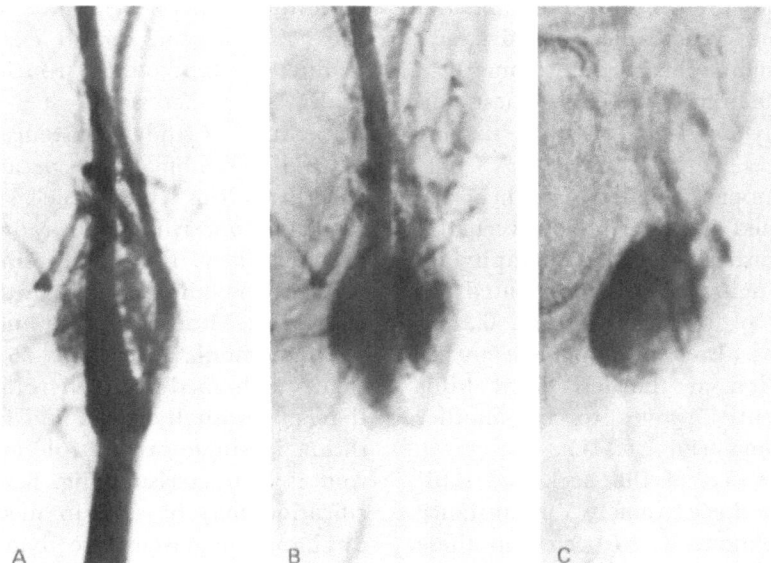

A   B   C

Fig. 6.32 Angiograms of carotid body paraganglioma. These angiograms of a right common carotid show timed filling and draining (A through C) of carotid vessels and carotid body paraganglioma vasculature. (Figures 3b, c, and d from Probst, F. P. Chemodectomas of the neck. Report of six cases with a review of the literature. *Radiologe 11:* 15-27, 1971, Springer-Verlag.) From Glenner, G. G. and Grimley, P. M. Tumors of the extra-adrenal paraganglion system (including chemoreceptors). In: *Atlas of Tumor Pathology,* second series, fascicle 9. Courtesy of Armed Forces Institute of Pathology, 1974, p. 57.

Fig. 6.33 Angiograms of vagal paraganglioma. These angiograms of a left common carotid demonstrate filling and draining (A to B) of a vagal paraganglioma vasculature during timed exposures. (Figures 7b and d from Probst, F. P. Chemodectomas of the neck. Report of six cases with a review of the literature. *Radiologe 11:* 15-27, 1971, Springer-Verlag.) From Glenner, G. G. and Grimley, P. M. Tumors of the extra-adrenal paraganglion system (including chemoreceptors). In: *Atlas of Tumor Pathology,* second series, fascicle 9. Courtesy of Armed Forces Institute of Pathology, 1974, p. 74.

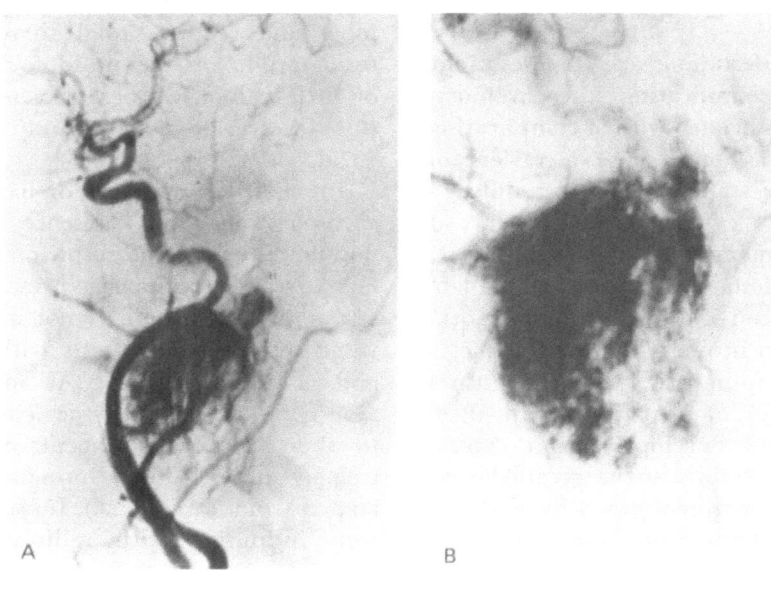

A   B

lesion may be obscured by the spine and not seen with routine stereoscopic PA and lateral films. A malignant pheochromocytoma can metastasize to the hilar nodes in the chest, and hilar adenopathy may be seen on a routine chest x-ray.

An extrapulmonary mediastinal pheochromocytoma situated in the left costovertebral angle is demonstrated by tomography in Figure 6.31A. Angiography demonstrated the vascular nature of this tumor (Fig. 6.31B). This patient was also found to have an abnormal circulation at the left renal hilus which subsequently proved to be another pheochromocytoma (Fig. 6.31C).

Appropriate x-rays of the neck and skull are indicated in the extremely rare instance when a chromaffinoma is suspected in these areas. A carotid arteriogram may be of value in detecting an intracranial tumor; it may also permit visualization of the internal jugular vein and jugular fossa in the venous phase and thus aid in excluding a chromaffin tumor, which on rare occasions has been reported in this region (571). An internal jugular venogram would, however, be more valuable in demonstrating a lesion of the jugular fossa. The diagnostic value of arteriograms of the common carotid arteries in localizing a carotid body and vagal paraganglioma is well illustrated by the radiographic findings revealed in Figures 6.32 and 6.33. Perhaps the most satisfactory method of delineating an intracranial neoplasm will prove to be computerized axial tomography.

Radiologic Manifestations of Diseases Associated with or Complicating Pheochromocytoma Diseases associated with or complicating pheochromocytoma may cause a variety of radiologic manifestations. For example, a neoplasm may be evident on skull x-ray if a cerebellar hemangioblastoma is present; radiologic manifestations of an aortic aneurysm may be seen if dissection of the aorta complicates pheochromocytoma; and megacolon or radiographic evidence of intestinal obstruction may occur in patients with pheochromocytoma who develop ischemic enterocolitis (953). It should also be recalled that patients with pheochromocytoma have a high incidence of cholelithiasis; hence, prior to surgery, a cholecystogram could be obtained on adults with pheochromocytoma. However, since the surgeon should examine the gallbladder at laparotomy, routine cholecystography is not necessary.

Because of the coexistence of medullary thyroid carcinoma and occasionally hyperparathyroidism with Sipple's syndrome, a few remarks concerning the radiologic features of medullary thyroid carcinoma (and its metastases) and hyperparathyroidism are warranted. Radiographic findings may be pathognomonic in perhaps 35 percent of patients with medullary thyroid carcinoma in that an unusually dense and irregular calcification in single or multiple areas of the thyroid is characteristic (Fig. 6.34). Similar calcification may be seen in medullary thyroid carcinoma metastases to lymph nodes and liver. Bone lesions caused by metastases are typically lytic, although in one patient both lytic and sclerotic spine lesions were noted. Metastases to the chest may present as mediastinal masses and/or an interstitial nodular pattern more suggestive of sarcoidosis than metastatic disease. Selective thyroid arteriography usually reveals multiple intrathyroidal avascular masses which appear as filling defects (Fig. 6.35A) and these probably represent deposits of amyloid. Calcified tumors in the thyroid always appear as avascular filling defects. Occasionally, when the lesions are small, multiple hypervascular areas may be seen in the thyroid (Fig. 6.35B) or in liver metastases. It appears that since medullary thyroid carcinoma invariably involves both lobes and requires total thyroidectomy, arteriographic or radioisotopic localization is of little value. Retrograde venograms of the thyroid are of no diagnostic value (503a, 737a).

In a patient who has, or has had, a pheochromocytoma, the presence of a thyroid nodule may raise the suspicion that a medullary thyroid carcinoma is present, even if the serum thyrocalcitonin is not abnormally elevated by provocative tests with pentagastrin and calcium infusion. (As mentioned previously, a negative thyrocalcitonin response to these provocative agents would be extremely unlikely in the presence of a medullary thyroid carcinoma.) In such a predicament, scanning with radioisotopes cannot segregate carcinomas from benign adenomas,

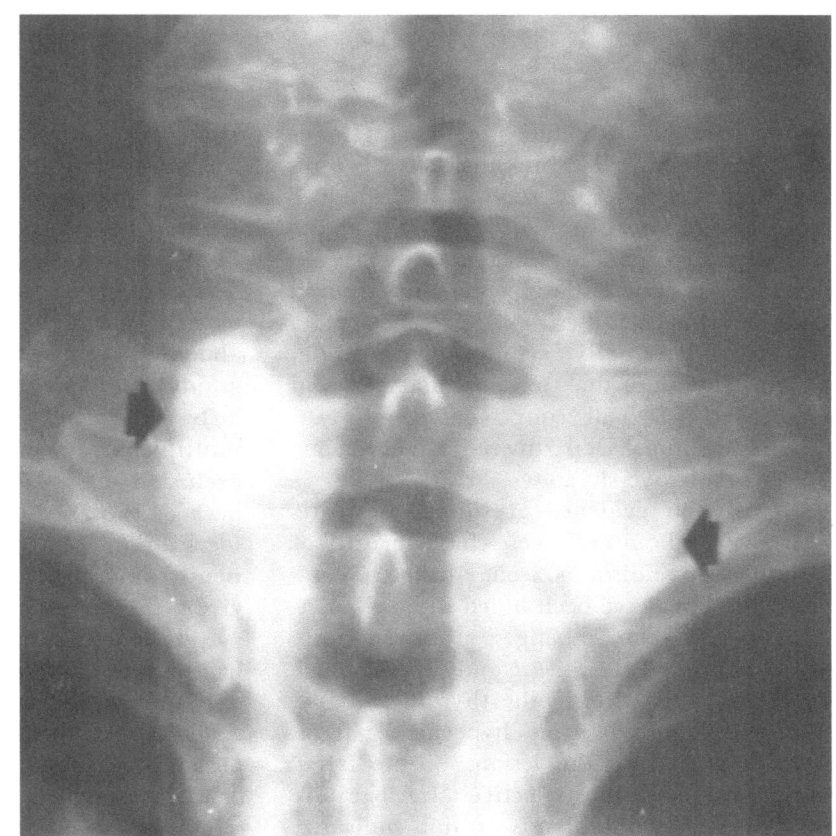

Fig. 6.34 Dense irregular
calcification (arrows)
in both thyroid lobes due to
medullary carcinoma. From
Keiser, H. R., Beaven, M. A.,
Doppman, J., Wells, S. Jr.,
and Buja, L. M., *Ann. Int.
Med. 78:* 568, 1973.

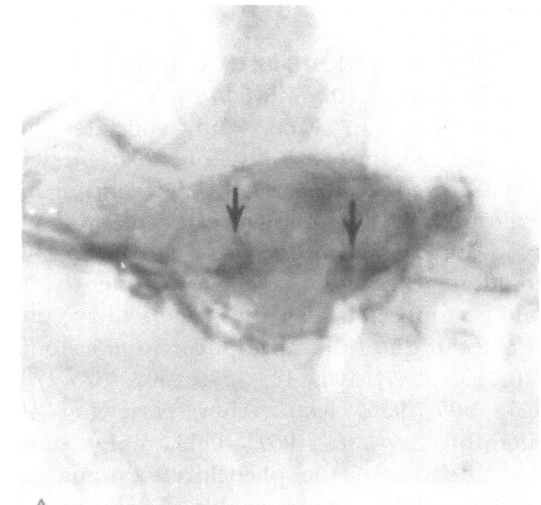

A

Fig. 6.35 Selective thyroid arteriography for
medullary carcinoma of the thyroid. A. Multiple areas
of abnormal staining indicating hypervascularity
(arrows) superimposed on thyroid lobe. B. Larger
medullary carcinoma masses presenting as
filling defects in opacified thyroid lobe (arrows).
From Keiser, H. R., Beaven, M. A., Doppman, J.,
Wells, S., Jr., and Buja, L. M, *Ann. Int. Med. 78:* 569,
1973.

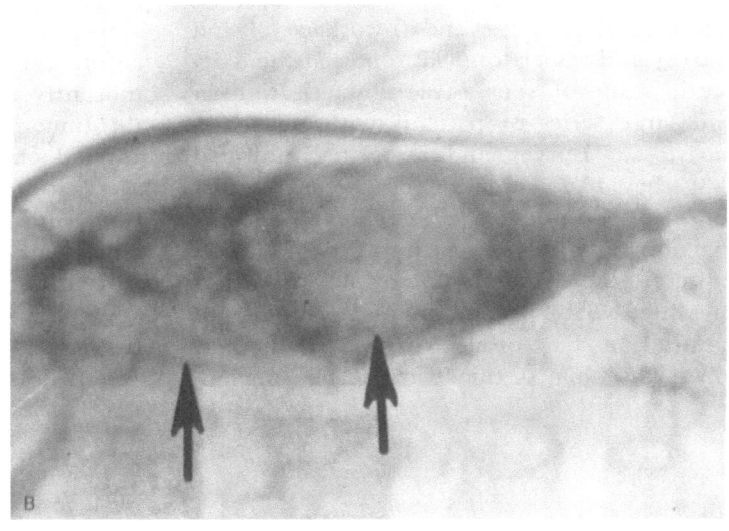

B

although a "cold" nodule is more apt to be malignant than a "hot" nodule. We are, however, unaware of any reports indicating a significant uptake of radioisotope by a medullary thyroid carcinoma. Echography may be valuable in differentiating a cystic from a solid thyroid nodule. The presence of a simple cyst essentially excludes the possibility that the nodule is due to a medullary thyroid carcinoma (personal conversation with Dr. Manfred Blum, Department of Medicine, New York University).

Usually no evidence of subperiosteal resorption or bone changes characteristic of hyperparathyroidism is seen, although occasional patients have been noted to have nephrocalcinosis, skeletal changes, and even chondrocalcinosis of the knees and wrists. Since small tumor deposits in the thyroid are difficult to differentiate from hyperplastic parathyroids and since the lesions of the latter are usually multiple, selective arteriography of the parathyroid glands is not indicated (503a, 737a).

CENTRAL VENOUS BLOOD SAMPLING FOR CATECHOLAMINE ASSAY

In 1955 von Euler and associates first catheterized the vena cava of a patient with pheochromocytoma, and, by determining the concentration of plasma catecholamines in blood obtained from various sites, were able to locate the tumor (294). Subsequently, we and a number of other investigators have used this technique to localize pheochromocytomas (76, 193, 267, 306, 423, 584, 602, 623, 703, 741, 905, 956, 992). After reviewing the literature up to 1967, Pekkarenin stated that the site of the pheochromocytoma was established by vena cava blood sampling in 26 out of 27 reported cases (741). More recently, in 1973, Agee and coworkers (2) and Lurvey and associates (596) reported the diagnostic value of vena cava catheterization in two large series of patients with pheochromocytoma. Lurvey and associates indicated that they had localized the pheochromocytoma in each of 14 patients in whom the diagnosis was proved by surgical exploration; however, the details of their study were not presented (596). At times this technique of localization has proved extremely helpful, especially when a tumor cannot be demon-

strated by other means. We recommend that central venous blood sampling, followed by adrenal phlebography, be performed on patients whose pheochromocytomas have not been localized by other radiographic procedures. Central venous sampling may prove extremely valuable in the face of a negative abdominal exploration and negative radiographic studies; moreover, it can be particularly helpful when tumors are very small, multiple, or metastatic, and it will permit exclusion of a pheochromocytoma in the neck or thorax. Accurate preoperative tumor localization is especially important in patients who are seriously ill and might not survive a prolonged surgical exploration.

Since plasma catecholamines may be within the normal range if the tumor secretes only intermittently or if the continuous secretion is very minimal, administration of a provocative drug (e.g., histamine) (193, 992) or the valsalva maneuver (741) may trigger release of catecholamines from the tumor and aid in identifying tumor location.

Vendsalu has found that central venous blood sampling with the catheter tip pointed in various directions can be of value in lateralizing the tumor site (992); however, some of our results, and those of Crout and Sjoerdsma (193) and others (423), indicate that venous drainage to sites somewhat removed from the tumor, or a "streaming" effect on blood draining the neoplasm, may cause an erroneous localization.

Crout and Sjoerdsma have stated that catheterization for preoperative localization is "indicated only when the tumor is a 'pure' norepinephrine producer and when the catecholamine secretion by the tumor appears to be continuous" (193). This opinion was based on their correlation of urinary catecholamines with tumor site in 75 cases of pheochromocytoma. When epinephrine was significantly elevated (42 percent of all cases), the tumor was found in, or adjacent to, an adrenal gland in about 95 percent of these cases; it was found in the organ of Zuckerkandl in about 5 percent. If the urine contained only elevations of norepinephrine (58 percent of all cases), the tumor occurred in an adrenal gland in about two-thirds of cases. It was extraadrenal in about one-third and extraabdominal in 6 percent of patients who had elevations of urinary norepinephrine alone (193). The possible value of elevated urine epinephrine concentrations in predicting that the pheochromocytoma is adrenal in location was first suggested by von Euler (285, 299).

Although increased concentrations of epinephrine in urine and plasma and increased urinary metanephrine have almost always signaled the presence of a pheochromocytoma in the adrenal areas or in the organ of Zuckerkandl, several exceptions to this rule have occurred. We believe that catheterization and central venous sampling are indicated whenever possible if other preoperative methods for determining the location of a continuously secreting pheochromocytoma have been unsuccessful. In our hands the procedure has been entirely safe and has not provoked any hypertensive paroxysms.

Preoperative localization of a tumor is of obvious importance to the surgeon, particularly when dealing with the pharmacologically explosive pheochromocytoma. Conceivably, a laparotomy may be inadvertently performed when, in fact, the pheochromocytoma is located in the thorax or neck. It is of considerable importance, and at times vital, that the surgeon promptly locate the tumor and ligate its blood supply, for prolonged operative delay in terminating recurrent massive release of catecholamines from a pheochromocytoma can be fatal.

With fluoroscopic guidance, we now usually sample from the following vena caval levels via femoral vein catheterization: Lumbar 4, 2, and 1; T12; and just above and below the entrance into the right atrium. The presence of a pheochromocytoma in the organ of Zuckerkandl, urinary bladder, or in other pelvic structures should cause higher concentrations of catecholamines in blood samples from L4 than in samples from other sites. We also sample blood from both renal veins (the left being usually located at L1 and the right at L2), and whenever possible from the adrenal veins Finally, if there is any suspicion of a chromaffinoma in the neck or head we sometimes sample blood from an internal jugular vein. The left adrenal vein drains into the left renal vein, whereas the right adrenal vein usually empties into the inferior vena cava approximately 4 cm cephalad to

the right renal vein and at about the level of the 12th thoracic vertebra (Fig. 6.24). At the latter level, some of the blood draining both the left and right adrenal will be sampled; however, this site is usually in very close proximity to blood draining from the right adrenal gland. Adrenal vein catheterization is usually possible on the left, but less frequently successful on the right; it is not always possible to obtain blood samples from the adrenal veins even if catheterized. Although blood sampling can usually be performed with ease from the left adrenal vein, sometimes only a few drops of blood are obtainable from the right adrenal vein.

We are aware of only one report (2) in the literature in which vena caval catheterization in a relatively large series of patients with pheochromocytoma has included adrenal vein sampling for plasma catecholamine determination. In the vast majority of adrenal pheochromocytomas, quantitation of adrenal venous blood should permit precise localization of the tumor. The presence of an elevated plasma catecholamine concentration in blood from the left renal vein will also strongly suggest a tumor in the left adrenal. However, since increased catecholamines have been found in adrenal blood following adrenal venography (225) in the absence of pheochromocytoma, blood sampling for diagnostic purposes should be performed prior to any angiographic studies. Others have also emphasized this latter point (423). At the present time we share the concern of Harrison and Freier (423), over the interpretation of elevated catecholamine concentrations in plasma obtained from the adrenal veins; adequate information is lacking regarding the normal catecholamine concentrations in blood draining the adrenals, and regarding the variability of these concentrations which may occur under a variety of circumstances. As this information becomes available, results may be interpreted with greater confidence.

We have sampled blood from various levels of the vena cava, and almost invariably this has proved extremely valuable in locating the approximate area of a catecholamine-secreting tumor. By comparing plasma catecholamine concentrations of blood collected from veins draining (a) the head and neck (internal jugular, innominate, or cephalad portion of the superior vena cava), (b) the thorax (superior vena cava at or below the junction of the azygos), and (c) the abdomen and pelvis (inferior vena cava), one should usually be able to distinguish whether the tumor is in the head or neck region, the thorax, or abdominopelvic region, respectively. The value of sampling blood drained by the azygos vein in detecting some thoracic tumors has been demonstrated (76).

It is imperative to monitor arterial blood pressure carefully by frequent measurements with a sphygmomanometer in an effort to recognize any instability suggesting variability in release of catecholamines by the tumor. Obviously, a significant variability in catecholamine secretion rate could vitiate the accuracy of this method of tumor localization and could mislead the physician. For example, if the rate of catecholamine secretion from an adrenal pheochromocytoma was minimal while sampling inferior vena cava blood, but markedly increased while sampling superior vena caval blood, one would be misled to conclude that the tumor was not in the abdomen. Pekkarinen reported that the valsalva maneuver triggered the release of catecholamines from a pheochromocytoma and was of aid in localizing a tumor of the organ of Zuckerkandl by central venous sampling in one patient (741). This latter finding emphasizes the importance of instructing the patient to avoid straining or any physical effort during sequential central venous sampling lest there be an inadvertent release of catecholamines which might lead to incorrect localization of the pheochromocytoma.

Inferior vena caval catheterization has not been accompanied by any morbidity in our hands. However, we have heard of a hypertensive crisis in a patient with pheochromocytoma in whom adrenal vein catheterization was performed for radiographic studies. Also, as mentioned above, Agee and coworkers (2) reported a hypertensive crisis following adrenal vein phlebography in a patient with pheochromocytoma. Although we have not found it necessary to use an α-adrenergic blocking agent prior to central venous sampling, we strongly urge that phentolamine, sodium nitroprusside, lidocaine, propranolol and levophed be available for immediate use

in case a severe hypertensive crisis, arrhythmia, or hypotension occur during vena caval and selective vein catheterization.

Some of our experience in vena caval and renal and neck vein catheterization in patients with pheochromocytoma is indicated in Figures 6.36–6.39; and the concentrations of

Fig. 6.36 Figures give concentration in μg/liter of epinephrine (E) and norepinephrine (N) drawn from various sites in the venous system. The patient was a 9-year-old black male with blood pressure of 150/90 mmHg, intermittent headaches, and diaphoresis. Urinary catecholamines were elevated. (Twenty months previously the patient had had total left adrenalectomy and subtotal right adrenalectomy for bilateral pheochromocytoma.) Radiographic studies: KUB, IVP, nephrotomograms, and presacral pneumogram were unremarkable. There was no angiographic evidence of tumor. Central venous blood sampling (via catheter in brachial vein) identified location of recurrent pheochromocytoma in right adrenal area. Tumor (20 g, 4×4×2 cm) was successfully removed and the patient (now 19½ years old) remains well and has developed normally on adrenal replacement therapy. This is patient No. 17 and 17a recorded in Figure 7.2 in Chapter 7. From Manger, W. M. and Wakim, K G. The role of norepinephrine and epinephrine in the etiology of diastolic hypertension. Chap. II In: *Hormones and Hypertension.* Courtesy of C. C. Thomas, 1966, p. 57.

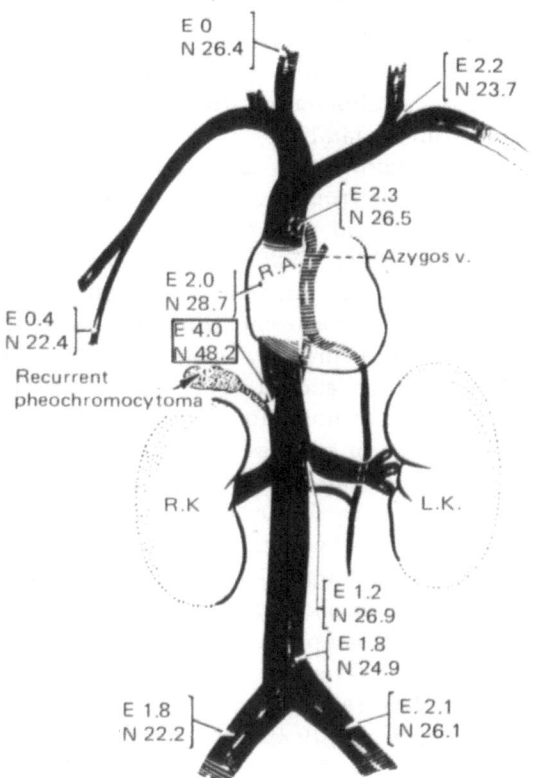

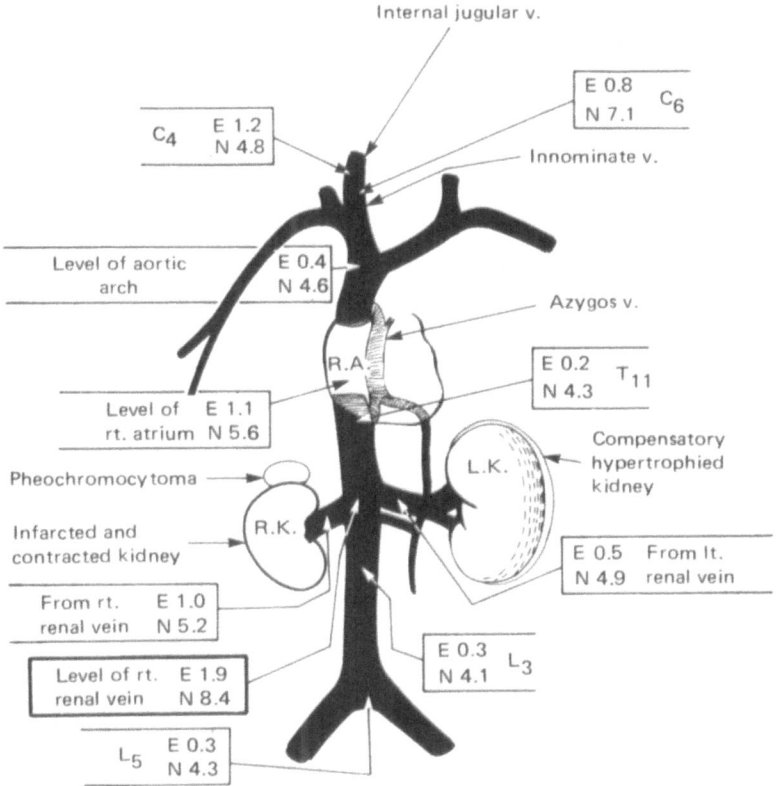

Fig. 6.37 Figures give concentration in μg/liter of epinephrine (E) and norepinephrine (N) in plasma drawn from various sites in the venous system. The patient was a 40-year-old white female who 1 year previously had had a right renal artery graft for renal artery stenosis and hypertension. Blood pressure elevation persisted and patient began noting episodes of hot sensations, epigastric pounding, pulsating headaches, diaphoresis, tremor, anxiety, weakness, blurred vision, and orthostatic hypotension. Urinary catecholamines, metanephrines, and VMA were elevated once but normal on another occasion. ECG showed prominent U waves and T-wave abnormalities. Serum cholesterol was 356 mg/dl. Peripheral venous plasma epinephrine: 1.2 and 1.5 μg/liter; norepinephrine: 8.0 and 8.6 μg/liter. Radiographic studies, including IVP and renal arteriograms, revealed a shrunken nonfunctioning right kidney, distal to an occluded graft, and compensatory hypertrophy of the left kidney. No pheochromocytoma was identified.

Central venous blood sampling (via transfemoral catheterization) revealed the highest plasma catecholamine concentrations to be at the level of the right renal artery. Explanation for the elevated norepinephrine value in blood obtained at level C6 is uncertain but might have resulted from an increased secretion of the tumor when this sample was collected. A right adrenal pheochromocytoma (20 g, 3×3×3 cm) was extirpated but hypertension persisted, requiring antihypertensive drugs. This is patient No. 20 recorded in Fig. 7.2 in Chapter 7.

epinephrine (E) and norepinephrine (N) in plasma sampled at various sites are recorded. We have employed central venous blood sampling as an aid in tumor localization in six patients with pheochromocytoma. In addition, central venous blood samples have been obtained on 10 patients with a variety of diseases without pheochromocytoma (W. M. Manger, M. Bosniak, and M. Madayag, unpublished data). The plasma catecholamine concentrations in this latter group of patients is recorded in Table 6.22 for comparison with the values obtained in the patients with pheochromocytoma. It should be noted, however, that some of these patients without pheochromocytoma had received diazepam (Valium) which may slightly lower plasma catecholamine concentrations.

It is particularly noteworthy that in patients Nos. 17, 20, and 35 (depicted in Figs. 6.36–6.38), pheochromocytomas were not detected by various radiographic examinations, whereas catecholamine assay of central venous blood established an intraabdominal location and identified the approximate level of each tumor.

The elevation of catecholamines in patient No. 20 (Fig. 6.37) was highest at the level of

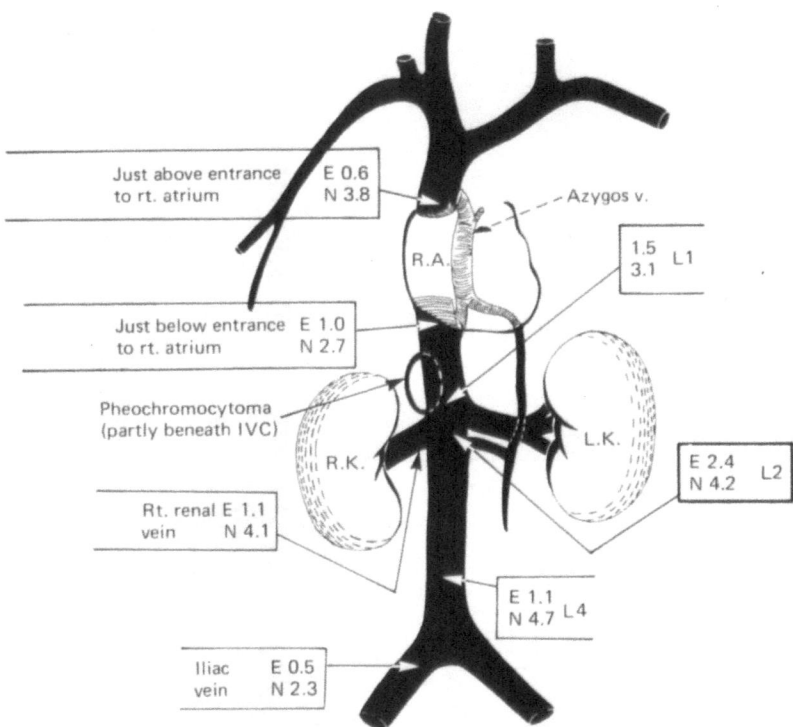

Just above entrance to rt. atrium E 0.6 N 3.8

Azygos v.

R.A.

1.5
3.1 L1

Just below entrance to rt. atrium E 1.0 N 2.7

L.K.

Pheochromocytoma (partly beneath IVC)

R.K.

E 2.4
N 4.2 L2

Rt. renal E 1.1 vein N 4.1

E 1.1
N 4.7 L4

Iliac vein E 0.5 N 2.3

Fig. 6.38 Figures give concentration in μg/liter of epinephrine (E) and norepinephrine (N) in plasma drawn from various sites in the venous system. Patient was a 41-year-old white male who for the last 1½ years had had labile hypertension and spontaneous hypertensive episodes (BP: normal to 240/140 and falling to 90/60 mmHg), sometimes precipitated by exercise, and with palpitations, pallor, diaphoresis, and headaches becoming more severe for the last 3 months.

Urinary catecholamines, metanephrines, and VMA were elevated and pheochromocytoma screening test was positive. Serum cholesterol: 248 mg/dl; triglycerides: 245 mg/dl, pre beta IV pattern. BUN: 55 mg/dl, returned to normal with hospitalization and hydration. ECG revealed left axis deviation and T-wave abnormalities. Radiographic studies, including tomograms and renal arteriograms, were normal. Central venous blood sampling, via transfemoral vein catheterization, identified the approximate vicinity of the tumor although only plasma epinephrine was minimally elevated. A pheochromocytoma (44 g, 8×7×1.5 cm) was successfully extirpated from beneath the inferior vena cava near the upper pole of the right kidney. This is patient No. 35 recorded in Table 7.1 and Fig. 7.3 in Chapter 7.

the right renal vein; however, norepinephrine was also somewhat elevated in blood sampled at the level of C6. The explanation of this latter finding is uncertain but might conceivably have resulted from an increased secretion of the adrenal tumor during sampling in the neck region. There was some concern that this patient might have a catecholamine-secreting tumor in her neck, similar to those reported by others (571), especially since a bruit was heard over the right neck area. Central venous sampling aided in eliminating this possibility.

In the patient depicted in Figure 6.38,

only a small increase in the concentration of epinephrine was detected at a level in the inferior vena cava slightly below the tumor; the concentration of epinephrine at the level of the pheochromocytoma was only at the upper limit of normal. The reason for this discrepancy is unclear; but drainage of blood from the tumor into the vena cava at a level below the lesion could explain these results.

Occasionally, patients with pheochromocytoma have been observed in whom plasma catecholamine concentrations in central venous samples have not differed significantly enough to indicate the location of a tumor.

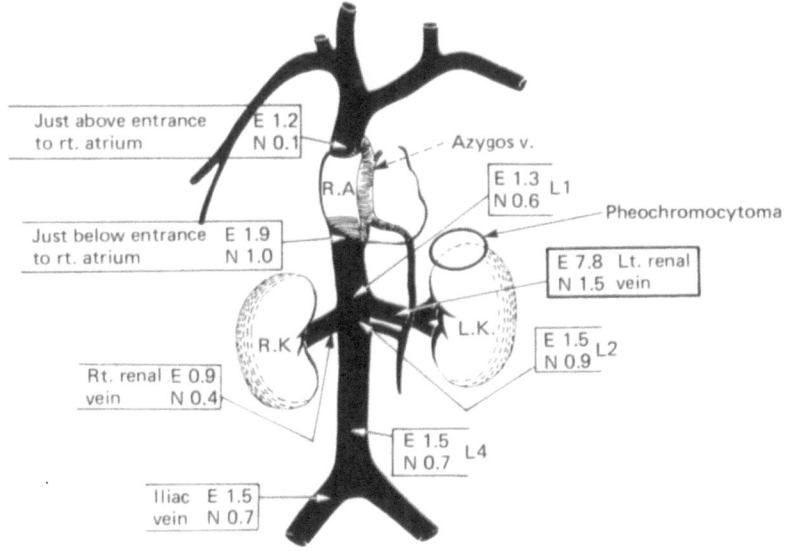

Fig. 6.39 Figures give concentration in μg/liter of epinephrine (E) and norepinephrine (N) in plasma drawn from various sites in the venous system. The patient was a 54-year-old white woman who for many years had had palpitations, becoming more severe and frequent for the last 1½ years, usually lasting 10 min, and with weakness and tingling in the extremities. BP: normal to 140/95–155/100 mmHg. Grade 2/6 precordial systolic murmur Urinary metanephrines and VMA were elevated.ECG: intermittent sinus node dysfunction, probably Mobitz type II AV block. Frequent APCs and VPCs in runs with tachycardia but generally periodic bradycardia with AV dissociation. Serum cholesterol: 266 mg/dl. Radiographic studies: ultrasonogram of abdomen, IVP, and nephrotomogram were negative. Arteriogram: 5 cm vascular tumor anterior and superior to upper pole of left kidney consistent with pheochromocytoma with vascular rim. No evidence of palpitations or attacks occurred during arteriography. Central venous blood sampling via transfemoral vein catheterization revealed highest concentration of catecholamines in left renal vein (epinephrine was significantly elevated) and established diagnosis and location of tumor. Left adrenal pheochromocytoma (30 g, 4×4.5×1.5 cm) was successfully extirpated. This is patient No. 37 recorded in Table 7.1 and Fig. 7.3 in Chapter 7.

The most likely explanation for paradoxical elevations of plasma catecholamines (i.e., elevations in sample sites quite distant from the tumor as well as in those close to the tumor) appears to be variations in catecholamine secretion rates by the pheochromocytoma during the central venous sampling, as mentioned above. However, secretion from more than one pheochromocytoma in the same patient (e.g., as occurred in patient No. 19—see case report in Chapter 7) could similarly result in elevated concentrations of plasma catecholamines at multiple sites in central venous blood.

Suffice it to reemphasize the importance of monitoring blood pressure and heart rate and carefully observing the patient for any alterations in symptoms or signs during sampling via a central venous catheter. These precautions may permit one to detect a deviation from the basal state, which might herald a change in the secretion rate of the tumor. If these latter points are kept in mind, confusion and erroneous conclusions from catheterization data should be minimized.

Finally, it should be mentioned that determination of catecholamine concentrations in vena caval blood may be helpful in establishing the diagnosis of pheochromocytoma in a patient who has normal concentrations of catecholamines and their metabolites in the urine and plasma. Patient No. 34, described earlier, had a normal excretion of urinary catecholamines, VMA, and total metanephrines (determined by a highly reliable laboratory). Catecholamine concentrations in ar-

Table 6.22 Concentrations of Plasma Catecholamines (μg/liter) in 10 patients Undergoing Renal Vein and Vena Caval Blood Sampling at Various Levels[a,b]

Patient	Age	Diagnosis	BP	IVC L-4		Renal veins Right		Renal veins Left		IVC L-2		IVC L-1		Just above right atrium	
				E	NE	E	NE	E	NE	E	NE	E	NE	E	NE
Hypertensives															
R.M.[c] ♂	50	Left renal artery stenosis; arteriosclerotic	180/105	0.6	1.1	0.4	1.2	0.3	1.7	0.4	1.7	0	1.4	0.3	1.3
S.M.[c] ♂	30	Right renal pyelonephritis	170/110	0	1.8	0.1	1.2	0	1.9	0	1.7	0	1.7	0.1	2.0
S.A. ♀	56	Right renal artery fibromuscular hyperplasia	170/95	0.2	1.0	0.3	2.0	0.4	2.5	0.6	1.7	0.4	1.7	0.3	1.9
T.A. ♂	56	Left renal artery graft stenosis	160/100	0.2	1.0	0.1	1.4	0	1.1	0.8	0	0.5	1.0	0	1.0
A.D. ♂	67	Right renal artery stenosis and nephrosclerosis	230/118	0.7	0.6	0.8	0.7	0.5	0.4	0.7	0.7	1.3	0.7	0.6	1.0
L.J. ♀	52	Left adrenal cortical adenoma	190/114	0.3	1.6	0.9	3.4	1.3	1.9	0.8	1.7	0.6	0.9	0.9	1.0
M.L.[c] ♀	47	Cushing's syndrome; bilateral adrenal hyperplasia	180/110	1.0	2.1	0.6	1.8	1.7	1.7	0.7	1.1	0.8	1.4	0.6	1.5
Mean	51		183/107	0.4	1.3	0.5	1.7	0.6	1.6	0.6	1.2	0.5	1.3	0.4	1.4
±SEm	±4		±9/±3	±0.1	±0.2	±0.1	±0.3	±0.2	±0.3	±0.1	±0.3	±0.2	±0.1	±0.1	±0.2

Normotensives

	Sex	Age	Diagnosis	BP												
R.P.[a]	♀	57	Right renal clear cell carcinoma; with metastases	$\frac{110}{70}$	0.3	0.9	0.2	1.0	0.4	0.5	0.3	0.9	0.3	1.0	0.3	1.5
N.M.[c]	♀	24	Cushing's syndrome	$\frac{135}{70}$	1.3	1.9	0.2	0.6	—	0	0.1	0.4	0.4	0.4	0.7	0.5
M.N.[c]	♀	52	Left adrenal cortical adenoma	$\frac{140}{80}$	0.5	0.5	0	0.9	2.7	1.6	0.5	0.3	0.9	0.9	1.0	0.4
Mean		44		$\frac{128}{73}$	0.7	1.1	0.1	0.8	1.6	1.1	0.3	0.4	0.8	0.8	0.7	0.8
±SEm		±10		$\frac{\pm9}{\pm3}$	±0.3	±0.4	±0.1	±0.1	±1.2	±0.5	±0.1	±0.2	±0.2	±0.2	±0.2	±0.4

[a] Courtesy of Manger, W. M., Bosniack, M. and Madayag, M. New York University Medical Center, New York. Unpublished.

[b] IVC = inferior vena cava; L-4 = level of 4th lumbar vertebra; L-2 = level of 2nd lumbar vertebra; L-1 = level of 1st lumbar vertebra; BP = blood pressure; E = epinephrine; NE = norepinephrine. Blood urea nitrogen values were normal in all subjects. There were no significant differences in concentrations of catecholamines between hypertensives and normotensives, or between the concentrations of catecholamines in blood sampled at various levels.

[c] Patient received Valium, which may lower plasma catecholamine concentrations.

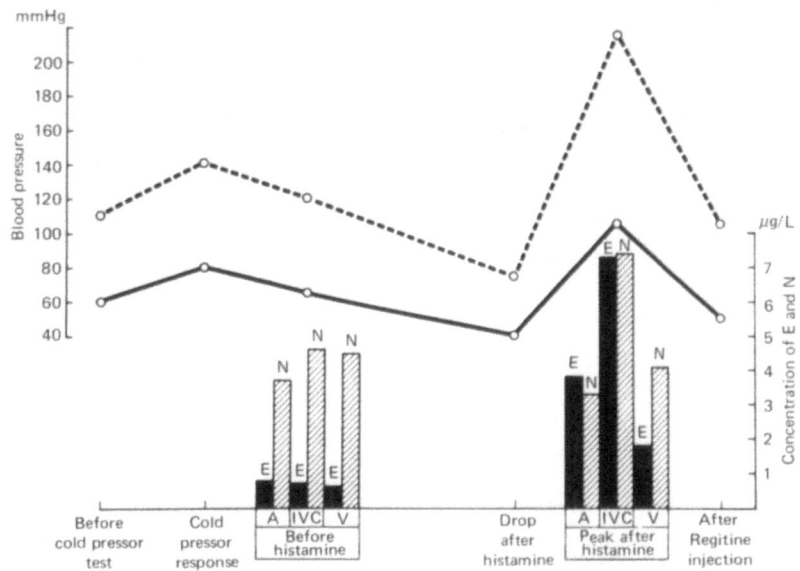

Fig. 6.40 This figure displays the results of a positive histamine provocative test in a 51-year-old white male commercial photographer who had recurrent "attacks" with hypertension for about 18 years. (The details of this case appear under "Patient No. 34" in Chapter 7.) The diagnosis of pheochromocytoma was established only by means of plasma catecholamine assays following a provocative test. Urine assays for catecholamines and their metabolites had been within normal limits. E = epinephrine; N = norepinephrine; A = arterial; IVC = inferior vena cava; V = venous.

Fig. 6.41 This 32-year-old white male gave a history of drug abuse [heroin, methadone, morphine, dilaudid, codeine sulfate, cocaine, pentazcine (Talwin), and marihuana] since 18 years of age. At 30 years of age he developed hypertension; there was no evidence of renal disease and no family history of hypertension. About 1 month later he had a myocardial infarction, and shortly thereafter, because of hypertension which precipitated angina, a coronary artery bypass was performed. Despite this latter procedure he had a second myocardial infarction approximately 4 months later. Catecholamines were quantitated in plasma obtained from an artery and the inferior vena cava before and after a cold pressor test and provocative tests with glucagon and histamine. The blood pressure responses and catecholamine changes following the provocative tests were within normal limits, which aided in excluding the presence of a pheochromocytoma. E = epinephrine; N = norepinephrine; A = arterial; IVC = inferior vena cava.

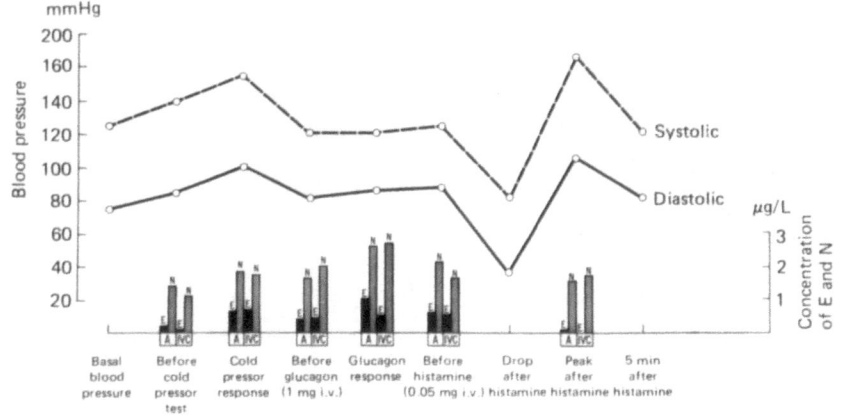

terial and peripheral venous plasma, and plasma collected from the inferior vena cava above the renal veins, were within the normal range (Fig. 6.40). Even at the time of the peak blood pressure response to a positive histamine (0.05 mg histamine base I.V.) provocative test (which reproduced typical symptoms of the attacks he had experienced spontaneously) the peripheral venous norepinephrine concentration was normal and the epinephrine concentration was only slightly above the normal range. On the other hand, the elevations of epinephrine and norepinephrine in plasma from the inferior vena cava were pronounced, and diagnostic of pheochromocytoma. Arterial plasma epineph-

rine, although much less than the level in the IVC, was also significantly elevated, but the norepinephrine concentration was within normal limits.

In patients without pheochromocytoma, cold pressor and provocative tests may cause changes in catecholamine concentrations in plasma collected from an artery, the IVC (Fig. 6.41), or a peripheral vein (180, 615, 621, 624), but these tests never cause catecholamine elevations into the range observed in patients with pheochromocytoma.

An outline of the techniques employed for preoperative localization of a pheochromocytoma by radiology and central venous blood sampling is depicted in Table 6.23.

Table 6.23 *Preoperative Localization of Pheochromocytoma*

I. Radiographic techniques
    Abdomen
        Survey (scout)
        IVP (23% positive)
        Laminography
        Nephrotomography (∼ 70% positive)
        Computerized axial tomography
        Ultrasonography (echography)
        Retroperitoneal pneumography (avoid!)
        Aortography (high; low)
        Selective arteriography: renal, adrenal, celiac, inferior mesenteric
        Adrenal phlebography
    Chest
        Include obliques
        Laminography
        Angiography
        Ultrasonography
        Computerized axial tomography
    Neck and/or head
        Scan
        Angiography
        Computerized axial tomography
        Cholecystography (for evidence of cholelithiasis)
II. Central venous blood sampling for catecholamine assay
    Catheterization of
        Inferior and superior vena cava at various levels
        Renal veins
        Adrenal veins
        Internal jugular vein

Studies on 38 Patients with Pheochromocytoma in Whom Catecholamines Were Determined

CHAPTER SEVEN

The value of our plasma and tumor catecholamine studies in a large series of patients with pheochromocytoma deserves special attention and merits this separate chapter. Relatively few studies of plasma catecholamines in patients with pheochromocytoma have been reported and we wish to emphasize the remarkable diagnostic value and accuracy of plasma catecholamine determinations in detecting patients with this tumor. In addition, correlative studies between blood pressure and plasma and tumor catecholamines may improve our understanding of the patterns of hypertension encountered, and may also shed light on secretion characteristics of these neoplasms.

CASE REPORTS

The relevant histories and findings in 38 patients with pheochromocytoma in whom we quantitated plasma catecholamines are recorded below.* It is hoped that the reader will become more alert to the various manifestations of pheochromocytoma, and that his or her index of suspicion for this potentially lethal tumor will be heightened by carefully studying these brief case reports.

* See pp. 282–295. For list of abbreviations see p. 295.

SPECIAL CASE REPORT—
PHEOCHROMOCYTOMA MASQUERADING
AS ECLAMPSIA

To "sensitize" the physician to the occasional difficulties in diagnosis and to the tragic consequences that can ensue when the diagnosis is missed, the following case of a patient seen in 1975 in a first-rate medical center is reported herein:

The patient was a 29-year-old black nurse and mother (gravida V, para III, abortus II). She had had two spontaneous abortions in 1969. In 1970 a normal baby was delivered by cesarean section because of cephalopelvic disproportion. Her blood pressure had always been normal; however, just prior to the cesarean section she experienced a severe pounding frontal and bifrontal headache and the blood pressure became transiently elevated to 180/110 mmHg. Headaches, which recurred periodically and were augmented by the valsalva maneuver, subsided several days post delivery.

In about the 36th week of a fourth pregnancy in 1973, her blood pressure was found to be 140/100 mmHg. Despite bed rest, sedation, and I.V. magnesium sulfate, she developed a grand mal seizure, following which her blood pressure rose to 200/140 but subsequently returned to 140/90 mmHg. It was presumed that these were manifestations of eclampsia. Urine metanephrines, VMA, and a pheoscreening test were normal. (During the period of urine collection the blood pressure had been relatively normal but had occasionally reached 160–170/100 mmHg.) Neurologic examination and echoencephalogram were normal, and nonspecific EEG changes were noted. The ECG was within normal limits. At 37 weeks gestation cesarean section was performed, and an apparently normal baby was delivered. Postoperatively the mother's blood pressure was very labile; she was treated with apresoline (Hydralazine) and chlorthalidone (Hygroton), and finally maintained on methyldopa (Aldomet) 250 mg twice daily, with reportedly fair control of her pressure. It is noteworthy that blood glucose concentrations fluctuated between normal levels and hyperglycemia up to 159 mg/dl. During the puerperium, a renal scan and IVP were normal. Subsequently, one ECG revealed a tachycardia of 105/min and T-wave

inversion in aVL, whereas another ECG revealed T wave inversions in lead I, aVL, and V_2, and low T waves in V_3 to V_6. (The infant did well initially but then developed hypertension and intractable heart failure and died on the 21st day of life; autopsy revealed bilateral renal vein thrombosis.)

During the first trimester of her fifth pregnancy, her blood pressure was minimally hypertensive. About the 35th week of gestation a mildly abnormal diabetic-type glucose intolerance was detected. The blood pressure varied between 150/100 and 160/110 mmHg. There had been a slight weight gain, and she had been experiencing daily headaches.

On May 6, 1975, at the 37th week of gestation, a cesarean section was performed and a normal baby delivered. Immediately postoperatively the mother developed acute pulmonary edema, supraventricular tachycardia, and hypotension, which required cardiopulmonary resuscitation. She was maintained on 100 percent O_2 via an endotracheal tube and was transferred to the intensive-care unit. Drug therapy included morphine, furosemide, Cedilanid (lanatoside C) I.V., steroids, and gentamicin. Heparin was also administered because of the chance that pulmonary emboli or amniotic fluid embolization had caused her pulmonary edema.

The possibility that the patient was harboring a pheochromocytoma was seriously considered; however, on May 8, 1975, another pheoscreening test of the urine was negative (B.P. was within normal limits except for two brief elevations to about 200/80 mmHg, and BUN and serum creatinine were normal on the day urine was collected). On May 13, 1975, the 24-hr urine volume was 1425 ml and the VMA was 6.0 mg (blood pressure was within normal limits and the BUN and creatinine were normal on the day urine was collected). Sodium nitroprusside infusion had to be used to control subsequent hypertensive episodes to 230/130 mmHg. Bilateral pneumothorax and pneumomediastinum appeared but were treated successfully. Ultimately, extracorporeal membrane oxygenation with partial circulatory bypass was employed and finally, on May 23, 1975, hemodialysis was required because of deterioration of renal function. On May 21, 1975, 24-hr urine volume was 2050 ml, total metanephrines was

0.07 mg (low normal), and total catecholamines was 82 µg (within normal limits); blood pressure varied from 150/100 to 200/110 mmHg, BUN was 98 mg/dl, serum creatinine was 7.2 mg/dl, and creatinine clearance was 2.2 ml/min during urine collection period.

Following a hypertensive episode to 240/130 mmHg, the patient became hypotensive and expired. Postmortem examination revealed: (1) pheochromocytoma (3×2×2.5 cm) in the right adrenal gland; (2) diffuse pulmonary fibrosis, possibly due to oxygen toxicity and/or amniotic fluid embolization; (3) CNS: recent subdural hemorrhages, recent left cerebellar hemorrhage, right frontal lobe encephalomalacia.

Comment: it is surprising that this patient invariably had repeatedly normal urinary assays for catecholamines and their metabolites. None of the drugs administered are known to suppress significantly the levels of excreted catecholamines or their metabolites, nor are the drugs known to interfere with any of the assays (methyldopa was not being administered when the catecholamines were quantitated). It is conceivable that the tumor was not secreting at the time urine was collected and when the blood pressure was relatively normal. Also, one might speculate that on May 21, 1975, when the blood pressure was at least somewhat elevated, the marked degree of renal insufficiency might have diminished the excretion of the total metanephrines and the catecholamines as well as the creatinine; however, we have no solid evidence to support this speculation.

Whatever the reason for the repeatedly normal urinary assays for the catecholamines and their metabolites, one must conclude that if a patient is strongly suspected of having a pheochromocytoma, every means available, including plasma catecholamine analysis (with central venous blood sampling) and extensive radiographic studies, may have to be used as an aid in establishing or excluding a diagnosis of this treacherous tumor. The performance of a provocative test during 1970 or the following years (performed, of course, when the patient was not in a precarious or terminal state, and with appropriate plasma and urine collection for catecholamine or metabolite assay), might have established the diagnosis of pheochromocytoma.

MAJOR COMPLAINTS AND FINDINGS AMONG PATIENTS WITH PHEOCHROMOCYTOMA

In our series, 21 patients presented with sustained, and 17 with paroxysmal, hypertension. There were 22 males and 16 females, with an age range from seven to 69 years. Only three were black. Because of the extraordinary interest and unusual findings in pa-

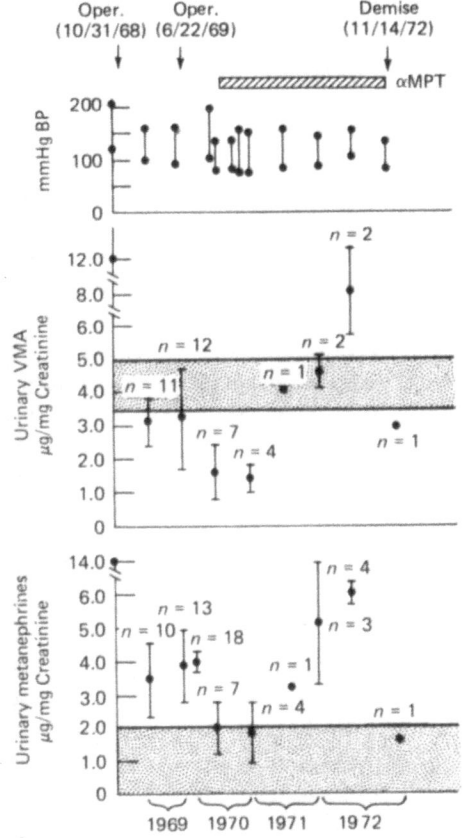

Fig. 7.1 Data on patient (No. 19) who developed 15 benign pheochromocytomas. A. Course of blood pressure and urinary catecholamine metabolites. B. Location of pheochromocytomas removed at the first operation (11/8/68). C. Effect of oral glucose tolerance test on blood glucose and growth hormone. (Normal basal serum growth hormone level is usually 15 µg/ml. In the normal subject growth hormone secretion is suppressed by elevation of the blood glucose whereas no suppression occurs in the acromegalic.) From Cobin, R., Pertsemlidis, D., Gitlow, S., and Krieger, D., *Am. J. Med.*, in press.

tient No. 19, this case is reported in considerable detail. This patient had the greatest number of pheochromocytomas ever reported, and in addition had a pituitary adenoma and parathyroid hyperplasia. The association of multiple benign pheochromocytomas and a pituitary tumor in this patient is particularly intriguing, since, as mentioned earlier, pheochromocytomas have been produced experimentally in rats by the chronic administration of growth hormone (675).

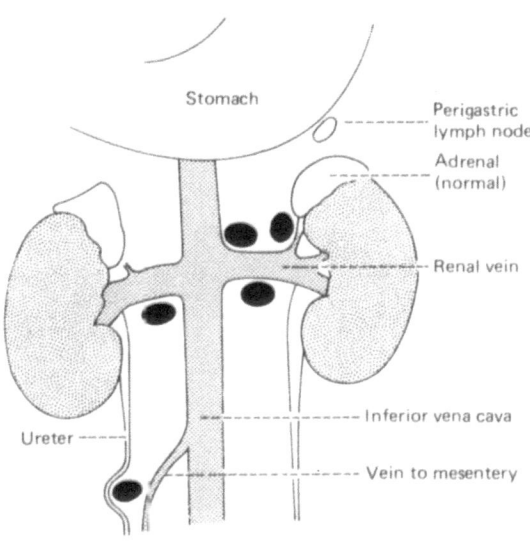

BLOOD PRESSURE AND CATECHOLAMINE CONCENTRATION IN PLASMA AND TUMORS OF PATIENTS WITH PHEOCHROMOCYTOMA

Figures 7.2 and 7.3 display the blood pressures and catecholamine concentrations in the plasma and tumors* of the patients with pheochromocytoma and sustained or paroxysmal hypertension just described under "Case Reports." The age, sex, and race of these patients are indicated; weights and locations of tumors are also included. The studies on the patients with paroxysmal hypertension were performed when paroxysms were absent and blood pressure was normal or minimally elevated. We have recently presented a preliminary report on the correlation between plasma and tumor catecholamines and blood pressure in 38 patients with pheochromocytoma (617a).

It is immediately evident that there is no close correlation between the levels of systolic or diastolic blood pressures and the concentrations of plasma catecholamines when patients are compared with each other. A reasonable correlation between blood pressures and plasma catecholamine concentrations was sometimes observed in the individual patient when samples were obtained on different days (patients No. 7, 10, 13, 25, 27, and 28), although this was not invariably so (patients No. 12, 15, and 22). The lack of correlation between blood pressures and plasma catecholamine concentrations when patients are compared with each other is not surprising, since the responsiveness of the cardiovascular system to circulating catecholamines is dependent on many factors, and varies widely from one patient to the next. For example, factors such as (a) the rate of catecholamine inactivation (by uptake mechanisms and enzymatic degradation), (b) the extent to which these amines

* The procedure which we usually used for preparing extracts of pheochromocytomas for the fluorometric determination of the catecholamines has been described elsewhere (624). The catecholamine concentrations in most of these tumors were also assayed by the method of paper chromotography (employing Whatman No. 4 Chromatographic paper and 75 percent phenol as the solvent; spraying with potassium ferricyanide permitted visual localization and quantitation of the catecholamines). Similar values obtained by the two methods lend support to the specificity of the fluorometric method.

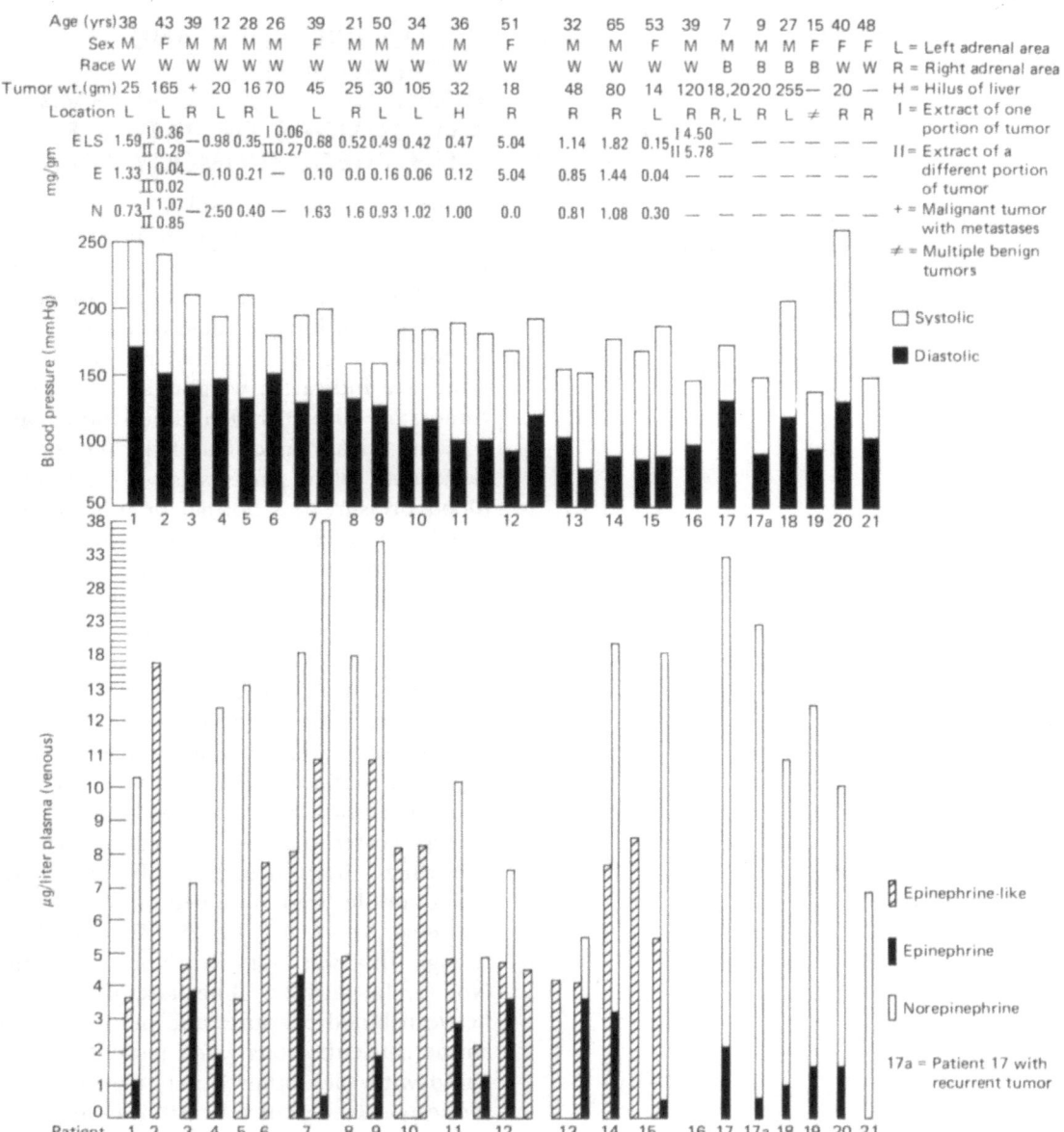

Fig. 7.2 Blood pressure and catecholamine concentrations in plasma and tumors of patients with pheochromocytoma and sustained hypertension. Note: In order to represent the total plasma catecholamine concentration the "clear" bar representing norepinephrine begins where the "black" bar, representing epinephrine ends (i.e., the concentration of norepinephrine would equal the total concentration minus the concentration of epinephrine). Upper limit of normal catecholamine concentrations: epinephrine-like substance (ELS) = 3.5 μg/liter, or less; epinephrine (E) = 1.3 μg/liter, or less; norepinephrine (N) = 6.3 μg/liter, or less.

diffuse and reach target cells (i.e., myocardial and vascular smooth muscle cells), (c) the inherent reactivity of myocardial and smooth muscle cells, and (d) the sensitivity of the baroreceptors are all involved in determining the magnitude of the blood pressure response resulting from activation of the adrenergic system and/or increased levels of circulating catecholamines. The age of the patient, the degree of atherosclerosis, and the severity and duration of hypertension (if present) may importantly influence some of these factors. Atherosclerosis can diminish the sensitivity of the baroreceptors (671), whereas hypertension can cause hypertrophy of the media of arterial resistance vessels (i.e., increase the wall-

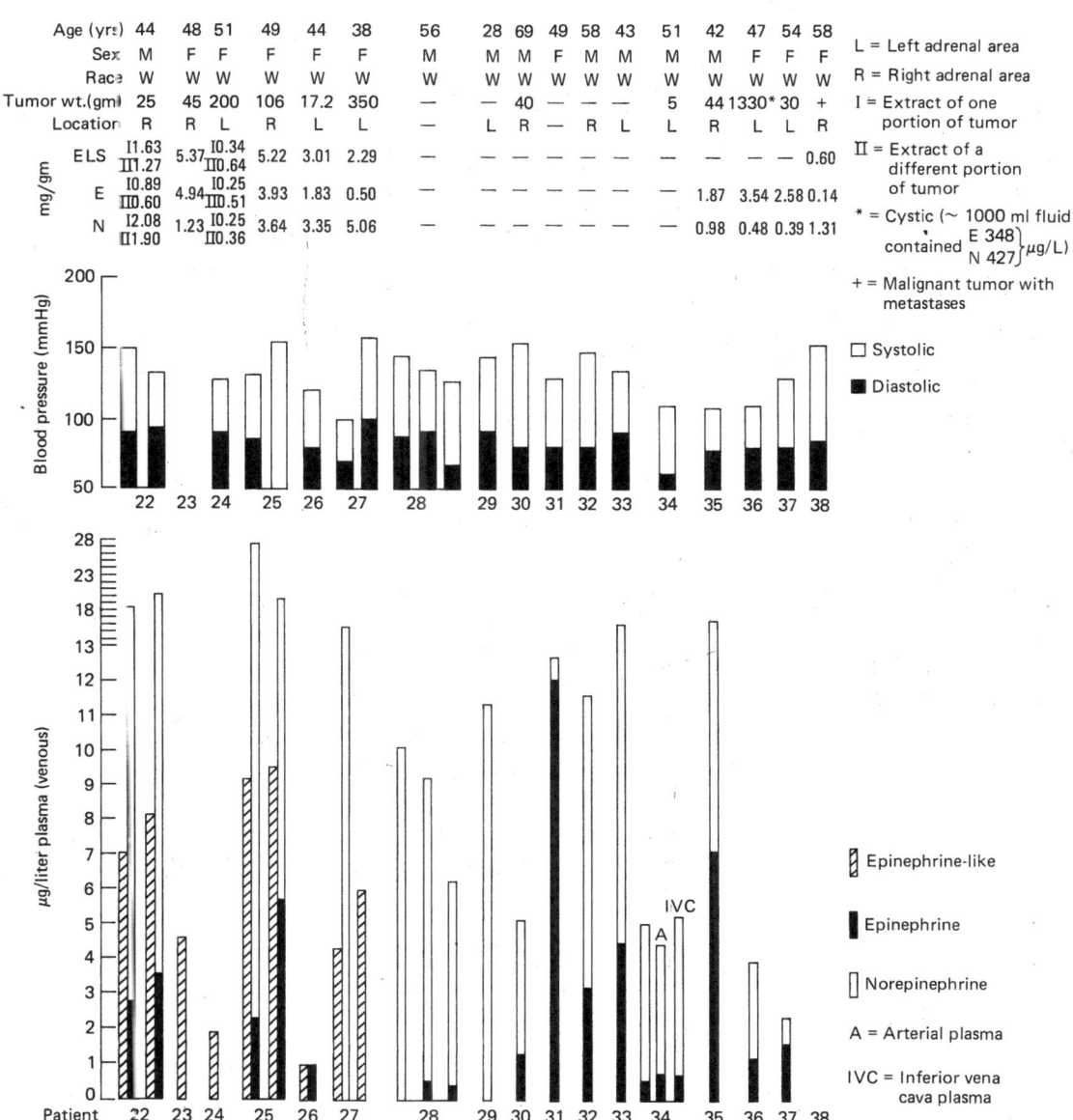

Fig. 7.3 Blood pressure and catecholamine concentrations in plasma and tumors of patients with pheochromocytoma and paroxysmal hypertension. (Patient studied when paroxysm was absent). Note: In order to represent the total plasma catecholamine concentration the "clear" bar representing norepinephrine begins where the "black" bar, representing epinephrine ends (i.e., the concentration of norepinephrine would equal the total concentration minus the concentration of epinephrine). Upper limit of normal catecholamine concentrations: epinephrine-like substance (ELS) = 3.5 μg/liter, or less; epinephrine (E) = 1.3 μg/liter, or less; norepinephrine (N) = 6.3 μg/liter, or less.

to-lumen ratio), and thereby enhance the blood pressure responsiveness to increased circulating catecholamines (321).

Recently we have shown that the variability and magnitude of the blood pressure response to infused norepinephrine in normotensive and hypertensive subjects was not correlated with the concentrations of plasma norepinephrine in the arterial blood (617). In fact, we suggested that hyperresponsiveness, at least in some of our patients with essential hypertension, was perhaps best explained by the hemodynamic response of structurally altered vessels, namely, an increased wall-to-lumen ratio, as proposed by Folkow (321).

Major Complaints and Findings among Patients with Pheochromocytoma

Patient No.[a]	Age in years, sex, race	Relevant history and major symptoms	Ophthalmoscopic findings[b]	Preoperative Laboratory Data			Urinary catecholamines[f] (μg/24 hr) and metabolites (mg/24 hr)
				BMR[c] (%)	Blood glucose[d] (mg/dl)	Blood urea[e] (mg/dl)	
1	38 ♂ W	Exertional dyspnea 18 months, headaches 14 months, hypertension known 12 months, blurred vision 6 months.	IV	+39	—	24	—
2	43 ♀ W	For 2 years: diminished vision, headaches, hypertension known, tachycardia, nervousness, wt. loss.	IV	+27	142	28	—
3	39 ♂ W	Thyroidectomy 8 years before examination because of enlarged thyroid, palpitations and nervousness but BMR = −6 preoperatively. Diabetes mellitus (moderately severe) 3 years. For 8 months, headaches and hypertension known, failing vision, 6 weeks.	IV	+49	358 256 238	26	—
4	12 ♂ W	Headaches, hypertension known 5 months, nosebleeds, easy sweating, and weight loss 3 months. One convulsion with high BP(190/150), tachycardia (172), and twitching left arm and leg 2 months before examination.	IV	+9	—	22	—
5	28 ♂ W	For 3.5 years: diminished vision, headaches, hypertension known, "jittery" feelings, easy sweating.	III	+21 +6 +6	107 109	24 38	—
6	26 ♂ W	For 5 months: headaches, easy sweating, palpitations, hypertension known.	IV	+13 +24	130 151	30 40	—
7	39 ♀ W	Attacks of sweating, headache, palpitation, shakiness, vomiting, wt. loss, blurring vision, fluctuating BP for 3.5 years. Attacks sometimes precipitated by quick movement of body.	III	+50	173	—	—
8	21 ♂ W	Hypertension known 12 years, cerebrovascular accident with hemiplegia and hemianopsia; pheochromocytoma and metastatic rib lesion removed 3 years before examination. For 1.5 years: "weak spells," excess sweating, headaches, epigastric discomfort.	II	+36 +20	111	20	—
9	50 ♂ W	Severe hypertension and recurrent episodes of nausea, vomiting, headaches, palpitation, sweating for 4 years. Bilateral thoracolumbar sympathectomy 3.5 years before examination: hypertension poorly controlled with antihypertensive treatment. Acrocyanosis noted.	II	—	—	44	—

Case	Age/Sex/Race	Clinical data					
10	34 ♂ W	Hypertension known since age 18. Used to have headaches but none for 10 years. Rejected by army at age 22 because of enlarged heart. Recently heart failure with nocturnal dyspnea and pink frothy sputum. Receiving antihypertensive medication.	I	+42 +39	115	26	—
11	36 ♂ W	Headaches 5 weeks, hypertension known 2 weeks.	Normal	+18	125	44 26	—
12	51 ♀ W	Chronic cholecystitis and mild hypertension 13 years before examination. Trembling, palpitation, weakness, pallor, headaches, intermittently 2.5 years. Occasional nausea and vomiting. (Cholecystectomy performed when pheochromocytoma removed.)	I	+3	190 153	30	—
13	32 ♂ W	Recurrent episodes of palpitation, dyspnea, weakness, headaches for 1.5 years. Several attacks of pulmonary edema. Has von Recklinghausen's disease and coronary sclerosis.	II	+28	135	26	—
14	65 ♂ W	For 1 year mentally depressed and nervous. Hypertension known 3–4 months. For 6 weeks, headaches, apprehension, dyspnea, perspiration, and palpitation. Myocardial infarct 3 years before examination with residual angina; duodenal ulcer on x-ray.	II	+23	113	42	—
15	53 ♀ W	Increased perspiration, heat intolerance, and weight loss for 2 years. 18 months ago BMR +27.	Normal	+86 +63 +66	115	—	—
16	39 ♂ W	For 3 years: epigastric pressure sensations extending to chest and throat. For 2 years: episodes of headache, shaking, pallor, slowing of pulse, and hypertension known.	I	+4	135	—	—
17	7 ♂ B	For 6 months: night sweats, 17 lb. weight loss, and cough. 5 months: polyuria and abdominal pain. 2.5 months: daily vomiting, fatigue, and headaches with sustained hypertension (up to 210/170) and heart rate 158. WBC 17,400, ESR 75, ECG T inverted in I, aVL, V1–V6. Retroperitoneal pneumogram (frontal and oblique views) showed enlarged right and left adrenals. Bilateral adrenal pheochromocytomas extirpated; placed on adrenal replacement therapy. Postoperative BP and lab studies normal.	Normal	—	112	17	NE 5690 E 876
17a	9 ♂ B	20 months after pheochromocytomas removed, returned with hypertension, intermittent headaches, and diaphoresis. WBC 19,000, ESR 62. Radiographic studies normal and pheochromocytoma localized by central venous sampling and extirpated from right adrenal area. Postoperative BP and lab studies normal; currently well at age 19.5.	Normal	—	105	29	NE 1726, 1322 E 0, 10

Major Complaints and Findings among Patients with Pheochromocytoma

Patient No.[a]	Age in years, sex, race	Relevant history and major symptoms	Ophthalmoscopic findings[b]	Preoperative Laboratory Data			Urinary catecholamines[f] (μg/24 hr) and metabolites (mg/24 hr)
				BMR[c] (%)	Blood glucose[d] (mg/dl)	Blood urea[e] (mg/dl)	
18	27 ♂ B	1–2 months: daily frontal headaches and hypertension (230/160). BP poorly controlled with antihypertensives. ECG: P-wave abnormalities; flat T waves II, III, aVF V5–V6. Rate 93. Cardiac catheterization: pulmonary artery pressure increased (23/12) and cardiac output increased (7.2 liters/min). Radiographic studies: IVP normal. Aortogram: normal renal arteries (during procedure BP decreased to 160/130 and pulse increased to 140). Nephrotomograms showed left suprarenal mass which was extirpated and postoperative BP normal.	III	—	108	22	E 94, 464, 60 NE 1166, 1775, 900 VMA 32, 50
19	15 ♀ B	[Data provided through courtesy of Drs. R. Cobin, D. Pertsemlidis, S. Gitlow, and D. Krieger (160a)]. Oct. 1968 (age 15): Right flank pain 3 days. [3 years prior back pain and dysuria transiently; and hypertension detected plus hyperpigmentation = incontinentia pigmenti (since birth) and spotty retinal depigmentation (flecked retina syndrome).] IVP normal. Urinary catecholamine metabolites elevated (course of BP and urinary catecholamine metabolites are recorded in Fig. 7.1A), serum cholesterol elevated (350 mg/dl), serum β-lipoprotein elevated and serum calcium variable (12, 11, and 9.8 mg/dl), alkaline phosphatase (80–220 IU/100 ml), serum parathormone normal. IVP revealed lateral displacement of proximal right ureter. x-Rays of chest, skeleton, skull negative. ECG normal. 5 benign (encapsulated) extraadrenal para-aortic pheochromocytomas (see Fig. 7.1B) were removed from abdomen. Shortly postoperative developed "dizziness," palpitations, and mild hypertension with orthostatic hypotension (70/50) and increased metanephrine but normal VMA. June 1969: right anterior chest pain and 3-cm mass seen in right superior mediastinum. Provocative tests with histamine and phentolamine test negative. Plasma E = 1.5 and NE = 11 μg/liter (both elevated). Benign mediastinal pheochromocytoma removed but no fall in BP. Nov. 1969: plasma catecholamine concentrations in blood obtained	Flecked retina, normal arteries	—	110	9	See Fig. 7.1

No.	Age/Sex/Race	Clinical features	ECG	BMR	BP		Catecholamines
10	34 ♂ W	Hypertension known since age 18. Used to have headaches but none for 10 years. Rejected by army at age 22 because of enlarged heart. Recently heart failure with nocturnal dyspnea and pink frothy sputum. Receiving antihypertensive medication.	I	+42 +39	115	26	—
11	36 ♂ W	Headaches 5 weeks, hypertension known 2 weeks.	Normal	+18	125	44 26	—
12	51 ♀ W	Chronic cholecystitis and mild hypertension 13 years before examination. Trembling, palpitation, weakness, pallor, headaches, intermittently 2.5 years. Occasional nausea and vomiting. (Cholecystectomy performed when pheochromocytoma removed.)	I	+3	190 153	30	—
13	32 ♂ W	Recurrent episodes of palpitation, dyspnea, weakness, headaches for 1.5 years. Several attacks of pulmonary edema. Has von Recklinghausen's disease and coronary sclerosis.	II	+28	135	26	—
14	65 ♂ W	For 1 year mentally depressed and nervous. Hypertension known 3–4 months. For 6 weeks, headaches, apprehension, dyspnea, perspiration, and palpitation. Myocardial infarct 3 years before examination with residual angina; duodenal ulcer on x-ray.	II	+23	113	42	—
15	53 ♀ W	Increased perspiration, heat intolerance, and weight loss for 2 years. 18 months ago BMR +27.	Normal	+86 +63 +66	115	—	—
16	39 ♂ W	For 3 years: epigastric pressure sensations extending to chest and throat. For 2 years: episodes of headache, shaking, pallor, slowing of pulse, and hypertension known.	I	+4	135	—	—
17	7 ♂ B	For 6 months: night sweats, 17 lb. weight loss, and cough. 5 months: polyuria and abdominal pain. 2.5 months: daily vomiting, fatigue, and headaches with sustained hypertension (up to 210/170) and heart rate 158. WBC 17,400, ESR 75, ECG T inverted in I, aVL, V1–V6. Retroperitoneal pneumogram (frontal and oblique views) showed enlarged right and left adrenals. Bilateral adrenal pheochromocytomas extirpated; placed on adrenal replacement therapy. Postoperative BP and lab studies normal.	Normal	—	112	17	NE 5690 E 876
17a	9 ♂ B	20 months after pheochromocytomas removed, returned with hypertension, intermittent headaches, and diaphoresis. WBC 19,000, ESR 62. Radiographic studies normal and pheochromocytoma localized by central venous sampling and extirpated from right adrenal area. Postoperative BP and lab studies normal; currently well at age 19.5.	Normal	—	105	29	NE 1726, 1822 E 0, 10

Major Complaints and Findings among Patients with Pheochromocytoma

vascular sinusoids (Zellballen pattern). Tumors were encapsulated by fibrous tissue but in some areas tumor cells had penetrated capsule and occasionally tumor cells replaced adjacent ganglion cells. (b) Pituitary adenoma (mixed chromophobe with predominantly acidophilic cells) about 2 cm diameter. (c) 3 parathyroids found—all hyperplastic mostly chief cells, nests of oxyphilic and water clear cells. (d) Ovaries—hyperplastic and multiple small follicular cysts. (e) Gastric ulcer 1.2 cm. (Combination of multi-extraadrenal pheochromocytoma, pituitary adenoma, and parathyroid hyperplasia has not been reported previously.) Note: This patient had the greatest number of benign tumors (15!) ever reported.

Patient No.[a]	Age in years, sex, race	Relevant history and major symptoms	Ophthalmoscopic findings[b]	Preoperative Laboratory Data			Urinary catecholamines[f] (μg/24 hr) and metabolites (mg/24 hr)
				BMR[c] (%)	Blood glucose[a] (mg/dl)	Blood urea[e] (mg/dl)	
20	40 ♀ W	1 year previously discovered to have severe hypertension (220/115) and right renal arterial graft performed because of moderate stenosis. Bilateral renal biopsies revealed nephrosclerosis. Hypertension persisted (220/100–240/130) and for past year experienced episodes of feeling hot, pounding in epigastrium, pulsating headaches, sweating on chest, tremor, anxiety, weakness. Also noted blurred vision and orthostatic hypotension occurred on several occasions. To and fro murmur heard in right neck. ECG: prominent U waves (interpreted as myocardial disease or electrolyte imbalance) and inferior lateral T-wave abnormalities. Phentolamine test positive (BP decreased from 220/120 to 150/70). Serum cholesterol: 356 mg/dl (normal up to 300 mg/dl). Radiographic studies: IVP—marked shrinkage of right kidney and compensatory hypertrophy of left. Renal arteriograms—practically no blood supply to right kidney, only collateral circulation. Stereoscopic, posterior, lateral, and oblique chest x-rays negative. Arteriogram (via brachial artery) of right internal carotid showed stenosis over several mm to ⅓ of normal diameter. Good filling of interior jugular vein. No abnormalities of jugular fossa or intracranial vessels.	II	—	99 100 156	10	Pheoscreen + NE 252 E 135 VMA 9.7, Metanephrine 3.5

	Age/Sex/Race	Clinical					Laboratory
21	48 ♀ W	Pheochromocytoma (3 cm diameter weighing 20 g) extirpated from right adrenal area along with infarcted right kidney. Postoperative BP 160/110–180/110 and pheochromocytoma screening test negative, ECG normal (no more U waves or T-wave abnormalities); serum cholesterol 306 and 246 mg/dl, 1 week and 7.5 months postoperative, respectively. Because of memory impairment, speech substitution and episodes of feeling faint and numbness in left hand, a medium-sized fibroatheromatous placque was removed from right internal carotid about 7.5 months after pheochromocytoma extirpated.	I	—	Variable 81 to 200	16	CA 1592, 256, 345 Total metanephrines 1.3, 4.3, 3.7, 3.8, 3.9 VMA 7.3, 8.2 Pheoscreen 1 + 1 −
		Life-long anxiety and labile hypertension with palpitations 8 years. 20 years ago: cholecystectomy for cholelithiasis. 3 years ago: work up for hypertension revealed 3 negative pheochromocytoma screening tests and negative IVP except for calcified stone in urethral diverticulum. Plasma renin activity was elevated, aldosterone normal. Treated with antihypertensives and estrogens several years but continued to experience emotional and BP lability and palpitations. BP 180/90–200/110. WBC 12,600. Glucose tolerance curve diabetic, uric acid 7.7 mg/dl (postoperative: 5.9). ECG: sinus bradycardia 52/min. LAD: some flat T waves and ST depression and diffuse U waves. Radiology: IVP normal. Abdominal aortography demonstrated neovascularity in right adrenal mass 4.5 cm diameter. When BP 150/103 plasma norepinephrine was elevated (7.2 μg/liter) on one occasion but normal on another (5.9 μg/liter). Epinephrine was within normal range. Pheochromocytoma with right adrenal extirpated and postoperative BP initially 160/110 normalized to 120/68 several days later.					
22	44 ♂ W	Headaches 2 years, accompanied for 2–3 months by sweating, palpitation, tachycardia, scotoma, nausea, vomiting, paroxysmal hypertension, weight loss. Symptoms aggravated by "desensitization" treatment with intravenous and subcutaneous histamine. Electroencephalogram evidenced left temporal abnormality.	II	—	115	22	—
23	48 ♀ W	For 7 years: hypertensive attacks with palpitation, dyspnea, cephalgia, nausea, vomiting, pallor, easy sweating, trembling, salivation.	I	+20	125	28	—

Major Complaints and Findings among Patients with Pheochromocytoma

Patient No.[a]	Age in years, sex, race	Relevant history and major symptoms	Ophthalmoscopic findings[b]	Preoperative Laboratory Data			Urinary catecholamines[f] (μg/24 hr) and metabolites (mg/24 hr)
				BMR[c] (%)	Blood glucose[d] (mg/dl)	Blood urea[e] (mg/dl)	
24	51 ♀ W	Hypertensive attacks, with headache, 4.5 months. Questionable myocardial infarction 1.5 years ago. For 4 months, easy sweating, weakness, weight loss.	Retinal hemorrhages possibly due to malnutrition	+21	198 226	—	—
25	49 ♀ W	Recurrent episodes of constriction in throat, palpitation, headache, sweating, for 2.5 years. Exertional dyspnea 6 months. Hypertension known 1 month. Firm round mass right hypochondrium and chronic cholecystitis. (Cholecystectomy performed when pheochromocytoma removed.)	I	+33	158 103	26	—
26	44 ♀ W	For 1 year: headache accompanied sometimes by black spots before eyes, unsteady gait, and hypertension known.	Normal	+2	100	—	—
27	38 ♀ W	Headaches 11 years, sometimes associated with sweating, tachycardia, vomiting, and hypertension. Left kidney easily palpable, and questionable left adrenal mass on x-ray.	Normal	−2	95	12 22	—
28	51 ♂ W	1958: recurrent episodes of hypertension, usually lasting several minutes and occurring up to 6 ×/day for 1 year. Sometimes associated with flushed face and facial warmth, pain in back of head, anxiety, apprehension, palpitations, transitory diminution of vision, numbness left side of face but no sweating. Severity of symptoms was correlated with height of BP elevation. Usually felt exhausted for 1 hr following attack. One attack occurred during palpation of abdomen and hyperventilation. BP rose to 200/100 and returned to 120/80. Carotid sinus pressure, neck pressure, or neck flexion sometimes increased BP. Gave history of migraine; also family history of hypertension and migraine. Lab: cholesterol 189 mg/dl, phospholipids 238 mg/dl, free fatty acids 358	I	+5	84	44	Bioassay for pressor substance in urine sometimes − sometimes +

mg/dl; and total lipids 747 mg/dl, 5-hydroxyindole acetic acid, uroporphyrin, and porphobilinogen all normal. Serum creatinine 1.8 mg/dl.

ECG rate varied 75–40/min; low amplitude QRS; minor T-wave abnormalities; Q waves III and aVF showed old posterior wall infarct. Bradycardia always observed during attacks; sometimes arrhythmias with 1st, 2nd, 3rd degree heart block, ventricular escape beats.

Radiographic studies: cervical spine hypertrophic changes C5, 6 and 7 with narrowed interspace between C6 and C7, chest normal. IVP and adrenal laminography normal.

One histamine test for pheochromocytoma negative and plasma catecholamines high normal. Subsequently, attacks provoked by IV histamine, norepinephrine, epinephrine, serotonin, angiotensin II, aramine, tetraethylammonium chloride. BP elevation reversed by Benzodioxone.

Found to be marked vascular hyperreactor (basal BP 136/86 increased to 215/150 with cold pressor test; 0.05 mg histamine I.V. caused BP increase from 140/90 to 172/114).

Antihypertensive therapy not beneficial but phenoxybenzamine reduced severity and frequency of attacks.

1959: symptoms continued.

1961: recurrent hypertensive paroxysms continued (sometimes induced by massaging back of neck) but less severe and less frequent. Developed anginal chest pain but did not occur during paroxysm. BP supine 140/84; standing 134/82. Aortic systolic murmur grade I. One histamine test was positive and one negative.

ECG as previously reported but shortly after being evaluated anteroseptal infarct noted and angina experienced on exertion, excitement, emotion, and at rest. Exertional dyspnea and ankle swelling noted.

1963: paroxysms continued but less when taking phenoxybenzamine, BP 134/82 supine, 126/87 standing. Two spontaneous episodes with BP to 170/105 noted during evaluation.

IVP and laminograms of adrenal areas normal. Chest x-rays normal.

Peripheral plasma catecholamines were elevated and diagnosis of pheochromocytoma appeared established but patient did not return for surgical exploration.

CA, 356, 660, 540

Slight VMA and normetanephrine elevations after histamine

Major Complaints and Findings among Patients with Pheochromocytoma

Patient No.[a]	Age in years, sex, race	Relevant history and major symptoms	Ophthalmoscopic findings[b]	Preoperative Laboratory Data			Urinary catecholamines[f] (µg/24 hr) and metabolites (mg/24 hr)
				BMR[c] (%)	Blood glucose[d] (mg/dl)	Blood urea[e] (mg/dl)	
29	28 ♂ W	1 year: hypertension 145/100, mild headaches, and excessive perspiration only with exercise, which he had always noted. Grade I/VI systolic murmur heard at left sternal border. 5 histamine tests performed on different dates were unremarkable, as were a glucagon and a tyramine test. Slightly abnormal glucose tolerance; plasma volume markedly diminished (2750 ml). Radiographic studies: IVP normal and renal arteriography unremarkable except for marked rise in BP during the procedure. Pheochromocytoma of left adrenal gland extirpated (some tumor cells noted invading adrenal vein) and left renal biopsy performed (no renal pathology noted). Since tumor removal, he has remained asymptomatic with a normal BP (120/80). Prior to operation orthostatic hypotension to tilt had been noted but this reaction disappeared postoperatively. Valsalva overshoot was greater postoperatively than preoperatively.	Normal	—3	101	36	CA in quinidine units 4.27, 1.76, 2.64, 4.28, 2.08, 4.98 (Normal ≤ 2.2 QU/24 hr) Total metanephrines 4.46, 5.11, 5.37, 4.15, 4.1 VMA, 8.0, 13, 15, 16, 7.1, 12
30	69 ♂ W	Discovered to have hypertension 6 months before admission. BP normalized on antihypertensive medication discontinued later. Intermittent forceful thumping in chest associated with substernal pressure developed 2 months later. These episodes recurred repeatedly and were often associated with light headedness, and on one occasion syncope occurred. While visiting his wife in hospital, he experienced nausea, substernal pain and palpitations; BP was 130/80 with regular pulse 140/min. ECG during recurrence of symptoms revealed sinus bradycardia with A-V dissociation and slow "nodal" junctional rhythm whereupon he was immediately admitted to coronary care unit with presumptive diagnosis of acute myocardial infarction. Physical examination was unremarkable on admission except for pulse of 110/min, soft apical systolic murmur, minimal retinal arteriolar narrowing, and	I	—	200 108	16	CA, 424, 312 Total metanephrine elevated MHPG elevated

pale (but dry) skin. BP was 140/80 mmHg. Lab findings were normal except for WBC of 12,000 and reduced plasma volume of 37 ml/kg (normal 45 ± 10 ml) and whole blood volume of 63 ml/kg (normal 70 ± 15 ml). During normotension, between attacks, cardiac index was 1.80 liters/min/m² and peripheral vascular resistance was 2000 dynes-sec-cm⁻⁵. Plasma catecholamines before and during attack (at which time only marked increase of epinephrine occurred) are indicated in Table 6.5, Case 1. A complete cycle of hypertension, A-V dissociation and return to normotension and regular sinus rhythm required 7 to 10 min (see Fig. 6.4). Attacks varied in frequency and were occasionally correlated with emotional stimulation.

Subsequently, with anesthesia induction, BP rose to 262/105 mmHg and was accompanied by A-V dissociation. During laparotomy, manipulation of right adrenal gland caused similar response; a 40-g pheochromocytoma was excised from this gland following which BP fell to 70/50 mmHg; I.V. norepinephrine caused rise in BP to 200/100 with transient reappearance of A-V dissociation. Postoperatively has remained normotensive and well. Urine catecholamines in µg for 24 hr: postoperatively 126, normal <250. Total metanephrines and MHPG normal postoperatively.

2 year: fluctuating BP with hypertensive periods associated with headaches. BP varied 130/70 to 170/100; ECG normal.

Radiology: IVP and retrograde pyelogram revealed diffuse dilatation of ureter and blunting of calyces on right, perhaps secondary to pyelonephritis. Abdominal aortogram unremarkable except for tiny aneurysm in right renal artery; vena caval catheterization revealed elevated plasma epinephrine concentrations varying from 9.4 to 12 µg/liter at all levels without definite tumor localization; norepinephrine was not elevated. Operation not performed. BP controlled at about 140/90 on medication up to present time.

In 1962 (several years postgastrectomy and shortly after vagectomy) noted palpitations and sweats ~45 min after eating. Thought to be related to postgastrectomy syndrome.

1963: abnormal glucose tolerance noted and treated with orinase or insulin.

31	49 ♀ W	I	—	75	20	CA 103, but elevated once; VMA 5.0, but elevated once
32	58 ♂ W	Normal	—	240 278	18	CA 54, 36, 73; VMA 10.8, 10, 21.6 (normal = 0–10 mg/24 hr)

Major Complaints and Findings among Patients with Pheochromocytoma

Patient No.[a]	Age in years, sex, race	Relevant history and major symptoms	Ophthalmoscopic findings[b]	Preoperative Laboratory Data			Urinary catecholamines[f] (μg/24 hr) and metabolites (mg/24 hr)
				BMR[c] (%)	Blood glucose[d] (mg/dl)	Blood urea[e] (mg/dl)	
		1964: noted transient spontaneous hypertensive attacks, also induced by left upper abdominal massage. VMA slightly elevated but histamine provocative test negative and selective arteriography of renal and pancreatic areas negative. I.V. tolbutamide test positive for diabetes. 1967: began complaining of intermittent attacks of palpitations with strong, slow heart beat, weakness, sweating, facial pallor, head and chest pressure, abdominal cramps, bitter taste in mouth. BP 180/70; pulse (62/min regular) grade 1/4 systolic murmur, loudest at pulmonic area. Multiple, nontender, small, mobile tumors of arms, back, and abdomen; angiolipoma on biopsy (some members of family had similar subcutaneous lesions but no hypertension). Right abdominal massage caused marked increase in BP lasting 2–7 min. (Attacks could be induced by left or right upper abdominal massage.) ECG during attacks: runs of nodal escape following periods of sinus bradycardia, occasional APC's and transient appearance of very tall T waves in many leads (see Figs. 6.5 and 6.6). Radiographic studies: renal arteriography negative but nephrotomogram revealed rounded density overlying upper pole right kidney; retroperitoneal air insufflation revealed superior pole enlarged but no tumor. Massage of right upper abdomen caused BP to rise from 158/80 to 300/160 and E and NE to increase markedly (see Table 6.5, Case 2). Placed on oral phentolamine with moderate relief of symptoms. A lemon-size, encapsulated, cystic pheochromocytoma was removed from right adrenal area. Postoperative BP normal.					Normetanephrine normal on 2 occasions, elevated on 2 occasions Metanephrine normal on 3 occasions, elevated on 1 occasion
33	43 ♂ W	6-7 years: episodes of palpitations, diaphoresis, tremor, pallor, epigastric pressure sensation, dyspnea, cough, urge to defecate, flushed feeling, known to be associated with elevated BP for 1 month (to 300/180). Attacks frequently induced by physical exertion; occur spontaneously	I	—	168 160	23 29 25	3 Pheoscreens tested + VMA 36.3

	Age/Sex/Race	Clinical					
34	51 ♂ W	and last 5–10 min but generalized sweats may persist 2 hr. Spells usually 3–5×/day becoming slightly more frequent but less severe. Precordial systolic ejection murmur. ECG: periods of A-V dissociation. Prominent U waves. Diabetic glucose tolerance test, serum cholesterol 480 mg/dl, uric acid 8.5 mg/dl. Radiographic studies: nephrotomogram negative. Aortogram suggested left adrenal mass. Left adrenal phlebogram demonstrated golf ball size tumor mass left adrenal. BP 135/90 increased to 190/120 on simulating shoveling motion and plasma E and NE simultaneously increased from 4.4 and 11.6 to 6.5 and 15.5 µg/liter, respectively, and noted palpitations, dyspnea, and warm feeling. 5.3-cm tumor extirpated. Postoperative BP 100/72.	Normal	—	84 95 97 74	19	CA 67 VMA 2 to 2.5 (normal < 3) Total metanephrine 1.65 (normal < 2.2)
35	42 ♂ W	16–18 years: episodes (usually at breakfast time) of apprehension, tachycardia, marked pallor, diaphoresis, dyspnea, tightness in chest, feeling as if head "exploding," sensation of impending syncope, weakness, tremor, cold extremities, and occasional nausea. Attacks becoming more frequent and severe past few months (initially episodes occurred every 3 weeks but recently several times each day), often followed by sensation of flushing. Occasionally spells precipitated by leaning forcefully on elevated left arm. Spells generally subside in 2–5 min. BP usually 110/70, pulse 80/min but during attack BP to 150/80 and 180/90 with slowing of pulse (74 to 56/min). (Recalls receiving E injection for allergy many years ago which caused somewhat similar symptoms to present attacks.) ECG normal except for rare PVC's. Serum cholesterol 248–295 mg/dl (normal < 275). Radiographic studies: IVP, abdominal and thoracic aortograms with good visualization of kidneys were negative. Histamine provocative test was positive, increasing BP from 120/60 to 215/110 and causing very severe headache, palpitation, and sweating. Phentolamine promptly caused marked and sustained BP reduction (a positive pharmacologic test for pheochromocytoma). Plasma catecholamines, initially normal, became significantly elevated after histamine I.V. and diagnosis of pheochromocytoma was established. A 5 g, 1.8 cm pheochromocytoma was extirpated from left adrenal. Postoperative BP 120/60–140/100. Remains well 6 years postoperative.	Normal except few hemor-	—	Variable 88 to 180	55 to 13	CA 926, 401 VMA 38, 18 Metanephrines

Major Complaints and Findings among Patients with Pheochromocytoma

Patient No.[a]	Age in years, sex, race	Relevant history and major symptoms	Ophthalmoscopic findings[b]	Preoperative Laboratory Data			Urinary catecholamines[f] and metabolites (μg/24 hr) (mg/24 hr)
				BMR[c] (%)	Blood glucose[a] (mg/dl)	Blood urea[e] (mg/dl)	
		tomograms and renal arteriograms) normal. Right-sided pheochromocytoma, localized in adrenal area by central venous blood sampling, extirpated. Postoperative BP normal.	rhages left fundus				19 Pheoscreen 2+
36	47 ♀ W	6 years: labile BP (54/? to 300/90) with attacks. 1 year ago: chest pain, palpitations, diaphoresis. ECG: prominent P wave, and Q waves in I, III, aVF, V1–V4 but only T waves abnormal 4 days later; with enzyme changes. 4 years ago: circumflex coronary artery stenosis 50–60% noted.

5–6 years: episodes of BP with throbbing headaches, palpitations, pallor, weakness, apprehension, diaphoresis, paresthesias, wt. loss, nausea, vomiting, sneezing. Attacks sometimes induced by standing or rolling on right side. Lab: diabetic glucose tolerance; periodic glycosuria 2.5 years.

ESR 72: WBC 12,000; creatinine, 2.8 reduced to 1.1 mg/dl (initially elevated BUN and creatinine ? due to poor renal perfusion during periods of hypotension). Serum cholesterol 306 mg/dl (normal < 255 mg/dl). Triglycerides 445 mg/dl (normal < 170 mg/dl), type IV pattern. Technetium thyroid scan showed slightly enlarged multinodular gland.

IVP, echogram, and arteriogram showed huge vascular cystic mass in left adrenal area. Extirpated along with spleen; kidney biopsied (only few sclerotic glomeruli seen with immunofluorescent glomeruli staining noted).

Spleen normal; cholelithiasis noted at operation. Postoperative BP normal.

Note: when BP normal, preoperative plasma catecholamines were normal (E = 1.1 and NE = 2.8 μg/liter), during operation they became elevated (E = 5.3 and NE = 7.3 μg/liter) with fairly stable BP but receiving phenoxybenzamine. | I | — | Variable 105–142 | 60 decreased to 16 | VMA 12.6, 22.2, 25.0 |
| 37 | 54 | Palpitations many years (worse 1.5 years): associated with weakness and | Normal | — | 110 | 20 | Pheoscreen |

38	58 ♀ W	Pheochromocytoma removed from right adrenal region 3 years before examination. Recurrence of symptoms (headache, palpitation, and warm feeling) for 4 months. Nausea and vomiting for 1 month.	I	120	+5	36	—

♀ W — tingling in extremities; spells lasted 10 min. BP 140/95–155/100; pulse 80/min. ECG: very high T waves in precordial and Leads I and II, later becoming flat; APC's, VPC's, occasional sinus tachycardia but generally bradycardia with periods of A-V dissociation and S-A arrest. Episodes of apparent Mobitz type II A-V block.

Abdominal ultrasonogram, IVP, nephrotomogram negative. Arteriogram showed tumor in left adrenal area; extirpated. Postoperative BP 150/80. — 107 — ? + Metanephrine 2.0, 1.3, 1.0 VMA 11.0, 9.5, 9.1

[a] Patients 1–21 had sustained hypertension and 22–38 had paroxysmal hypertension.

[b] Grouping according to Keith, Wagener, and Barker (504).

[c] BMR = basal metabolic rate.

[d] Normal blood glucose range in fasting state at Mayo Clinic = 80 to 120 mg/dl of blood.

[e] Normal blood urea range at Mayo Clinic = 10 to 40 mg/dl of blood.

[f] Normal urine values for catecholamines and metabolites (unless otherwise indicated):

CA = Catecholamines (total) = up to ∼135 μg/24 hr urine.

E = Epinephrine up to ∼25 μg/24 hr urine or less.

NE = Norepinephrine up to ∼100 μg/24 hr urine or less.

Total metanephrines (metanephrine + normetanephrine) = up to 0.9 mg/24 hr urine; 2.2 μg/mg creatinine.

VMA = up to 6.8 mg/24 hr urine; 3.5 μg or less/mg creatinine.

MHPG = 3-Methoxy-4-hydroxyphenylglycol = 1.8 mg/24 hr urine or less; 2.0 μg/mg creatinine.

Pheoscreen: positive (+) if metanephrine, VMA or phenylglycol are increased; negative (−) if metabolites not increased.

Note: In a number of cases no catecholamine or metabolite determinations were performed since these urinary assays were not available when some of these patients were examined.

[g] Normal serum cholesterol concentrations varied among laboratories.

Of paramount significance is the fact that, in all the patients with pheochromocytoma and sustained hypertension in whom plasma catecholamines were determined, the concentration of catecholamines was invariably elevated on one or more determinations. However, it is noteworthy that in one of three samples obtained from patient No. 12 the catecholamine concentration was within normal limits even when the blood pressure was 182/100 mmHg. This latter experience, although extremely unusual, emphasizes the importance of *repeating* any catecholamine assay yielding normal or borderline results in any patient suspected of harboring a pheochromocytoma, even if the blood sample was taken during a period of hypertension. In our experience, plasma catecholamine determinations in a patient with hypertension due to a functioning pheochromocytoma have been exceedingly reliable, if not foolproof, in detecting these tumors.

On the other hand, six out of 16 patients (37.5 percent) with pheochromocytoma but with blood pressures relatively normal (i.e., in the absence of a paroxysmal attack) when the blood was sampled, had plasma catecholamine concentrations within normal limits. This observation once again reemphasizes the crucial point that the presence of a pheochromocytoma in some of these patients can be detected only by determining plasma catecholamine concentrations in blood obtained during a paroxysmal attack, either occurring spontaneously or induced by a physical maneuver or by intravenous injection of a provocative drug.

It is also evident in Figures 7.2 and 7.3 that there was no good correlation between the size of the tumors or their contents of catecholamines, and the blood pressures of the patients harboring these tumors. Although the catecholamine concentrations varied somewhat when different parts of the same tumors were analyzed, the percentages of epinephrine and norepinephrine did not change very markedly. For example, in the three pheochromocytomas in which two different parts of the tumors were analyzed, the percentages of epinephrine varied from 2.3 to 3.6 percent in patient No. 2, from 24.0 to 30 percent in patient No. 22, and from 50 to 58.6 percent in patient No. 24. The concentrations of epinephrine-like substance in two different portions of the pheochromocytomas differed by about 24, 28, and 28 percent in the tumors of patients No. 2, 16, and 22, respectively. However, it is noteworthy that in patients No. 24 and 6 the difference in concentration of epinephrine-like substance in two portions analyzed was considerable, i.e., 88 and 350 percent respectively.

CORRELATION BETWEEN CATECHOLAMINES IN PHEOCHROMOCYTOMAS AND ELEVATIONS OF PLASMA CATECHOLAMINES DUE TO ACTIVELY SECRETING TUMORS

Of particular interest was a correlative analysis of the tumor and plasma concentrations of catecholamines. The correlation was considered "complete" if the catecholamine most concentrated in the tumor was also most elevated in the plasma, and the correlation was considered "partial" if the catecholamine most concentrated in the tumor was the only elevated catecholamine in the plasma. On the other hand, a "reverse" correlation was considered to exist if the catecholamine most concentrated in the tumor either was not elevated in the plasma or was elevated less than the other plasma catecholamine. Table 7.1 reveals that out of 11 patients with sustained hypertension, the correlation was "complete" in four, "partial" in three, and "reverse" in three; in patient No. 7 there was "complete" correlation on one occasion and "partial" on another day. A correlative analysis of seven patients with paroxysmal hypertension who had elevated plasma catecholamines revealed "complete" correlation in three, "partial" correlation in three, and "reverse" in one. [Note: the four patients in Figure 7.3, whose tumor and plasma concentrations of epinephrine and norepinephrine were determined and in whom the plasma catecholamines were elevated, were included in this correlative analysis. In addition, patient No. 36 (who had a greater elevation of plasma epinephrine than norepinephrine during laparotomy), patient No. 37 (who had only plasma epinephrine elevated during central venous catheterization), and patient No. 38 (who had only plasma norepinephrine elevated during a spontaneous hypertensive crisis) were also

Table 7.1 *Correlation between Catecholamines in Pheochromocytomas and Elevations of Plasma Catecholamines due to Actively Secreting Tumors*[a]

Patient	CA in tumor	Elevated plasma CA[b]	Correlation[c]
1 S	E $\gg$ NE	Only NE	Reverse
4 S	NE $\ggg$ E	NE $\gg$ E	Complete
5 S	NE $\gg$ E	Only NE	Partial
7 S	NE $\ggg$ E	NE $\gg$ E	Complete
		Only NE	Partial
8 S	Only NE	Only NE	Complete
9 S	NE $\ggg$ E	NE $\ggg$ E	Complete
11 S	NE $\ggg$ E	E $>$ NE	Reverse
12 S	Only E	Only E	Complete
13 S	E $>$ NE	Only E	Partial
14 S	E $\gg$ NE	NE $>$ E	Reverse
15 S	NE $\ggg$ E	Only NE	Partial
22 P	NE $\gg$ E	NE $>$ E	Complete
25 P	E $>$ NE	NE $\gg$ E	Reverse
27 P	NE $\ggg$ E	Only NE	Partial
35 P	E $\gg$ NE	E $\ggg$ NE	Complete
36 P	E $\ggg$ NE	E $\gg$ NE[d]	Complete
37 P	E $\ggg$ NE	Only E[e]	Partial
38 P	NE $\ggg$ E	Only NE[f]	Partial

[a] CA = catecholamines; E = epinephrine; NE = norepinephrine; $\ggg$ = markedly greater; $\gg$ = moderately greater; $>$ = slightly greater; S = sustained hypertension; P = paroxysmal hypertension.

[b] Elevated above upper limit of normal.

[c] Complete (7 patients) = catecholamine most concentrated in tumor was most elevated in plasma. Partial (6 patients) = catecholamine most concentrated in tumor was only elevated plasma catecholamine. Reverse (4 patients) = catecholamine most concentrated in tumor was not elevated or elevated $<$ other plasma catecholamine. Complete or partial (1 patient).

[d] Plasma catecholamines during laparotomy.

[e] Plasma catecholamines from left renal vein.

[f] Plasma catecholamines during spontaneous attack.

included in this correlative analysis which relates the concentration of tumor catecholamines to the catecholamines which they release into the circulation.]

The finding of only a "partial" or even "reverse" correlation between tumor and plasma catecholamine concentrations is intriguing, since it indicates that in about 61.1 percent of patients, whose pheochromocytomas are secreting at the time of blood sampling, the ratio of plasma catecholamines does not precisely reflect the ratio of the catecholamine content of the tumors. The conclusion must be drawn that secretion of one catecholamine from some of these tumors may occur selectively, while the other amine remains sequestered in the tumors. Hypothetically, in some tumors norepinephrine might

not be released but serve only as the precursor for epinephrine; however, we have no evidence to support this concept. On the other hand, it should be mentioned that Goldfien and coworkers (using essentially the same fluorometric assay which we employed) found high correlation between the proportions of epinephrine and norepinephrine in the plasma and pheochromocytoma of seven patients (382a).

The explanation for the lack of "complete" correlation between tumor catecholamine content and the elevations of these amines in the plasma of 61.1 percent of our patients with actively secreting tumors remains unclear. Despite our findings that analysis of different sites of a pheochromocytoma did not in general reveal marked variations in the percentage of epinephrine and norepinephrine concentration, it is conceivable that the samples of the tumor assayed were not always representative of the major portion of the tumor. It is interesting that two different patterns of tumor secretion occurred in patient No. 7, suggesting that in this pheochromocytoma the secretion of catecholamines did not represent a uniform discharge from the entire tumor. Equally interesting is the finding that, although 88 percent of the tumor catecholamines in patient No. 36 was epinephrine, and only epinephrine was elevated in the plasma obtained from the left renal vein, yet 55 percent of the catecholamine content of the cystic fluid was norepinephrine (norepinephrine $= 427$ μg/liter and epinephrine $= 347$ μg/liter). This paradoxical finding suggests that different portions of the same tumor may secrete significantly different proportions of the catecholamines.

We found no correlation between the tumor weight and the concentration of plasma catecholamines, a finding in keeping with the statement of Goodall and Stone that the amounts of catecholamines excreted in the urine had no relationship to the size of the pheochromocytomas in their patients (385). Hermann and Mornex have also indicated that in a number of case reports tumors contained high concentrations of catecholamines whereas urinary catecholamines were low; in other reports the reverse occurred (437, p 141).

Goodall and Stone found that the catecholamine content in the urine closely reflected the catecholamines present in the tumors, although the ratios of epinephrine to norepinephrine excreted varied markedly in several of their patients. Blaschko and coworkers performed biochemical studies on five patients with pheochromocytomas and found that in all but one there was no correlation between the ratios of epinephrine and norepinephrine in the tumors with these ratios in the urines (82). Of considerable interest was a study of 35 patients with pheochromocytoma reported by von Euler and Ström (299). Of the 17 tumors analyzed, all contained norepinephrine and 15 also contained epinephrine. Increased urinary excretion of norepinephrine was invariably found; however, epinephrine was not elevated in the urine of about one-third of patients whose tumors contained

both catecholamines. This latter finding is consistent with our observation that some tumors containing both epinephrine and norepinephrine may, at least on some occasions, release only one of these amines into the circulation.

ANALYSIS OF FINDINGS ON 38 PATIENTS WITH PHEOCHROMOCYTOMA

Table 7.2 reveals mean values of the data appearing in Figures 7.2 and 7.3. Approximately 55 percent of the tumors caused sustained hypertension; this occurred twice as often in males as in females. No sex predilection was evident in the patients with paroxysmal hypertension. Pheochromocytoma was encountered in only three blacks, all of whom had sustained hypertension. One of the black patients (No. 17 and 17a) was a boy who originally had had bilateral adrenal pheochromocytomas removed but who returned for removal of a recurrent tumor near the region of the right adrenal gland. The race distribution is probably not representative, since more than half of our patients were studied at the Mayo Clinic (where a relatively small segment of the patients examined were black) and none of these was black. In the New York area, 20 percent of our patients with pheochromocytoma were black, which suggests that there is no race predilection for this tumor (as judged by the racial distribution in the New York area, which has a black population of about 16 percent). Others have reported the incidence of pheochromocytoma in blacks as comparable to that in whites (155).

The mean age of male patients with paroxysmal hypertension was greater ($p < 0.025$) than that of those with sustained hypertension. This age difference was also true for the females but the difference was not statistically significant. When the mean age for the total group with sustained hypertension (35 ± 3 years) was compared with that for the total group with paroxysmal hypertension (49 ± 2 years), it was found that the difference was highly significant ($p < 0.005$). The greatest number of patients (seven) with sustained hypertension were in the fourth decade, whereas the greatest number of patients (eight) with paroxysmal hypertension were in

Table 7.2 *Mean Values of Data on Patients with Sustained and Paroxysmal Hypertension due to Pheochromocytoma Depicted in Figures 7.2 and 7.3*[a]

	Hypertension		p value for difference
	Sustained	Paroxysmal	
No. of patients (W = white; B = black)			
Total	21	17	
Male	14 (12W; 2B)	8 (8W; 0B)	
Female	7 (6W; 1B)	9 (9W; 0B)	
Age (years $\pm$ SE$_m$)			
Total	35 $\pm$ 3	49 $\pm$ 2	<0.005
Male	33 $\pm$ 4	49 $\pm$ 4	<0.025
Female	41 $\pm$ 5	49 $\pm$ 2	NS
BP (mmHg) $\left(\dfrac{\text{systolic} \pm \text{SE}_m}{\text{diastolic} \pm \text{SE}_m}\right)$			
Total	$\dfrac{187 \pm 7}{120 \pm 5}$	$\dfrac{133 \pm 4}{81 \pm 2}$	<0.001 <0.001
Male	$\dfrac{185 \pm 8}{122 \pm 6}$	$\dfrac{136 \pm 6}{82 \pm 4}$	<0.001 <0.001
Female	$\dfrac{191 \pm 16}{115 \pm 9}$	$\dfrac{130 \pm 5}{81 \pm 2}$	<0.005 <0.005
Tumor location (R = right adrenal; L = left adrenal; H = liver hilus; M = multiple benign)			
Total	10R, 10L, 1H, 1M	7R, 8L	
Male	7R, 7L, 1H	4R, 3L	
Female	3R, 3L, 1M	3R, 5L	
Tumor weight (g $\pm$ SE$_m$)			
Total	62 $\pm$ 15 (18)	108 $\pm$ 34 (11)	NS
Male	65 $\pm$ 18 (13)	29 $\pm$ 9 (4)	NS
Female	52 $\pm$ 29 (5)	154 $\pm$ 53 (7)	NS
Tumor catecholamines (mg/g)			
ELS	1.29 $\pm$ 0.42 (15)	2.63 $\pm$ 0.76 (7)	NS
E	0.73 $\pm$ 0.39 (13)	2.05 $\pm$ 0.53 (10)	NS
NE	1.00 $\pm$ 0.18 (13)	1.87 $\pm$ 0.51 (10)	NS
Total catecholamines (E + NE)	1.73 $\pm$ 0.33 (13)	3.92 $\pm$ 0.69 (10)	<0.02
Plasma catecholamines (μg/liter)			
ELS	6.8 $\pm$ 0.9 (15)	4.9 $\pm$ 1.3 (7)	NS
E	1.7 $\pm$ 0.3 (17)	2.8 $\pm$ 0.9 (14)	NS
NE	13.4 $\pm$ 2.2 (17)	8.1 $\pm$ 1.7 (14)	NS
Total catecholamines (E + NE)	14.5 $\pm$ 2.1 (17)	11.0 $\pm$ 1.8 (14)	NS

[a] E = epinephrine; ELS = epinephrine-like substance; NE = norepinephrine; NS = not significant.

the fifth decade of life. The three patients 15 years of age and younger all had sustained hypertension. It seems possible that the patients with sustained hypertension were recognized earlier, since their hypertension was constantly manifest and therefore easier to detect than when it occurred intermittently. Paroxysmal manifestations, on the other hand, are perhaps more easily misinterpreted or missed. The diagnosis of pheochromocytoma in patients with paroxysmal hypertension may, therefore, elude the clinician for a longer period of time than the diagnosis in those patients with sustained hypertension and other clinical manifestations of persistently elevated levels of circulating catecholamines. Yet, if paroxysmal manifestations are pronounced, one would suspect that the physician would be promptly alerted to consider a diagnosis of pheochromocytoma.

Average systolic and diastolic blood pressure for the total group of patients with sustained hypertension ($187 \pm 7/120 \pm 5$ mmHg) was almost identical with the values for males and females. The average blood pressure for the entire group of patients with paroxysmal hypertension was normotensive ($133 \pm 4/81 \pm 2$ mmHg) and almost identical with values for males and females in this group. The blood pressures for this latter group were, of course, recorded in the absence of a paroxysmal attack and were therefore almost invariably normotensive and hence significantly lower ($p < 0.001$) than the values for the group with sustained hypertension.

About 94 percent of all patients (in whom the sites of the pheochromocytomas were known) had tumors located in the adrenal areas. There was no predilection for the right or the left side in this series. Patient No. 19 had multiple (15 tumors) benign pheochromocytomas located in the abdomen, chest, and neck. The pheochromocytoma of patient No. 11 originated in a most unusual location—the hilus of the liver.

When tumor weights from all patients with sustained hypertension were compared with those from patients with paroxysmal hypertension, the mean weight in the group with paroxysmal hypertension was greater (108 ± 34 g vs. 62 ± 15 g), but not statistically significant. [The total weight of the

tumor removed from patient No. 36 was not included in these calculations since the weight of this tumor (1330 g) was due mainly to a huge cyst which contained about 1000 ml of fluid; the actual tumor weight was considered to be approximately 330 g.] Differences in tumor weights between males, and also between females, with sustained or with paroxysmal hypertension were not significant. The mean tumor weight of the females (154 ± 53 g) was significantly greater ($p < 0.01$) than that of the males (29 ± 9 g) in the paroxysmal hypertensive group; however, tumors from only four males were included in this comparison.

Table 7.3 is a summary of the data presented in Figures 7.2 and 7.3 for tumor and plasma catecholamines. Epinephrine and norepinephrine were present in all tumors causing paroxysmal hypertension and in 84.6 percent of tumors causing sustained hypertension. Of note is the fact that the tumor concentration of epinephrine was greater than that of norepinephrine in 60 percent of the tumors causing paroxysmal hypertension. In 69.2 percent of tumors from patients with sustained hypertension, norepinephrine concentration was greater than that of epinephrine (or norepinephrine was the only catecholamine present).

As mentioned previously, the plasma catecholamines were elevated in all patients with sustained hypertension but in only 62.5 percent of those with paroxysmal hypertension. As can be seen in Table 7.3, norepinephrine predominated as the elevated plasma catecholamine in 77.6 percent of patients with sustained and 50.0 percent of those with paroxysmal hypertension. Only norepinephrine was elevated in the plasma of seven patients with sustained and three patients with paroxysmal hypertension, whereas epinephrine alone was elevated in the plasma of three patients with sustained and two patients with paroxysmal hypertension.

It has been reported by others that there was no correlation between the concentration of catecholamines or the ratio of epinephrine to norepinephrine in pheochromocytomas, and the presence of sustained or paroxysmal hypertension (377, 466). In our series, the mean concentrations of epinephrine-like substance (2.63 ± 0.76 mg/g), epinephrine (2.05

Table 7.3 *Summary Table of Data on Tumor and Plasma Catechol-amines in Patients with Sustained and Paroxysmal Hyper-tension due to Pheochromocytoma Depicted in Figures 7.2 and 7.3[a]*

| | Hypertension | | | |
| | Sustained | | Paroxysmal | |
	No.	%	No.	%
Tumor catecholamines present and relative amounts				
Tumors analyzed for E and NE	13		10	
E and NE present	11	84.6	10	100
NE > E	8	61.5[d]	4	40[d]
E > NE	3	23.1	6	60
NE only present	1	7.7[d]	0	0[d]
E only present	1	7.7	0	0
Plasma catecholamines elevated and relative elevations				
Total CA determined (patients)	20		16	
Total CA elevated	20	100	10[e]	62.5
E and NE determined	18		14	
E and NE elevated[b]	8	44.4	5	35.7
NE > E	7	38.8[e]	4	28.6[e]
E > NE	1	5.6	1	7.1
NE only elevated[b]	7	38.8[e]	3	21.4[e]
E only elevated[b]	3	16.8	2	14.3

[a] E = Epinephrine; NE = norepinephrine.
[b] Elevated above upper limit of normal.
[c] One borderline elevation.
[d] Note: NE > E in 69.2% of tumors causing sustained hypertension and in 40.0% of tumors causing paroxysmal hypertension.
[e] Note: NE > E in plasma of 77.6% of patients with sustained hypertension and 50.0% of patients with paroxysmal hypertension.

± 0.53 mg/g), norepinephrine (1.87 ± 0.51 mg/g), and total catecholamines (3.92 ± 0.69 mg/g) in the tumors of the patients with paroxysmal hypertension were greater than the concentrations for epinephrine-like substance (1.29 ± 0.42 mg/g), epinephrine (0.73 ± 0.39 mg/g), norepinephrine (1.00 ± 0.18 mg/g), and total catecholamines (1.73 ± 0.33 mg/g) in the tumors of patients with sustained hypertension. However, only the concentration of total catecholamines was significantly greater ($p < 0.02$) in the patients with paroxysmal hypertension (see Table 7.2). The finding of greater concentrations of catechol-amines in tumors of patients with paroxysmal hypertension, when compared to tumors from patients with sustained hypertension, is particularly interesting. It seems reasonable to speculate that tumors which cause paroxysmal

hypertension and secrete only periodically are more likely to accumulate greater concentrations of catecholamines (at least between paroxysms) than are tumors which are constantly secreting. The ratios of epinephrine to norepinephrine in the tumors from patients with sustained and with paroxysmal hypertension were, respectively, 0.73 and 1.1; however, the difference between these ratios was not statistically significant when analyzed according to the Wilcoxon rank sum test. This test was also employed to analyze the statistical significance of differences in the concentrations of tumor and plasma catecholamines in these patients.

Although the mean concentrations of plasma epinephrine (2.8 ± 0.9 μg/liter), norepinephrine (8.1 ± 1.7 μg/liter), and total catecholamines (11.0 ± 1.8 μg/liter) in the patients with paroxysmal hypertension were abnormally elevated, their blood pressures were relatively normal. The mean concentrations of epinephrine (1.7 $\pm$ 0.3 μg/liter), norepinephrine (13.4 $\pm$ 2.2 μg/liter), and total catecholamines (14.5 $\pm$ 2.1 μg/liter) in the patients with sustained hypertension were not significantly different from those of patients in the paroxysmal group; however, there was a tendency for the plasma concentration of norepinephrine to be greater, and that of epinephrine to be less, in patients with sustained rather than paroxysmal hypertension. The ratios of the mean plasma concentrations of epinephrine to norepinephrine in the group with sustained hypertension was about 0.13, whereas in the paroxysmal group it was 0.35. Although the difference between these ratios is not statistically significant, it is conceivable that whether a patient with pheochromocytoma has sustained or paroxysmal hypertension may depend, at least in part, not only on an elevated concentration of catecholamines in the plasma but also on the ratio of epinephrine to norepinephrine.

DISCUSSION

We are unaware of other studies in which the concentrations of catecholamines in pheochromocytomas and in plasma have been determined and correlated with the presence of paroxysmal or sustained hypertension.

Hermann and Mornex have reported an interesting correlation between tumor catecholamine concentrations and clinical manifestations (437, pp. 146–150). They reviewed the findings in 82 patients and found that tumors containing the highest concentrations of catecholamines were those responsible for paroxysmal hypertension, whereas the concentrations were relatively low in patients with sustained hypertension (less than 400 mg of total catecholamine per tumor). It was also evident that tumors in patients with intermittent manifestations generally contained relatively high percentages of epinephrine, whereas practically all the tumors in patients with permanent hypertension contained relatively low percentages of epinephrine (less than 30 percent).

Studies similar to ours must be performed

to further test the speculation that the ratio of epinephrine to norepinephrine in the plasma may be one of the determinants of the level of the blood pressure in patients with pheochromocytoma. Our results (depicted in Figs. 7.2 and 7.3) do not strongly support this speculation; however, the hypothesis is consistent with the findings of Goldenberg and coworkers that, in normal subjects, infusion of a mixture of equal amounts of epinephrine and norepinephrine caused a slight fall of mean arterial pressure, a striking increase of cardiac output, and a sharp fall in total peripheral resistance from the elevated levels found during infusion of norepinephrine alone (378). The hypothesis is also consistent with the reports by several investigators that predominantly epinephrine-secreting pheochromocytomas may produce primarily β-adrenergic effects and a distinctive clinical syndrome of paroxysms of hypotension, or of hypertension alternating with hypotension (329, 417, 492, 730, 780, 791).

Why some pheochromocytomas paroxysmally release catecholamines into the blood and cause crises of hypertension, but remain relatively quiescent at other times, remains an enigma. One might postulate that the storage mechanism in tumors causing paroxysmal hypertension is nearly normal, whereas in tumors causing sustained hypertension the storage mechanism may be partially defective and thereby permit newly synthesized catecholamines to be released continuously from the tumor. On the other hand, some of the tumors in our patients with paroxysmal hypertension were, in fact, continuously secreting catecholamines even when the blood pressure was normal. This finding again suggests that the ratio of epinephrine to norepinephrine which pheochromocytomas contain and secrete may play a role in determining whether a patient manifests paroxysmal or sustained hypertension.

These various speculations have not yet been tested, since in previous biochemical studies by other investigators pheochromocytomas have not been adequately differentiated into those causing paroxysmal and those causing sustained hypertension. Additional analyses of tumor and plasma catecholamines in patients with paroxysmal and sustained hypertension are needed; a comparative reexamination of ATP concentrations in chromaffin granules, and also of the exocytosis mechanism in pheochromocytomas with different patterns of secretion, might shed additional light on the mechanism of secretion in these tumors. [Lovenberg recently commented that significant elevations of serum DBH occurred in some of his patients with pheochromocytoma and that these elevations returned to normal levels after tumor extirpation; however, no difference was observed in the pattern or degree of exocytosis between patients with paroxysmal or sustained hypertension due to pheochromocytoma (personal communication from Dr. Walter M. Lovenberg, Head, Section on Biochemical Pharmacology, National Heart and Lung Institute, Bethesda, Md.).]

A final point of interest is that the pheochromocytoma of patient No. 8 contained only norepinephrine and that of patient No. 12 contained only epinephrine. These findings suggest that these tumors originated from a single parent cell, i.e., one that produces only norepinephrine or one that produces only epinephrine. On the other hand, all the other tumors we analyzed contained both epinephrine and norepinephrine and it seems reasonable to speculate that these latter tumors might have originated from a cell capable of elaborating both norepinephrine and epinephrine. Whether such a cell exists in the normal adrenal medulla has never been established. It may seem unlikely that sporadic pheochromocytomas containing both epinephrine and norepinephrine originate from two or more parent cells, i.e., some producing only epinephrine and others only norepinephrine (such a possibility seems more plausible in familial pheochromocytomas where the tumor origin appears to be multicentric). However, it is conceivable that a mutagenic agent may stimulate abnormal growth in cells containing only epinephrine and also in cells containing only norepinephrine; a tumor containing both cells would then result.

It is somewhat paradoxical that most adrenal pheochromocytomas are composed of predominantly norepinephrine-containing cells whereas the normal adrenal medulla is composed of predominantly epinephrine-containing cells. This paradox raises the speculation that the cell or cells of tumor origin may have a defect or deletion in the methylating enzyme (PNMT) normally present in epinephrine secreting cells.

Treatment

CHAPTER EIGHT

INTRODUCTION

The importance of expertise and teamwork for the successful management of pheochromocytoma cannot be overstated. Surgical removal, which is the only curative form of therapy, should be performed expeditiously in all patients in whom operation is not contraindicated. There is no substitute for experience in the treatment of patients harboring this pharmacologically explosive and potentially lethal tumor. In order to provide the greatest degree of safety for the patient, it is essential that the internist, surgeon, and anesthesiologist fully understand the pathophysiology of these catecholamine-secreting neoplasms. Judicious use of adrenergic blockade and/or volume replacement preoperatively and intraoperatively, the routine use of a transabdominal (transperitoneal) surgical approach, careful monitoring of arterial blood pressure and the ECG intraoperatively, and the prompt control of blood pressure elevations and arrhythmias have all significantly reduced the hazards of surgical exploration and tumor extirpation. When discussing various aspects of treatment, we have usually referred only to those studies which report results on a reasonably large number of patients with pheochromocytoma.

PREOPERATIVE EVALUATION

At this point it is worthwhile to recapitulate briefly some of the important points regarding preoperative evaluation.

RECOGNITION AND EXCLUSION OF OTHER CONDITIONS

Once the chemical diagnosis of a neural crest tumor has been suggested, one must exclude the presence of other conditions which may cause increased excretion of catecholamines and their metabolites. (These conditions and also the differential diagnosis have been considered in detail earlier.) The possibility must also be kept in mind that the clinical manifestations of pheochromocytoma may occasionally be mimicked by other neural crest tumors.

A thorough history and careful physical examination, in addition to appropriate laboratory studies, are essential in order to ascertain whether any other disease entity coexists with the pheochromocytoma, and to assess whether the pheochromocytoma may be familial. If one elicits a history which confirms or suggests that the pheochromocytoma is familial, it is *essential* to determine whether there is any evidence of medullary thyroid carcinoma or hyperparathyroidism, since the association of these conditions with familial pheochromocytoma is not uncommon.

An attempt to detect the presence of a medullary thyroid carcinoma by demonstrating abnormal elevations of serum calcitonin (under basal conditions or following intravenous administration of pentagastrin, glucagon, or calcium) can be delayed until after pheochromocytoma removal. If a calcitonin provocative test is performed in any patient harboring or suspected of harboring a pheochromocytoma, it should be performed with adequate precautions to counteract the possible occurrence of any untoward hypertensive or hypotensive reaction. (Should a pheochromocytoma appear to be familial, it is encumbent upon the physician to screen the patient's primary relatives carefully, whenever possible, for evidence of pheochromocytoma, medullary thyroid carcinoma, and hyperparathyroidism. Such screening is mandatory in close relatives, and the physician must be committed to a periodic search every 1 or 2 years for any

evidence of this syndrome throughout their lifetimes. In addition, any patient with MEN–type 2 or –type 3 should receive genetic counselling.)

A patient with pheochromocytoma who has any manifestations of Cushing's syndrome should be thoroughly evaluated before extirpation of the pheochromocytoma. Conceivably, this syndrome may be due to Cushing's disease with bilateral adrenocortical hyperplasia, to adrenal adenomas, or to adrenal carcinoma (i.e., the manifestations may not be the result of excess ACTH-like substance elaborated by a coexisting pheochromocytoma). If the syndrome is due to bilateral adrenocortical hyperplasia one must consider bilateral adrenalectomy for Cushing's disease, in addition to removal of the pheochromocytoma. Also, it is important to establish whether Cushing's disease coexists, since wound healing is notoriously delayed in patients with this disease, a factor which dictates a delay in postoperative suture removal by the surgeon.

Since pheochromocytoma is malignant in about 10 percent of cases, the possible existence of metastatic lesions should be seriously considered and evaluated where indicated, prior to surgery.

PREOPERATIVE LOCATION OF THE TUMOR

Quantitation of both epinephrine (or metanephrine) and norepinephrine (or normetanephrine) in urine and/or plasma should be performed if possible, particularly in patients whose pheochromocytomas have not been localized. The presence of increased concentrations of epinephrine or metanephrine strongly suggests that the tumor is located in the adrenal region, although a few extraadrenal pheochromocytomas which secrete epinephrine have been reported.

Occasionally, if a pheochromocytoma is quiescent and not spontaneously secreting catecholamines, it will be necessary to collect blood or urine following a maneuver (e.g., massage of the abdomen or a provocative test) which causes a release of catecholamines from the tumor. Although a blood pressure elevation during a careful and systematic palpation and massage of the abdomen and flanks may be a valuable guide in establishing the location of a tumor, occasionally it may be misleading. Similarly, a history of induction of clinical manifestations by the patient's lying on or bending to one side is not always a reliable guide in localizing the side on which the tumor is present.

Central venous catheterization and sampling of blood from various sites in the vena cava for catecholamine assay is not essential in the usual patient whose pheochromocytoma has been identified; it can, however, be of great help in localizing a pheochromocytoma which has not been located by other means. Moreover, it may be of value in establishing the presence of multiple tumors, and it is particularly indicated in any patient harboring a pheochromocytoma who has had a negative abdominal exploration. Sampling blood from the adrenal veins may also prove particularly valuable in detecting pheochromocytoma in patients with MEN–type 2 or –type 3. In these syndromes, peripheral plasma catecholamines and urinary catecholamines and their metabolites are not infrequently in the normal range and are not elevated by provocative tests. Therefore, it is reasonable to speculate that the chances of detecting any abnormal elevation of plasma catecholamines would be maximized if the venous effluent from the adrenals (where familial pheochromocytomas invariably arise) were assayed.

All patients should have a nephrotomogram when possible, since this radiographic technique localizes an adrenal pheochromocytoma in more than two-thirds of the cases. In addition, it permits one to establish the presence of bilateral renal function (748), information of vital importance in the event that one kidney may have to be sacrificed during tumor removal. If no lesion is apparent on nephrotomography, we believe that preoperative angiographic localization of pheochromocytomas is indicated whenever possible. Angiographic studies can be of considerable value and provide a vascular "road map" to the surgeon which permits a more rapid and effective removal of the tumor.

One must never forget that a pheochromocytoma may arise in the urinary bladder and, therefore, that if there is evidence of hematuria or any suggestion that hypertensive attacks occur with micturition or distension of the bladder, cystoscopy should be performed preoperatively. Prior to cystoscopy, it is preferable to administer phenoxybenzamine and induce α-adrenergic blockade in any patient suspected of harboring a pheochromocytoma. The same precautions taken with arteriography should be observed during cystoscopy.

During the preoperative evaluation, it is well to remember that *any diagnostic procedure which entails even a minor degree of trauma and stress should be performed with caution and with drugs available to combat a hypertensive crisis and arrhythmia and hypotension.* Certainly any elective surgery should be postponed and, as mentioned earlier, thyroid or parathyroid surgery, if indicated, should be delayed until the pheochromocytoma has been removed. In the event that functioning malignant metastases are present and cannot be resected, then an adequate α- (and sometimes also a β-) blockade should be induced prior to any surgery. Finally, it is valuable, when feasible, to measure the total blood volume and plasma volume in all patients with pheochromocytoma, since not infrequently these volumes may be significantly decreased. A moderate deficit in total volume due to a decreased plasma volume is frequently found and this should be corrected prior to, or at the time of, surgery.

PREOPERATIVE PREPARATION

With a thorough preoperative evaluation completed and the preoperative diagnosis of pheochromocytoma established, the patient should be expeditiously prepared for removal of the tumor. Only very rarely will a patient refuse surgery or appear with other medical problems which preclude operation (364). We and others have found that age is no barrier to surgery. Gitlow and associates reported a 72-year-old man with Group IV retinopathy, cardiac enlargement, and left bundle branch block whose surgical course was uneventful, and who postoperatively became normotensive and regained his eyesight (364). It has been correctly emphasized that all patients with pheochromocytoma should be considered urgent surgical problems, and that surgery should not be delayed unnecessarily. Dr. Robert M. Miles cited the case of one patient who died the night before surgery was to be performed, and of another who required emergency surgery at 2 A.M. because of rapidly progressing hemiplegia (cited in 875a).

Very rarely, when a patient with pheochromocytoma presents with acceleration in frequency and severity of hypertensive crises (so-called "acute pheochromocytoma"), administration of adrenergic blocking agents and semi-emergency surgical removal of the tumor may be necessary to prevent life-threatening complications (254). Egdahl and Chobanian have described two such patients: one was a patient with severe hypertensive and hypotensive crises in whom emergency removal of an adrenal pheochromocytoma was performed without the use of blocking drugs; the other was a patient in whom phenoxybenzamine therapy was instituted but on whom semi-emergency removal of an adrenal pheochromocytoma was performed because of increasing hypertensive attacks associated with manifestations of cerebrovascular insufficiency (254). Operation was uncomplicated in both patients. Postoperatively, however, the second patient, while normotensive, became comatose, with findings suggesting herniation of the temporal lobe of the brain; ventriculostomy relieved the increased intracranial pressure and the patient regained consciousness and improved.

Certain rare complications (e.g., hemorrhage within a pheochromocytoma with resultant abdominal pain and shock, ischemic enterocolitis, acute urinary tract obstruction, spinal cord compression, and occasionally a dissecting aneurysm) may require emergency surgery; however, since these are indeed unusual complications, almost all patients with pheochromocytoma can be thoroughly evaluated before surgical intervention.

Rarely, a patient may present during a prolonged hypertensive crisis or with malignant hypertension (sometimes accompanied by acute hypertensive encephalopathy with confusion, somnolence, headache, nausea, vomiting, and occasionally convulsions and coma). Under these circumstances, as mentioned earlier, the intravenous administration of 5 mg of phentolamine may cause a significant and prolonged hypotensive response suggesting the diagnosis of pheochromocytoma; however, false positive phentolamine tests may occur in some patients with malignant hypertension, with or without encephalopathy, and especially in the presence of uremia. [In such circumstances some have suggested use of a modified phentolamine test as an aid in diagnosis and in detecting false positive tests (see Chapter 6).] Treatment of the hypertensive emergency with the intravenous infusion of phentolamine (20 to 40 mg/liter of 5 percent dextrose in water) or sodium nitroprusside (50 to 150 mg/liter of 5 percent dextrose in water) is indicated to normalize and control the blood pressure until the diagnosis of pheochromocytoma can be confirmed or excluded. Sodium nitroprusside should be administered cautiously in the presence of renal insufficiency since this drug can accumulate and be converted to thiocyanate. In the presence of impaired renal function or with prolonged infusion of nitroprusside, the thiocyanate level in the blood should be monitored, since concentrations greater than 10 mg/dl may cause toxic psychosis.

In the event that a β-adrenergic blocking agent is also indicated in order to control tachycardia and arrhythmias, oral propranolol should be administered in a dosage of about 40 mg per day (10 mg every 6 hr) and increased as necessary every 3 to 4 days until adequate blockade is achieved. As will be discussed subsequently, *it is mandatory that α-blockade be performed before β-blockade.*

After confirmation of the diagnosis of pheochromocytoma by assay of plasma or urinary catecholamines or their metabolites, phenoxybenzamine should also be administered orally 2 to 4 times daily (usually in a total daily dosage of 20 to 40 mg) as soon as possible in order to control the blood pressure constantly without intravenous medication. Phenoxybenzamine has a prolonged duration of action and is preferable to oral phentolamine, which has a short duration (2 to 4 hr) and is considerably more expensive. If adequate reduction in blood pressure is not achieved or if side effects (particularly nausea and vomiting despite administration of the drug with meals) make it difficult or impossible to control the blood pressure with phenoxybenzamine alone, then phentolamine may be administered orally in a dose of 50 mg 4 times per day or as needed. However, since phentolamine in this latter dosage frequently causes intolerable gastrointestinal symptoms (e.g., nausea, vomiting, diarrhea, and abdominal pains), it may occasionally be worthwhile to try a combination of both drugs but with a reduced dosage for each.

Since sodium nitroprusside is light-sensitive and since it will decay significantly if exposed to strong light, it is advisable to wrap (with aluminum foil or paper) the bottle and tubing utilized for intravenous administration of this drug. For prolonged administration it is also probably wise to replace the nitroprusside solution with a freshly prepared one every 4 hr.

The antihypertensive drugs used in the treatment of essential hypertension are rarely of help in controlling the blood pressure of a patient with pheochromocytoma. Frequently they cause paradoxical blood pressure responses, perhaps by liberation of catecholamines directly from the tumors and/or by a displacement of excessive stores of catecholamines from sympathetic nerves. Paradoxical blood pressure responses have been observed particularly when ganglionic blocking drugs are used. Some investigators have reported, however, that oral administration of ganglionic blocking drugs or bretylium or guanethidine usually causes a decrease in the blood pressure of patients with pheochromocytoma, whereas sometimes a hypertensive response may be observed if these drugs are given intravenously (813).

It should also be mentioned that if digitalis is indicated it should be administered with caution, since myocardial irritability may be considerably augmented by excessive circulating catecholamines. A point worth recalling is that digoxin and deacetyl-lanatoside C are eliminated mainly by renal excretion whereas digitoxin is eliminated primarily by hepatic degradation. Hence, before administering any of these commonly used digitalis preparations, it is valuable to ascertain whether a significant degree of renal insufficiency or hepatic dysfunction exists, especially in patients with pheochromocytoma.

PREPARATION: TO BLOCK OR NOT TO BLOCK—THAT IS THE QUESTION

Controversy continues to revolve around the preoperative preparation and intraoperative treatment of patients with pheochromocytoma. We have adopted the philosophy that the preoperative therapeutic approach to a patient with pheochromocytoma has to be somewhat flexible and individualized. Preoperative management will depend somewhat on (1) the severity and/or frequency of manifesta-

tions, (2) whether preoperative localization of the tumor or tumors has been possible, (3) whether multiple tumors are anticipated, (4) whether a particularly large tumor is present which may be especially difficult to remove, and (5) the age and preoperative condition of the patient.

It is not our intent to state emphatically that one approach to management is far superior to another. It appears that once the preoperative diagnosis of pheochromocytoma has been made, the operative morbidity and mortality *in highly experienced hands* is *equally* good *whether or not* preoperative α- and β-adrenergic blockade is induced. It is implicit in this statement that the physician, the surgeon, and the anesthesiologist all are highly skilled and have considerable expertise in the management of pheochromocytoma. Certainly, the hazards faced by the surgeon and the anesthesiologist during removal of a pheochromocytoma are so serious that it is in the best interest of the patient that he be referred to a qualified team of experts for appropriate management. A novice should never tackle the problem without the supervision and assistance of the experts.

In general, with minor variations, the following basic approaches to the preoperative use of α- and β-blocking agents in patients with pheochromocytoma have been suggested:

1. In all patients with pheochromocytoma use phenoxybenzamine (Dibenzyline) in moderate to large dosage preoperatively and up to the time of operation so that the α-blocking effect of this drug continues during surgery.

2. Use phenoxybenzamine in moderate to large dosage preoperatively in patients with sustained hypertension or in patients having paroxysmal hypertensive crises. Discontinue phenoxybenzamine (whenever there is no serious hazard to the patient) about 72 to 48 hr before laparotomy so that the patient is not significantly blocked with a long-acting α-blocker during surgical exploration.

3. Only very rarely use phenoxybenzamine preoperatively, and only in patients with severe sustained hypertension (e.g., 250/150 mmHg) and/or severe hypertensive crises. (Some physicians prefer to use intravenous

sodium nitroprusside or phentolamine to control severe manifestations preoperatively; these drugs may be used alone or they may be used preoperatively for at least 72 hr after phenoxybenzamine has been discontinued.)

4. Some physicians feel that in addition to α-blockade, the routine use of propranolol (a β-blocking agent) is indicated preoperatively up to the time of surgery in most if not all patients with pheochromocytoma, whereas others feel it is indicated only in those demonstrating significant arrhythmias and/or tachycardia.

A number of physicians, surgeons, and anesthesiologists recommend the administration of α- and β-blocking agents preoperatively to patients with pheochromocytoma (179, 190, 219, 249, 367, 421, 489, 718, 721, 747, 784, 813, 909, 990). Their choices of drug dosage and of mode of administration differ considerably, and no precise formulation of an ideal approach to adrenergic blockade is possible because of the variability of manifestations in patients with pheochromocytoma and their variability in responsiveness to adrenergic blocking agents.

α-**Adrenergic Blockade**   The use of *phenoxybenzamine* in the preoperative management of patients with pheochromocytoma was first suggested in 1962 by Johns and Brunjes (489) and subsequently by Sjoerdsma and associates (909).

Therapy with phenoxybenzamine is usually started 1 to 3 weeks before operation. To obtain a moderate α-blockade, 20 to 40 mg per day is administered in divided doses (2 to 4 times daily). If necessary this dosage may be increased by increments of 10 to 20 mg per day until clinical manifestations are controlled and the blood pressure is reduced to normal. The half-life of intravenously administered phenoxybenzamine is about 24 hr (1069). The peak blockade, which is much less and more variable after oral administration, probably occurs 3 to 4 hr after administration. The duration of therapeutic action after the peak effect should be about 24 hr—the same as the half-life (personal communication from Dr. Mark Nickerson, Professor of Pharmacology, McGill University). Because of this prolonged duration of action, only one

daily dose of phenoxybenzamine would probably be therapeutically sufficient; however, it is prudent to divide even moderately large doses and administer the drug several times per day in order to avoid or minimize any gastrointestinal intolerance.

The effect of phenoxybenzamine administered intravenously* is probably not maximal in less than 1 hr; the blockade is very persistent and, after only a single dose of phenoxybenzamine, significant blockade may be evident for 3 to 4 days (708, p. 549). A strong α-blockade can usually be induced by increasing the daily dosage up to 100 mg per day or until gastrointestinal side effects are experienced. Some prefer to administer phenoxybenzamine both orally and intravenously (1 mg/kg) (813). It is noteworthy that one patient with pheochromocytoma who was given phenoxybenzamine intravenously to control a hypertensive crisis lost consciousness and developed profound shock. Consciousness did not return until 6 hr after infusion of this agent was terminated (52). According to Nickerson, the usual α-blocking dose of phenoxybenzamine in man is 1 mg/kg I.V. (708, p. 536). Nickerson has personally managed 11 patients with pheochromocytoma during operation and has been involved with the management of about a dozen other patients. In all of these cases approximately 1.0 mg/kg of phenoxybenzamine was given intravenously 36 hr before operation and again about 12 hr prior to operation. (Since the onset of action is slow, it is not a suitable drug to give during operations.) His experience was uniformly excellent; there were no hypertensive episodes and no cardiac arrhythmias except for a few premature ventricular contractions in two or three cases. He did not combine a β-adrenoceptor blocking agent with phenoxybenzamine and, although several patients had considerable tachycardia, this did not cause any real problem.

Nickerson has never observed significant postoperative hypotension (systolic pressure <100 mmHg), and these blocked patients always had a wide pulse pressure. He recounted the dramatic case of a boy with bilateral adrenal pheochromocytomas in whom the surgeons performed extensive dissection prior to

* Intravenous preparation of phenoxybenzamine is not available in the U.S.A.

clamping the blood supply in order to preserve adrenal cortical tissue. Analysis of his operative and postoperative urine indicated that nearly 40 mg of norepinephrine were released during the operation, but his blood pressure varied a total of only 20 mmHg and a continuous ECG showed only three premature contractions.

Nickerson suggested that in patients under α-blockade with phenoxybenzamine careful monitoring of the heart rate might adequately substitute for blood pressure as a guide for tumor location during palpation of areas suspected of harboring a pheochromocytoma; the β-adrenergic effects of catecholamines are not blocked by this drug. (We have not assessed the value of monitoring heart rate under these circumstances.) The only missed tumor in their series was a case in which the surgeons were so sure of the location that they performed a lumbar approach and did not look further.

As an interesting sidelight, Nickerson mentioned a case of pheochromocytoma recently presented to him at the Capital Hospital in Peking. Phenoxybenzamine was administered as recommended by Nickerson and the operation (under acupuncture anesthesia) and postoperative course were entirely uneventful (personal communication from Dr. M. Nickerson).

One of us (R.W.G.) observed that, following the intravenous administration of 100 mg of phenoxybenzamine to a woman (weighing about 60 kg) who had a pheochromocytoma, the infusion of high concentrations of norepinephrine had no pressor effect; however, infusion of angiotensin caused the usual pressor effect. The oral dosage required to create an α-blockade may vary considerably because of differences in the rate and completeness of absorption from the gastrointestinal tract. Side effects of α-blockade with phenoxybenzamine include postural hypotension and reflex tachycardia, miosis, nasal stuffiness, and inhibition of ejaculation. Postural hypotension may at times be severe enough to require the patient to remain in bed if the α-blockade is complete. In addition, symptoms unrelated to α-blockade (e.g., nausea, vomiting, sedation, weakness, and tiredness) may occur (708, pp. 539, 540). Some caution must be exercised when administering phenoxybenzamine to patients with severe cerebral atherosclerosis or with reduced renal blood flow, since the flow to the brain may be further compromised. It is worth noting that sudden death was reported when phenoxybenzamine was given to a patient who was being treated with quinidine (682).

α-Blockade can also be accomplished by oral administration of *phentolamine* (about 50 mg every 4 hr); however, as mentioned earlier, gastrointestinal side effects frequently limit the usefulness of this drug when given orally. Alarming tachycardia, arrhythmias, and anginal pain may occur, particularly after parenteral administration; it has even been implicated as a precipitating factor in myocardial infarction (708, p. 543). Blockade may be effectively accomplished by infusing phentolamine for a prolonged period without side effects. We are aware of a patient with sustained hypertension and a cerebrovascular accident due to a pheochromocytoma whose precarious condition precluded early removal of the tumor. The patient was maintained on a constant intravenous infusion of phentolamine (approximately 100 mg/hr) for 1 month before the pheochromocytoma was successfully removed. This mode of therapy, although extremely expensive (1 mg of phentolamine costs approximately one dollar), was highly effective in this particular patient, who subsequently has shown a remarkable recovery (personal communication from Dr. Demetrius Pertsemlidis and Dr. Stanley E. Gitlow, Mt. Sinai Hospital, New York).

Advocates of preoperative blockade with phenoxybenzamine that is continued to the time of operation argue that blockade with this drug (a) prevents severe clinical manifestations in the preoperative period; (b) reverses hypovolemia which is frequently present; and (c) promotes a smooth anesthetic induction and operation. Those who oppose the routine preoperative use of phenoxybenzamine up to the time of operation feel that if the α-blockade is complete, the surgeon will not have the advantage of (a) utilizing increases in blood pressure as a guide to tumor location, or of (b) immediately recognizing (by the persistence of hypertension) that another tumor may exist in the patient following pheochromocytoma removal. It has further been argued that complete blockade with phenoxybenzamine may occasionally result in a pronounced hypotensive period following removal of the tumor; however, such a hypotensive event should not present a major problem, since it can almost invariably be prevented or adequately treated by volume replacement preoperatively or intraoperatively.

Except in rare circumstances with very severe sustained or paroxysmal hypertension, we have not found it necessary to administer phenoxybenzamine preoperatively to patients with pheochromocytoma. On the other hand, we do not strongly oppose the preoperative use of phenoxybenzamine in *moderate* dosage, especially if the sustained or paroxysmal hypertension is very severe or if the patient is precariously ill. The important point is that it is preferable that during surgery no patient be *fully* blocked with a prolonged α-adrenergic blocking drug such as phenoxybenzamine. Our feeling on this point is even stronger when there is uncertainty as to the location of a pheochromocytoma and/or when the likelihood of encountering more than one tumor is increased. For example, in the event that an extensive radiographic investigation, central venous blood sampling for catecholamine assay, and/or a preceding laparotomy have failed to localize a pheochromocytoma, then an elevation of blood pressure during manipulation of a tumor may prove to be an invaluable guide for localizing a small and inconspicuous lesion. We are personally aware of several very small pheochromocytomas which would not have been detected had it not been for the increase in blood pressure which accompanied palpation of these tumors.

Complete α-blockade with phenoxybenzamine is also undesirable when operating on children and on subjects with familial pheochromocytoma, since these patients have an increased prevalence of multiple tumors. The persistence of hypertension following tumor removal is a valuable indication that one or more additional tumors are present. Since α-blockade normalizes blood pressure and hypertension is absent, the blood pressure is no longer an index of excessive circulating catecholamines caused by a residual functioning tumor.

Administration of phenoxybenzamine in moderate dosage which does not cause complete blockade may not prevent some rise in blood pressure during manipulation of a pheochromocytoma. However, even incomplete blockade caused by phenoxybenzamine in moderate dosage can normalize the blood pressure preoperatively so that the level of the blood pressure following removal of a pheochromocytoma is of no value in assessing whether one or more tumors are still present in the patient.

Occasionally, phenoxybenzamine may cause hypotension and tachycardia in a patient with a pheochromocytoma which is secreting predominantly epinephrine (249, 730). In this situation, α-blockade may unmask the vasodilating β-adrenergic activity of epinephrine and reflexly augment the heart rate. These latter manifestations of excessive α-adrenergic activity can be controlled by the administration of a β-blocking agent such as propranolol (Inderal). It must be constantly kept in mind, however, that *β-blockade should never be induced without initially inducing α-blockade.* Creation of β-blockade in the absence of α-blockade will overcome any vasodilating effect caused by epinephrine, if present, and may thereby result in an augmentation of the hypertension.

Very rarely, complete bed rest may be indicated prior to operation if the patient experiences severe postural hypotension or recurrent paroxysmal hypertension despite careful management with adrenergic receptor blockade.

β-Adrenergic Blockade When there exists a significant persistent tachycardia (i.e., a heart rate felt to be hazardous to the patient), and/or when arrhythmias (e.g., premature ventricular contractions or ventricular bigeminy) recur frequently, a β-adrenergic blocking agent is indicated. The presence of angina pectoris may also be an indication for using a β-blocker. Theoretically, a pheochromocytoma which secretes primarily epinephrine could also be considered an indication for β-blockade.

Given intravenously, the half-life of propranolol is of the order of 1.5 to 3 hr, whereas, when given orally, it is 3.5 to 6 hr (879). In the presence of heart failure, or of cirrhosis with portacaval anastomoses and/or hypoproteinemia, the half-life may be markedly prolonged.

Since β-adrenergic blockade with propranolol can aggravate bronchial constriction and block compensatory reflexes which maintain cardiac output, it is not surprising that this drug can aggravate or precipitate heart failure and asthma in susceptible patients. Propranolol may also produce profound bradycardia and heart block, which may require treatment with atropine, glucagon, or isoproterenol. Other side effects reported are fatigue, anorexia, nausea, vomiting, diarrhea, cold extremities, Raynaud's phenomenon, depression, insomnia, and vivid dreams. Rarely, rashes, thrombocytopenia, and alopecia occur (879). Its use is contraindicated in heart failure, second or third degree heart block, marked bradycardia, and asthma; Raynaud's disease is a relative contraindication to using the drug. A point to be kept in mind is that although the inotropic action of digitalis is not prevented by propranolol, both drugs depress A-V conduction. "Propranolol can cause A-V dissociation and cardiac arrest in patients with preexisting partial heart block due to digitalis or other factors" (708, p. 552). Caution should be exercised whenever both digitalis and propranolol are used in any patient. Some feel that since cardiac glycosides sensitize the myocardium to catecholamines, they should be avoided preoperatively in patients with pheochromocytoma.

It would seem that propranolol, which reduces sinus rate, decreases rate of depolarization of ectopic pacemakers (i.e., automaticity), and slows conduction (particularly in the atria and the A-V node), is the drug of choice in treating supraventricular and ventricular arrhythmias due to excessive circulating catecholamines (879).

As mentioned above, propranolol should *never be given to patients with pheochromocytoma without first creating an α-blockade*. Administration of a β-blocking agent, even in the presence of α-blockade, may significantly elevate blood pressure and require an increase in dosage of the α-blocker. The use of propranolol in conjunction with α-receptor blocking drugs in the treatment of pheochromocytoma was first suggested by Prichard and Ross (770, 813).

It has been demonstrated that propranolol can aggravate myocardial depression caused by anesthesia (993). Some anesthetic agents have sympathomimetic activity which counteracts myocardial depression, but thiopental, halothane, methoxyflurane, and enflurane lack this activity. In a recent medical letter (647) concern was expressed regarding continuing β-receptor blockade up to the time of operation when dealing with surgical problems other than pheochromocytoma, because of the possibility of severe myocardial depression, bradycardia, and hypotension. One report was cited indicating an inability to resuscitate four of five patients who, while receiving propranolol, developed cardiac failure immediately following cardiac by-pass operations; however, other surgeons have not encountered this problem. Finally, it was noted that abrupt withdrawal of propranolol medication in some patients with angina may precipitate myocardial infarction. It is important for physicians utilizing propranolol to be fully aware of its potential side effects and hazards.

Shand has stated that a plasma concentration of about 100 ng of propranolol per ml at the end of the usual 6-hr dosage interval indicates that a high degree of β-blockade is probably present in most patients (879). He suggested that patients be started on low doses (40 mg/day) and that the dose be cautiously increased as necessary every 3 to 4 days until tachycardia and/or arrhythmias are controlled. If no response to therapy is evident despite increasing dosage and/or if the plasma concentration does not increase commensurately with the dosage, then one must consider the likelihood that the patient is not taking all the medication. However, one of us (R.W.G.) has observed that the minimally effective dosage of propranolol for controlling tachycardia or arrhythmias is 20 mg given 4 times per day.

Guidelines to Adequate α- and β-Blockade
The guidelines to adequate α- and β-blockade in patients harboring pheochromocytoma are, of course, control of clinical manifestations, blood pressure, pulse rate, electrocardiographic alterations, and the return of blood volume changes toward normal. Diminished sensitivity to intravenously administered tyramine has been used by Crago and coworkers to assess the degree of α- and β-adrenergic blockade (179); however, we do not feel testing with tyramine is indicated or necessary.

In addition to the disadvantages of complete α-blockade (with regard to changes in blood pressure as a guide to tumor location and detection of residual tumors) mentioned earlier, other problems of adrenergic blockade may be encountered. Ross and associates have pointed out that for the following reasons complete α- and β-blockade can add to the difficulties of anesthetic and surgical management of patients with pheochromocytoma: (1) the patient may become very sensitive to the hypotensive effect of thiopental or of hemorrhage; (2) venous oozing may be more pronounced; and (3) the tachycardia of hemorrhage is more readily apparent (813).

None of the 69 patients operated upon at the Mayo Clinic up to 1960 (352), and only one of 45 patients operated upon at the Cleveland Clinic up to 1973 (223), received phenoxybenzamine. It is noteworthy that there was only one operative death (Mayo series), and none of the patients had any intraoperative or postoperative morbidity ascribable to the fact that phenoxybenzamine had not been used (223).

At the Mayo Clinic between 1965 and 1969 the effect of preoperative adrenergic blocking drugs was studied in three groups of patients with pheochromocytoma. Six patients received no adrenergic blocking drug, 20 patients received 30 to 60 mg of phenoxybenzamine orally per day for 7 to 14 days, and seven patients received the same schedule of phenoxybenzamine but, in addition, were given 30 mg of propranolol orally for 2 days prior to surgery. All 33 patients were adults and all tumors were intraabdominal. [Nineteen were in the right adrenal, 12 in the left, and two in the organ of Zuckerkandl. The average duration of anesthesia (nitrous oxide and ether) was 2 hr and 35 min (range: 1 hr and 50 min to 4 hr).] The events occurring during surgery are given in Table 8.1. As can be seen, significant hypertension (>250 mmHg) occurred in three patients despite α-blockade, and in another patient despite administration of both α- and β-adrenergic blocking agents. Phentolamine had to be administered more frequently in the unblocked patients than in patients with adrenergic blockade. Acute hypotension (<80 mmHg) occurred in one patient receiving no drugs but not in any of the patients taking adrenergic blocking agents. Tachycardia developed in five of six patients receiving no drugs but in only five of 20 patients taking phenoxybenzamine. It is noteworthy, however, that three of the seven patients receiving both phenoxybenzamine and propranolol developed tachycardia. Only one patient required lidocaine and none received

Table 8.1   *Results of Preoperative Preparation and Anesthetic Management in 33 Patients Undergoing Operation for Removal of Pheochromocytoma[a]*

	Group 1 (6 patients)[b]		Group 2 (20 patients)[c]		Group 3 (7 patients)[d]	
	No. of patients	%	No. of patients	%	No. of patients	%
With blood pressure						
>250 mmHg	1	17	3	15	1	14
<80 mm Hg	1	17	0	0	0	0
With pulse rate						
>120/min	5	83	5	25	3	43
Needing phentolamine	4	67	5	25	1	14
Developing arrhythmia	1	17	2	10	3	43

[a] From Perry, L. B. and Gould, A. B., Jr. *Anesth. Analg. 51:* 37, 1972.

[b] No adrenergic blocking agent before operation.

[c] Phenoxybenzamine (30 to 60 mg orally per day) 7 to 10 days before operation.

[d] Phenoxybenzamine (30 to 60 mg orally per day) plus propranolol (30 mg orally per day) before operation.

propranolol intravenously. Perry and Gould felt that in their series of patients no benefit occurred from the use of propranolol (747); however, the dosage they used was relatively small and may not have been effective for that reason. A subsequent report by Remine and coworkers from the Mayo Clinic stated that they believed that adding propranolol to the preoperative regimen decreased the incidence of cardiac arrhythmias during the surgical procedure (784).

Ross and associates reported their opera-

tive experience with 27 patients harboring pheochromocytoma who had been prepared preoperatively with various α- and β-adrenergic blocking agents given both orally and intravenously in variable dosage. They concluded that adequate α-blockade controlled blood pressure and permitted reexpansion of blood volume, thereby preventing hypotension following tumor removal, provided blood loss was replaced. Moreover, pressor agents were not needed. Tachycardia and arrhythmias were controlled by β-blockers given

Fig. 8.1 Fluctuations of blood pressure and pulse rate during operation.
A. No preoperative preparation with adrenergic blocking agents was given.
B. Accidentally undertreated with α-adrenergic blocking agent. C. Preoperative preparation with both α- and β-adrenergic blocking agents. D. Preoperative preparation with both α- and β-adrenergic blocking agents. Hypotensive effect of induction and of hemorrhage is shown. From Ross, E. J., Prichard, B. N. C., Kaufman, L., Robertson, A. I. G., and Harries, B. J., *Br. Med. J. 1:* 191-194, 1967.

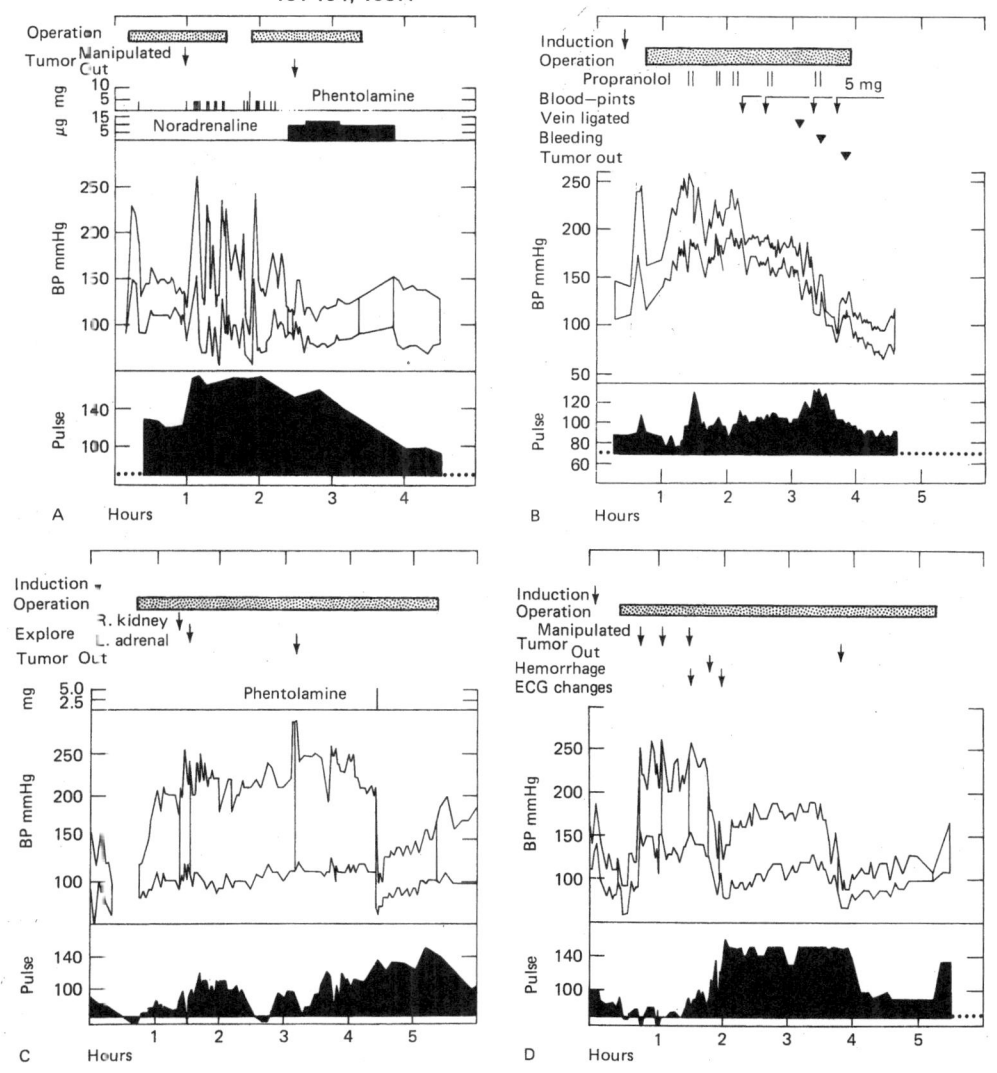

orally preoperatively and intravenously during operation. They did not, however, feel that complete α- and β-blockade was desirable, since it could negate the value of blood pressure response as a guide to tumor location.

Figure 8.1 reveals the fluctuations of blood pressure and pulse and certain other events occurring during four operations for pheochromocytoma reported by Ross and coworkers (813). Blood pressures showed wide fluctuations and pulse rates were not well controlled in the patient receiving no preoperative drugs and in the patient undertreated with phenoxybenzamine (cases A and B, respectively). The blood pressures also became markedly elevated, especially during tumor manipulation, in both patients (cases C and D) who had preoperatively received what were thought to be adequate doses of α- and β-adrenergic blocking agents. (Note: Case C had a recurrent malignant pheochromocytoma and is the same patient as case A.) A hypotensive effect of induction and of hemorrhage was also observed in case D. Case A required repeated intravenous injections of phentolamine intraoperatively to control the wide swings of blood pressure; furthermore, a norepinephrine infusion was necessary for 4 hr following tumor removal to maintain blood pressure (blood transfusion for this patient was not mentioned). Case B required repeated intravenous injections of propranolol to control the tachycardia; extrasystoles and left bundle branch block occurred following a hemorrhage, but they disappeared with blood replacement. In cases C and D the only significant tachycardia occurred after a sudden reduction of blood pressure following phentolamine injection or hemorrhage.

STEROID REPLACEMENT THERAPY

It is essential to provide the patient with appropriate replacement therapy if bilateral adrenalectomy is contemplated, e.g., in the presence of MEN–type 2 or –type 3, or if large bilateral adrenal pheochromocytomas are evident, or even in the conceivable circumstance of there being a pheochromocytoma in addition to an unrelated Cushing's disease, or in the rare event that the patient's only adrenal gland is removed with the pheochromocytoma. Except in these circumstances, steroid therapy is not indicated.

We suggest the following schedule:

1. Just before anesthetic induction and throughout the operative period administer hydrocortisone (Solucortef) intravenously at a rate of 20 to 25 mg per hr as a steady drip (from a bottle containing 100 mg/liter) until the patient regains consciousness in the recovery room. Then immediately administer 50 mg of hydrocortisone in about 50 ml of saline intravenously over a period of 15 to 30 min and repeat every 6 hr. This solution can be conveniently prepared and administered in a Solu Set connected in tandem to an intravenous infusion line that has previously been established. If there is any suspicion of adrenal insufficiency it is important that steroid be administered before anesthesia is begun, since anesthesia per se is a stressful procedure.
2. On the first postoperative day give 50 mg hydrocortisone intravenously every 6 hr in a similar way.
3. On the second postoperative day give 25 mg hydrocortisone intravenously every 6 hr in a similar way.
4. On the third postoperative day start the oral administration of 75 to 100 mg cortisone acetate daily in divided doses given every 8 hr. (If for some reason the patient is unable to take medication orally at this point, intravenous administration may be continued in progressively reduced dosage until oral medication is feasible.)
5. At the end of the first postoperative week, in addition to 30 to 40 mg of cortisone acetate given daily in divided doses every 8 hr, administer 0.1 mg of fludrocortisone (Florinef) daily.
6. During the second week, the dosage of cortisone acetate should be reduced to 12.5 mg given twice daily, and this dosage and 0.1 mg of fludrocortisone should be continued thereafter indefinitely.

(The above schedule for steroid replacement is essentially that of Dr. Donald A. Holub, endocrinologist and Associate Professor of Clinical Medicine at Columbia Medical Center in New York City.)

Others (249) have recommended a comparable regimen for replacement therapy post-adrenalectomy, with the variation that hydrocortisone be given intramuscularly for the first 5 postoperative days. Since postoperative hypotension and circulatory insufficiency may occasionally occur and impair the absorption of intramuscular medication, we prefer to administer hydrocortisone intravenously, at least during the first few days following surgery.

All patients who have undergone bilateral adrenalectomy should initially be followed closely at weekly intervals. After several weeks the intervals may become monthly, and after about 1 year the patient should be seen every 6 months.

PREMEDICATION

Premedication with tranquilizers (e.g., diazepam or droperidol) and a barbiturate (preferably secobarbital) is routinely carried out, primarily to allay any anxiety and emotional upset of the patient which might trigger release of catecholamines into the circulation. Some prefer to administer meperidine (Demerol) routinely. Morphine should not be used since it may cause release of catecholamines from pheochromocytomas. The virtue of administrating atropine is questionable, since it may cause tachycardia; we prefer to avoid its use, since it seems reasonable to assume that an intact parasympathetic system may act somewhat to counterbalance some of the effects of excessive circulating catecholamines in patients with pheochromocytoma. As mentioned earlier, phenothiazines should be avoided since they have occasionally caused profound hypotensive reactions in patients with pheochromocytoma. In one patient with pheochromocytoma, diamorphine caused hypertensive crises, indicating the inadvisability of using any narcotics which have the capacity to liberate histamine (149). Hypnosis was found to aid in abating one patient's hypertensive paroxysms, and induction of a trance facilitated her immediate preoperative preparation (498).

MONITORING SYSTEMS AND INFUSION LINES

Before anesthetic induction the following monitoring devices and infusion lines should be in place:

1. An arterial catheter (usually placed in an artery of the arm) attached to a strain gauge in order to permit continuous recording of the systolic and diastolic blood pressures on a direct-writing oscillograph, easily visible to the anesthesiologist. Measurements of the blood pressure with a sphygmomanometer and stethoscope are undesirable, not only because of the time delays in recording, but also because with severe vasoconstriction a pressure reading may sometimes be unobtainable, and this may be misinterpreted as being due to circulatory shock. Since it is important to avoid hypercarbia and acidosis, arterial blood may be drawn if desired for analysis of blood gasses and pH.

2. An electrocardiogram which records standard Lead II and is constantly displayed on an oscilloscope which is easily visible to the anesthesiologist.

3. A venous catheter which has been passed (usually through an arm vein) into the superior vena cava for central venous pressure (CVP) measurement by means of a strain gauge to permit continuous recording on a direct-writing oscillograph which is easily visible to the anesthesiologist.

4. A stethescope attached to the precordium as an additional method for measuring heart rate. (After anesthetic induction, some anesthesiologists employ an esophageal stethoscope and an esophageal thermometer, which are conveniently passed into place.)

5. After anesthetic induction, a Foley catheter is inserted in order to monitor urine output. [Some anesthesiologists monitor the effects of both succinylcholine and *d*-tubocurarine with the aid of a nerve stimulator (498).]

OPERATIVE MANAGEMENT*

INTUBATION

Unless the patient with pheochromocytoma is properly prepared with muscle relaxants

---

* Since many unrecognized pheochromocytomas have become manifest during intubation, anesthetic administration, operation, or parturition, it is a worthy precaution to have drugs immediately available for appropriate treatment of hypertensive crises, arrhythmias, and hypotension during any operation. This precaution is especially important if any tumor of unknown origin in the adrenal gland or in the posterior mediastinum is to be removed.

and anesthesia, intubation may sometimes induce a severe hypertensive crisis. *d*-Tubocurarine (a curare alkaloid) or pancuronium (a synthetic steroid), competitive neuromuscular blocking agents, is administered intravenously. Although *d*-tubocurarine may release histamine and theoretically provoke release of tumor catecholamines into the circulation, this has not proved to be a problem. Pancuronium, which is about five times as potent as *d*-tubocurarine, may cause tachycardia, but it has minimal cardiovascular actions and it does not release histamine (386, pp. 576, 577). Some prefer not to use pancuronium because of its tendency to cause tachycardia and elevated blood pressure.

Approximately 5 min after administration of one of these nondepolarizing muscle relaxants (a small dose is used so that neuromuscular blockade is not complete), induction of anesthesia with the intravenous administration of a small amount of thiopental (3 to 4 mg/kg, individual doses) is accomplished, and this is followed by administration of a general anesthetic and succinylcholine (Anectine). Succinylcholine is a depolarizing agent causing muscle relaxation. (Usual fasiculation noted with this drug is prevented because of prior neuromuscular blockade.) Succinylcholine can be of value for continuous muscle relaxation and intubation. The trachea is then sprayed with 4 percent lidocaine (Xylocaine) and intubated. Under these circumstances, if the patient is lightly anesthetized before succinylcholine is given and before intubation, there should be no untoward hypertensive reaction to intubation. During the operation, muscle relaxation is maintained with *d*-tubocurarine (498).

GENERAL ANESTHESIA

It may be said that in highly competent hands a number of different anesthetics have been used as the primary agent with equal success. However, certain restrictions on and limitations of some anesthetics should be mentioned.

For example, *diethyl ether*, one of the oldest anesthetic agents, was previously often used in patients with pheochromocytoma. It proved to be an excellent anesthetic, and by 1965 it had been used with great success at the Mayo Clinic in 78 cases (868). Its explosive property has, however, precluded its use when cautery is employed or when electrical equipment (e.g., that required for cardioversion) may be needed.

Cyclopropane sensitizes the myocardium to catecholamines and therefore should not be used in patients with pheochromocytoma, despite the fact that it has been used for removal of such tumors without untoward effects (470).

Halothane (Fluothane) may exert an effect somewhat similar to that of cyclopropane but this myocardial sensitization is relatively mild. It also exerts an antiadrenergic effect. Some feel halothane is contraindicated in patients with pheochromocytoma (206). The slightly increased incidence of cardiac arrhythmias encountered during use of halothane in patients with pheochromocytoma has not frequently been a serious problem, and this anesthetic has been employed in many centers, usually with great success (73, 170, 282, 332, 382, 494, 513, 690, 799, 803, 807). Untoward incidents occurred in two cases at the Mayo Clinic during operation when this agent was used. Development of bigeminy required discontinuance of halothane in one patient; cardiac resuscitation was required in the other patient but the operation was completed with halothane (868).

Methoxyflurane (Penthrane) also has an antiadrenergic effect and it has been advocated as a particularly suitable anesthetic agent for use in patients with pheochromocytoma (73, 77, 179, 190, 223, 308, 721, 837, 838, 1010). It does not sensitize the myocardium to catecholamines to the same degree as do other halogenated agents in use. Unfortunately, since this anesthetic occasionally causes significant nephrotoxicity (637a) with deposition of calcium oxalate crystals in renal tubules, tubular necrosis, and persistent renal dysfunction (156), it has lost its popularity.

Thiopental (Pentothal) was administered in 82 cases of pheochromocytoma at the Mayo Clinic, often as the primary agent; however, when used as the primary agent, this short-acting barbiturate has to be injected repeatedly to maintain anesthesia. Since it accumulates in the body, recovery from anesthesia may be prolonged. Certain adverse respiratory actions (apnea, coughing, laryngospasm, and bronchospasm) and myocardial depression may occur. It is also a poor analgesic (386, pp. 99, 100).

Epidural blockade has apparently been used successfully on at least one patient with pheochromocytoma (178a); however, experience with this modality of anesthesia is lacking, and it seems to us that difficulties with hypotension might be compounded by a sympathetic blockade induced by epidural or spinal anesthesia.

Currently the most popular anesthetic is *enflurane* (Ethrane), which was introduced for human use in 1973. It is a member of the ether family but nonexplosive and with relatively few side effects and no serious toxicity. Enflurane affords adequate muscular relaxation for intraabdominal procedures. The clinical effects of this anesthetic are similar to those of halothane and methoxyflurane, except that muscular relaxation is greater and tachypnea is uncommon when spontaneous ventilation is permitted during surgery. Enflurane is, therefore, superior to halothane or methoxyflurane under these conditions during abdominal surgery (386, p. 95). Excessive concentrations of enflurane and hypocarbia should be avoided since under these circumstances seizure-like activity may appear.

Since enflurane, like halothane, sensitizes the myocardium (particularly the cardiac conducting system) to the arrhythmogenic actions of the catecholamines (386, p. 95), ventricular extrasystoles may be expected in some patients with pheochromocytoma, during anesthesia with this agent. No reports of renal toxicity definitely attributable to enflurane have appeared; however, it may be capable of producing nephrotoxicity in patients with renal transplants and severe renal disease (582). A recent report of hepatic necrosis associated with viral infection after enflurane anesthesia concluded that the hepatic pathology was probably unrelated to the anesthetic (233a). Enflurane has all the advantages of halothane and fewer of the disadvantages. Only occasional reports of the virtues of using this anesthetic agent in patients with pheochromocytoma have appeared in the literature (525, 528a, 724), but at the present time, in many medical centers it has already replaced other anesthetics in the management of pheochromocytoma.

Finally, it should be mentioned that practically all anesthesiologists routinely use a *combination of one of the volatile anesthetics and nitrous oxide*. With careful administration, the potential hazard of hypoxia when the latter agent is employed is usually not a problem. It is especially important that adequate ventilation be maintained at all times during operation of patients with pheochromocytoma. As mentioned above, at the Mayo Clinic, the average duration of anesthesia in 33 patients with pheochromocytoma operated upon between 1965 and 1969 was 2 hr 35 min, with a range of 1 hr 50 min to 4 hr (747).

MANAGEMENT OF HYPERTENSIVE CRISES AND ARRHYTHMIAS

It is important to stress that an effort should be made to avoid any undue anxiety, excessive noise, and any physical maneuvers during transportation of the patient from his bed to the operating table which might cause release of catecholamines from the pheochromocytoma. Questioning and observing the patient closely, and recording the pulse and blood pressure, will detect such an event in an unblocked or partially blocked patient. One should be aware that even abdominal pressure during a slightly vigorous cleansing preparation of the abdomen may be enough to trigger catecholamine secretion from a tumor. Any hypertensive crises should be immediately treated with an intravenous bolus of phentolamine or sodium nitroprusside, followed by repeated injections or infusions of these agents if necessary.

Once the monitoring systems are in place and operative, it is the anesthesiologist's constant duty to scan the blood pressure recording and the ECG. He must be acutely alert at all times to any change in blood pressure or cardiac rhythm which requires prompt therapy. The major problems encountered by the anesthesiologist during operation are hypertension, arrhythmias, and hypotension. A plastic venous catheter, with a rubber-capped side arm for delivery of drugs, should be placed in an arm vein and connected to a bottle of 5 percent dextrose in water for maintaining a slow drip infusion. To control hypertensive episodes a solution of 100 mg of sodium nitroprusside in 500 ml of 5 percent dextrose in water can be used for infusion into the side arm of the plastic venous catheter as desired. Several syringes containing some of the solution of sodium nitroprusside should be available for prompt and rapid injection through the side arm to control sudden and severe elevations of blood pressure. A bolus of 250 μg (i.e., 0.25 mg) of sodium nitroprusside may be sufficient to abort an elevation of blood pressure promptly (personal communication from Dr. Lubos Triner, anesthesiologist, Columbia Medical Center, New York City). However, the number of injections of nitroprusside required and the rate of infusion of this drug which may be needed to control blood pressure vary from patient to patient. The effect of a bolus of nitroprusside is so evanescent that an infusion of this agent must also be administered to control properly the blood pressure. Occasionally it may be necessary to infuse a drip containing as much as 500 μg of nitroprusside per ml. Some recommend that a test dose of 500 μg of sodium nitroprusside be given intravenously before starting treatment with this drug. The onset of the antihypertensive action of nitroprusside is almost immediate and its duration of action is very short—about 3 min. This drug is apparently an extremely potent vasodilator and acts directly on vascular smooth muscle. Tachycardia is usually not caused by administration of nitroprusside and tachyphylaxis does not occur (498).

Phentolamine, a blocker of α-adrenergic receptors, can be administered by infusion to control blood pressure effectively. It can also be given by bolus in a dose of 1 to 5 mg (1 mg/ml), but this must be adjusted to the needs of the patient. Pertsemlidis, Gitlow, and associates have recommended that two bottles, containing phentolamine concentrations of 10 μg/ml (5 mg in 500 ml of 5 percent dextrose and water), and 80 μg/ml (40 mg in 500 ml of 5 percent dextrose and water), respectively, be connected to an intravenous line so that either concentration can be infused at the desired rate. They have further stated that during manipulation of very active tumors, concentrations up to 160 μg/ml (40 mg in 250 ml of 5 percent dextrose and water) will be necessary (748). As mentioned earlier, they used a constant infusion of phentolamine in high concentration in one of their patients for 1 month preoperatively without any side effects.

In order to avoid prolonged α-blockade with phenoxybenzamine, Gitlow and associates generally prefer to control the blood pressure of their patients who have pheochromocytoma with intravenous phentolamine intraoperatively and, if necessary, for 1 or more days preoperatively. Their desire to avoid use of phenoxybenzamine is based on the fact, previously mentioned, that the blood pressure cannot be used as a guide to tumor location or as an indication of residual tumor in the presence of marked α-blockade.

Although the onset of action of intravenously administered phentolamine is almost as prompt as that of sodium nitroprusside, the duration of action of phentolamine may persist for 5 to 10 min, and sometimes longer. Rarely, a profound hypotensive response to phentolamine has been observed in patients with pheochromocytoma, and one patient was reported whose blood pressure was not reduced by phentolamine but was promptly controlled with sodium nitroprusside. Although either phentolamine or nitroprusside can be used effectively to control blood pressure in practically all patients with pheochromocytoma, we and others (498) prefer to use nitroprusside.

It has become apparent that during anesthesia and operation arrhythmias are apt to appear when sudden increases in blood pressure occur (especially when the systolic pressure exceeds 170 mmHg), at least during anesthesia with halothane (498). Usually these arrhythmias disappear as soon as the blood pressure is lowered; consequently, prompt lowering of the blood pressure with nitroprusside or phentolamine is mandatory and is the first step in combatting arrhythmias. (Regarding arrhythmias encountered with pheochromocytoma, see Chapter 6 under Electrocardiographic Changes.) Sometimes the frequency of severe blood pressure elevations and arrhythmias can be reduced by increasing the depth of anesthesia.

If the arrhythmia continues despite reduction of the blood pressure below the arrythmogenic threshold, the intravenous administration of a bolus of lidocaine (50 to 100 mg) or propranolol (0.1 to 0.25 mg) is indicated. Lidocaine has proved particularly effective in controlling ventricular extrasystoles or ventricular tachycardia; its onset of action following intravenous administration is very rapid and its effect disappears within 10 to 20 min. It depresses automaticity; however, it has little effect on the electrophysiologic properties of atrial muscle and is ineffective in atrial arrhythmias. It may cause alarming ventricular acceleration during atrial flutter and it should not be used for treatment of supraventricular arrhythmias. S-A nodal arrest has occurred when lidocaine was used with quinidine. Since convulsions may occasionally occur, a suitable barbiturate and diazepam should be available for prompt intravenous injection (386, p. 697). Finally, since lidocaine can lower blood pressure further, it should not be given in the presence of profound hypotension.

Two patients operated upon at Columbia Medical Center developed marked decreases in diastolic blood pressure which resulted from ventricular arrhythmias; both arrhythmias reverted to normal sinus rhythm with injections of less than 0.3 mg of propranolol (personal communication from Dr. Charles E. Wolf, Professor of Anesthesiology, University of Texas). Since propranolol can cause significant myocardial depression, it is preferable that the total dose administered during operation should not exceed 5 mg. Arrhythmias due to excessive circulating catecholamines will usually respond to either propranolol or lidocaine; however, occasionally arrhythmias will respond to only one of these drugs and not to the other. Sjoerdsma and coworkers have used propranolol in doses of 2 to 5 mg (0.05 to 0.1 mg/kg), which they found was much more successful than 50 mg of lidocaine in correcting significant ventricular arrhythmias, such as bigeminy (six cases), multifocal ventricular premature contractions (four), and ventricular tachycardia (one); however, they suggested that their dose of lidocaine may have been too small and that 100 mg should be used if 50 mg is ineffective. Ventricular arrhythmias are usually reversed by adequate doses of either propranolol or lidocaine within 30 sec. If no response from one of these agents is observed, the dose should be repeated. If with repeated doses there is still no response to one of these agents, then the other agent should be tried. We prefer to start with 0.5 mg or less of propranolol or 50 mg of lidocaine and repeat and increase dosage as necessary. Cardioversion equipment should always be available for immediate use if needed.

HYPOTENSION: PREVENTION AND TREATMENT

The importance of volume replacement, both preoperatively and intraoperatively, in patients with pheochromocytoma has become increasingly apparent during the past decade. Ideally, it would be desirable to know preoperatively the total blood volume and also the plasma volume and the red cell mass, particularly in those patients with sustained hypertension due to pheochromocytoma. Patients with sustained hypertension usually have the most pronounced changes in blood volume, although patients with frequent and severe bouts of paroxysmal hypertension may also have decreased blood volumes. If one determines the various volume parameters, replacement of the precise volume deficit can be accomplished with blood, red blood cells, 6 percent Albumisol, or dextran (Macrodex) a day before the operation. Usually, a deficit of plasma volume is evident in patients with sustained hypertension due to pheochromocytoma. Tarazi and associates have observed a predictable inverse relationship between plasma volume and diastolic blood pressure in patients with pheochromocytomas as well as in those with essential or renovascular hypertension (966).

In a series of 92 patients with pheochromocytoma treated at the Mayo Clinic up to 1965, Schnelle and associates found differences in the response to anesthesia and surgery between patients with sustained and those with paroxysmal hypertension (868). For example, 38 percent of patients with sustained hypertension developed a systolic pressure of 250 mmHg or greater as compared with 21 percent of those with paroxysmal hypertension. Furthermore, almost 9 percent of patients with sustained hypertension reached systolic pressures of 300 mmHg or greater, whereas none of those with paroxysmal hypertension had elevations of this magnitude. Also, the systolic blood pressure fell below 80 mmHg in 31 percent of patients with sustained hypertension, as compared with 12 percent in the paroxysmal group. Finally, it was noted that 90 percent of patients who had a particularly stormy course of anesthesia, and all those who died, had sustained hypertension. They concluded that patients with sustained hypertension are more likely to present greater difficulties during anesthesia than patients with paroxysmal hypertension (868).

As we previously demonstrated, patients with sustained hypertension due to pheochromocytoma continuously secrete catecholamines into the circulation, whereas some patients with paroxysmal hypertension may release catecholamines from their tumors only during paroxysms (616, 624, 823). Schnelle and coworkers pointed out that alterations in blood volume are more likely to be present in patients with sustained hypertension who have a persistently constricted vascular bed than in those with paroxysmal hypertension; consequently, there was a lower incidence of severe hypotension in the latter group following tumor extirpation (868). They found that the degree of difficulties encountered during anesthesia could be roughly predicted from the preoperative levels of plasma catecholamines (determined by the ethylenediamine fluorometric method as modified by Manger). As can be seen in Table 8.2, there was an inverse relationship between the basal concentrations of plasma catecholamines and the average minimal systolic blood pressure observed following tumor removal. A similar relationship between urinary levels of catecholamines or their metabolites and the blood pressure response after tumor removal was less reliable.

One of the virtues of normalizing blood pressure by α-adrenergic blockade with phenoxybenzamine for a week or more prior to operation is that the blood volume returns to normal. On the other hand, long-term β-adrenergic blockade is not associated with volume expansion in essential hypertension (967).

Table 8.2 *Relationship between Levels of Catecholamines and Blood Pressure*[a]

Basal plasma catecholamines (µg/liter)	No. of patients	Average minimal systolic blood pressure after removal of tumor (mmHg)
<6 (normal)	8	105
10–20	10	88
>20 (maximal, 213)	6	64

[a] From Schnelle, N., Carney, F. M. T., Didier, E. P., and Faulconer, A., Jr. *Surg. Clin. North Am. 45:* 997, 1965.

Usually, blood loss during operative removal of a pheochromocytoma is relatively minor; however, occasionally damage to a major vessel, such as the inferior vena cava, can occur during dissection of an adherent tumor, and blood loss may then become a major problem, requiring transfusion of large amounts of whole blood. The average amount of intraoperative fluids given to a series of patients at the Mayo Clinic was 2 units (2 pints) of blood and 2800 ml of electrolyte solution per patient. It is always best to transfuse considerably more than the blood lost at operation (747). Scott and associates also recommend aggressive blood and fluid replacement (usually 50 to 70 g of albumin and 2 to 3 liters of Ringer's lactate) during operation (875a).

In past years, before preoperative volume replacement or α-adrenergic blockade was performed, it was recognized that even in the uncomplicated case (i.e., without any major hemorrhage), there was often a profound and prolonged drop in blood pressure immediately following tumor removal, and sometimes for several days postoperatively. Apparently this was due, in part at least, to a disparity between the decreased blood volume and the expansion of the vascular space which occurred after tumor removal, and the accompanying marked decrease in circulating catecholamines. It was concluded that hypotension following tumor removal was more appropriately treated with intraoperative blood transfusion than with administration of vasopressor agents (489, 909).

Prior to routine adequate blood replacement preoperatively and intraoperatively, patients not infrequently had to be maintained on constant infusions of norepinephrine for several days postoperatively in order to prevent hypotension. Today intra- and postoperative infusion of pressor agents is rarely necessary. It is, however, still an important precaution to prepare a solution of norepinephrine (Levophed) in 5 percent dextrose and water for immediate use in the presence of a severe hypotensive crisis which does not respond to volume replacement. Pertsemlidis, Gitlow, and associates (748) recommend the preparation of two dilutions of norepinephrine (8 µg/ml and 64 µg/ml) so that either concentration can be infused through the venous infusion catheter, according to the needs of the patient. (If a norepinephrine infusion is administered it is extremely important to avoid extravasation of this solution into the tissues; it is well known that the intensity of the vasoconstriction caused by this pressor agent may result in tissue ischemia, necrosis, and sloughing.)

In an effort to demonstrate the importance of preoperative blood transfusion in reducing the incidence of hypotension postoperatively, 46 patients with pheochromocytoma were studied at the Cleveland Clinic (223). Of the 24 patients who received no preoperative blood transfusion, 17 (71 percent) required vasopressors in the operative or postoperative management, only four (18 percent) of the 22 patients who received 2 units of blood preoperatively on an empirical basis (i.e., not based on blood volume determinations) required vasopressors (Table 8.3). Continuous vasopressor treatment was required for 24 to 48 hr postoperatively in four of the patients who received no preoperative transfusion, whereas this prolonged duration of treatment was never required in the patients who received 2 units of blood preoperatively (Table 8.3).

We are convinced of the importance of

volume replacement preoperatively and intraoperatively in preventing postoperative hypotension: we feel it is of fundamental importance in the operative management of patients with pheochromocytoma. Whether routine empirical volume replacement (e.g., with 2 units of blood) is performed or whether replacement is precisely tailored to the patient's deficits (based on volume measurements) is probably not of crucial importance.

SURGICAL TECHNIQUES AND STRATEGY

The operative technique utilizing the anterior approach to adrenalectomy for pheochromocytoma has been elegantly presented in color figures by Edis, Ayala, and Egdahl (249). "The artwork represents the distillation of twelve months of intensive collaboration between the authors and a staff of medical illustrators to ensure anatomic fidelity and clarity" (249). We are particularly grateful for permission to reproduce a series of color illustrations and accompanying commentary (with minimal alteration), which we believe will be especially appreciated by surgeons involved with adrenal surgery.

We feel strongly that an anterior transabdominal (i.e., transperitoneal) approach is virtually mandatory when operating for a

Table 8.3   *Vasopressors in Operative and Postoperative Management of 46 Patients with Pheochromocytoma[a]*

Vasopressor treatment	No. of patients	
	No preoperative transfusion— 1952 to 1967 (24 patients)	2 Units of blood preoperatively— 1966 to 1972 (22 patients)
Vasopressor required		
Intraoperative only	3	2
Postoperative		
0–8 hr	5	1
8–24 hr	5	1
24–48 hr	4	0
Total	17 (71%)[b]	4 (18%)[b]
No vasopressor required	7	18

[a] After Deoreo, G. A., Jr., Stewart, B. H., Tarazi, R. C., and Gifford, R. W., Jr. *J. Urol. 111:* 719, 1974.

[b] This difference is significant at $p < 0.005$; chi-square with Yates' correction is 10.79.

pheochromocytoma. Several strong arguments for the anterior approach can be made. First, approximately 10 percent of the patients have their tumor in an extraadrenal location. Certainly the entire abdomen must be carefully explored at every operation. Second, despite almost certainty of the preoperative location of one pheochromocytoma, about 8 percent of adults, and 35 percent of children, have multiple tumors. Third, associated pathology (e.g., cholelithiasis, intraabdominal neurofibromatosis, and vascular abnormalities) may be corrected at operation. A final compelling reason for an anterior approach is the occasional need for cardiac massage and resuscitation. (This is based upon a personal comment by Dr. Peter J. Puchner, Assistant Professor of Clinical Urology at Columbia Medical Center, who has had extensive experience in removing pheochromocytomas.) Resuscitation is accomplished much more readily if the patient is on his back rather than on his side, as, for example, in a lumbodorsal retroperitoneal approach; turning the patient from his side onto his back during a surgical exploration is indeed undesirable but the supine position is required for the most effective resuscitation.

We and our colleagues do not feel it is "necessary or even wise to transgress the integrity of the pleural cavity" (784) when removing an intraabdominal pheochromocytoma. The anterior abdominal approach is generally made through a bilateral subcostal incision—particularly where the angle of the costal margin is wide and there is a flaring rib cage. On the other hand, a long midline incision may be preferred in thin patients where the costal margins form an acute angle (Fig. 8.2). Since the adrenal glands usually "sit high" in the abdomen, the long midline incision extending from the xyphoid downward may permit better exposure in the thin patient. Most patients with pheochromocytoma are, in fact, thin, since many of them have lost a considerable amount of weight. A vertical midline incision is also preferred if the pheochromocytoma is located in the organ of Zuckerkandl, bladder, or pelvis, or if multiple extraadrenal tumors are anticipated.

Dr. James T. Priestley (Emeritus Chairman of the Surgical Section at the Mayo Clinic, whose experience removing intraabdominal pheochromocytomas has been one of the most extensive) stated that it is his impression that the anterior approach is not accompanied by any significant increase in morbidity as compared with the posterolumbar approach. He noted, however, that exposure of the left adrenal gland through an anterior approach requires some mobilization of the spleen, which may result in trauma and bleeding, thus making splenectomy necessary; however, this occurrence is uncommon (personal communication). Occasionally technical difficulties, particularly with an invasive or large tumor, may require splenectomy or nephrectomy or even both (869).

After the peritoneal cavity has been entered, the routine procedure is first to examine all viscera and then to concentrate on the sites where chromaffin tissue occurs, i.e., the adrenal glands, para-aortic and lumbar ganglia, the perirenal area, the region of the organ of Zuckerkandl, the pelvic area, and the bladder. Most surgeons prefer to explore the region where the tumor is thought to exist last of all, since palpation can cause hypertensive crises that make further examination difficult or hazardous (784).

When the tumor has been exposed, its venous drainage should be promptly ligated. The vascular architecture and large vessels of a pheochromocytoma may be readily apparent on previously obtained angiographic studies, and this knowledge may facilitate and expedite ligation of the tumor's blood vessels. Manipulation of the tumor should be minimized in order to avoid releasing massive quantities of the catecholamines into the circulation. If nitroprusside (or phentolamine) infusion is being administered it should be discontinued a few minutes before tumor removal; some suggest that the primary anesthetic agent be discontinued at the same time and that anesthesia then be maintained with nitrous oxide and d-tubocurarine (498).

When a single adrenal pheochromocytoma is present, adrenalectomy should be performed, with removal of adjacent fatty tissue. In the presence of bilateral pheochromocytoma, Remine and coworkers recommend that a small portion of the normal adrenal gland be left behind in the gland with the smaller tumor (784). On the other hand, Edis, Ayala, and Egdahl prefer to perform bilateral total adrenalectomy when tumors are bilateral; they point out that there have been several instances where inadvertent rupture of an apparently benign encapsulated tumor during dissection has resulted in a spread and recurrence of the tumor (249).

Recently, Carney and coworkers have recommended that once the diagnosis of adrenal medullary disease is made in a patient with MEN–type 2 syndrome (symptomatic or asymptomatic) bilateral total adrenalectomy be performed. To support their recommendation they cited the fact that in this syndrome there is (a) great likelihood of synchronous bilateral involvement, (b) a risk of local recurrence if the entire adrenal is not removed, and (c) a high mortality from the adrenal component of the syndrome (135b). Admittedly, this recommendation of Carney and coworkers is controversial and must await additional experience to establish its validity. One might be tempted to conclude that total bilateral adrenalectomy may similarly be indicated in patients with the MEN–type 3 syndrome; however, such a conclusion cannot be justified or rejected until adrenal medullary pathology in this particular syndrome is adequately evaluated. Finally, it has been pointed out that patients with familial pheochromocytoma that is unassociated with medullary thyroid carcinoma may not show a greater propensity to have multiple chromaffin tumor foci (631a). Adrenal medullary biopsy and the demonstration of a pheochromocytoma or medullary hyperplasia on frozen section could aid in deciding whether bilateral adrenalectomy is indicated in some patients with the MEN–type 2 and –type 3 syndromes; the diagnostic value of adrenal medullary biopsy and its risks have not been assessed.

It is suggested that following tumor extirpation, the entire abdominal cavity should be thoroughly reexplored and any suspicious nodules be biopsied. Bloom and Fonkalsrud suggested that in children, because of the high incidence of bilateral pheochromocytomas, a biopsy be considered on the contralateral gland—even if it appears normal at operation (84). To support this suggestion they cited the observation of Stefanini and associates that the tumor in the adrenal gland is nonpalpable and the gland appears normal in 5 percent of patients (937).

It is worth mentioning that in one patient a pheochromocytoma of the right adrenal was not detected by the surgeon and, unfortunately, an enlarged left adrenal gland was removed. The enlargement was due to adrenal cortical hyperplasia which was compensatory for cortical atrophy caused by pressure from the medullary tumor in the opposite gland (462).

The presence of tumor in liver and lymph nodes and in sites distant from the primary tumor, where chromaffin tissue does not ordinarily occur, suggests metastatic disease. There seems to be general agreement that "metastatic tumor should be removed where feasible to reduce the bulk of functioning tissue and thereby facilitate pharmacologic therapy" (249).

Puchner has remarked that it is well for the surgeon to recall that the vascular supply of the adrenal glands is "consistently inconsistent" (personal comment). He has cautioned that removal of a pheochromocytoma in the right adrenal area is particularly hazardous since one may inadvertently damage the connection of the right middle adrenal vein to the inferior vena cava and thus produce a massive hemorrhage. Tumors in the right adrenal are apt to lie behind the vena cava in a less accessible region than on the left side. A left adrenal pheochromocytoma may be more readily seen, since a portion of the tumor may overlie the aorta; the adrenal vein can usually be easily identified entering the left renal vein. Another important point stressed by Dr. Puchner is that dissection of these tumors from adjacent tissue may cause considerable hemorrhage. Even when they are approached laterally, there may be considerable bleeding since these tumors can grow and rotate in such a manner as to displace some of the major vasculature into a lateral aspect. An uncomplicated removal of a single pheochromocytoma requires approximately 2 to 3 hr and usually does not entail much blood loss.

The following surgical color illustrations and commentary by Edis, Ayala, and Egdahl very clearly depict the operative technique and strategy used to expose and remove adrenal pheochromocytomas (Figs. 8.2–8.13, pp. 328–334).

Regarding exploration for extraadrenal

pheochromocytomas, Edis, Ayala, and Egdahl have stated that

Exploration of the para-aortic sympathetic chains, the opposite adrenal, and the perihilar zones of each kidney must be carried out in every case to exclude supernumerary extraadrenal pheochromocytomas. Failure to register a decrease in blood pressure after an adrenal medullary tumor is removed should alert the surgeon to the possibility that a second lesion is present.

Preoperative alpha-adrenergic blockade is seldom complete so that manipulation of a tumor is often associated with a transient elevation in blood pressure due to the release of catecholamines into the circulation. This phenomenon may be used as a guide to the location of extraadrenal pheochromocytomas.

Closure of the abdomen is performed in the usual way (249).

The operative technique of adrenal exposure described by Edis, Ayala, and Egdahl is similar to that utilized at the Mayo Clinic, Cleveland Clinic, and Columbia Medical Center. However, the surgical strategy of immediate ligation of the tumor vasculature practiced by the Cleveland surgeons differs from that of the other groups. Our associates at the Cleveland Clinic stress that good preoperative localization of pheochromocytomas simplifies and expedites the isolation and ligation of the blood supply of these tumors immediately after the abdomen is opened. They prefer to delay collateral exploration of the abdomen and pelvis until the tumor is removed. They have observed that blood pressure fluctuations during exploration are more reliable as a guide to residual tumors once the preoperatively localized pheochromocytoma has been removed, whereas falsely positive blood pressure elevations often occur with the latter in situ (223).

With the previously localized tumor removed and with the patient in a nonblocked state, exploration and palpation of the contralateral adrenal gland and all accessible sites where extraadrenal chromaffin tissue ordinarily occurs (e.g., the aorta, para-aortic regions, the organ of Zuckerkandl, iliac vessels, pelvis, renal pedicles) should be performed. During this procedure a valid blood pressure response can then be observed. As mentioned earlier, a decrease in blood pressure after tumor removal and the lack of a hypertensive response

to palpation in various areas help to exclude the presence of residual pheochromocytomas. Our associates at the Cleveland Clinic have found that a self-retaining ring retractor is particularly helpful in surgical exploration and extirpation of some abdominal pheochromocytomas (Fig. 8.12).

Although most surgeons today agree that the anterior transperitoneal approach is the most desirable, some recommend an extension of the incision into the thorax for improved exposure of pheochromocytomas arising in the adrenal glands. In order to minimize manipulation of the tumors, Scott and associates recommend that adrenal pheochromocytomas first be localized through an abdominal approach followed by removal through a wide thoracoabdominal incision (876). They par-

Fig. 8.12 A. Exposure gained by use of Smith ring retractor. Right subcostal incision is used. B. Large right pheochromocytoma is evident. Vena cava is retracted to expose arterial blood supply of gland. Clip and ligature secure major inferior adrenal artery arising from aorta. Suction tip points to hilus of right kidney. From Deoreo, G. A., Jr., Stewart, B. H., Tarazi, R. C., and Gifford, R. W., Jr., *J. Urol. 111:* 720, 1974. By permission of Williams & Wilkins Co.

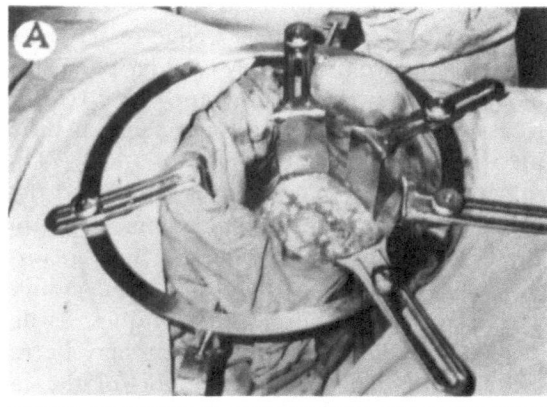

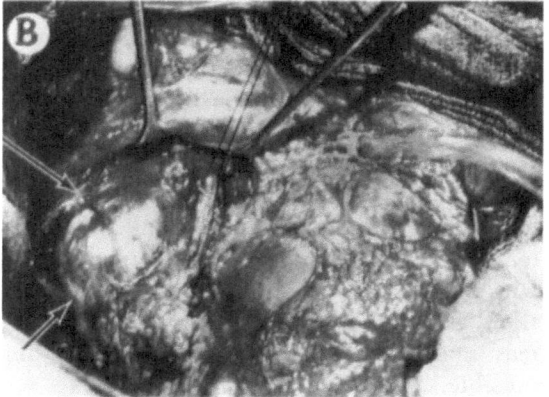

ticularly recommend extending the anterior transperitoneal incision across the costal margin into the eighth and ninth intercostal space in order to improve exposure of tumors greater than 6 cm in diameter (875a). We and our surgical colleagues at the Mayo and Cleveland Clinics and at Columbia Medical Center, however, feel this approach is rarely indicated.

MANAGEMENT OF EXTRAADRENAL PHEOCHROMOCYTOMAS

Extraadrenal pheochromocytomas in the abdomen, thorax, or neck must be removed completely for complete cure. The surgical approach will be dictated by their anatomic locations, and the same precautions with preoperative and intraoperative management should be observed in all patients with functioning pheochromocytomas. A point to remember when dissecting and removing any pheochromocytoma is that a reasonably wide excision of the tumor and its surrounding tissue is indicated. Some reports indicate that fragmentation of a pheochromocytoma during its removal can result in implants and recurrence of the tumor (878, 900).

Partial cystectomy (or a wedge resection) is usually curative for urinary bladder pheochromocytoma; however, malignancy may require total cystectomy, prostatectomy, seminal vesiculectomy, and urinary diversion (877). The routine thoracic approach is employed for extirpation of pheochromocytomas in the chest. For lesions in the neck, which in rare instances may even extend into the cranial cavity, specialized surgical techniques, as described by Glenner and Grimley, may be required (370). For example, tumors of the carotid body may be intimately connected with the common carotid artery and may require vascular reconstruction. Glomus jugulare tumors (which arise from the tympanic branch of the glossopharyngeal nerve or from the auricular branch of the vagus nerve) may require hypotympanotomy, radical mastoidectomy, or a combined suboccipital and transtemporal approach; extension intracranially, with involvement of cranial nerves, bone erosion, and impingement on vital structures, may make removal of the entire tumor impossible.

MANAGEMENT OF PHEOCHROMOCYTOMAS DURING PREGNANCY

The seriousness of pheochromocytoma, especially if unrecognized, as a life-threatening condition for both mother and fetus cannot be over emphasized. Every pregnant patient with hypertension of unknown etiology must be screened for the possible presence of a pheochromocytoma.

It has been suggested that if a pheochromocytoma is detected during the first 5 months of pregnancy, it is preferable to control the blood pressure and return any blood volume deficit toward normal by the use of α-adrenergic blocking agents, and, shortly thereafter, remove the tumor (324). Since it is undesirable to expose the fetus to excessive x-ray radiation, preoperative location of the pheochromocytoma by radiologic means is not recommended. As mentioned earlier, however, the demonstration of significant quantities of epinephrine in the urine or plasma, or of metanephrine (its metabolite) in the urine, strongly suggests that the tumor arises from the adrenal gland. In addition, catheterization of the vena cava and blood sampling from various sites is a relatively benign procedure which may help localize a pheochromocytoma. Unless abortion is contemplated, fluoroscopy should not be used for catheter localization in the pregnant patient. Despite the risk of abortion, the seriousness of pheochromocytoma in pregnancy makes it essential that the tumor be removed expeditiously. Gentle abdominal exploration during laparotomies in pregnant patients is considered important (260). Finally, an important point to be kept in mind when treating any pregnant patient is that hypotension (401) can compromise placental blood flow and thereby cause fetal distress and possibly death of the fetus. One must, therefore, exercise extreme caution in treating pregnant patients and constantly strive to avoid hypotensive as well as hypertensive crises.

In 1971 Schenker and Chowers reported a review of 86 cases of pheochromocytoma occurring in pregnancy (863). [A total of 96 cases of pheochromocytoma associated with pregnancy have been reported (46).] Again, the seriousness of this condition was emphasized. If the pheochromocytoma was undiagnosed,

58 percent of reported cases proved fatal to the mothers and 56 percent to the fetus. On the other hand, if the diagnosis was made during pregnancy, the maternal mortality was 17.3 percent but the fetal mortality was only slightly decreased. They cited evidence indicating the occurrence of enzymatic degradation of the catecholamines by COMT in the placenta; this would explain why the plasma catecholamines are much lower in cord blood than in the mother's blood. A marked differential between plasma catecholamine concentrations in cord and maternal blood has also been noted by others (46). Nevertheless, it is possible that detrimental elevations of circulating catecholamines may occur in the fetus during a hypertensive crisis in the mother. Chronic or acute oxygen deprivation may occur in the fetus and be related to excessive vasoconstriction in the fetus and/or the placenta; separation of the placenta may also occur during a hypertensive crisis.

Schenker and Chowers found 43 women who died as a result of their pheochromocytoma; 10 died before term, 3 died during labor, and 30 succumbed within 72 hr of vaginal delivery or cesarean section (863). Of the 62 fetal deaths studied, 16 pregnancies terminated in spontaneous abortion, 23 fetal deaths occurred in utero before term, and 23 of the newborn died during birth or early in the postpartum period.

It is imperative that the diagnosis of pheochromocytoma be confirmed or excluded in all pregnant patients with sustained or paroxysmal hypertension of uncertain etiology. Even in the absence of hypertension, patients with clinical manifestations suggesting pheochromocytoma should be thoroughly investigated. Early and proper management is crucial for the safety of both the mother and fetus.

If a pheochromocytoma is detected in the latter months of pregnancy, it has been recommended that the blood pressure be controlled with blocking agents until fetal maturity is reached, at which time vaginal delivery be permitted (260); or, with adequate preoperative preparation, cesarean section and removal of the pheochromocytoma can be performed at the same time (324, 402, 917). Despite α- and β-adrenergic blockade, the condition of a pregnant patient with pheochro-

mocytoma may deteriorate and require cesarean section before term (154). Infusion of phentolamine can be of value in controlling hypertensive crises (100). Again, measurement of epinephrine or its metabolite (metanephrine) in urine or plasma, and vena cava sampling without fluoroscopy (159), as mentioned above, may help localize the tumor preoperatively. Fetal maturity can be gauged by measuring the lecithin/sphingomyelin ratio; maturity is sufficient if the ratio in the amniotic fluid is two or greater. It should be kept in mind that even amniocentesis may conceivably trigger a massive release of catecholamines into the circulation.

In general, we believe it is desirable to remove a pheochromocytoma as soon as it is discovered, no matter what the stage of pregnancy. A transverse upper abdominal incision is usually desirable. It must be appreciated that in the third trimester surgical exploration may be somewhat limited and excision of the tumor may be difficult, if not impossible, without prior delivery. Therefore, if manifestations caused by excessive circulating catecholamines can be satisfactorily controlled with α- and β-adrenergic blocking agents, it may be preferable in certain instances to delay surgical intervention until the fetus reaches adequate maturity. If the fetus is mature, we believe it is preferable to perform a cesarean section, and remove the tumor at the same operation, rather than to permit the patient to deliver by the vaginal route; the stress of labor in patients with pheochromocytoma is indeed hazardous. These views are in agreement with those of Schenker and Chowers (863).

EFFECT OF ANESTHESIA AND TUMOR PALPATION ON BLOOD PRESSURE AND PLASMA CATECHOLAMINES

The effect of anesthesia with thiopental (Pentothal) sodium or ether as the major anesthetic agent, and nitrous oxide as basal anesthesia, on blood pressure and plasma catecholamine concentrations (usually venous but in some instances arterial) is displayed in Figures 8.13 and 8.14. In addition, the effect of tumor palpation and manipulation during

328

Fig. 8.2 Incision A. A bilateral subcostal incision provides excellent exposure. However, a transverse upper abdominal incision or a long midline incision may be preferred in some patients. B. The abdomen is opened and routine inspection and palpation of the abdominal contents is carried out. At this time the surgeon quickly confirms the presence of adrenal tumor and takes note of any other pathology. From Edis, J. A., Ayala, L. A., and Egdahl, R. H. *Manual of Endocrine Surgery*. Courtesy of Springer-Verlag, 1975, p. 189.

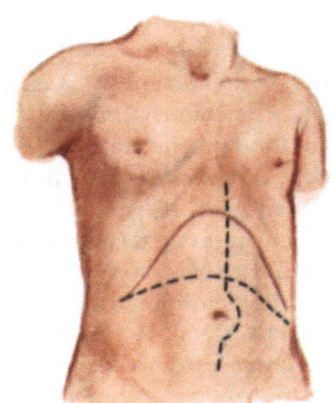

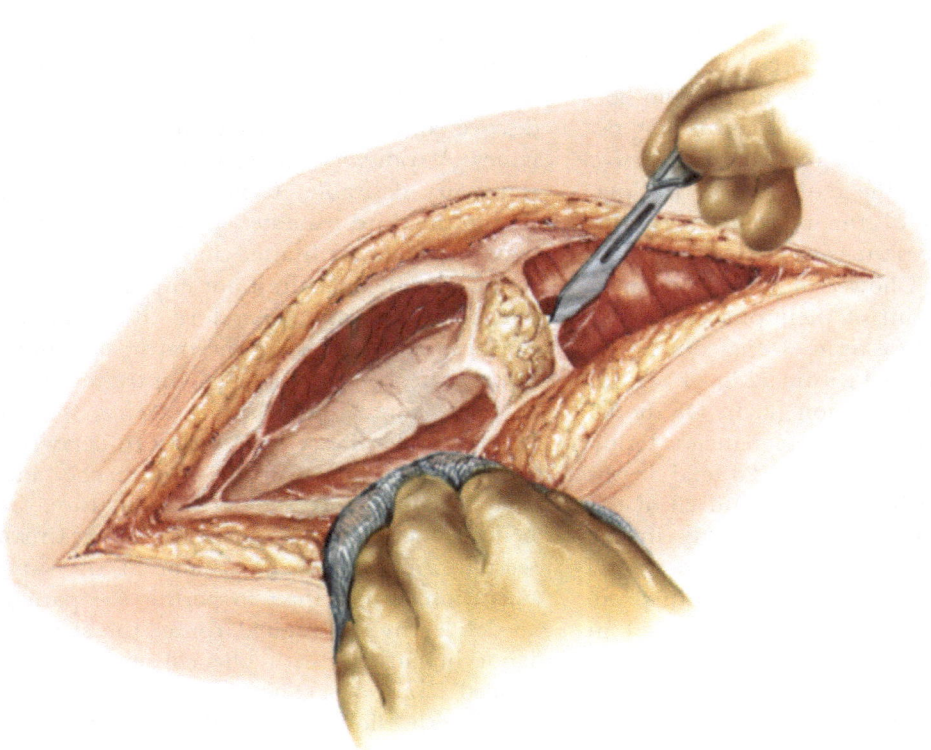

Fig. 8.3 Exposure of a tumor of the right adrenal gland. The technique is depicted in this and the following illustrations.

The hepatic flexure of the colon has been mobilized and retracted downward to expose the duodenal loop. The second portion of the duodenum is freed by dividing its lateral avascular peritoneal reflection with scissors (Kocher maneuver). The right lobe of the liver is retracted upward. From Edis, J. A., Ayala, L. A., and Egdahl, R. H. *Manual of Endocrine Surgery*. Courtesy of Springer-Verlag, 1975, p. 190.

Fig. 8.4 The descending duodenum is separated from the retroperitoneal structures posteriorly by blunt and sharp dissection and is then turned forward and to the left. This maneuver exposes the underlying vena cava and a pheochromocytoma of the right adrenal gland overlying the superior pole of the kidney. From Edis, J. A., Ayala, L. A., and Egdahl, R. H. *Manual of Endocrine Surgery*. Courtesy of Springer-Verlag, 1975, p. 191.

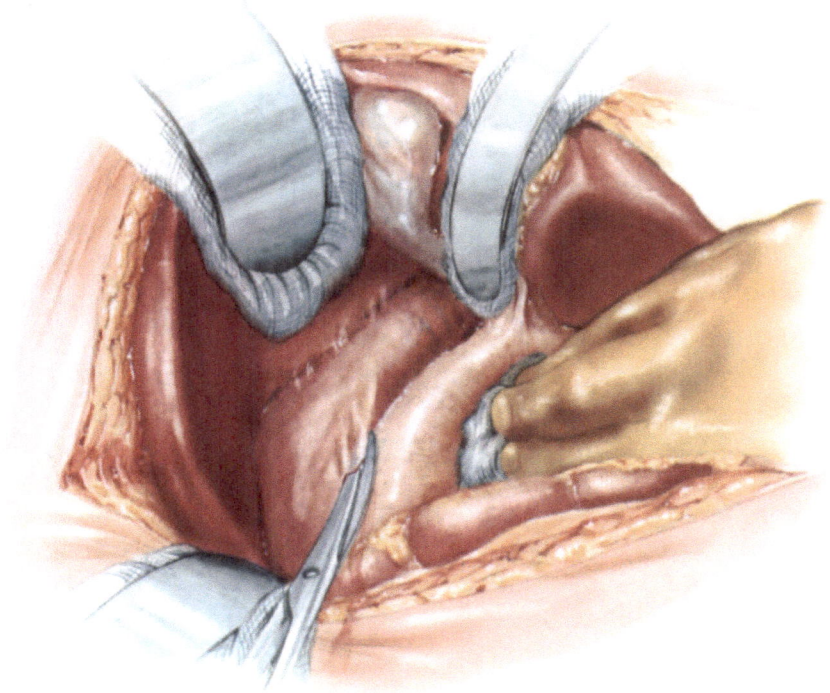

Figure 8.3

Figure 8.4

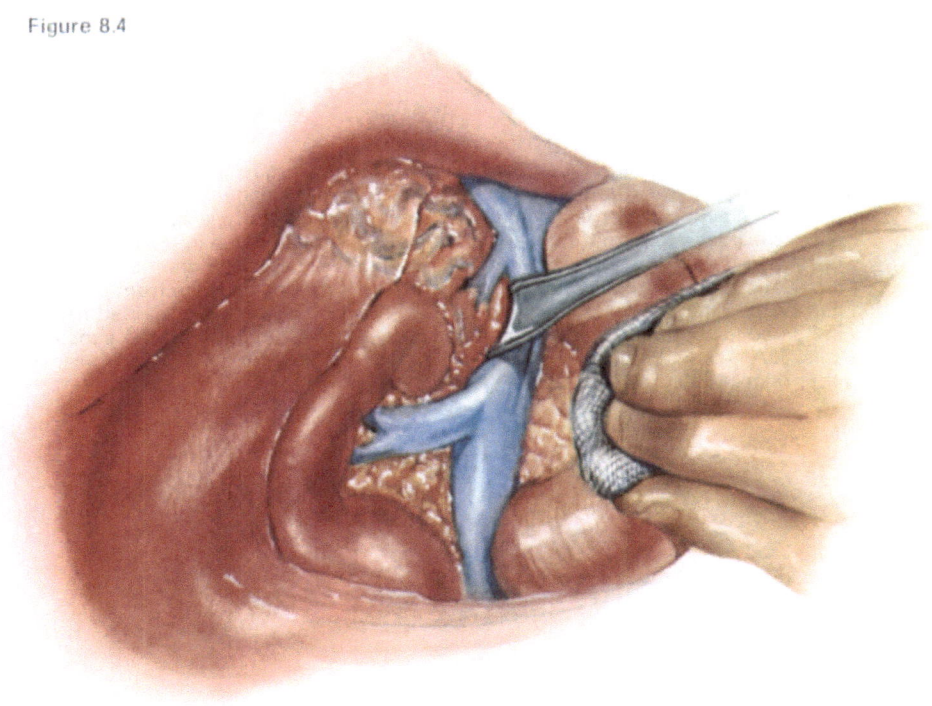

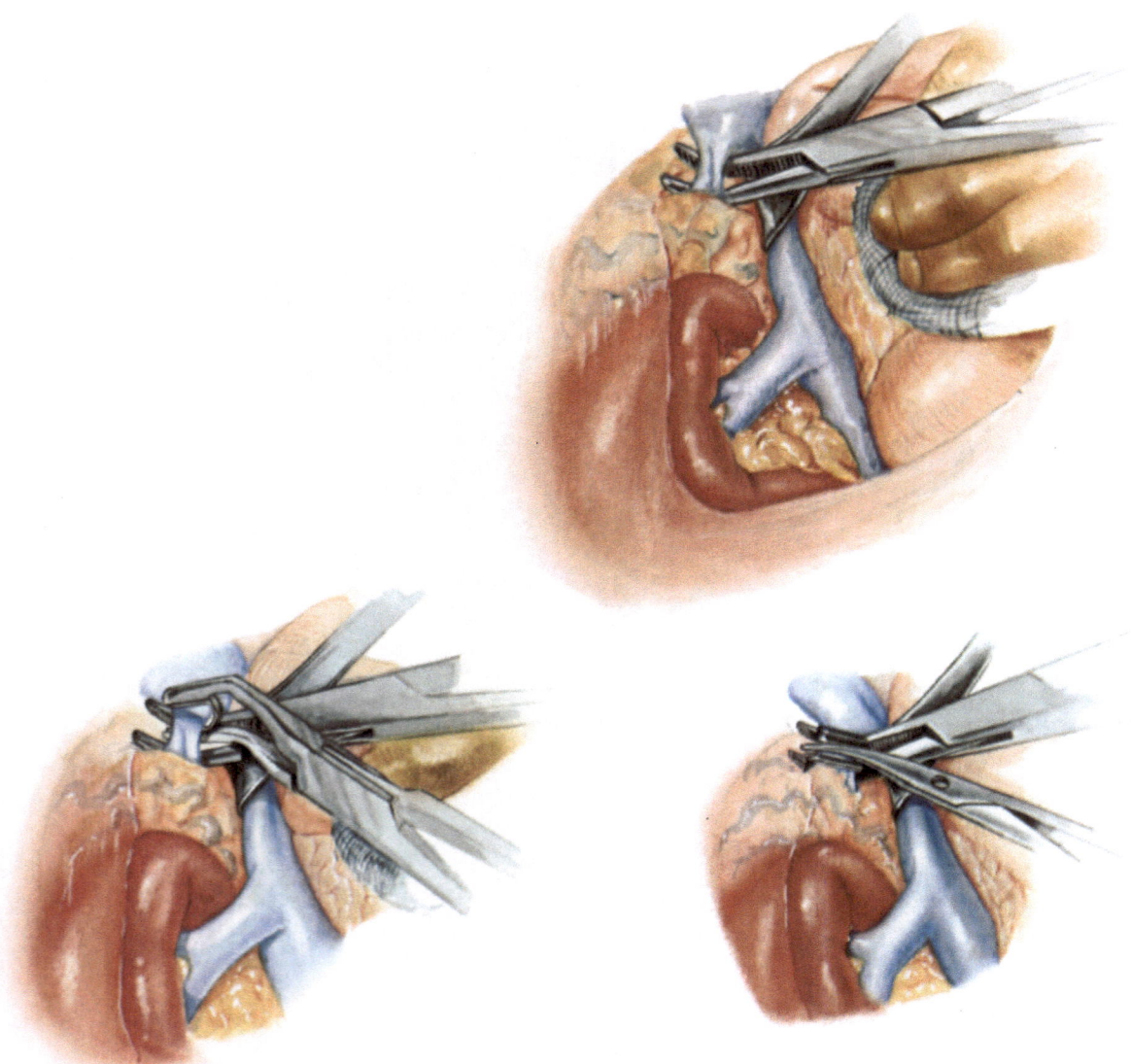

Fig. 8.5 Ligation of the right adrenal vein. The venous drainage of the tumor should be ligated as the next step to prevent release of catecholamines into the general circulation as the tumor is manipulated. Proceeding carefully, a sufficient length of vena cava is exposed to permit side application of a vascular clamp in the event of a caval tear during attempts to control the venous drainage from the tumor. In this case, the short, wide right adrenal vein is seen clearly as it passes over the front of the medial part of the tumor to reach the vena cava. A. The adrenal vein is dissected free, B. ligated in continuity using large metal clips, C. severed between the clips. From Edis, J. A., Ayala, L. A., and Egdahl, R. H. *Manual of Endocrine Surgery.* Courtesy of Springer-Verlag, 1975, p. 192.

Fig. 8.6 With the pheochromocytoma effectively isolated from the venous side of the circulation, the process of freeing it from its bed can proceed with less concern for the occurrence of paroxysms of hypertension or cardiac irregularities. The entire tumor is dissected free from above downward using metal clips for hemostasis. The authors prefer not to dissect out the lower pole of the tumor until the upper, lateral, and medial borders have been freed. From Edis, J. A., Ayala, L. A., and Egdahl, R. H. *Manual of Endocrine Surgery.* Courtesy of Springer-Verlag, 1975, p. 193.

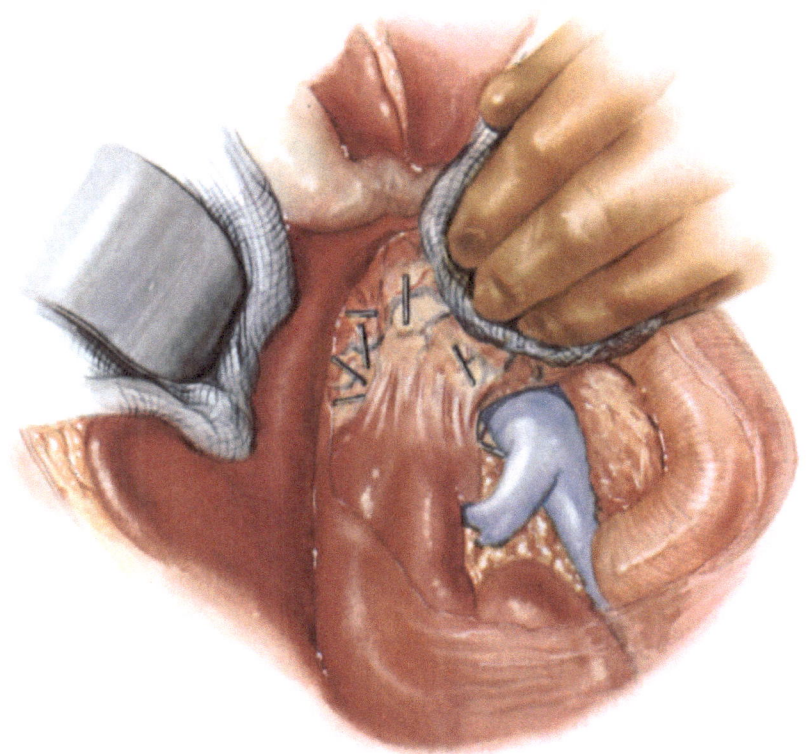

Fig. 8.7 Quite frequently a tumor of the right adrenal gland will extend upward behind the right edge of the vena cava. However, it usually is easily separated from the vena cava by retracting the latter as shown. Finally, the fascial attachments to the kidney are divided and the tumor removed. From Edis, J. A., Ayala, L. A., and Egdahl, R. H. *Manual of Endocrine Surgery.* Courtesy of Springer-Verlag, 1975, p. 193.

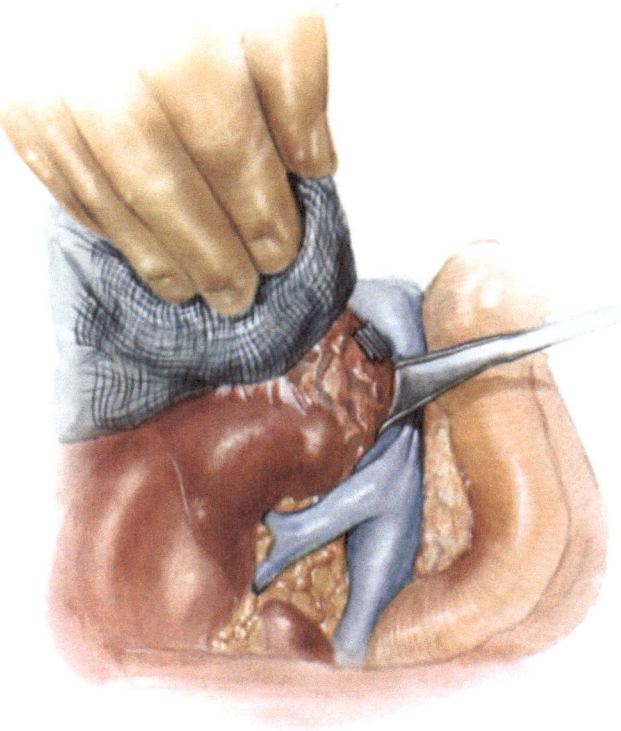

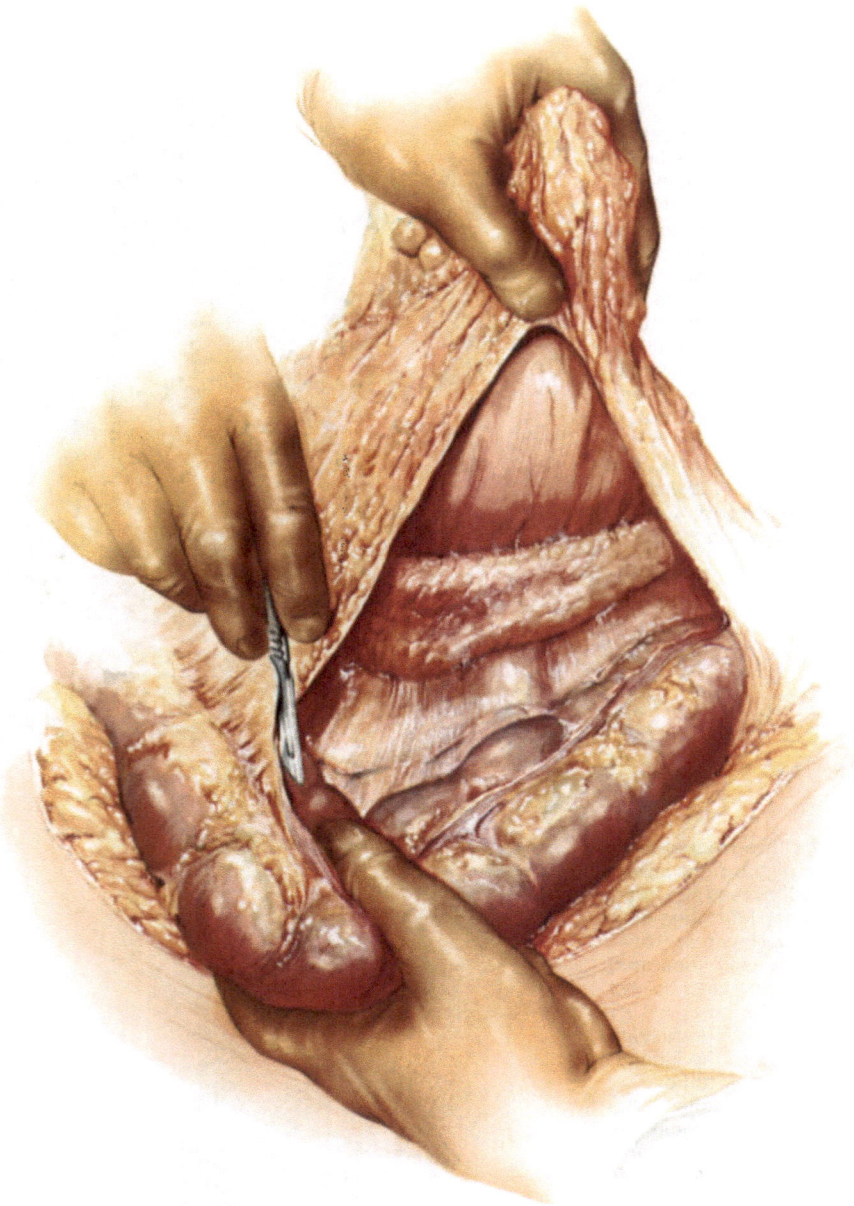

Fig. 8.8 Exposure of a tumor of the left adrenal gland. The left adrenal gland can be exposed safely and conveniently via the lesser sac. Using gentle upward traction on the greater omentum, its avascular attachment to the distal transverse colon is divided to give direct access into the lesser sac. Care is taken to avoid excessive traction of the splenocolic ligament for fear of tearing the splenic capsule. If exposure is not adequate, it is sometimes helpful to mobilize the splenic flexure of the colon. From Edis, J. A., Ayala, L. A., and Egdahl, R. H. *Manual of Endocrine Surgery.* Courtesy of Springer-Verlag, 1975, p. 194.

333

Fig. 8.9 With the stomach retracted superiorly and the transverse colon inferiorly the pancreas comes into view. The peritoneum along the inferior border of the body and tail of the pancreas is incised (broken line). From Edis, J. A., Ayala, L. and Egdahl, R. H. *Manual of Endocrine Surgery.* Courtesy of Springer-Verlag, 1975, p. 195.

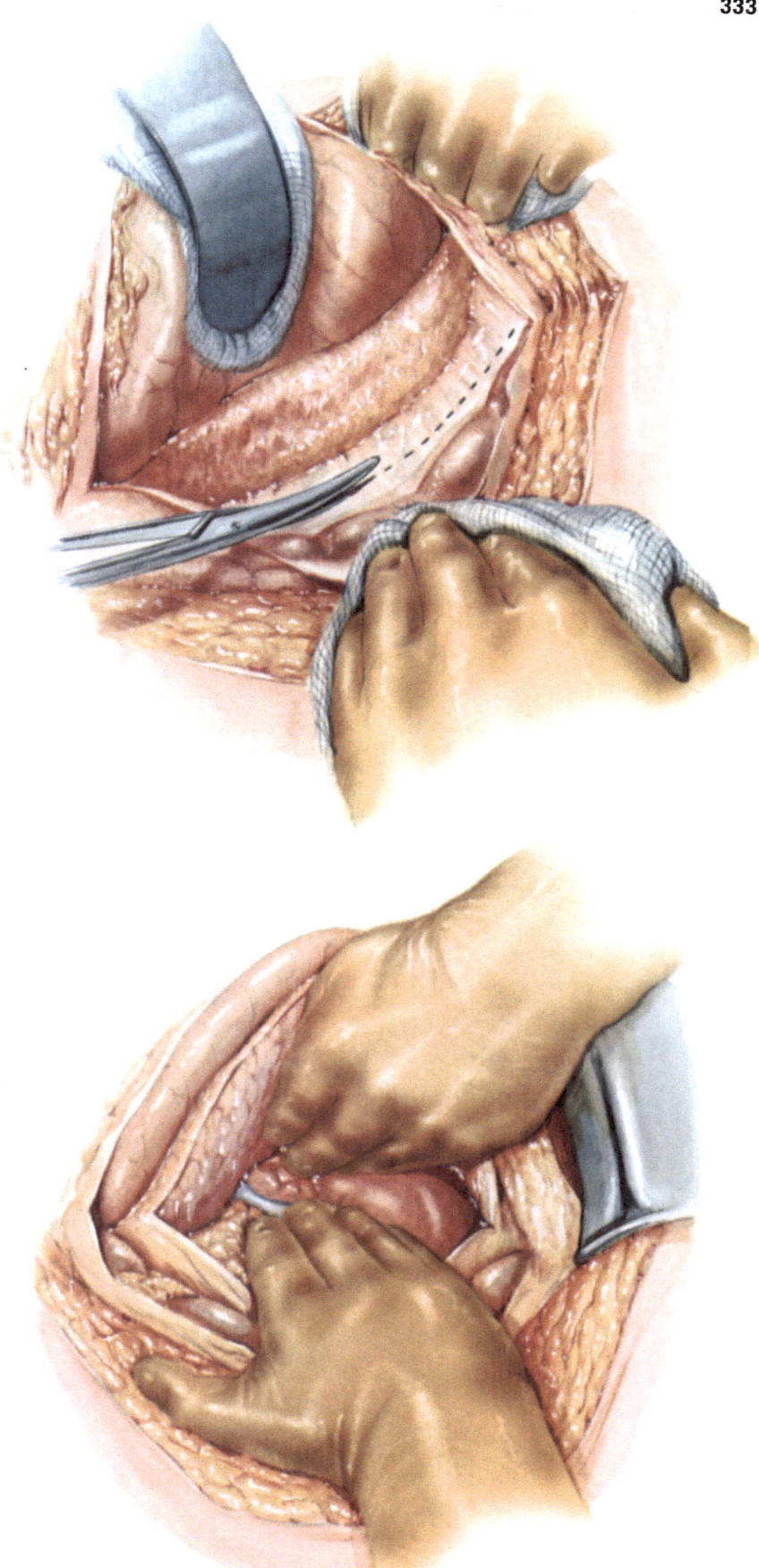

Fig. 8.10 The areolar plane deep to the pancreas is opened by blunt finger dissection, as depicted. The crooked fingers of the left hand elevate the tail of the pancreas and work in gentle motion, with the fingers of the right hand providing counteraction, to separate the areolar tissue and progressively free the gland. From Edis, J. A., Ayala, L. A., and Egdahl, R. *Manual of Endocrine Surgery.* Courtesy of Springer-Verlag, 1975, p. 195.

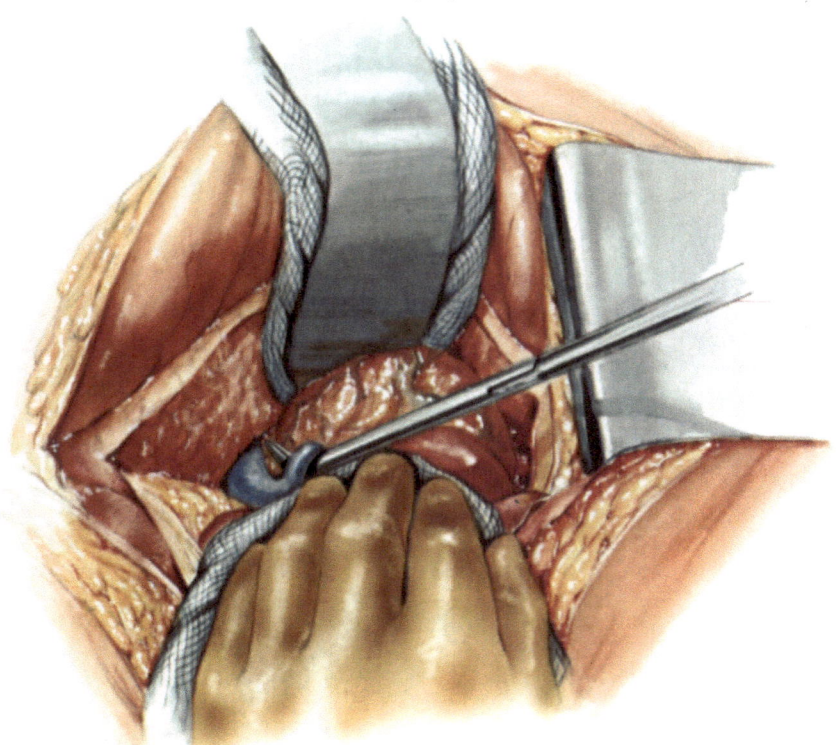

Fig. 8.11 With the pancreas freed and retracted upward out of the way, the kidney and a left adrenal tumor lie exposed. The left adrenal vein can be seen entering the left renal vein. It is isolated over a right angled clamp, clipped in continuity, and divided. As before the tumor is dissected free from the retroperitoneal fat and finally, from the kidney, using multiple small metal clips for hemostasis. From Edis, J. A., Ayala, L. A., and Egdahl, R. H. *Manual of Endocrine Surgery*. Courtesy of Springer-Verlag, 1975, p. 196.

Medical illustrations (Figs. 8.2 to 8.11 drawn under the direction of Jerome T. Glickman, Team Administrator, Educational Media Support Center, Boston University Medical Center, Boston, Massachusetts 02118

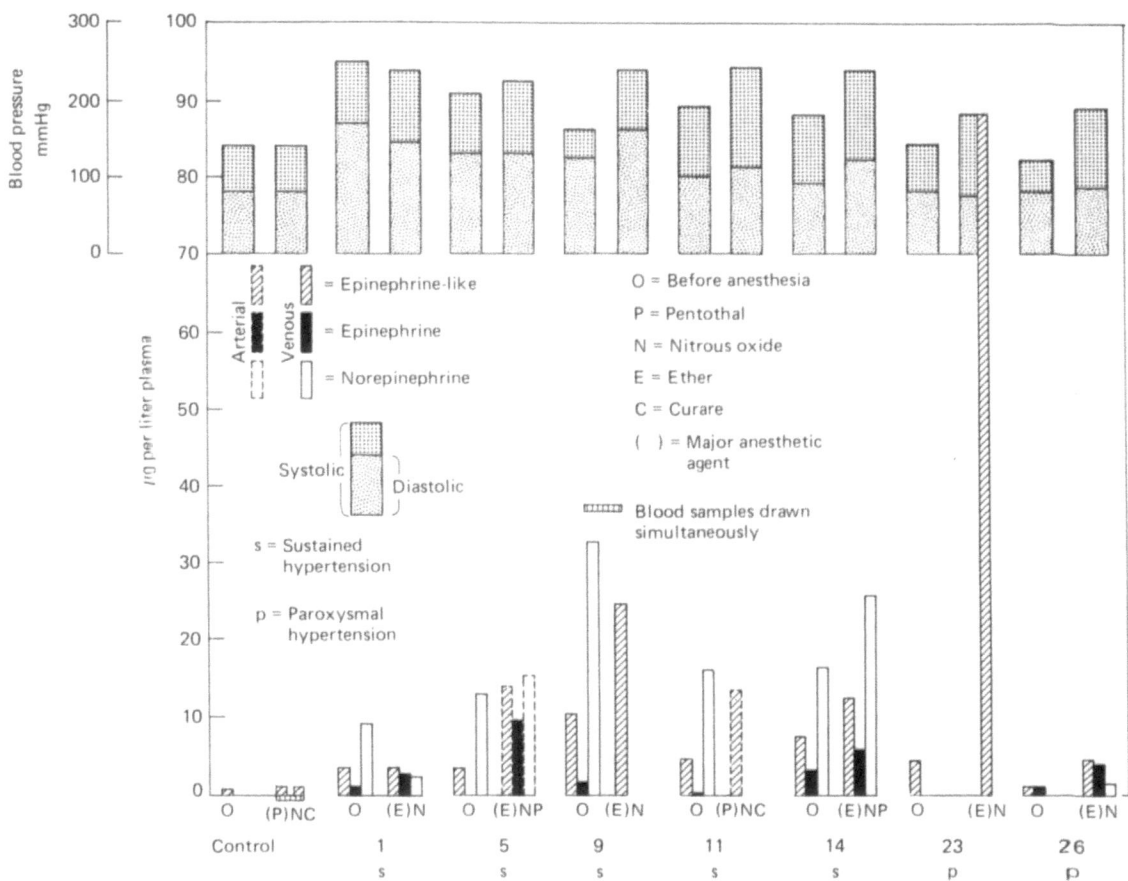

Fig. 8.13 Effect of anesthesia on plasma catecholamines and blood pressure in patients with pheochromocytoma. From Manger, W. M., Wakim, K. G., and Bollman, L. J. *Chemical Quantitation of Epinephrine and Norepinephrine in Plasma.* Courtesy of C. C. Thomas, 1959, p. 99.

operation is shown in Figure 8.14. These data have been previously reported (624). Except in patients 1,s, 7,s, 12,s, and 24,p, concentration of epinephrine-like substance in the course of anesthesia was significantly increased, particularly in patients 3,s, 13,s, and 23,p. It is not known whether the transitory anoxia sometimes associated with induction of anesthesia is responsible for stimulation of the adrenergic system and of the pheochromocytoma, with associated liberation of catecholamines.

Epinephrine and norepinephrine were quantitated prior to and during anesthesia in eight of the 16 patients. Elevation of both catecholamines occurred in five patients (5,s; 13,s; 14,s; 26,p; 27,p); epinephrine was decreased and norepinephrine increased in two (12,s; 22,p), whereas epinephrine was increased and norepinephrine decreased in one patient (1,s). The blood pressure of all but one patient (1,s) with pheochromocytoma rose slightly or

distinctly during anesthesia. The blood pressure of patient 7,s during anesthesia was lower than the preanesthesia value, but this drop in pressure resulted from phentolamine administration.

When ether or thiopental was used as the major anesthetic agent, in combination with nitrous oxide, and with or without use of a muscle relaxant, there appeared to be no correlation between the type of anesthetic agent used and the magnitude of catecholamine or blood pressure elevation. Neither of the control patients (without pheochromocytoma) had any remarkable increase in blood pressure or plasma catecholamines during anesthesia.

In patient 3,s the concentration of epinephrine-like substance increased from the effect of anesthesia and then greatly increased after palpation and operative manipulation of the tumor. Concentrations were determined on plasma obtained simultaneously from venous

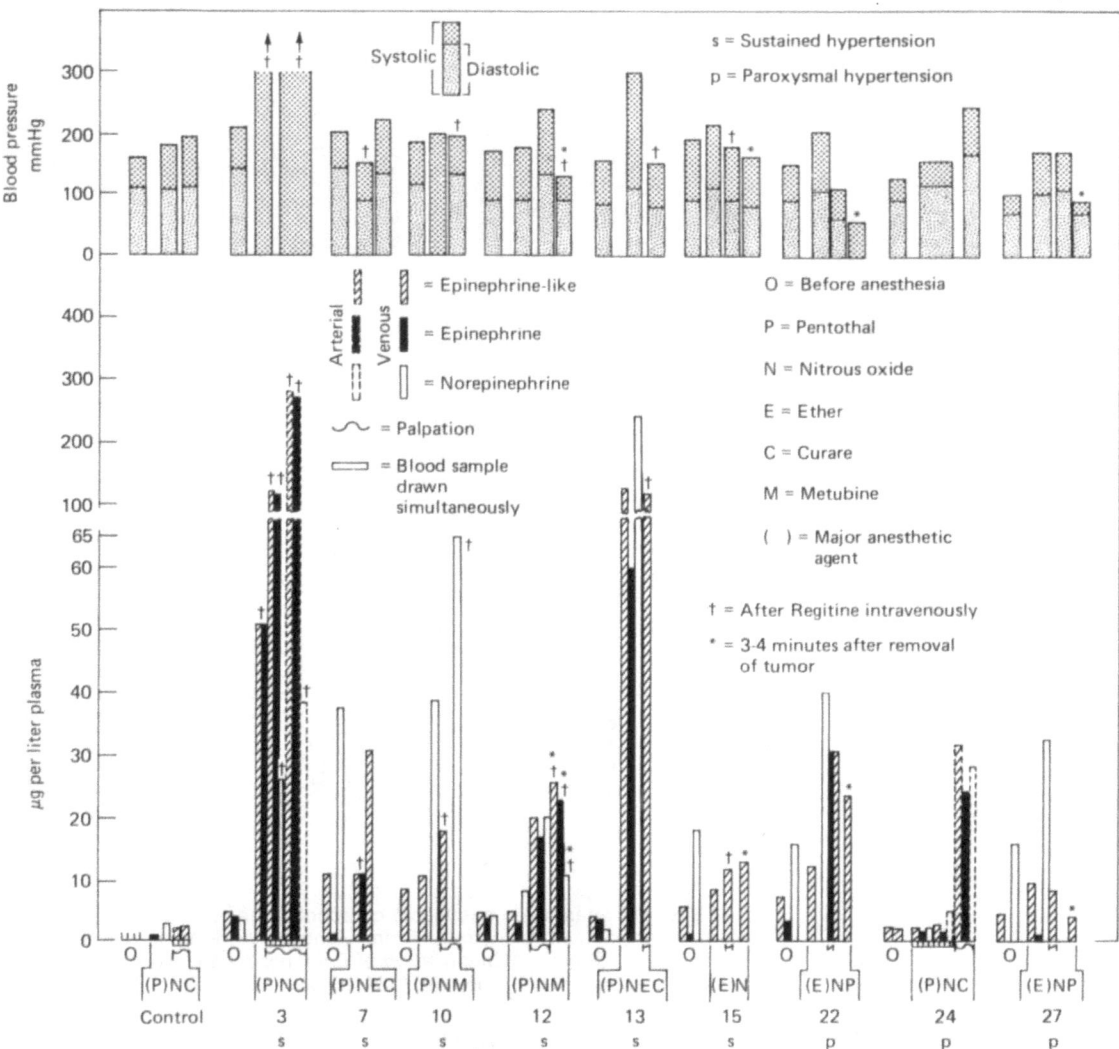

Fig. 8.14 Effect of anesthesia and operative manipulation on plasma catecholamines and blood pressure in patients with pheochromocytoma. From Manger, W. M., Wakim, K. G., and Bollman, L. J., *Chemical Quantitation of Epinephrine and Norepinephrine in Plasma.* Courtesy of C. C. Thomas, 1959, p. 100.

and arterial blood of the same arm. The concentration of epinephrine in arterial plasma was more than twice that in venous plasma. The difference indicates a considerable loss of epinephrine (about 58 percent) in the forearm, secondary to neuronal and extraneuronal uptake, metabolic degradation, and diffusion. The concentration of norepinephrine was also less in venous than in arterial plasma, but the decrease in concentration was only about 28 percent. The greater reduction of epinephrine as compared with norepinephrine could possibly be explained by a greater metabolic degradation of epinephrine than of norepinephrine in the arm. (This patient had a ma-

lignant pheochromocytoma with extensive metastases and no tissue was resected.)

In patient 24,p, anesthesia had no effect on either venous or arterial concentrations of epinephrine-like substance; however, palpation and operative manipulation caused considerable increase in plasma catecholamines. In the great majority of patients with pheochromocytoma, anesthesia alone or anesthesia with palpation and operative manipulation of the tumor caused considerable increase in the plasma concentration of epinephrine-like substance. Only a slight increase in concentration of this substance was noted in the plasma of the control (no pheochromocytoma) during anesthesia and palpation of adrenal glands. In another patient with paroxysmal hypertension, who had no evidence of pheochromocytoma on abdominal exploration, the concentration of epinephrine-like substance during palpation of the adrenal glands was slightly elevated above the normal range (4.1 μg per liter); all preoperative concentrations had been normal.

Plasma catecholamines of four of the patients (12,s; 15,s; 22,p; 27,p) were quantitated 3 to 4 min after tumor removal and were still elevated in all but patient 27,p. It appears that in these patients either the excessive circulating catecholamines were only gradually inactivated, or, perhaps, excessive stores in their sympathetic nerves continued to be released into the circulation. (Neither thiopental nor ether produced any interfering fluorescence with use of our catecholamine assay.)

It is noteworthy that anesthesia and tumor manipulation are not the only causes for release of catecholamines and hypertensive crises immediately prior to and during operation. In 33 cases of pheochromocytoma studied at the Mayo Clinic, Perry and Gould listed several activities sometimes associated with maximal systolic blood pressure during anesthesia (Table 8.4). Tumor manipulation was the most common cause of a hypertensive crisis. Most patients also had bouts of hypertension that probably were related to mechani-

cal stimulation of the tumor from increased intraabdominal pressure (e.g., straining while being moved to the operating table, coughing during intubation, or even, having the abdomen scrubbed). They stated that "These episodes may be avoided by having the patient well sedated, by moving him gently, by having him well relaxed and well anesthetized during intubation, and by reminding the surgical team to prepare the patient gently" (747).

OPERATIVE MORTALITY AND MORBIDITY

In the largest series of patients with pheochromocytoma reported (138 cases at the Mayo Clinic), it was indicated that the operative mortality can be kept below 3 percent (784). Four deaths occurred prior to 1965, two were due to massive uncontrollable bleeding resulting from trauma to the inferior vena cava and common iliac veins, and two resulted from cardiac arrest complicating hypertension at the time of operation.

Mortality rate at the Mayo Clinic is very similar to that experienced in the past 15 years at Columbia Medical Center, where only one operative death has occurred in 30 patients (3.3 percent) operated upon for pheochromocytoma (Dr. Meyer M. Melicow, unpublished data). At the Cleveland Clinic 46 consecutive cases were operated upon between 1952 and 1973, without any operative mortality. During the past decade others have reported relatively low mortality rates (170, 190, 861). It should be pointed out that the preoperative diagnosis was suspected or known in all of these patients on whom these mortality figures are based and that they pertain to abdominal pheochromocytomas. Furthermore, these centers have special expertise in handling patients with pheochromocytoma. If the diagnosis is unsuspected and operation for some other reason is performed, the operative mortality may be as high as 50 percent (382).

The surgical morbidity at the Mayo and Cleveland Clinics and at Columbia Medical Center has been minimal. The causes of the morbidity experienced in 17.4 percent of 46 cases at the Cleveland Clinic are listed in Table 8.5.

At the Vanderbilt University Medical Cen-

Table 8.4 *Position of Patient and Activity Related to Maximal Systolic Blood Pressure Obtained during Anesthesia in 33 Cases of Pheochromocytoma[a]*

Activity	No. of patients	
	Lateral position	Supine position
Induction and intubation	1	6
Positioning	1	0
Skin preparation	0	3
Incision	0	1
Tumor manipulation	1	20
Total	3	30

[a] From Perry, L. B. and Gould, A. B., Jr., *Anesth. Analg. 51:* 38, 1972.

Table 8.5 *Surgical Mortality and Morbidity in 46 Cases of Pheochromocytoma[a]*

	No. of Cases
Mortality	0
Morbidity	8 (17.4%)
Wound seroma or sepsis	2
Pulmonary, with fever	3
Congestive heart failure	1
Hypotension with azotemia	1
Thrombophlebitis with possible pulmonary embolus	1

[a] From Deoreo, G. A., Jr., Stewart, B. H., Tarazi, R. C., and Gifford, R. W., Jr., *J. Urol. 111:* 721, 1974.

ter, where the thoracoabdominal incision is usually employed, atelectasis and pneumonitis occurred in five of 31 patients who had had removal of a pheochromocytoma; in addition, one of these had a persistent pleural effusion and another required a thoracotomy tube because of a pneumothorax. There were isolated instances of wound infection, urinary tract infection, thromboembolism, bleeding from stress ulcers, and transient hemiparesis. Six patients (in the early years of the study) required postoperative infusions of norepinephrine for from 1 to 3 days to maintain the blood pressure; two of these patients developed sloughs at the site of infusion. One of the 31 patients died 4 weeks postoperatively in oliguric renal failure, which might have been related to the use of methoxyflurane (Penthrane) anesthesia (875a).

RECOVERY ROOM OBSERVATIONS

Postoperatively, monitoring should continue, and the patient should be observed very closely, since during this period severe hypotension may develop and volume replacement may be needed. Occasionally it may be desirable to continue intraarterial monitoring for a day or more if the blood pressure remains unstable. The urine output is of value in assessing renal perfusion. It should be emphasized that the primary management of postoperative hypotension is usually fluid administration with volume replacement. The objective should be, not to normalize the blood pressure, but simply to keep the systolic pressure between 90 and 100 mmHg, provided

the condition of the patient is satisfactory and the urine output is adequate. Attempts to raise the blood pressure above 100 mmHg may lead to fluid overload or to the unnecessary and injudicious use of pressor agents.

As mentioned by Edis, Ayala, and Egdahl, "persistent hypotension in the immediate postoperative period, in the presence of apparently adequate volume replacement suggests bleeding at the operative site" (249). They and others have pointed out that venous oozing can be a problem with adrenergic blockade. Myocardial infarction or inadequate steroid replacement following bilateral adrenalectomy can also cause persistent postoperative hypotension; however, if the steroid therapy recommended above has been utilized, then inadequate steroid replacement as a cause of hypotension would be extremely unlikely. It has been stated that in some cases acute adrenal insufficiency may be the cause of collapse after removal of pheochromocytomas (838); however, this must indeed be an extremely rare cause of postoperative hypotension.

The occurrence of hypertension in the recovery room may signify one of the following three situations: the presence of pain (which will respond in most instances to an analgesic); the presence of a residual pheochromocytoma (either tumors unrecognized at operation or metastatic disease); or the presence of an inadvertently ligated renal artery. The latter two possibilities can be confirmed or excluded by subsequent plasma and urine catecholamine or metabolite assay, and by appropriate radiographic studies. Every means available for localizing residual functioning tissue should be utilized before reexploring the patient.

POSTOPERATIVE FOLLOW-UP

SURVIVAL

At the Mayo Clinic the tumor recurrence rate following pheochromocytoma removal was 9.8 percent. Five-year survival following operation was 96 percent for patients with benign tumors, whereas it was 44 percent for those with malignant pheochromocytomas.

Of 18 patients with malignant pheochromocytomas, five had palliative procedures, and on 13 curative resections were attempted. Twelve of these 18 patients died of the disease within 1 month to 17 years after the primary operation (median survival time being 5.6 years); two apparently had no evidence of recurrence, and four were alive, but with evidence of pheochromocytoma 5, 20, 20, and 21 years after primary surgical treatment (784). Malignancy appeared more virulent and occurred more commonly in their patients with extraadrenal pheochromocytomas (28.6 percent) than in those with intraadrenal tumors (11.3 percent). Remine and associates also pointed out that patients with pulmonary metastases have a poorer prognosis than do other patients (784).

BLOOD PRESSURE AND PLASMA CATECHOLAMINES

Of 103 patients examined 1 year following surgical removal of a benign pheochromocytoma, 75 were normotensive and 28 had persistent hypertension. Preoperatively, 18 of these 28 patients had sustained hypertension, whereas nine had paroxysmal hypertension, and one patient, with Sipple's syndrome, was normotensive (784). Tcherdakoff and coworkers reported that in their series of 42 patients, one-third continued to have hypertension following pheochromocytoma removal (972). Four of 17 patients (23.5 percent) reported by Ohman and coworkers were hypertensive following extirpation of the tumor; it was their impression that sustained hypertension may persist after operation, whereas the paroxysmal form is usually cured (718). Scott and associates found that 18 of 27 patients with benign pheochromocytoma remained normotensive during follow-up periods of from 1 to 20 years after tumor removal (875a).

After removal of a pheochromocytoma from a patient having paroxysmal hypertension, paroxysms disappear unless there is a recurrence of the tumor. On the other hand, from most reports where there has been a follow-up, about 20 to 30 percent of patients who had sustained hypertension continue to have sustained systolic and diastolic hypertension. We lack an explanation for the latter phenomenon. It is possible that some of these patients also have essential hypertension, or even renal hypertension unrelated to the effects of the pheochromocytoma; however, it

seems conceivable that vascular lesions might have developed during the period of sustained hypertension from excessive circulating catecholamines, and that such lesions might possibly perpetuate the hypertension. In practically all patients in whom hypertension persists despite complete removal of the pheochromocytomas, we and our associates, as well as others (cited in 875a), have been able to satisfactorily manage their hypertension with antihypertensive drugs. On a rare occasion, resection of a pheochromocytoma may have no beneficial effect on the patient's blood pressure and on the progress of the hypertensive complications. One woman with malignant hypertension (with severe and diffuse arteriosclerosis and nitrogen retention) sustained no improvement following removal of a small para-aortic pheochromocytoma; she died in uremia 3 months postoperatively (875a).

Renovascular hypertension has been reported in four patients shortly after excision of pheochromocytomas in the vicinity of the renal vasculature. In one patient the hypertension, which resulted from retroperitoneal fibrosis, gradually obstructed renal blood flow to one kidney; in the other patients the hypertension resulted from the inadvertent ligation of some of the renal arterial supply. Nephrectomy is usually necessary for cure of the hypertension; however, in one patient, resection of the ischemic portion of the kidney was sufficient to interrupt the renin–angiotensin system and permit the blood pressure to return to normal (142, 491). One should always consider the possibility that iatrogenic renovascular hypertension may occur postoperatively.

In Table 8.6 are recorded preoperative and postoperative (at least 3 days after all pressor medication had been discontinued) blood pressures and plasma concentrations of epinephrine-like substance, epinephrine, and norepinephrine in 16 patients with sustained, and seven patients with paroxysmal, hypertension. The preoperative concentrations in these patients have been discussed earlier but they are recorded again in this table for comparison with postoperative values. One value for preoperative plasma epinephrine-like substance of one of the patients with sustained hypertension and pheochromocytoma (12,s)

Table 8.6 *Catecholamines in Peripheral Venous Plasma of Patients with Pheochromocytoma, before and after Removal of the Tumors[a]*

Patient	Preoperative BP (mmHg)	Concentration (µg/liter of plasma) Preoperative			Concentration (µg/liter of plasma) Postoperative			Postoperative BP (mmHg)
		ELS	E	NE	ELS	E	NE	
1,s	270/170	3.6	1.1	9.2	1.2	0.0	4.4	185/125
2,s	240/150	17.7; 15.4	—[b]	—	2.1	—	—	150/100
3,s	210/140	4.7	3.8	3.4	Not estimated; tumor not removed			
4,s	195/145	4.8	1.9	10.5	1.2	0.1	3.9	130/85
5,s	210/130	3.6	0.0	13.2	1.3	0.0	4.8	186/132
6,s	180/150	7.8	—	—	3.4	—	—	120/80
7,s	194/128	8.1	4.2	14.3	2.1	0.4	6.3	128/85
	200/140	10.9	0.7	37.4				
8,s[c]	160/130	4.9	0.0	18.0	3.1	0.9	8.1	166/100
9,s	160/125	10.8	1.8	33.0	1.4	0.0	5.1	144/92
10,s	185/110	8.2	—	—	1.3	1.0	1.2	98/56
	185/115	8.3	—	—	1.6[d]	—	—	124/90[d]
11,s	190/100	4.8	2.8	7.4	1.9	0.7	4.5	150/100
12,s	182/100	2.2	1.2	3.7	3.4[e]	—	—	178/100
	[170/90]	[4.7]	[3.6]	[4.0]	7.3[f]	—	—	170/98
	[194/120]	[4.5]	—	—				
13,s	156/106	4.2	—	—				
	154/80	4.1	3.6	1.8	1.6	0.7	3.2	118/80
14,s	180/90	7.7	3.2	16.6	2.0	1.2	2.9	150/80
15,s	170/88	8.5	—	—	1.8	0.7	4.0	130/80
	190/90	5.4	0.5	17.9				
16,s	148/98	—	—	—	1.0	—	—	132/96
	194/124*	4.7*	—	—				
22,p	150/90	7.0	2.7	15.8	1.0	0.0	3.7	105/70
	134/94	8.1	3.5	16.7				
	244/164*	15.7*	4.9*	39.5*				
23,p		4.6	—	—	0.7	0.0	2.6	100/74
24,p	128/90	1.9; (2.1)	—	—	0.0	0.0	0.0	105/70
	250/160*	9.5*	—	—				
25,p	132/85	9.2	2.3	25.3	1.6	0.7	3.4	130/85
	155/?	9.5	5.7	13.9				
26,p	120/80	1.0	1.0	0.0	0.5	0.5	0.0	130/75
27,p	100/70	4.3	0.0	15.8	0.9	0.0	3.3	110/84
	158/100	6.0	—	—				
	194/114*	7.2*	—	—				
38,p	156/80	—	—	—	6.0	—	—	140/75
	230/110[g]	6.6[g]	0.0[g]	24.2[g]				

[a] ELS = epinephrine-like substance; E = epinephrine; NE = norepinephrine; s = sustained hypertension; p = paroxysmal hypertension; ( ) = arterial plasma. Note: Quantities between brackets are values determined 6 months after the first values determined in the case. Upper limit of normal for: ELS = 3.5 µg/liter; E = 1.3 µg/liter; NE = 6.3 µg/liter.

[b] Not estimated.

[c] Receiving cortisone.

[d] 8 months postoperative.

[e] 6 days postoperative.

[f] 10 days postoperative.

[g] During spontaneous paroxysm of hypertension.

* During provocative test with histamine (see table 6.20).

was within normal limits (2.2 μg/liter); however, two other determinations on the same patient, 6 months later, gave definitely elevated values (4.7 and 4.5 μg/liter) for plasma epinephrine-like substance. (This case indicates the importance of following a patient and of making repeated determinations of the concentration of plasma catecholamines when pheochromocytoma is suspected.) In two of the cases of paroxysmal hypertension, the preoperative concentrations of epinephrine-like substance were not elevated when the blood pressures were normal.

Following removal of the pheochromocytoma, the concentrations of epinephrine-like substance were less than 3.5 μg/liter in all the patients who had sustained hypertension, except in case 12,s, where a value on the 10th postoperative day was 7.3 μg/liter. Whether this patient had residual functional tumor tissue is uncertain; on examination 25 months postoperatively, the hypertension was found to be persistent although, in the interval, the patient had not experienced symptoms suggestive of pheochromocytoma. Pharmacologic tests for pheochromocytoma in this patient gave negative results, and the concentration of plasma catecholamines was within normal limits.

Because of the presence of malignant pheochromocytomas and metastasis, removal of the tumor from patient 3,s (Table 8.6) was not attempted, and only part of the recurrent tumor was removed from patient 38,p. The postoperative concentration of epinephrine-like substance in patient 8,s was considered to be in the "high normal" range (3.1 μg/liter) and, a year later, the patient was found to have metastatic pheochromocytoma. At that time the plasma concentrations of epinephrine-like substance and norepinephrine were elevated (3.6 and 13.2 μg/liter, respectively). However, despite the "high normal" postoperative concentration of plasma epinephrine-like substance in patient 6,s (3.4 μg/liter), recurrence did not become evident.

It is mandatory that all patients be followed rather closely two or three times a year for several years and at yearly intervals for at least 5 to 10 years postoperatively. Patients suspected of having had familial pheochromocytomas should be followed throughout their lifetimes. In addition to a careful history and physical examination to elicit or exclude any clinical manifestations suggesting a recurrence of a pheochromocytoma, 24-hr urine metanephrines should be determined. Quantitation of plasma and/or urine catecholamines or metabolites before and after a provocative test may be indicated in some patients who have only paroxysmal symptoms and in whom the values for urinary catecholamines and their metabolites are normal or borderline.

It is noteworthy that we and others (299, 437, p. 125; 807) have occasionally observed that the plasma catecholamines or the urinary catecholamines and their metabolites may not immediately return to normal after pheochromocytoma removal. Since some have reported that the urinary catecholamines may not return to a normal range for 1 or 2 weeks (299), or even a month or two, postoperative (806), one should be cautious in concluding that an elevation of plasma or urinary catecholamines or their metabolites in the *immediate* postoperative period *invariably* indicates the presence of a residual tumor or metastatic disease.

Two of 15 patients (13.3 percent) who had sustained hypertension preoperatively continued to have severe hypertension after tumor removal. (The tumor was not removed from one of the 16 patients with sustained hypertension.) Four more of the 15 (26.6 percent) continued to have mild diastolic hypertension. The postoperative blood pressures were normal in all the patients with paroxysmal hypertension, despite the fact that case 38,p had a residual functioning tumor (Table 8.6).

Finally, it is imperative to evaluate periodically, for evidence of medullary thyroid carcinoma and hyperparathyroidism, all patients and their primary relatives in whom the pheochromocytoma may have been familial. Because of the difficulty in identifying all patients with familial pheochromocytoma or the MEN–type 2 and –type 3 syndromes, there is some evidence suggesting that even patients thought to have sporadic pheochromocytoma should be screened for evidence of medullary thyroid carcinoma (personal communication from Dr. Glen W. Sizemore, endocrinologist, Mayo Clinic).

CHRONIC MEDICAL MANAGEMENT

In the event that a pheochromocytoma has metastasized or is not totally resectable, one must endeavor to remove as much tumor as possible in order to reduce functioning tissue to a minimum. By so doing, pharmacologic control of the clinical manifestations may be facilitated. Chemotherapy has been of no help, since such tumors are insensitive to these cytotoxic agents. They are also quite resistant to radiation therapy, although some benefit in palliation has been reported (483).

α-Methyl-*p*-tyrosine has been used effectively to decrease the synthesis of catecholamines and it has been used in the treatment of pheochromocytoma (775, 908, 909, 929). It is known to inhibit tyrosine hydroxylase, the rate-limiting enzyme for catecholamine biosynthesis. In 17 patients with pheochromocytoma treated by Sjoerdsma and coworkers (909), a reduction of as much as 70 to 80 percent in the urinary excretion of catecholamines and their metabolites occurred. In addition, a reduction in blood pressure, pulse rate, sweating, and metabolic rate was observed. Unfortunately this drug has caused significant renal damage, which has precluded its use, except as an experimental drug. Other side effects, such as frequent severe nausea, anorexia, and occasionally a Parkinsonism-like syndrome, have also been noted in some patients taking it (908). Furthermore, blood pressure may not be adequately controlled by α-methyl-*p*-tyrosine alone (775).

Administration of α-methyldopa (an inhibitor of aromatic amino acid decarboxylase) has also been found to reduce the urinary excretion of catecholamines or their metabolites and to decrease the blood pressure in some patients with pheochromocytoma (884, 906), but this has not proved to be particularly effective in the routine management of these patients. In two patients with pheochromocytoma Crout observed that although α-methyldopa reduced the production of VMA by as much as 20 percent, this was insufficient to have any beneficial effect; moreover, the increase in orthostatic hypotension induced by the drug made its use intolerable (cited in 275).

Therapy with Phenoxybenzamine If it is impossible to totally resect a pheochromocytoma for technical reasons, or because of the presence of functioning metastatic disease which is causing clinical manifestations, then chronic medical treatment with phenoxybenzamine is indicated. Therapy with this α-blocker can also be used very effectively to control manifestations when operation has to be deferred temporarily or even permanently because the precarious condition of a patient could significantly increase the risk of surgery (e.g., intercurrent infection, recent myocardial infarction or cerebrovascular accident, severe congestive heart failure, or very advanced age with marked disability), or because of the patient's refusal to undergo surgery.

Phenoxybenzamine was first used in the management of pheochromocytoma at the Mayo Clinic shortly after the drug became available. Allen and coworkers demonstrated that, when given chronically, this drug could effectively control the manifestations of a malignant pheochromocytoma (7). The prolonged successful control of physiologic and metabolic alterations with phenoxybenzamine was subsequently reported in four patients with pheochromocytoma who were extensively studied by Engelman and Sjoerdsma (275). Two of these patients were 12-year-old girls with metastatic pheochromocytoma. A remarkable normalization of the manifestations of pheochromocytoma was accomplished in both patients by the administration of 30 and 40 mg orally twice daily, and this regimen had been continued for over 1 year at the time of reporting. A third patient was a 70-year-old woman with severe recurrent angina pectoris requiring 8 to 12 nitroglycerine tablets per day; operation was not performed since she was considered too poor an operative risk. Phenoxybenzamine (given orally 40 mg in the morning and 20 mg in the afternoon) had been administered for over 1 year, with normalization of the blood pressure, elimination of the wide variations in blood pressure, and diminution of the orthostatic fall in blood pressure observed prior to this medication. The fourth patient was a 23-year-old black woman who probably had a catecholamine cardiomyopathy which caused cardiomegaly with congestive heart failure, pleural effusions, and 3 to 4+ proteinuria. Since at that time she was being treated with digitalis, diuretics, and salt restriction, it was felt that she could not survive surgery to remove her pheochromocytoma; however, within 1 week after institution of treatment with phenoxybenzamine

Table 8.7 *Treatment*

Team effort: Internist, surgeon, anesthetist

Preoperative

Evaluation and recognition of associated conditions

Location of tumor

Preparation

    To block or not to block?

        α-Adrenergic blockade (oral phenoxybenzamine, ⌣40 mg/day; increase as indicated)
            Prevents severe symptoms and BP swings
            Promotes smooth induction and operation
            Reverses hypovolemia
            But may obscure location of tumor or detection of residual tumor
        β-Adrenergic blockade (oral propranolol, ⌣40 mg/day; increase as indicated)
    Expand intravascular volume with whole blood (1000 ml) or Albumisol
    Steroids, if bilateral adrenectomy anticipated
    Premedication
    Monitor
      Arterial BP
      ECG
      CVP
      Temperature
      Urine output

Operative

Intubation—after neuromuscular blocking agents and induction

Anesthesia—enflurane, 1st choice; halothane, 2nd choice

Operative technique and strategy
    Anterior transperitoneal incision *mandatory*

Intraoperative management
    Hypertensive crises: nitroprusside; phentolamine
    Arrhythmias: propranolol; lidocaine
    Hypotension: blood replacement (vasopressors, rarely)
    (Death usually from hemorrhage or cardiac arrest)

Postoperative

Recovery room—continue monitoring closely

    If hypertensive, may be due to:
      Pain
      Residual tumor
      Renal artery ligation
      Fluid overload
    If hypotensive, may be due to:
      Internal bleeding or inadequate volume replacement

Follow-up examination and assay for catecholamines (and medullary thyroid carcinoma and hyperparathyroidism if familial)

Chronic medical management if operation contraindicated or metastatic disease
    (use phenoxybenzamine and propranolol as indicated)

(given orally 30 mg daily) excessive sweating disappeared and the patient's condition improved remarkably. Within 1 month pleural effusions had disappeared, the heart size had decreased slightly, and diuretics were no longer required. Approximately 11 months later a 35 g pheochromocytoma was removed from the area of the lower pole of the left kidney (275). Engelman and Sjoerdsma emphasized that their results indicate that the entire clinical status of a patient with pheochromocytoma can be normalized, regardless of whether a tumor is benign or malignant. In their patients the pulse and supine and standing blood pressures became normal and pressor crises were eliminated. Furthermore, excessive sweating, anxiety, hypermetabolism, and elevated free fatty acids were eliminated or returned toward normal, and the deleterious effects of the catecholamines on the cardiovascular system were sufficiently inhibited to improve myocardial function.

Phenoxybenzamine does not appear to influence the growth or metabolism of a pheochromocytoma. This long-acting α-adrenergic blocking agent exerts its therapeutic effect by blocking the peripheral effects of the catecholamines. It was recommended that for chronic use it be given orally twice daily. The only side effect noted by the patients reported was slight sedation (275).

Phentolamine has been used in chronic therapy of patients with pheochromocytoma (54); however, because of its short duration of action, the need to give it frequently, and the side effects (tachycardia and gastrointestinal upset), it is unsatisfactory for use in chronic treatment. Other antihypertensive drugs (e.g., hydralazine, reserpine, and guanethidine) have proved unsatisfactory in the management of patients with pheochromocytoma (275).

β-Adrenergic blockade with propranolol should be used as necessary to control tachycardia and arrhythmias.

It would be preferable to have a nontoxic drug which could effectively eliminate the synthesis of catecholamines by a pheochromocytoma in patients with metastatic disease or in patients where surgery is contraindicated; however, such a drug is not available, and phenoxybenzamine is currently the drug of choice in managing these patients.

Table 8.7 gives a summary outline for treatment of patients with pheochromocytoma.

Comments and Conclusions

CHAPTER NINE

In this monograph we have attempted, whenever possible, to deal in depth with every clinical and experimental facet and ramification of pheochromocytoma. In conclusion, we emphasize some of the more important aspects of this disease.

Above all, the physician must heighten his index of suspicion and his acumen for recognizing, in the vast crowd of hypertensive patients, the occasional patient with pheochromocytoma. His ability to detect that occasional patient may, in fact, determine whether that person survives. The point to stress is that with surgical removal of the pheochromocytoma about 90 percent of such patients can be cured. Tragically, although the tumor is pathologically malignant in only 10 percent of cases, patients in whom the diagnosis is missed are doomed to the morbid—and ultimately lethal—effects of excessive circulating catecholamines.

The physician who understands pheochromocytoma will know *what* the manifestations are, *why* and *when* these manifestations are apt to occur, *where* these tumors arise, *whom* to suspect in the differential diagnosis, and *how* to approach diagnosis and treatment skillfully.

It is fitting to recall that familiar and relevant verse by Rudyard Kipling:

I keep six honest serving men
They taught me all I knew,
Their names are What and Why and When
And How and Where and Who.
(From "The Elephant Child" in the
Just So Stories)

These "six honest serving men" have previously been recommended to serve the clinician; they are especially appropriate guides for the clinician confronted with a patient suspected of harboring a pheochromocytoma.

From our experience and that of our colleagues, coupled with an extensive review of the literature and countless discussions and debates, we have endeavored to present an exhaustive study of pheochromocytoma. (We have become weary and "exhausted" in the process!) We feel that the effort has been well worthwhile, particularly since we have introduced many facts and concepts regarding pheochromocytoma not previously published. Furthermore, unlike other investigators, we have *separately* analyzed our studies on the basis of whether patients had sustained *or* paroxysmal hypertension. In patients with paroxysmal hypertension due to pheochromocytoma some of the manifestations differ considerably from those in patients with sustained hypertension; we do not yet clearly understand what biochemical factors determine whether the hypertension is sustained or paroxysmal.

The teaching tables and selected figures should make the physician more familiar with the fascinating characteristics and vagaries of this catecholamine-producing neoplasm.

Certain facts in this monograph particularly merit recapitulation:

CHAPTER 1   It may seem surprising that perhaps 36,000 persons in the United States harbor a pheochromocytoma. Yet this seems a fair and conservative estimate, assuming 0.1 percent incidence in 18 million persons with sustained diastolic hypertension, and assuming further that about 50 percent of patients with pheochromocytoma have paroxysmal rather than sustained hypertension.

CHAPTER 2   Most pheochromocytomas have a markedly increased rate of catecholamine synthesis compared to that of the normal adrenal medulla. It appears that these tumors have the various enzymes necessary for the conversion of tyrosine to the catecholamines (i.e., dopamine, norephinephrine, and epinephrine); some tumors contain enzymes necessary for catecholamine degradation, although the degradative enzymes have not been well studied. It seems likely that release of catecholamines from these tumors occurs mainly by diffusion and not by a process of exocytosis. However, the mechanism whereby a massive discharge of catecholamines is triggered (other than by mechanical compression) remains obscure. In contrast to the normal adrenal medulla, there is no evidence for a nervous innervation in pheochromocytomas; hence, it is unlikely that activation of the adrenergic nervous system can cause a direct stimulation of the tumor and, thereby, secretion of catecholamines.

Some investigators have found that small tumors with a low catecholamine content have a rapid turnover of catecholamines and secrete a relatively large amount of unmetabolized catecholamines directly into the circulation. On the other hand, large tumors with a high content of catecholamines and a slow turnover rate release a relatively large amount of catecholamine metabolites. The precise biochemical differences between these two types of tumors are not clear, but they may be partly related to differences in storage and binding of the catecholamines.

CHAPTER 3   Pheochromocytomas can arise wherever chromaffin tissue exists, either in intraadrenal or extraadrenal locations. The chromaffin cell is of neuroectodermal origin. The major sites where pheochromocytomas occur are in the adrenal medulla (90 percent), in paraganglia cells of the sympathetic nervous system, and in the organ of Zuckerkandl. Less commonly, they arise from chromaffin tissue in the wall of the urinary bladder, in para-aortic regions, behind the liver, in the hilus of the liver or kidney, in the chest (<2 percent), and in the neck (<0.1 percent). Multiple and extraadrenal tumors are far more common in children than in adults. For some unknown reason, tumors occur more commonly in the right adrenal medulla than in the left. Tumors of the chemoreceptors have, on occasion, been reported to secrete catecholamines; however, the classification of chemodectomas is unsettled.

Pheochromocytomas may occur at any age, the greatest frequency being in the fourth and fifth decades. There is no distinct sex predilection in adults, but before puberty the tumor occurs more commonly in boys than girls.

The etiology of pheochromocytoma remains unknown. It is relatively rare in both man and animal. Particularly intriguing is a familial incidence, perhaps 10 percent, which is transmitted with a high penetrance by a dominant autosomal mode of inheritance. Familial pheochromocytomas are most often located in the adrenal glands and are very frequently bilateral and multicentric. They may have a higher incidence of malignancy than the nonfamilial (sporadic) tumor. Diffuse or nodular adrenal medullary hyperplasia appears to be a precursor of familial pheochromocytoma in the MEN–type 2 and –type 3 syndromes.

Most pheochromocytomas weigh less than 70 g, but they may vary from microscopic size to 3600 g. Not infrequently they contain hemorrhagic and cystic areas, which may be very large. Cells are generally polygonal or spheroidal, with multiple minute granules. Both cytoplasm and intracytoplasmic secretory granules, which contain catecholamines, can be stained characteristically brown with chromium salts. Frequently an alveolar arrangement of cells is evident, but cellular patterns are quite variable. Approximately 10 percent of tumors are malignant, but it is impossible to determine whether a tumor is benign or malignant from the histopathology alone. Only the presence of metastases or extensive invasion of adjacent tissue will establish that the tumor is malignant. There are no biochemical features that identify a pheochromocytoma as malignant; however, a relatively greater proportion of malignant tumors, as compared with benign ones, secrete dopamine.

Ultrastructurally, cells of the normal adrenal medulla and pheochromocytomas contain either norepinephrine granules (very dark electron-dense contents bounded by electron-lucent zones) or epinephrine granules (completely filled with lighter electron-dense material, and with few, if any, electron-lucent zones). There is fair correlation between the number and size of these granules and the concentration of catecholamines.

Pathologic complications of pheochromocytoma are primarily those caused by hypertension; however, increased concentrations of circulating catecholamines can inhibit gastrointestinal motility and, rarely, cause severe ileus. Very rarely, ischemic enterocolitis may also occur, perhaps as a consequence of intense splanchnic vasoconstriction. A catecholamine cardiomyopathy has also occasionally been observed; characteristic pathologic lesions of the myocardium have been identified in a significant number of patients dying from pheochromocytoma and its complications.

Of particular significance is the rare occurrence of hemorrhagic necrosis in a pheochromocytoma, which may simulate an acute abdomen.

Shock may follow prolonged hypertensive crises, during anesthesia and operation, or even following minor trauma. Occasionally it results from hemorrhage within a pheochromocytoma, or even from a ruptured adrenal gland.

Other complications result from compression of structures adjacent to a pheochromocytoma, or from the metastases if the tumor is malignant.

CHAPTER 4   The clinical manifestations encountered in patients with pheochromocytoma consist of such a large variety of symptoms that they have been described as kaleidoscopic. Symptoms and signs result primarily from the hemodynamic and metabolic effects of excessive circulating catecholamines. Of particular note is the frequent occurrence of severe headaches, excess generalized sweating, and palpitations (with or without tachycardia). These are the most common symptoms occurring in patients with either paroxysmal or sustained hypertension. About 50 percent of adult patients with pheochromocytoma have sustained hypertension; most of the remainder have paroxysmal hypertension. Rarely, patients present with symptomatic episodes without hypertension. Orthostatic hypotension occurring in a hypertensive patient who is not being treated with antihypertensive medications suggests pheochromocytoma. Patients may occasionally present with manifestations due to complications of hypertension or with other consequences of excessive circulating catecholamines (e.g., arrhythmias, cardiomyopathy, ischemic enterocolitis). Manifestations may also appear of conditions which sometimes coexist with pheochromocytoma (e.g., cholelithiasis, neurofibromatosis or other neurocutaneous lesions, medullary thyroid carcinoma, hyperparathyroidism, Cushing's syndrome, von Hippel-Lindau disease, and acromegaly).

Familial pheochromocytoma in association with multiple endocrine tumors (e.g., medullary thyroid carcinoma and hyperparathyroidism) has been classified as "multiple endocrine neoplasia type 2 and type 3." Hyperparathyroidism, although common in MEN–type 2, occurs only rarely in MEN–type 3; furthermore, the latter syndrome is characterized by the presence of mucosal neuromas, thickened lips, thickened corneal nerves, decreased tear flow (sometimes producing symptoms of keratoconjunctivitis sicca), and frequently a marfanoid habitus and alimentary-tract ganglioneuromatosis.

It is noteworthy that hypertension in members of a family affected with pheochromocytoma tends to be consistent, i.e., all members of a family will have sustained, or all will have paroxysmal, hypertension; however, it should be appreciated that a relatively high percentage of patients with familial pheochromocytomas in the MEN–type 2 and –type 3 syndromes are normotensive and/or asymptomatic.

On rare occasions, clinical manifestations may result from compression of adjacent structures by the tumor or from invasion and compression of distant structures if the tumor is malignant and metastasizes.

Symptomatic attacks may vary from once every few months to 25 times daily, and may last from less than 1 min up to 1 week. Usually one or more attacks occur weekly and last for less than 15 min. Attacks may occur spontaneously or be produced by a variety of drugs (e.g., histamine, glucagon, tyramine, tetraethylammonium, methacholine, ACTH, saralasin and other angiotensin analogues, nicotine, anectine, and phenothiazines), by physical maneuvers, and even by psychic stimulation. Precipitation of an attack by micturition or bladder distention suggests a pheochromocytoma of the urinary bladder. Of interest is the finding that the highest incidence of urinary bladder pheochromocytoma occurs in patients between 10 and 19 years of age.

It is vitally important to suspect pheochromocytoma as the cause of hypertension in all pregnant patients. Some have reported a maternal and fetal mortality rate of 58 and 56 percent, respectively, when pheochromocytoma was unrecognized at the time of delivery. Manifestations of pheochromocytoma may appear as (a) severe preeclampsia, (b) paroxysmal hypertension, (c) typical symptoms without hypertension, (d) sudden shock and death in the antepartum period, (e) hyperpyrexia after delivery, or (f) shock after delivery.

Manifestations of pheochromocytoma in children differ in certain ways from those in adults. For example, 90 percent of children with pheochromocytoma have sustained hypertension. Polydipsia, polyuria, and convulsions occurred more commonly in children than in adults. Occasionally a reddish-blue mottling of the skin, or a red, cyanotic appearance of the hands, has been described in children, but not in adults.

CHAPTER 5 Pheochromocytoma has rightfully acquired the title of the "great mimic," and the "great masquerader." Because this "impostor" may appear in so many different disguises, the clinican should thoroughly familiarize himself with the long list of unrelated disease entities presented under "Differential Diagnosis" in Chapter 5. In the final analysis, of course, the preoperative diagnosis of pheochromocytoma must be confirmed by demonstrating significant elevations of catecholamines or their metabolites in the urine or plasma. A careful history and physical examination can be of great value in deciding which patients with sustained or paroxysmal hypertension to screen for pheochromocytoma, since approximately 95 percent of patients with this tumor are symptomatic.

It is strongly urged that all symptomatic patients with sustained or paroxysmal hypertension be screened for pheochromocytoma unless the cause of their hypertension is known. Even asymptomatic patients with hypertension of unknown etiology should be screened if they have diseases known occasionally to coexist with pheochromocytoma, or if they have laboratory abnormalities which may be caused by increased circulating catecholamines. In addition, all patients with MEN–type 2 and –type 3 (and their first degree relatives) should be carefully screened for adrenal medullary hyperfunction, even if they are asymptomatic and normotensive.

The diseases and conditions which may be accompanied by an increased urinary excretion of catecholamines and/or their metabolites have been listed and italicized in Table 5.1, and they have been discussed in detail under "Differential Diagnosis." It is worth repeating that if the physican encounters clinical manifestations suggesting pheochromocytoma in a person having access to a variety of drugs, the remote possibility of factitious production of symptoms (i.e., pseudopheochromocytoma) must always be considered.

Finally, the extreme importance of recognizing the clinical picture of hemorrhagic necrosis in a pheochromocytoma cannot be overstated. This condition may present as an acute abdomen or a cardiovascular catastrophe, and without prompt institution of appropriate therapy and extirpation of the tumor, the patient will almost certainly die. A high index of suspicion is fundamental in the diagnosis of this rare complication.

CHAPTER 6   If the guidelines outlined in Table 6.1 are utilized by the physician to screen hypertensive patients, we feel confident that the diagnosis of pheochromocytoma will rarely if ever be missed.

The following laboratory abnormalities which have been observed in some patients with pheochromocytoma may sometimes be helpful clues in the diagnosis: hyperglycemia, impaired glucose tolerance, glycosuria, hypermetabolism, and increased free fatty acids. On rare occasions polycythemia or a transitory leukocytosis may occur, and occasionally hyperreninemia may be found. Finally, it must be appreciated that when a patient with pheochromocytoma has an associated condition, other laboratory abnormalities may occur. For example, the presence of Cushing's syndrome is accompanied by elevations of serum ACTH (elaborated by the pheochromocytoma), plasma cortisol, and urinary steroids; hyperparathyroidism is accompanied

by elevations of serum calcium and parathyroid hormone and sometimes by a decreased serum phosphate. Medullary thyroid carcinoma can cause elevations in serum prostaglandin, ACTH-like substances, and serotonin, and an increase in urinary excretion of 5-HIAA; the presence of this thyroid carcinoma (or its precursor, C-cell hyperplasia) can be detected by an elevated serum thyrocalcitonin.

A wide variety of ECG abnormalities which have been reported in patients with pheochromocytoma have been enumerated in Table 6.6. Unfortunately, there is a lack of specificity of the ECG changes occurring in patients with pheochromocytoma; however, reversibility of ECG abnormalities (in the absence of an etiologic explanation) in hypertensive subjects suggests pheochromocytoma.

Since the advent of chemical methods for detecting excess quantities of catecholamines or their metabolites in urine or blood, pharmacologic tests are rarely utilized for diagnostic purposes. There is now almost no need for performing a phentolamine test, since the diagnosis of pheochromocytoma can always be made in patients with sustained hypertension by urinary or plasma assays for catecholamines or their metabolites. In the rare situation when a patient presents in a hypertensive crisis or in a sustained malignant hypertensive state, the blood pressure response to intravenous administration of phentolamine may be of great value in the differential diagnosis. However, false positive phentolamine tests may occur in some patients with malignant hypertension.

Occasionally, a provocative test (with glucagon or histamine), when combined with chemical quantitation of urine or plasma catecholamines or their metabolites, can prove indispensable in the diagnosis of a paroxysmally secreting pheochromocytoma. Adequate precautions to counteract hypertensive crises must always be observed in performing provocative tests.

Our experience has indicated that histamine is the most reliable drug in provoking a hypertensive response in patients with pheochromocytoma. However, since side effects are more pronounced with histamine than glucagon, we perform a glucagon test initially; if the response to glucagon is negative, then we perform a histamine test, since some patients with pheochromocytoma may respond to one of these drugs and not the other. Our experience and the vast experience at the Mayo Clinic has indicated that provocative tests are safe if performed correctly and with the proper precautions.

The sine qua non for the preoperative diagnosis of pheochromocytoma is the demonstration of elevated concentrations of catecholamines and/or their metabolites in the urine, and/or the demonstration of elevated plasma catecholamines. Obviously, the reliability of the assay is mandatory. Any operation in search of a catecholamine secreting tumor without chemical confirmation or radiologic evidence of a tumor's presence is indefensible.

There should be no problem in detecting the patient with pheochromocytoma who has sustained hypertension due to excess circulating catecholamines; such a patient will invariably have elevated plasma and urinary concentrations of catecholamines or their metabolites. In rare cases, however, some patients with pheochromocytoma do have normal urinary excretions of catecholamines and their metabolites, as well as normal plasma concentrations of catecholamines when their blood pressure is normal. When evaluating these latter patients it is imperative that plasma and/or urine be obtained for catecholamine and metabolite determinations during a hypertensive period (either occurring spontaneously or induced by a provocative agent), since occasionally a definite preoperative diagnosis can be made only through this approach.

The measurement of total urinary metanephrines is favored for screening patients since it has proved to be the single most reliable test for detecting the presence of pheochromocytoma: more than 95 percent of patients with pheochromocytoma will have elevated excretions of total metanephrines. Furthermore, quantitation of the total metanephrines is comparatively easy, and fewer drugs interfere with its measurement as compared to the determination of urinary catecholamines or VMA. The substances which can interfere with quantitation of urinary catecholamines or their metabolites are listed

in Table 6.14, and those which may create problems in the diagnosis of pheochromocytoma have been indicated. It is essential that all drugs which significantly alter these urinary assays be avoided, preferably for one week, before a urine specimen is collected for analysis. Yet, we are not aware of any patient with a pheochromocytoma in whom drug therapy lowered the excretion rate of the catecholamines or their metabolites to a normal range. On the other hand, severe renal insufficiency may conceivably result in a marked impairment of the excretion of catecholamines and their metabolites. We observed one hypertensive patient with a pheochromocytoma and marked renal insufficiency whose urinary excretion of catecholamines and total metanephrines was normal.

Conditions (other than pheochromocytoma) which may be accompanied by significantly increased or decreased excretion of catecholamines and their metabolites are indicated in Table 6.15. These conditions must always be kept in mind when evaluating a patient suspected of having a pheochromocytoma. A point worth emphasizing is that a patient who is requested to collect a 24-hr urine specimen for assay of catecholamines or their metabolites should be instructed to avoid severe stress (e.g., prolonged strenuous physical activity, exposure to extreme cold) during the period of collection, since this may result in significantly elevated levels of the substances assayed.

The diagnostic accuracy of identifying patients with pheochromocytoma by determining plasma catecholamines has been substantiated. Our experience has indicated that the patient with sustained hypertension due to excessive circulating catecholamines from a pheochromocytoma can invariably be detected by plasma catecholamine assay. Since some patients with paroxysmal hypertension due to pheochromocytoma have normal plasma catecholamines when their blood pressures are relatively normal, it is essential that quantitation of plasma catecholamines be performed on blood sampled during a paroxysm (either one spontaneously occurring or one induced by a physical maneuver or a provocative drug).

An increased concentration of epinephrine or its metabolite (metanephrine) in the urine, and/or an elevated plasma epinephrine concentration, strongly suggests that the pheochromocytoma is located in the adrenal area. (Rarely, tumors secreting significant concentrations of epinephrine have occurred in extraadrenal sites, e.g., in the organ of Zuckerkandl, the urinary bladder, the hilus of the liver, and the thorax.)

Certain stressful conditions and diseases which cause significant changes in the urinary excretion of catecholamines (Table 6.15) can, of course, cause similar changes in the concentration of plasma catecholamines. Table 6.19 indicates the drugs and fluorescent substances which may significantly interfere with the fluorometric or double isotope assays in such a way as to cause erroneous results and possibly diagnostic errors.

Preoperative localization of one or more pheochromocytomas can be of considerable help and at times invaluable to the surgeon. In addition to demonstrating increased concentrations of epinephrine (or metanephrine) in the urine or plasma (which suggests an intraadrenal pheochromocytoma), radiography and central venous blood sampling for catecholamine assay can be of great value in localizing pheochromocytomas.

Nephrotomography was successful in localizing about 67 percent of intraabdominal pheochromocytomas, of which 90 percent were intraadrenal. Initial experience suggests that computerized axial tomography may prove valuable in detecting retroperitoneal tumors. Angiography (aortography, selective arteriography, and adrenal phlebography) is an exceptionally valuable radiographic technique for localizing pheochromocytomas. This technique has the advantage of demonstrating vascular abnormalities in both intraadrenal as well as many extraadrenal tumors. Aortography will almost invariably demonstrate tumors which are large and well-vascularized. However, in some cases, only selective arteriography or adrenal phlebography will demonstrate the tumor. Angiography and computerized axial tomography may be of great value in localizing tumors in the thorax and neck. Oblique chest x-rays should be routinely obtained in any patient suspected of having an intrathoracic pheochromocytoma.

Controversy exists as to whether an α-adre-nergic blockade should be induced in all patients suspected of having a pheochromocytoma prior to angiography, in order to avoid hypertensive crises which may be precipitated by the injection of contrast media. In most instances we see no great advantage in having a patient unblocked during angiographic studies, since, in the vast majority of patients, the location of an abdominal tumor will be detected by aortography and selective arteriography. However, a previous negative exploration of the abdomen is an indication for avoiding adrenergic blockade, since a hypertensive response during selective arteriography can sometimes be an important aid in confirming the diagnosis and in localizing a pheochromocytoma. Appropriate precautions to combat hypertensive crises, hypotension, and arrhythmias must be taken if angiography is performed in the unblocked patient suspected of harboring a pheochromocytoma.

When feasible, vena caval catheterization and central venous blood sampling for catecholamine assay, followed by adrenal phlebography, should be performed on patients whose pheochromocytomas have not been localized by other radiographic procedures. Central venous sampling can be particularly helpful when tumors are very small, multiple, or metastatic, and it will usually permit exclusion of cervical or intrathoracic pheochromocytomas. Although we have not found it necessary to induce α-adrenergic blockade prior to venous catheterization for the purpose of blood sampling, the precautions recommended for angiography in the unblocked patient should be observed. Very rarely, to establish the diagnosis of pheochromocytoma it may prove crucial to assay the plasma catecholamines in the inferior vena cava (above the level of the tumor), or in arterial blood during a hypertensive crisis induced by a provocative drug.

CHAPTER 7   To alert and sensitize the reader to the vagaries of pheochromocytoma, the relevant histories, physical findings, and laboratory studies of 38 patients were reported. In addition, the catecholamine concentrations in plasma and tumors of patients with sporadic (nonfamilial) pheochromocytoma were analyzed. When patients were compared with each other, no close correlation between levels of systolic and diastolic pressure and the concentrations of plasma catecholamines was observed. However, in the individual patient a reasonably good correlation between blood pressure and plasma catecholamine concentrations was sometimes observed when samples were obtained on different days.

Concentration of plasma catecholamines was invariably elevated on one or more determinations in patients with pheochromocytoma and sustained hypertension. On the other hand, 37.5 percent of patients with pheochromocytoma but with blood pressures relatively normal when blood samples were obtained, had normal plasma catecholamine concentrations. This observation points out again the importance of determining catecholamine concentrations in blood obtained during a paroxysmal attack to detect the presence of pheochromocytoma in some of these patients.

The mean age for patients with paroxysmal hypertension (49 years) was significantly older than that (35 years) for patients with sustained hypertension, perhaps because patients with sustained hypertension were recognized earlier than those with paroxysmal symptoms.

There was no good correlation between the size of pheochromocytomas or their contents of catecholamines, and the blood pressures of patients with these tumors.

It was intriguing that the ratio of plasma catecholamines did not always precisely reflect the ratio of the catecholamine content of the tumors. The conclusion must be drawn that secretion of one catecholamine from some of these tumors may occur selectively, while the other amine remains sequestered in the tumors. It is noteworthy that in 60 percent of the tumors causing paroxysmal hypertension, the tumor concentration of epinephrine was greater than that of norepinephrine; whereas in 69.2 percent of tumors from patients with sustained hypertension, norepinephrine concentration was greater than that of epinephrine (or norepinephrine was the only catecholamine present).

The mean concentration of total catecholamines in tumors of patients with paroxysmal hypertension was significantly greater than that in patients with sustained hypertension.

Possibly, tumors which cause paroxysmal hypertension and secrete only periodically are more likely to accumulate greater concentrations of catecholamines than are tumors which are constantly secreting. Although the ratios of epinephrine to norepinephrine in the tumors and plasma of patients with paroxysmal hypertension were higher than those in patients with sustained hypertension, the differences were not statistically significant. It remains unclear whether the ratio of epinephrine to norepinephrine which pheochromocytomas secrete plays a role in determining whether a patient manifests paroxysmal or sustained hypertension.

Why some pheochromocytomas paroxysmally release catecholamines into the blood and cause crises of hypertension but are relatively quiescent at other times remains an enigma. It is conceivable that in tumors causing paroxysmal hypertension the storage mechanism is nearly normal, whereas in tumors causing sustained hypertension the storage mechanism may be partially defective and thereby permit newly synthesized catecholamines to be released continuously from the tumor.

CHAPTER 8   Expertise and teamwork are essential for the successful management of pheochromocytoma. Surgical removal is the only curative therapy.

Preoperatively, one must exclude the presence of other conditions which may cause increased excretion of catecholamines and their metabolites. If there is any evidence suggesting that a patient has familial pheochromocytoma, it is mandatory to ascertain whether medullary thyroid carcinoma or hyperparathyroidism is also present. Although these two latter conditions rarely occur in patients with nonfamilial (sporadic) pheochromocytoma, the combination of these conditions is most often familial. (These conditions should be treated appropriately after the pheochromocytoma has been removed.)

The very rare occurrence of Cushing's syndrome in patients with pheochromocytoma requires preoperative evaluation, but ACTH infusion tests, if ever indicated, should be performed with extreme caution, since serious hypertensive crises and a fatality have been reported.

The possibility that malignant pheochromocytomas may metastasize must be kept in mind, and the presence of metastatic lesions excluded or identified when possible.

Preoperative location of a pheochromocytoma by the modalities mentioned above can be of great help to the surgeon. Angiographic studies can provide the surgeon with a vascular "road map" which permits a more rapid and effective removal of the tumor. If there is any indication that a pheochromocytoma is in the urinary bladder, cystoscopy (with the patient in an α-adrenergic blocked state) should be performed.

It is well to remember that *any diagnostic procedure which entails even a minor degree of trauma or stress should be performed with caution and with drugs available to combat a hypertensive crisis and arrhythmia or hypotension.*

Occasionally patients with pheochromocytoma may appear with acute or malignant hypertension or with acute abdominal or cardiovascular complications. The need for immediate medical and surgical therapy has been discussed.

Controversy continues to revolve around the preoperative and intraoperative management of patients with pheochromocytoma. Advocates of preoperative blockade with phenoxybenzamine (an α-adrenergic blocker) which is continued to the time of operation argue that blockade with this drug (a) prevents severe clinical manifestations in the preoperative period, (b) reverses hypovolemia which is frequently present, and (c) promotes a smooth anesthetic induction and operation. Those who oppose the routine preoperative use of phenoxybenzamine up to the time of operation feel that, if the α-blockade is complete, the surgeon will not have the advantage of (a) utilizing increases in blood pressure as a guide to tumor location, and (b) immediately recognizing (by persistence of hypertension) that another tumor may exist in the patient following pheochromocytoma removal. Except in rare circumstances with very severe sustained or paroxysmal hypertension, we have not found it necessary to administer phenoxybenzamine preoperatively to patients with pheochromocytoma. Although we do not strongly oppose the preoperative use of phenoxybenzamine in moderate dosage (especially if sustained hypertension or paroxysmal attacks are very severe or if the patient is precariously ill), we feel complete α-blockade is contraindicated when the location of a pheochromocytoma is uncertain or when the likelihood of encountering more than one tumor is anticipated.

Preoperative β-adrenergic blockade (with propranolol) is indicated in the presence of persistent tachycardia or arrhythmias felt to be hazardous to the patient or in the presence of angina pectoris (provided there are no contraindications to the use of this drug). However, *propranolol or other β-adrenergic blocking drugs should never be given to patients with pheochromocytoma without first creating α-blockade.* It should be mentioned that *in expert hands* the operative mortality (which has ranged from 0 to 3.3 percent) does not appear to have been influenced by preoperative α- and β-adrenergic blockade.

Certain drugs (e.g., morphine, phenothiazines) should be avoided in patients with pheochromocytoma, since they may precipitate hypertensive crises and/or hypotension. In the event that bilateral adrenalectomy is anticipated, appropriate steroid replacement therapy should be instituted before the patient is anesthetized.

Careful monitoring is crucial to successful intraoperative management. Intubation must be performed with appropriate premedication. Currently enflurane (Enthrane) appears to be the most desirable anesthetic agent.

Prompt control of hypertensive crises and arrhythmias during operation is critical to the safety and successful management of the patient. The appropriate use of sodium nitroprusside, propranolol, lidocaine, and volume expanders has been discussed in detail. Of paramount importance in preventing postoperative hypotension is the preoperative and intraoperative correction of any blood volume deficit. Vasopressor agents are only rarely indicated for the treatment of postoperative hypotension.

The anterior (transperitoneal) approach is mandatory when operating for an intraabdominal pheochromocytoma since these tumors may be multiple and extraadrenal in location. Although operative techniques of exposure and tumor removal are quite similar, surgical strategy varies somewhat. We believe the desirable strategy is one of immediate ligation of the tumor vasculature followed by extirpation and a thorough exploration for any residual tumors. Because of the high incidence of coexisting cholelithiasis, the gallbladder should be carefully examined during exploration.

Extraadrenal pheochromocytomas of the neck and chest require specialized surgical techniques, but preoperative, intraoperative, and postoperative management is similar to that already described for tumors located intraabdominally. Management of the pregnant patient depends somewhat on the duration of the pregnancy at the time a diagnosis of pheochromocytoma is made. In the early months of pregnancy, extirpation of a pheochromocytoma has been recommended, whereas, after the fifth month of pregnancy it has been suggested that the patient may be treated with adrenergic blocking agents as indicated until close to term. In general, we believe it is desirable to remove a pheochromocytoma as soon as it is discovered, no matter what the stage of the pregnancy. In the third trimester, if the manifestations of excessive circulating catecholamines can be satisfactorily controlled by adrenergic blockade, it may sometimes be preferable to delay tumor removal until the fetus is mature. When the fetus is adequately mature, we believe cesarean section with tumor extirpation is superior to permitting the patient to undergo the stressful procedure of vaginal delivery.

Monitoring and close observation should be continued postoperatively until the patient's condition is felt to be stable. One should consider bleeding at the operative site as a cause of postoperative hypotension. Postoperative hypertension may result from fluid overload, pain, a residual pheochromocytoma, or the inadvertent ligation of a renal artery.

The 5-year survival rate of patients with benign tumors is approximately 96 percent, whereas it is about 44 percent for patients with malignant pheochromocytomas. Approximately three-fourths of patients are normotensive following surgical removal of their pheochromocytomas, while the remainder has sustained or paroxysmal hypertension. Ordinarily patients should be followed for any evidence of recurrence for 5 to 10 years postoperatively; patients suspected of having familial pheochromocytoma should be followed throughout their lifetimes.

In the event that a pheochromocytoma has metastasized or is not totally resectable, one must endeavor to remove as much tumor as possible in order to reduce functioning tissue to a minimum. Radiotherapy and chemotherapy have been relatively ineffective. By blocking the peripheral effects of the catecholamines, chronic medical treatment with phenoxybenzamine has proved very successful in controlling the blood pressure and the manifestations of excessive circulating catecholamines, although it does not influence the growth of a pheochromocytoma. It would be more rational to use a drug which would prevent or markedly decrease the synthesis of catecholamines in the tumor; unfortunately, a drug with this therapeutic effect and devoid of serious side effects is not yet available.

Bibliography

A

1. Adicoff, A., Alexander, C. S., and Davis, R. B.: Malignant carcinoid syndrome. *Arch. Intern. Med. 117*: 250–255, 1966.
2. Agee, O. F., Kaude, J., and Lepasoon, J.: Preoperative localization of pheochromocytoma. *Acta Radiol. Diagn. 14*: 545–560, 1973.
3. Ainley-Walker, J. C. S., and Woodward, J. W.: Acute hypertension developing under anesthesia: a near fatality. *Br. J. Anaesth. 31*: 167–170, 1959.
4. Albers, D. D., Kalmon, E. H., and Back, K. C.: Pheochromocytoma: Report of 5 cases, one a spontaneous cure. *J. Urol. 78*: 301–308, 1957.
5. Albores-Saavedra, J., Maldonado, M. E., Ibarra, J., and Rodriguez, H. A.: Pheochromocytoma of the urinary bladder. *Cancer 23*: 1110–1118, 1969.
6. Alezais, and Peyron: Un groupe nouveau de tumeurs epithéliales: les paraganglions. *C. R. Seances Soc. Biol. Paris 65*: 745–747, 1908.
7. Allen. E. V., Bannon, W. G., Upson, M., Jr., Huizenga, K. A., Bastron, J. A., and Waugh, J. M.: A new sympatholytic and adrenolytic drug. Clinical studies on pheochromocytoma and essential hypertension. *Trans Assoc. Am. Physicians 64*: 109–121, 1951.
8. Allen, J. A., and Raddie, I. C.: The role of circulating catecholamines in sweat production in man. *J. Physiol. (London) 227*: 801–814, 1972.
9. Almqvist, S., Berg-Telenius, M., and Wästhed, B.: Serum calcitonin in medullary thyroid carcinoma. Radioimmunoassay technique and diagnostic value. *Acta Med. Scand. 196*: 177–180, 1974.
10. Amar-Costesec, A., Bohuon, C., and Schweisguth, O.: Activité mono amine oxydase dans les tumeurs de la crete nuerale. *Eur. J. Cancer 1*: 225–231, 1965.
11. Amery, A., and Conway, J.: A critical review of diagnostic tests for pheochromocytoma. *Am. Heart J. 73*: 129–133, 1967.

12. Anderson, A. B., and Anderson, M. D.: The effect of adrenaline on ketosis in phloridzinised and normal rats. *Biochem. J. 21*: 1398–1403, 1927.
13. Anderson, B. G., Beierwaltes, W. H., Harrison, T. S., Ansari, A. N., Buswink, A. A., and Ice, R. D.: Labeled dopamine concentration in pheochromocytomas. *J. Nucl. Med. 14*: 781–784, 1973.
14. Andreassen, A. K.: Phaeocromocytoma with metastases and endocrine activity. *Acta Chir. Scand. 107*; 214–217, 1954.
15. Andruff, M., and Kuhn, E.: Diastolic murmur caused by a pheochromocytoma. *Dtsch. Med. Wochenschr. 100*: 1530–1531, 1975.
16. Anton, A. H., Greer, M., Sayre, D. F., and Williams, C. M.: Dihydroxyphenylalanine secretion in a malignant pheochromocytoma. *Am. J. Med. 42*: 469–475, 1967.
17. Anton, A. H., and Sayre, D. F.: A study of the factors affecting the aluminum oxide–trihydroxyindole procedure for the analysis of catecholamines. *J. Pharmacol. Exp. Ther. 138*: 360–375, 1962.
18. Apgar, V., and Papper, E. M.: Pheochromocytoma—anesthetic management during surgical treatment. *Arch. Surg. (Chicago) 62*: 634–648, 1951.
19. Aranow, H., Jr.: Differential diagnosis of pheochromocytoma: *Med. Clin. North Am. 34*: 757–767, 1950.
20. Aranow, H., Jr.: Pheochromocytoma. *In*: Bean, W. B., ed., *Monographs in Medicine. Series 1*. Baltimore, Williams and Wilkins, 1952, pp. 179–224.
20a. Arendt, A. and Herrmann, W.: Phäochromocytom des Nebennierenmarkes bei Neurofibromatose mit Spongioblastom. *Z. Allg. Pathol. 101*: 243–249. 1960.
21. Arias-Stella, J.: Human carotid body at high altitudes. *Am. J. Pathol. 55*: 82a, 1969.
22. Armstrong, M. D., and McMillan, A.: Studies on

the formation of 3–methoxy–4–hydroxy–D–mandelic acid, a urinary metabolite of norepinephrine and epinephrine. *Pharmacol. Rev. 11*: 394–401, 1959.

23. Armstrong, M. D., McMillan, A., and Shaw, N. F.: 3–methoxy–4–hydroxy–D–mandelic acid, a urinary metabolite of norepinephrine. *Biochim. Biophys. Acta 25*: 422–423, 1957.

24. Atkins, F. L., Beaven, M. A., and Keiser, H. R.: Dopa decarboxylase in medullary carcinoma of the thyroid. *N. Engl. J. Med. 289*: 545–548, 1973.

25. Atuk, N. O., Owen, J. A., Jr., and Westfall, T. C.: Acute intermittent porphyria: Altered catecholamine metabolism and response to propanolol. Abstract presented at the American College of Clinical Pharmacology, May 3, 1975, Atlantic City, New Jersey.

26. Avakian, O. V. and Gillespie, J. S.: The relationship between the development of fluorescence on and the response of arterial smooth muscle perfused with noradrenaline. *J. Physiol. 191*: 71P–72P, 1967.

27. Avakian, O. V., and Gillespie, J. S. Uptake of noradrenaline by adrenergic nerves, smooth muscle and connective tissue in isolated perfused arteries and its correlation with the vasoconstrictor response. *Br. J. Pharmacol. 32*: 168–184, 1968.

28. Axelrod, J.: O–Methylation of epinephrine and other catechols *in vitro* and *in vivo*. *Science 126*: 400–401, 1957.

29. Axelrod, J.: Purification and properties of phenylethanolamine–N–methyl transferase. *J. Biol. Chem. 237*: 1657–1660, 1962.

30. Axelrod, J.: The fate of noradrenaline in the sympathetic neurone. *In: The Harvey Lectures*, New York and London, Academic Press, 1972, pp. 175–197.

31. Axelrod, J.: The formation, metabolism, uptake and release of noradrenaline and adrenaline. *In:* Variey, H., and Goweniock, A. H. eds., *Symposium on the Clinical Chemistry of Monoamines*. Amsterdam, Elsevier Publishing Co., 1963, pp. 5–18.

32. Axelrod, J.: The metabolism of catecholamines *in vivo* and *in vitro*. *Pharmacol. Rev. 11*: 402–408, 1959.

33. Axelrod, J., Inscoe, J. K., Senoh, S., and Witkop, B.: O–Methylation, the principle pathway for the metabolism of epinephrine and norepinephrine in the rat. *Biochim. Biophys. Acta 27*: 210–211, 1958.

34. Axelrod, J., Kopin, I. J., and Mann, J. D.: 3–methoxy–4–hydroxyphenylglycol sulfate: A new metabolite of epinephrine and norepinephrine. *Biochim. Biophys. Acta 36*: 576–577, 1959.

35. Axelrod, J., Weil-Malherbe, H., and Tomchick, R.: Physiological disposition of H3–Epinephrine and its metabolite metanephrine. *J. Pharmacol. Exp. Ther. 127*: 251–256, 1959.

B

36. Baird, I. M., and Cohen, H.: Pheochromocytoma: a case with hypotension, paroxysmal hypertension and urinary retention. *Lancet 2*: 270–272, 1954.

37. Balogh, K. J., Jr., Draskóczy, P. R., and Caulfield, J. B.: Norepinephrine in tumors of the jugular glomus. *Am. J. Pathol. 48*: 40a, 1966.

38. Baltaxe, H. A., Levin, D. C., and Imperato, J. L.: The angiographic demonstration of partially infarcted pheochromocytomas of the adrenal gland. *Am. J. Roentgenol. Radium Ther. Nucl. Med. 119*: 793–795, 1973.

39. Barbeau, A.: Le pheochromocytome: Une revue générale du sujet. *Union Med. Can. 86*: 1045–1081, 1957.

40. Barger, A. C., Herd, J. A., and Liebowitz, M. R.: Chronic catheterization of coronary artery: Induction of ECG pattern of myocardial ischemia by intracoronary epinephrine. *Proc. Soc. Exp. Biol. Med. 107*: 474–477, 1961.

41. Barnard, P. J., and Jacobson, L.: Malignant phaeochromocytoma associated with argentaffinoma and hypotensive crises; report of a case. *Cent. Afri. J. Med. 11*: 185–190, 1965.

42. Barnett, A. J., Blacket, R. B., DePoorter, A. E., Sanderson, P. H., and Wilson, G. M.: The action of noradrenaline in man and its relation to pheochromocytoma and hypertension. *Clin. Sci. 9*: 151–179, 1950.

43. Bartels, E. C.: Malignant pheochromocytoma. *Surg. Clin. North Am. 39*: 805–808, 1959.

44. Bartels, E. C., and Cattell, R. B.: Pheochromocytoma: Its diagnosis and treatment. *Ann. Surg. 131*: 903–916, 1950.

44a. Bartsch, G., Hörtnagl, H., and Winkler, H.: Electron micrographs of a cromaffin granule fraction isolated from a phaeochromocytoma. *Beitr. Pathol. 143*: 312–315, 1971.

45. Bässler, R., and Habighorst, L. V.: Vergleichende licht- und elektronenmikroskopische Untersuchungen am Nebennierenmark und Phäochromocytom. *Beitr. Pathol. Anat. Allg. Pathol. 130*: 446–488, 1964.

46. Batta, J. A., Jr., Tchilinguirian, N. G. O., and Passmore, J.: Pheochromocytoma in pregnancy: A case report and review of the pathophysiology. *Am. J. Obstet. Gynecol. 118*: 576–577, 1974.

47. Bauer, J., and Belt, E.: Paroxysmal hypertension with concomitant swelling of the thyroid due to pheochromocytoma of the right adrenal gland. Cure by surgical removal of the pheochromocytoma. *J. Clin. Endocrinol. Metab. 7*: 30–46, 1947.

47a. Baum, J. L. and Adler, M. E.: Pheochromocytoma, medullary thyroid carcinoma, multiple mucosal neuroma. *Arch. Ophthalmol. 87*: 574-584, 1972.

48. Baumgarten, E. C., and Cantor, M. O.: Pheochromocytoma: Case report. *Ann. Surg. 111*: 112–116, 1940.

49. Baylin, S. B.: Ectopic production of hormones and other proteins by tumors. *Hospital Practice 10* (10): 117–126, 1975.

50. Baylin, S. B., Beaven, M. A., Engelman, K., and Sjoerdsma, A.: Elevated histaminase activity in medullary carcinoma of the thyroid gland. *N. Engl. J. Med. 283*: 1239–1244, 1970.

51. Baylin, S. B., Gann, D. S., and Hsu, S. H.: Clonal origin of inherited medullary thyroid carcinoma and pheochromocytoma. *Science 193*: 321–323, 1976.

52. Baylis, P. H.: Reaction to phenoxybenzamine. *Lancet 2*: 1514–1515, 1974.

53. Beer, E., King, F. H., and Prinzmetal, M.: Pheochromocytoma with demonstration of pressor (adren-

alin) substance in blood preoperatively during hypertensive crises. *Ann. Surg. 106*: 85–91, 1937.

54. Bellas, J. E.: Nonsurgical pheochromocytoma. *J. Am. Med. Assoc. 185*: 601–602, 1963.

55. Belt, A. E., and Powell, T. O.: Clinical manifestations of chromaffin cell tumors arising from suprarenal medulla. *Surg. Gynecol. Obstet. 59*: 9–24, 1934.

56. Benedeczky, I., and Lapis, K.: Vergleichende elektronenmikroskopische Untersuchungen am Nebennierenmark und Phäochromocytom des Menschen. *Beitr. Pathol. Anat. 137*: 403–438, 1968.

57. Benfey, B. G., Ledoux, G., and Segal, M.: The action of antisympathomimetic drugs on the urinary excretion of adrenaline and noradrenaline. *Br. J. Pharmacol. 14*: 380–384, 1959.

58. Bennett, I. L., Jr., and Hyman, A.: Paroxysmal hypertension associated with tabes dorsalis: Report of 3 cases. *Am. J. Med. 5*: 729–735, 1948.

59. Bennett, M., and Mather, G.: Pheochromocytoma in pregnancy. *Lancet 1*: 811–812, 1959.

60. Berdal, P., Braaten, M., Cappelen, C., Jr., Mylius, E. A., and Walaas, O.: Noradrenaline–adrenaline producing nonchromaffin paraganglioma. *Acta Med. Scand. 172*: 249–257, 1962.

61. Berkheiser, S. W., and Rappoport, A. E.: Unsuspected pheochromocytoma of the adrenal: Report of 5 cases. *Am. J. Clin. Path. 21*: 657–665, 1951.

62. Berl, S., Puszkin, S., and Nicklas, W. J.: Actomyosin-like protein in brain. *Science 179*: 441–446, 1973.

63. Berlin, L., Guthrie, T. C., Goodell, H., and Wolff, H. G.: Studies on the central excitatory state. Factors responsible for the variability of the motor response to cutaneous stimulation in human subjects with isolated spinal cords. *Arch. Neurol. Psychiatry 72*: 764–779, 1954.

64. Bernal, P.: *Crises Hypertensives*. Thesis, G. Doin, Paris, 1933.

65. Bernal, P. *Crises Hypertensives; etude clinique, pathogenique et therapeutique*. Paris, G. Doin, 1934.

66. Berne, R. M., Hoffman, W. K., Jr., Kagan, A., and Levy, M. N.: Response of the normal and denervated kidney to l'epinephrine and l'nor-epinephrine, *Am. J. Physiol. 171*: 564–571, 1952.

67. Bernheimer, H., Ehringer, H., Heistracher, P., Kraupp, O., Lachnit, V., Obiditsch-Mayer, I., and Wenzl, M.: Biologisch aktives, nicht metastasierendes Bronchuscarcinoid mit Linksherzsyndrom. *Wien. Klin. Wochenschr. 72*: 867–873, 1960.

68. Bernier, J. J., Rambaud, J. C., Cattan, D., and Prost, A.: Diarrhea associated with medullary carcinoma of the thyroid. *Gut 10*: 980–985, 1969.

69. Bernstein, A., Wright, A. C., and Spencer, D.: Pheochromocytoma as a cause of gastrointestinal distension. *Postgrad. Med. J. 43*: 180–183, 1967.

70. Besterman, E., Bromley, L. L., and Peart, W. S.: An intrapericardial pheochromocytoma. *Br. Heart J. 36*: 318–320, 1974.

71. Bialestock, D.: Hyperplasia of the adrenal medulla in hypertension of children. *Arch. Dis. Child. 36*: 465–473, 1961.

72. Binger, M. W. and Craig, W. McK.: An atypical case of hypertension with a tumor of the adrenal gland. *Mayo Clinic Proc. 13*: 17–20, 1938.

73. Bingham, W., Elliott, J., and Lyons, S. M.: Management of anaesthesia for phaeochromocytoma. *Anaesthesia 27*: 49–60, 1972.

74. Biscol, T. J.: Carotid body: Structure and function. *Physiol. Rev. 51*: 437–495, 1971.

75. Biserte, G.: Présence d'homocystine dans les extraits de surrénales humaines. *Bull. Soc. Chim. Biol. 39*: 549–552, 1957.

76. Björk, V. O., Linderholm, H., Lublin, H., Pernow, B., and Törnberg, B.: Malignant intrathoracic pheochromocytoma with lung metastases and raised noradrenaline concentration in superior vena cava blood: Report of a case. *Acta Chir. Scand. 116*: 411–422,, 1959.

77. Black, G. W., Glasgow, J. F. T., and Smyth, B. T.: Management of a phaeochromocytoma in a child. *Br. J. Anaesth. 41*: 184–187, 1969.

78. Blacket, R. B., Pickering, G. W., and Wilson, G. M.: The effects of prolonged infusions of noradrenaline on the arterial pressure of the rabbit. *Clin. Sci. 9*: 247–257, 1950.

79. Blacklock, J. W. S., Ferguson, J. W., Mack, W. S., Shafar, J., and Symington, T.: Phaeochromocytoma. *Br. J. Surg. 35*: 179–197, 1947.

80. Blackwell, B. Marley, E., Price, J., and Taylor, D.: Hypertensive interactions between monoamine oxidase inhibitors and foodstuffs, *Br. J. Psychiatry 113*: 349–365, 1967.

81. Blaschko, H., Born, G. V. R., D'Iorio, A., and Eade, N. R.: Observations on the distribution of catecholamines and adenosinetriphosphate in the bovine adrenal medulla. *J. Physiol. 133*: 548–557, 1956.

82. Blaschko, H., Jerrome, D. W., Robb-Smith, A. H. T., Smith, A. D., and Winkler, H.: Biochemical and morphological studies on catecholamine storage in human phaeochromocytoma. *Clin. Sci. 34*: 453–465, 1968.

83. Blaschko, H., Richter, D., and Schlossmann, H.: The oxidation of adrenaline and other amines. *Biochem. J. 31*: 2187–2196, 1937.

83a. Block, M. A., Jackson, C. E., and Tashjian, A. H., Jr.: Medullary thyroid carcinoma detected by serum calcitonin assay. *Arch. Surg. 104*: 579–586, 1972.

84. Bloom, D. A., and Fonkalsrud, E. W.: Surgical management of pheochromocytoma in children. *J. Pediatr. Surg. 9*: 179–184, 1974.

85. Bogaert, M. G. and Vermeulen, A.: Pheochromocytoma of the urinary bladder, with inconclusive chemical and pharmacologic tests. *Am. J. Med. 53*: 797–800, 1972.

86. Bohuon, C.: Catecholamine metabolism in neuroblastoma. *J. Pediatr. Surg. 3*: 114–118, 1968.

87. Bohuon, C., and Guérinot, F.: Dopamine-β-hydroxylase dans les tumeurs d'origine sympathique. *Clin. Chim. Acta 14*: 414–416, 1966.

88. Bohuon, C., Guérinot, F., Tcherdakoff, P. H., and Bonnay, M.: Dopamine-β-hydroxylase activity in five cases of pheochromocytoma. *Biochem. Soc. Trans. 1*: 152–153, 1973.

89. Boijsen, E., Williams, C. M., and Judkins, M. P.: Angiography of pheochromocytoma. *Am. J. Roentgenol. Radium Ther. Nucl. Med. 98*: 225–232, 1966.

90. Bolande, R. P.: The neurocristopathies. A unifying

concept of disease arising in neural crest maldevelopment. *Hum. Pathol. 5:* 409–429, 1974.

91. Bollman, J. L., Flock, E. V., Roth, G. M., and Kvale, W. F.: Catecholamines in patients with pheochromocytoma. *J. Lab. Clin. Med. 56:* 506–519, 1960.

92. Bondy, P. K.: Hypoglycemic states. *In:* Beeson, P. B., and McDermott, W., eds. *Cecil-Loeb Textbook of Medicine.* 13th edition. Philadelphia, W. B. Saunders, 1971, pp. 1656–1659.

93. Borello, E. D., and Gorlin, R. J.: Melanotic neuroectodermal tumor of infancy: A neoplasm of neural crest origin. Cancer, *19:* 196–206, 1966.

94. Bosniak, M. A., Siegelman, S. S., and Evans, J. A.: *Tumors of the Adrenal, Retroperitoneum and Lower Urinary Tract (An atlas of Tumor Radiology).* Chicago, Year Book Medical Publishers, 1976.

95. Bourne, R. B., and Beltaos, E.: Pheochromocytoma of the bladder. Case report and summary of the literature. *J. Urol. 98:* 361–364, 1967.

96. Bradley, J. E., Young, J. D., Jr., and Lentz, G.: Polycythemia secondary to pheochromocytoma. *J. Urol. 86:* 1–6, 1961.

97. Braley, A. E.: Medullated corneal nerves and plexiform neuroma associated with pheochromocytoma. *Trans. Am. Ophthalmol. Soc. 52:* 189–197, 1954.

98. Brann, W. C., Puryear, W. G., and Landes, R. R.: Pheochromocytoma in pregnancy, *J. Urol. 76:* 323–329, 1956.

99. Brasfield, R. D. and Das Gupta, T. K.: von Recklinghausen's Disease: A clinico-pathological study. *Ann. Surg., 175:* 86–104, 1972.

100. Brenner, W. E., Yen, S. S. C., Dingfelder, J. R., and Anton, A. H.: Pheochromocytoma: Serial studies during pregnancy. *Am. J. Obstet. Gynecol. 113:* 779–788, 1972.

101. Brewer, G., Larson, P. S., and Schroeder, A. R.: On the effect of the epinephrine on blood potassium. *Am. J. Physiol. 126:* 708–712, 1939.

102. Brody, I. A.: Shock after administration of prochlorperazine in patient with pheochromocytoma. *J. Am. Med. Assoc. 169:* 1749–1752, 1959.

103. Brown, J. J., Davies, D. L., Lever, A. F., and Robertson, J. I. S.: Plasma renin concentration in human hypertension. II: Renin in relation to aetiology. *Br. Med. J. 2:* 1215–1219, 1965.

104. Brown, J. W., Burton, R. C., and Dahlin, D. C.: Chemodectoma with skeletal metastasis: Report of two cases. *Mayo Clin. Proc. 42:* 551–555, 1967.

105. Brown, R. B. and Borowsky, M.: Further observations on intestinal lesions associated with pheochromocytomas. A case of malignant pheochromocytoma in pregnancy. *Ann. Surg. 151:* 683–692, 1960.

106. Brown, R. B., Rice, B. H., and Szakas, J. E.: Intestinal bleeding and perforation complicating treatment with vasoconstrictors. *Ann. Surg. 150:* 790–798, 1959.

107. Bruce, G. M.: Changes in the ocular fundus associated with pheochromocytoma of the adrenal gland. *Arch. Ophthalmol. 39:* 707–730, 1948.

108. Bruce, G. M.: The ocular fundus in pheochromocytoma of the adrenal gland: Report of three cases. *Trans. Am. Ophthalmol. Soc. 45:* 201–228, 1947.

109. Brundin, J., and Engstrom, L.: Urinary excretion of free catecholamines during spontaneous and oxytocin-induced labor. *Obstet. Gynecol. 17:* 99–102, 1961.

110. Brunjes, S., Johns, V. J., Jr., and Crane, M. G.: Pheochromocytoma: Postoperative shock and blood volume. *N. Eng. J. Med. 262:* 393–396, 1960.

111. Burack, W. R., and Draskóczy, P. R.: The turnover of endogenously labeled catecholamine in several regions of the sympathetic nervous system. *J. Pharmacol. Exp. Ther. 144:* 66–75, 1964.

112. Burak, N., Loesch, J., and Costa, J.: Adrenocortical adenoma, clinically simulating pheochromocytoma. *N.Y. State J. Med. 59:* 1849–1851, 1959.

113. Burch, G. E.: Pork and hypertension. *Am. Heart J. 86:* 713–714, 1973.

114. Burch, G. E., and Phillips, J. H.: The large upright T-wave as an electrocardiographic manifestation of intracranial disease. *South. Med. J. 61:* 331–336, 1968.

115. Burger, M., and Langermann, H.: Bestimmungen von Adrenalin und Noradrenalin sowie von Decarboxylase- und Aminoxydase-Aktivitaten in Zellfranktionen van Phäochromocytomen. *Klin. Wochenschr. 34:* 941–944, 1956.

116. Burgess, A. M., Waterman, G. W., and Cutts, F. B.: Adrenal sympathetic syndrome with unusual variations in cardiac rhythm. *Arch. Int. Med. Exp. 58:* 433–447, 1936.

117. Burn, G. P.: Urinary excretion of pressor amines in relation to pheochromocytoma. *Br. Med. J. 1:* 697–699, 1953.

118. Burns, A. B., Tesluk, H., and Palmer, J. M.: Hypertension associated with vascular lesions of neurofibromatosis. *J. Urol. 108:* 676–679, 1972.

C

119. Cabañas, V. Y., Faulconer, R. J., and Fekete, A. M.: Pheochromocytoma presenting as a ureterocele. *J. Urol. 110:* 389–390, 1973.

120. Cadman, E. F. B., and Tinckler, L. F.: Localization of phaeochromocytomas. *J. Fac. Radiol. (London) 4:* 211–215, 1953.

121. Cahill, G. F.: Hormonal tumors of the adrenal. *Surgery 16:* 233–265, 1944.

122. Cahill, G. F.: Pheochromocytoma. *Bull. N. Y. Acad. Med. 29:* 749–764, 1953.

123. Cahill, G. F., and Melicow, M. M.: Tumors of the adrenal gland. *J. Urol. 64:* 1–25, 1950.

124. Cahill, G. F., and Monteith, J. C.: The use of dibenamine and norepinephrine in the operative management of pheochromocytoma. Report of two cases. *N. Engl. J. Med. 244:* 657–661, 1951.

125. Cahill, G. F. and Papper, E. M.: Techniques involved in surgical removal of pheochromocytoma. *J. Urol. 76:* 467–477, 1956.

126. Calkins, E., and Howard, J. E.: Bilateral familial phaeochromocytoma with paroxysmal hypertension: successful removal of tumors in two cases, with discussion of certain diagnostic procedures and physiological considerations. *J. Clin. Endocrinol., 7:* 475–492, 1947.

127. Cameron, D. G., Warner, H. A., and Szabo, A. J.:

Chronic diarrhea in an adult with hypokalemic nephropathy and osteomalacia due to a functioning ganglioneuroblastoma. *Am. J. Med. Sci. 253*: 417–424, 1967.

128. Cameron, S. J., and Doig, A.: Cerebellar tumours presenting with clinical features of phaeochromocytoma. *Lancet 1*: 492–494, 1970.

129. Campbell, D. J., Sherbamisek, R., and Rigby, J.: False positive reaction due to methocarbamol in the screening test for vanilmandelic acid. *Clin. Chem. 10*: 447–450, 1964.

130. Cannon, F. J.: Some newer aspects of electrocardiography: Study of 16 cases of phaeochromocytoma. *Irish J. Med. Sci. 359*: 499–511, 1955.

131. Cannon, P., and Sjöstrand, T.: ECG—Changes seen in cases of pheochromocytoma compared with changes experimentally evoked by adrenaline. *Scand. J. Clin. Lab. Invest. 4*: 266–267, 1952.

132. Cantu, R. C., Correll, J. W., and Manger, W. M.: Reassessment of central neural pathways necessary for adrenal catecholamine output in response to hypoglycemia. *Proc. Soc. Exp. Biol. Med. 129*: 155–161, 1968.

133. Cantu, R. C., Nahas, G. G., and Manger, W. M.: Effect of hypercapnic acidosis and hypoxia on adrenal catecholamine output of the spinal dog. *Proc. Soc. Exp. Biol. Med. 122*: 434–437, 1966.

134. Capella, C., and Solcia, E.: Optical and electron microscopical study of cytoplasmic granules in human carotid body, carotid body tumours and glomus jugulare tumours. *Virchows Arch. B. 7*: 37–52, 1971.

134a. Capen, C. C., Young, D. M.: The ultrastructure of the parathyroid glands and thyroid parafollicular cells of cows with parturient paresis and hypocalcemia. *Lab. Invest. 17*: 717–737, 1967.

135. Carney, J. A., Go, V. L. W., Sizemore, G. W., and Hayles, A. B.: Alimentary-tract ganglioneuromatosis. A major component of the syndrome of multiple neoplasia, type 2b. *N. Engl. J. Med.* 295: 1287–1291, 1976.

135a. Carney, J. A., Sizemore, G. W., and Lovestedt, S. A.: Mucosal ganglioneuromatosis, medullary thyroid carcinoma, and pheochromocytoma: Multiple endocrine neoplasia, type 2b. *Oral Surg. 41*: 739–752, 1976.

135b. Carney, A., Sizemore, G. W., and Sheps, S. G.: Adrenal medullary disease in multiple endocrine neoplasia, type 2. Pheochromocytoma and its precursors. *Am. J. Clin. Pathol. 66*: 279–290, 1976.

136. Carney, J. A., Sizemore, G. W., and Tyce, G. M.: Bilateral adrenal medullary hyperplasia in multiple endocrine neoplasia, type II. The precursor of bilateral pheochromocytoma. *Mayo Clinic Proc. 50*: 3–10, 1975.

137. Case records of the Massachusetts General Hospital: Case Report: 27022–1941. Dissecting aneurysm of ascending aorta with rupture into pericardium. Pheochromocytoma of the adrenal gland. *N. Engl. J. Med. 224*: 77–79, 1941.

138. Case Records of the Massachusetts General Hospital: Pheochromocytoma of adrenal gland, bilateral, with cyst formation, marked, left. *N. Engl. J. Med. 268*: 894–898, 1963.

139. Case Records of the Massachusetts General Hospital: Case Report: 35–1973. Medullary carcinoma of thyroid gland, bilateral, pheochromocytoma of right adrenal gland and parathyroid hyperplasia (Sipple's syndrome). *N. Engl. J. Med. 289*: 472–479, 1973.

140. Case Records of the Massachusetts General Hospital: Case Report: 3. Pheochromocytoma, right, secreting epinephrine and norepinephrine. *N. Engl. J. Med. 292*: 151–156, 1975.

141. Case Records of the Massachusetts General Hospital: Pheochromocytoma (three), of adrenal glands and ectopic adrenal gland. Parathyroid hyperplasia. Medullary carcinoma of thyroid gland, with metastases to liver. *N. Engl. J. Med. 293*: 1085–1092, 1975.

142. Castle, C. H.: Iatrogenic renal hypertension: two unusual complications of surgery for familial pheochromocytoma. *J. Am. Med. Assoc. 225*: 1085–1088, 1973.

143. Castleden, L. I. M.: The effect of adrenalin on the serum potassium level in man. *Clin. Sci. 3*: 241–245, 1938.

144. Catalona, W. J., Engelman, K., Ketcham, A. S., and Hammond, W. G.: Familial medullary thyroid carcinoma, pheochromocytoma, and parathyroid adenoma (Sipple's Syndrome). *Cancer 28*: 1245–1254, 1971.

145. Chamovitz, J. and Fanger, H.: Malignant pheochromocytoma and hypertension. A case report. *Am. J. Clin. Path. 19*: 243–251, 1949.

146. Chapman, R. C. and Diaz-Perez, R.: Pheochromocytoma associated with cerebellar hemangioblastoma. Familial occurrence. *J. Am. Med. Assoc. 182*: 1014–1017, 1962.

147. Chapman, R. C., Kemp, V. E., and Taliaferro, I.: Pheochromocytoma associated with multiple neurofibromatosis and intracranial hemangioma. *Am. J. Med. 26*: 883–890, 1959.

148. Chasis, H., Ranges, H. A., Goldring, W., and Smith, H. W.: The control of renal blood flow and glomerular filtration in normal man. *J. Clin. Invest. 17*: 683–697, 1938.

149. Chaturvedi, N. C., Walsh, M. J., Boyle, D. McC., and Barber, J. M.: Diamorphine-induced attack of paroxysmal hypertension in pheochromocytoma. *Br. Med. J. 2*: 538, 1974.

149a. Cheng, T. O., and Bashour, T. T.: Striking cardiographic changes associated with pheochromocytoma masquerading as ischemic heart disease. *Chest 70*: 397–399, 1976.

150. Chesley, L. C., Markowitz, I., and Wetchler, B. B.: Proteinuria following momentary vascular constriction. *J. Clin. Invest. 18*: 51–58, 1939.

150a. Chong, G. C., Beahrs, O. H., Sizemore, G. W., and Woolner, L. H.: Medullary carcinoma of the thyroid gland. *Cancer 35*: 695–704, 1975.

151. Chretien, P. B., Engelman, K., Hoye, R. C., and Geelhold, G. W.: Surgical management of intravascular glomus jugulare tumor. *Am. J. Surg. 122*: 740–743, 1971.

152. Christensen, M. S., and Christensen, N. J.: Plasma catecholamines in hypertension. *Scand. J. Clin. Lab. Invest. 30*: 169–173, 1972.

153, Christensen, N. J.: A sensitive assay for the determination of dopamine in plasma. *Scand. J. Clin. Lab. Invest. 31*: 343–346, 1973.

153a. Christensen, N.J.: Plasma nonadrenaline and adrenaline in patients with thyrotoxicosis and myxoedema. *Clin. Sci. Mol. Med. 45*: 163–171, 1973.

154. Chukwuemeka, A. C., Paton, A. M., Gebbie, D. A. M., Ayim, E. N., and Dhall, D. P.: Phaeochromocytoma in pregnancy. *East Afr. Med. J. 51*: 496–499, 1974.

155. Chung, E. B. and Pressoir, R.: Pheochromocytoma in blacks. *J. Nat. Med. Assoc. 67*: 22–26, 1975.

156. Churchill, D., Knaack, J., Chirito, E., Barré, P., Cole, C., Muehrcke, R., and Gault, M. H.: Persisting renal insufficiency after methoxyflurane anesthesia. Report of two cases and review of literature. *Am. J. Med. 56*: 575–582, 1974.

157. Churchill-Davidson, H. C., Wylie, W. D., Miles, B. E., and De Wardener, H. E.: The effects of adrenaline, noradrenaline, and methedrine on the renal circulation during anaesthesia. *Lancet 2*: 803–805, 1951.

158. Clausen, E. G.: Pheochromocytoma in children: Review of significant surgical aspects and report of 3 additional cases. *Am. J. Surg. 94*: 409–416, 1957.

159. Cleveland, B. R., Lawhon, J., and Cunningham, P. J.: Pheochromocytoma simulating toxemia in pregnancy. *Tex. Med. 69*: 70–73, 1973.

160. Coates, P. A., and Rigal, W. M.: Postanaesthetic death from pheochromocytoma without hypertension. *Lancet 1*: 1374–1375, 1961.

160a. Cobin, R. Pertsemlidis, D., Gitlow, S., and Krieger, D.: Coexistence of multiple pheochromocytomas, acromegaly, and hyperparathyroidism. *Am. J. Med.* In press.

161. Coggin, M. J., Adamson, A. R., Finberg, J., and Joekes, A. M.: Pheochromocytoma of the urinary bladder with acute oliguric renal failure: The use of a plasma catecholamine assay in diagnosis. *Postgrad. Med. J. 47*: 238–242, 1971.

162. Cohen, G., and Goldenberg, M.: The simultaneous fluorimetric determination of adrenaline and noradrenaline in plasma-II. Peripheral venous plasma concentrations in normal subjects and in patients with pheochromocytoma. *J. Neurochem. 2*: 71–80, 1957.

163. Cohn, J. N.: Paroxysmal hypertension and hypovolemia. *N. Engl. J. Med. 275*: 643–646, 1966.

164. Cohn, J. N., and Daddario, R. C.: Mechanism of disappearance of Korotkoff sounds in clinical shock. *Circulation, 32 (Suppl. 2)*: 69, 1965

165. Colcock, B. P., and Hull, J. E.: Pheochromocytoma as a massive abdominal tumor. *J. Indiana State Med. Assoc. 48*: 955–957, 1955.

166. Cole, L.: Early diagnosis of pheochromocytoma. *Br. Heart J. 12*: 232–238, 1950.

167. Comroe, J. H., Jr.: The peripheral chemoreceptors. *In*: Fenn, W. O., and Rahn, H., eds., *Handbook of Physiology: Respiration, Sect. 3, Vol. 1.* Washington, American Physiological Society, 1964, pp. 557–583.

168. Cone, T. E., Jr.: Recurrent pheochromocytoma; report of a case in a previously treated child. *Pediatrics 21*: 994–999, 1958.

169. Cone, T. E. Jr., Allen, M. S., and Pearson, H. A.: Pheochromocytoma in children: Report of three familial cases in two unrelated families. *Pediatrics 19*: 44–56, 1957.

170. Cooperman, L. H., Engelman, K., and Mann, P. E. G.: Anesthetic management of pheochromocytoma employing halothane and beta-adrenergic blockade. A report of fourteen cases. *Anesthesiology 28*: 575–582, 1967.

171. Cope, O., Keynes, W. M., Roth, S. I., and Castleman, B.: Primary chief-cell hyperplasia of parathyroid glands: new entity in surgery of hyperparathyroidism. *Ann. Surg. 148*: 375–388, 1958.

172. Corbett, J. L., Kerr, J. H., Prys-Roberts C., Crampton-Smith, A., and Spalding, J. M. K.: Cardiovascular disturbances in severe tetanus due to overactivity of the sympathetic nervous system. *Anesthesia 24*: 198–212, 1969.

173. Corday, E., and Williams, J. H.: Effect of shock and of vasopressor drugs on the regional circulation of the brain, heart, kidney and liver. *Am. J. Med. 29*: 228–241, 1960.

174. Cornell, S. H., and Kirkendall, W. M.: Neurofibromatosis of the renal artery: An unusual cause of hypertension. *Radiology 88*: 24–28, 1967.

175. Cornog, J. L., Wilkinson, J. H., Arvan, D. A., Freed, R. M., Sellers, A. M., and Barker, C.: Extraadrenal pheochromocytoma: Some electron microscopic and biochemical studies. *Am. J. Med. 48*: 654–660, 1970.

176. Coupland, R. E.: Electron microscopic observations on the structure of the rat adrenal medulla. I: The ultrastructure and organization of chromaffin cells in the normal adrenal medulla. *J. Anat. 99*: 231–254, 1965.

177. Coupland, R. E.: Post-natal fate of the abdominal para-aortic bodies in man. *J. Anat. 88*: 455–464, 1954.

178. Coupland, R. E.: *The Natural History of the Chromaffin Cell.* London, Longmans, Green and Co., Ltd., 1965, 279 pp.

178a. Cousins, M. J., and Rubin, R. B.: The intraoperative management of phaeochromocytoma with total epidural sympathetic blockade. *Br. J. Anaesth. 46*: 78–81, 1974.

178b. Cragg, R. W.: Concurrent tumors of the left carotid body and both Zuckerkandl bodies. *Arch. Pathol. 18*: 635–645, 1934.

179. Crago, R. M., Eckholdt, J. W., and Wisnell, J. G.: Pheochromocytoma. Treatment with alpha and beta-adrenergic blocking drugs. *J. Am. Med. Assoc. 202*: 870–874, 1967.

180. Cremer, G. M., Molnar, G. D., Moxness, K. E., Shep, S. G., Maher, F. T., and Jones, J. D.: Hormonal and biochemical response to glucagon administration in patients with pheochromocytoma and in control subjects. *Mayo Clin. Proc. 43*: 161–176, 1968.

181. Critchley, J. A. H. J., West, C. P., and Waite, J.: Dangers of corticotropin in phaeochromocytoma. *Lancet 2*: 782, 1974.

182. Crockett, K. A., Snow, E., and Rees, V. L.: Pheochromocytomas as cause of unexpected operating room deaths. *Amer. Surg. 27*: 395–399, 1969.

183. Crockford, P. M., Port, D., Jr., Woods, F. C., Jr.,

and Williams, R. H.: Effect of glucagon on serum insulin, plasma glucose and free fatty acids in man. *Metabolism 15:* 114–122, 1966.

184. Cross, G. O., and Pace, J. W.: Malignant pheochromocytoma with paroxysmal hypertension and metastasis to the cervical spine. *J. Am. Med. Assoc. 142:* 1068–1070, 1950.

185. Crout, J. R.: Catecholamine metabolism in pheochromocytoma and essential hypertension. *In:* Manger, W. M. ed., *Hormones and Hypertension.* Chap. I. Springfield, Ill., C. C. Thomas, 1966, pp. 3–40.

186. Crout, J. R.: Pheochromocytoma. *Pharmacol. Rev. 18:* 651–657, 1966.

187. Crout, J. R.: Sampling and analysis of catecholamines and metabolites. *Anesthesiology 29:* 661–669, 1968.

188. Crout, J. R.: Some spectrophotofluorimetric observations on blood and urine catecholamine assays. *Pharmacol. Rev. 11:* 296–299, 1959.

189. Crout, J. R.: *Standard Methods of Clinical Chemistry,* Vol. III. New York, Academic Press, 1960.

190. Crout, J. R., and Brown, B. R., Jr.: Anesthetic management of pheochromocytoma: The value of phenoxybenzamine and methoxyflurane. *Anesthesiology 30:* 29–36, 1969.

191. Crout, J. R., Pisano, J. J., and Sjoerdsma, A.: Urinary excretion of catecholamines and their metabolites in pheochromocytoma. *Am. Heart J. 61:* 375–381, 1961.

192. Crout, J. R., and Sjoerdsma, A.: Catecholamine excretion after banana feeding. *J. Pharm. Pharmacol. 11:* 190–191, 1959.

193. Crout, J. R., and Sjoerdsma, A.: Catecholamines in the localization of pheochromocytoma. *Circulation 22:* 516–525, 1960.

194. Crout, J. R., and Sjoerdsma, A.: The clinical and laboratory significance of serotonin and catecholamines in bananas. *N. Engl. J. Med. 261:* 23–26, 1959.

195. Crout, J. R., and Sjoerdsma, A.: Turnover and metabolism of catecholamine in patients with pheochromocytoma. *J. Clin. Invest. 43:* 94–102, 1964.

196. Crowther, K. V.: Two cases of phaeochromocytoma. *Br. Med. J. 1:* 445–448, 1951.

197. Cruz, S. R., and Colwell, J. A.: Pheochromocytoma and ileus. *J. Am. Med. Assoc. 219:* 1050–1051, 1972.

198. Cunliffe, W. J., Black, M. M., Hall, R., Johnston, I. D. A., Hudgson, P., Schuster, S., Gudmundsson, T. V., Joplin, G. F., Williams, E. D., Woodhouse, N. J. Y., Galante, L., and MacIntyre, I. A.: A calcitonin-secreting thyroid carcinoma. *Lancet 2:* 63–66, 1968.

198a. Cunliffe, W. J., Hudgdon, P., Fulthorpe, J. J., Black, M. M., Hall, R., Johnston, I. D. A., and Shuster, S.: A calcitonin-secreting medullary thyroid carcinoma associated with mucosal neuromas, Marfanoid features, myopathy, and pigmentation. *Am. J. Med. 48:* 120–126, 1970.

199. Cushman, P.: Familial endocrine tumors. *Am. J. Med. 32:* 352–360, 1962.

D

200. Dahlström, A.: Adrenergic neurons (with special reference to fluorescence microscopical studies in mammals). *In:* Bargmann, W., and Scharrer, E., eds., *Aspects of Neuroendocrinology. V. International Symposium on Neurosecretion.* Berlin, Heidelberg, New York, Springer-Verlag, 1970, pp. 55–78.

201. Dahlström, A., and Fuxe, K.: A method for the demonstration of adrenergic nerve fibres in peripheral nerves. *Z. Zellforsch. Mikrosk. Anat. 62:* 602–607, 1964.

202. Dale, H. H.: Nomenclature of fibres in autonomic system and their effects. *J. Physiol. 80:* 10–11, 1933.

203. Dalessio, D. J.: *Wolff's Headache and Other Head Pain.* 3rd ed. Oxford University Press, New York, 1972, 688 pp.

204. Dancis, J., and Smith, A. A.: Familial dysautonomia. *N. Engl. J. Med. 274:* 207–209, 1966.

205. Daugherty, G., Manger, W. M., Roth, G. M., Flock, E. V., Childs, D. S., Jr., and Waugh, J. M.: Malignant carcinoid with hyperserotonemia occurring spontaneously or induced by palpation of the tumor or by intravenous histamine: Report of case. *Mayo Clin. Proc. 30:* 595–601, 1955.

206. Davies, D. M., Ross, J. H., Richardson, J. E., and Brown, A. I.: Experience with phaeochromocytoma. *Postgrad. Med. J. 39:* 337–347, 1963.

206a. Davis, F. W., Jr., Hull, J. G., and Vardell, J. C., Jr.: Pheochromocytoma with neurofibromatosis. *Am. J. Med. 8:* 131–135, 1950.

206b. Davis, J. O.: The control of renin release. *Am. J. Med. 55:* 333–350, 1973.

207. Davis, J. O.: The Control of Renin Release: The Renal Sympathetic Nerves and Catecholamines in Renin Release. *In:* J. H. Laragh, ed., *Hypertension Manual.* New York, Dun-Donnelley, 1974, pp. 175–181.

208. Davis, P., Peart, W. S., and van't Hoff, W.: Malignant phaeochromocytoma with functioning metastases. *Lancet 2:* 274–275, 1955.

209. Dawson, D. W., and Tapp, E.: A compound tumor of the adrenal medulla. *J. Pathol. 97:* 231–233, 1969.

210. Dawson, J., and Bone, A.: The relationship between urine volume and urinary adrenaline and noradrenaline excretion in a group of psychotic patients. *Br. J. Psychiat. 109:* 629–630, 1963.

211. Day, R., Smith, J. R., and Klingman, W. O.: Tests of function of vegetative nervous system in acrodynia. *Am. J. Dis. Child. 57:* 269–277, 1939.

212. Dean, R. E.: Pheochromocytoma and pregnancy. *Obstet. Gynecol. 11:* 35–42, 1958.

213. Dearborn, E. H., and Lasagna, L.: The antidiuretic action of epinephrine and norepinephrine. *J. Pharmacol. Exp. Ther. 106:* 122–128, 1952.

214. De Champlain, J., Farley, L., Cousineau, D., and van Amerigen, M-R.: Circulating catecholamine levels in human and experimental hypertension. *Circ. Res. 38:* 109–114, 1976.

215. DeCourcy, J. L., and DeCourcy, C. B.: *Pheochromocytomas and The General Practitioner.* Cincinnati, Barclay Newman, 1952, 163 pp.

216. DeDuve, C.: Endocytosis. *In:* De Renck, A. V. S., and Cameron, M. P., eds., *Lysosomes.* CIBA Foundation Symposium. London, Churchill, 1963, p. 126.

217. Deftos, L. J., Bury, A. E., Haebner, J. F., Singer, F. R., and Potts, J. T., Jr.: Immunoassay for human

calcitonin. II. Clinical studies. *Metabolism 20*: 1129–1137, 1971.

218. DeGraeff, J., and Horak, B. J. V.: The incidence of pheochromocytoma in the Netherlands. *Acta Med. Scand. 176*: 583–593, 1964.

218a. DeGraeff, J., Muller, H., and Moolenaar, A. J.: Phaeochromocytoma. A report of seven cases. *Acta. Med. Scand. 164*: 419–430, 1959.

219. Delaney, J. P.: Management of pheochromocytoma. *Minn. Med. 57*: 553–557, 1974.

220. Delaney, P. V., and Mungall, I. F.: Bilateral malignant pheochromocytomas presenting as massive retroperitoneal hemorrhage. *J. Indian Med. Assoc. 64*: 428–429, 1971.

221. DeLellis, R. A.: Formaldehyde-induced fluorescence technique for the demonstration of biogenic amines in diagnostic histopathology. *Cancer 28*: 1704–1710, 1971.

222. Demole, M., and Rutishauser, E.: Hypertension paroxystique dans un cas de tuberculose d'une surrénale. *Presse Med. 47*: 747–749, 1939.

223. Deoreo, G. A., Jr., Stewart, B. H., Tarazi, R. C., and Gifford, R. W., Jr.: Preoperative blood transfusion in the safe surgical management of pheochromocytoma: A review of 46 cases. *J. Urol. 111*: 715–721, 1974.

224. DeQuattro, V., and Chan, S.: Raised plasma catecholamines in some patients with primary hypertension. *Lancet 1*: 806–809, 1972.

225. DeQuattro, V., Margolin, A. H., and Stocks, L. O.: Pseudopheochromocytoma: Adrenomedullary response to venography. *J. Clin. Endocrinol. Metab. 30*: 138–140, 1970.

226. De Robertis, E., and Vaz Ferreira, A.: Electron microscope study of the excretion of catechol-containing droplets in the adrenal medulla. *Exp. Cell. Res. 12*: 568–574, 1957.

227. Desai, P. B.: Microscopic phaeochromocytoma of the adrenal. *Indian J. Surg. 21*: 1–7, 1959.

228. De Villiers, J. C.: Intracranial haemorrhage in patients treated with monoamineoxidase inhibitors. *Br. J. Psychiatry 112*: 109–118, 1966.

229. De Vries, A., Rachmilewitz, M., and Schumert, M.: Pheochromocytoma with diabetes and hypertension. *Am. J. Med. 6*: 51–59, 1949.

230. Diner, O.: L'Expulsion des granules de la medullosurrenale chez le hamster. *C. R. Acad. Sci., ser. D 265*: 616–619, 1967.

231. Donahower, G., Schumacher, O. P., and Hazard, J. B.: Two cases of medullary thyroid carcinoma causing Cushing's syndrome. *Clin. Res. 14*: 430, 1966 (abstr.).

232. Donath, A., Käser, H., Ross, B., Ziegler, W., Oetliker, O., Colombo, J. P., and Bettex, M.: Le phéochromocytome familial. Discussion de la malignité et du mode héréditaire; à propos d'un cas chez l'enfant à sécrétion particulière. *Helv. Paediat. Acta 20*: 1–18, 1965.

233. Donati, R. M., McCarthy, J. M., Lange, R. D., and Gallagher, N. I.: Erythrocythemia and neoplastic tumors. *Ann. Intern. Med. 58*: 47–55, 1963.

233a. Douglas, H. J., Eger, E. I., II, Biava, C. G., and Renzi, C.: Hepatic necrosis associated with viral infection after enflurane anesthesia. *N. Engl. J. Med. 296*: 553–555, 1977.

234. Douglas, W. W.: Stimulus-secretion coupling: The concept and clues from cromaffin and other cells. *Br. J. Pharmacol. 34*: 451–474, 1968.

235. Douglas, W. W., Kanno, T., and Sampson, S. R.: Effects on acetylcholine and other medullary secretagogues and antagonists on the membrane potential of adrenal chromaffin cells: an analysis employing techniques of tissue culture. *J. Physiol. 188*: 107–120, 1967.

236. Drake, F. R. and Ebaugh, E. G.: Pheochromocytoma and electroconvulsive therapy. *Am. J. Psychiatry 113*: 295–301, 1956.

237. Drill, V. A.: Reactions from the use of Benzodioxane (933F) in the diagnosis of pheochromocytoma. *N. Engl. J. Med. 241*: 777–779, 1949.

238. Drukker, W., Formijne, P., and van der Schoot, J. B.: Hyperplasia of adrenal medulla. *Br. Med. J. 1*: 186–189, 1957.

239. Duke, W. W., Boshell, B. R., Soteres, P., and Carr, J. H.: A norepinephrine-secreting glomus jugulare tumor presenting as a pheochromocytoma. *Ann. Intern. Med. 60*: 1040–1047, 1964.

240. Duke, W. M., Phillips, M. W., Donald, J. M., Jr., and Boshell, B. R.: A norepinephrine-secreting glomic tissue tumor (chemodectoma). *J. Am. Med. Assoc. 193*: 20–22, 1965.

241. Dunn, F. G., De Garvalho, J. G. R., Kern, D. C., Higgins, J. R., and Frohlich, E. D.: Pheochromocytoma crisis induced by saralasin. Relation of angiotensin analogue to catecholamine release. *N. Engl. J. Med. 295*: 605–607, 1976.

242. Durant, J., and Soloff, L. A.: Arrhythmic crisis of phaeochromocytoma. *Lancet 2*: 124–126, 1962.

243. Dury, A.: The effect of epinephrine and insulin on the plasma potassium level. *Endocrinol. 49*: 663–670, 1951.

244. Dustan, H. P., Tarazi, R. C., and Bravo, E. L.: Physiologic Characteristics of Hypertension. *In*: Laragh, J. H., ed., *Hypertension Manual*. New York, Dun-Donnelley, 1974, pp. 232, 233.

245. Dyck, P. J.: Diseases of Nerve Roots, Plexuses and Peripheral Nerves. *In*: Beeson, P. B., and McDermott, W., eds., *Cecil-Loeb Textbook of Medicine*, 13th ed. Phila., London, Toronto, W. B. Saunders, 1971, pp. 333–334.

246. Dyke, P. C., and Mulkey, D. A.: Maturation of ganglioneuroblastoma to ganglioneuroma. *Cancer 20*: 1343–1349, 1967.

E

247. Eade, N. R.: The distribution of the catecholamines in homogenates of the bovine adrenal medulla. *J. Physiol. 141*: 183–192, 1958.

248. Eaton, P., and Steinberg, D.: Effects of medium fatty acid concentration, epinephrine, and glucose on palmitate-1-C^{14} oxidation and incorporation into neutral lipids by skeletal muscle *in vitro*. *J. Lipid Res. 2*: 376–382, 1961.

249. Edis, J. A., Ayala, L. A., and Egdahl, R. H.: *Manual of Endocrine Surgery*. New York, Heidelberg, Berlin, Springer-Verlag, 1975.

250. Edwards, C., Heath, D., and Harris P.: The carotid body in emphysema and left ventricular hypertrophy. *J. Pathol. 104*: 1–13, 1971.

251. Edwards, C., Heath, D., and Harris, P.: Ultrastructure of the carotid body in high-altitude guinea-pigs. *J. Pathol. 107*: 131–136, 1972.

252. Edwards, C., Heath, D., Harris, P., Costillo, Y., Kruger, H., and Arias-Stella, J.: The carotid body in animals at high altitude. *J. Pathol. 104*: 231–238, 1971.

253. Egdahl, R. H.: Surgery of the adrenal gland. *N. Engl. J. Med. 278*: 939–949, 1968.

254. Egdahl, R. H., and Chobanian, A. V.: Acute pheochromocytoma. *Surg. Clin. North Am. 46*: 645–652, 1966.

255. Ehinger, B., Genneser, G., Owman, C., Persson, H., and Sjöberg, N.-O.: Histochemical and pharmacological studies of amine mechanisms in the umbilical cord, umbilical vein and ductus venosus of the human fetus. *Acta Physiol. Scand. 72*: 15–24, 1968.

256. Eisenberg, A. A., and Wallerstein, H.: Pheochromocytoma of the suprarenal medulla (paraganglioma) . *Arch. Pathol. 14*: 818–836, 1932.

257. Ekbom, K.: Prophylactic treatment of cluster headache with a new serotonin antagonist, BC-105. *Acta Neurol. Scand. 45*: 601–610, 1969.

258. Ekbom, K.: *Studies on Cluster Headache.* Stockholm, 1970. Cited in Dalessio, D. J. Wolff's Headache and Other Head Pain. Oxford University Press, New York, 1972.

259. Ellis, F. H., Jr., Dawe, C. J., and Claggett, O. T.: Cysts of the adrenal glands. *Ann. Surg. 136*: 217–227, 1952.

260. El-Minawi, M. F., Paulino, E., Cuesta, M., and Ceballos, J.: Pheochromocytoma masquerading as pre-eclamptic toxemia. *Am. J. Obstet. Gynecol. 109*: 389–395, 1971.

261. Emlet, J. R., Grimson, K. S., Bell, D. M., and Orgain, E. S.: Use of Piperoxan and Regitine as routine tests in patients with hypertension. *J. Am. Med. Assoc. 146*: 1383–1386, 1951.

262. Emmanuel, D. A., Rowe, G. G., Musser, M. J., and Philpot, V. B. Jr.: Prolonged hypotension with fatal termination after a phentolamine (Regitine) methanesulfonate test. *J. Am. Med. Assoc. 161*: 436–439, 1956.

263. Engel, A., and von Euler, U. S.: Diagnostic value of increased urinary output of noradrenaline and adrenaline in pheochromocytoma. *Lancet 2*: 387, 1950.

264. Engel, F. L., Mencher, W. H., and Engel, G. L.: "Epinephrine shock" as a manifestation of pheochromocytoma of the adrenal medulla; Report of a case with successful removal of the tumor. *Am. J. Med. Sci. 204*: 649–661, 1942.

265. Engel, G. L., and Aring, C. D.: Hypothalamic attacks with thalamic lesions. *Arch. Neurol. and Psychiatry 54*: 37–43, 1945.

266. Engelman, K.: Assay of Plasma Catecholamines. An Approach to Evaluating Altered Sympathetic Activity in Essential Hypertension. *In*: Laragh, J. H., ed., *Hypertension Manual.* New York, Dunnelley, Yorke Medical Books, 1974, pp. 605–619.

267. Engelman, K.: Principles in the diagnosis of pheochromocytoma. *Bull. N. Y. Acad. Med. 45*: 851–858, 1969.

268. Engelman, K., and Hammond, W. G.: Adrenaline production by an intrathoracic pheochromocytoma. *Lancet 1*: 609–611, 1968.

269. Engelman, K., Horwitz, D., Jéquier, E., and Sjoerdsma, A.: Biochemical and pharmacologic effects of α-methyltyrosine in man. *J. Clin. Invest. 47*: 577–594, 1968.

270. Engelman, K., Mueller, P. S., and Sjoerdsma, A.: Elevated plasma free fatty acid concentrations in patients with pheochromocytoma: Changes with therapy and correlations with the basal metabolic rate. *N. Eng. J. Med. 270*: 865–870, 1964.

271. Engelman, K., and Portnoy, B.: A sensitive double-isotope derivative assay for norepinephrine and epinephrine. *Circ. Res. 26*: 53–57, 1970.

272. Engelman, K., Portnoy, B., and Lovenberg, W.: A sensitive and specific double-isotope derivative method for the determination of catecholamines in biological specimens. *Am. J. Med. Sci. 255*: 259–268, 1968.

273. Engelman, K., Portnoy, B., and Sjoerdsma, A.: Plasma catecholamine concentrations in patients with hypertension. *Circ. Res. 27 (Suppl. 1)*: 141–146, 1970.

274. Engelman, K., and Sjoerdsma, A.: A new test for pheochromocytoma: pressor responsiveness to tyramine. *J. Am. Med. Assoc. 189*: 81–86, 1964.

275. Engelman, K., and Sjoerdsma, A.: Chronic medical therapy for pheochromocytoma: A report of four cases. *Ann. Intern. Med. 61*: 229–241, 1964.

276. Engelman, K., Zelis, R., Waldmann, T., Mason, D. T., and Sjoerdsma, A. M.: Mechanism of orthostatic hypotension in pheochromocytoma. *Circulation 38 (Suppl. 6)*: VI-72, 1968.

277. Eränko, O.: Cell types in the adrenal medulla. *In*: Vone, J. R., Wolstenholme, G. E. W., and O'Connor, M., eds. *Adrenergic Mechanisms.* Boston, Little, Brown, 1960, pp. 103–108.

278. Eränko, O.: Nodular hyperplasia and increase of noradrenaline content in the adrenal medulla of nicotine-treated rats. *Acta Pathol. Microbiol. Scand. 36*: 210–218, 1955.

279. Eriksen N., Martin, G. M., and Benditt, E. P.: Oxidation of the indole nucleus of 5-hydroxytryptamine and the formation of pigments: isolation and partial characterization of a dimer of 5-hydroxytryptamine. *J. Biol. Chem. 235*: 1662–1667, 1960.

280. Esperson, T., and Dahl-Iversen, E.: The clinical picture and treatment of pheocromocytomas of the suprarenal. *Acta Chir. Scand. 94*: 271–290, 1946.

281. Espersen, T., and Jørgensen, J.: Electrocardiographic changes in paroxysmal hypertension due to chromaffin adrenal tumor. *Acta Med. Scand. 127*: 494–500, 1947.

282. Etsten, B. E., and Shimosato, S.: Halothane anesthesia and catecholamine levels in a patient with pheochromocytoma. *Anesthesiology 26*: 688–691, 1965.

283. Euler, C. von, Euler, U. S. von, and Floding, I.: Biologically inactive catechol derivatives in urine. *Acta Physiol. Scand. 33 (Suppl. 118)*: 32, 1955.

283a. Euler, U. S., von: Adrenal medullary and other chromaffin cell tumours. *Ciba Found. Coll. on Endocrinol. 12*: 268–277, 1958.

284. Euler, U. S. von.: III. Epinephrine and norepinephrine: Adrenaline and noradrenaline. Distribution and action. *Pharmacol. Rev. 6*: 15–22, 1954.

285. Euler, U. S. von: Increased urinary excretion of noradrenaline and adrenaline in cases of pheochromocytoma. *Ann. Surg. 134*: 929–933, 1951.

286. Euler, U. S. von: *Noradrenaline.* Springfield, Ill., C. C. Thomas, 1956, 382 pp.

287. Euler, U. S. von: Presence of a substance with sympathin E properties in spleen extracts. *Acta Physiol. Scand. 11*: 168–186, 1946.

288. Euler, U. S. von: The presence of a sympathomimetic substance in extracts of mammalian heart. *J. Physiol. 105*: 38–44, 1946.

289. Euler, U. S. von, and Floding, I.: A fluorimetric micromethod for differential estimation of adrenaline and noradrenaline. *Acta Physiol. Scand. 33 (Suppl. 118)* : 45–56, 1955.

290. Euler, U. S. von, and Floding, J.: Diagnosis of phaeochromocytoma by fluorimetric estimation of adrenaline and noradrenaline in urine. *Scand. J. Clin. Lab. Invest. 8*: 288–295, 1956.

291. Euler, U. S. von, Floding, I., and Lishajko, F.: The presence of free and conjugated 3,4: dihydroxyphenylacetic acid (dopac) in urine and blood plasma. *Acta Soc. Med. Ups. 64*: 217–225, 1959.

292. Euler, U. S. von, Franksson, C., and Hellström, J.: Adrenaline and noradrenaline content of surgically removed human suprarenal glands. *Acta Physiol. Scand. 31*: 6–8, 1954.

293. Euler, U. S. von, Franksson, C., and Hellström, J.: Adrenaline and noradrenaline output in urine after unilateral and bilateral adrenalectomy in man. *Acta Physiol. Scand. 31*: 1–5, 1954.

294. Euler, U. S. von, Germzell, C. A., Ström, G., and Westman, A.: Report of a case of pheochromocytoma, with special regard to preoperative diagnostic problems. *Acta Med. Scand. 153*: 127–136, 1955.

295. Euler, U. S. von, and Hellner, S.: Excretion of noradrenaline, adrenaline and hydroxytyramine in urine. *Acta Physiol. Scand. 22*: 161–167, 1951.

296. Euler, U. S. von, Ikkos, D., and Luft, R.: Adrenaline excretion during resting conditions and after insulin in adrenalectomized human subjects. *Acta Endocrinol. 38*: 441–448, 1961.

297. Euler U. S. von, and Lishajko, F.: Improved technique for the fluorimetric estimation of catecholamines. *Acta Physiol. Scand. 51*: 348–355, 1961.

298. Euler, U. S. von, Lund, A., Olsson, A., and Sandblom, P. H.: Noradrenaline and adrenaline in blood and urine in a case of pheochromocytoma. *Scand. J. Clin. Lab. Invest. 5*: 122–128, 1953.

299. Euler, U. S. von, and Ström, G.: Present status of diagnosis and treatment of pheochromocytoma. *Circulation 15*: 5–13, 1957.

300. Eusebi, V., and Massarelli, G.: Phaeochromocytoma of the spermatic cord: Report of case. *J. Pathol. 105*: 283–284, 1971.

301. Evans, C. H., Westfall, V., and Atuk, N. O.: Astrocytoma mimicking the features of pheochromocytoma. *N. Eng. J. Med. 286*: 1397–1399, 1972.

302. Evans, R. W.: *Histological Appearance of Tumours: With a Consideration of Their Histogenesis and Certain Aspects of Their Clinical Features and Behaviour,* 2nd ed. Baltimore, Williams and Wilkins, 1966, 1255 pp.

303. Evans, W. F., and Stewart, H. J.: The peripheral blood flow in a case of adrenal pheochromocytoma before and after operation. *Am. Heart J. 24*: 835–842, 1942.

304. Evans, W. H., and Mueller, P. S.: Effects of palmitate on the metabolism of leukocytes from guinea pig exudate. *J. Lipid Res. 4*: 39–45, 1963.

305. Evarts, E. V., Gillespie, L., Fleming, T. C., and Sjoerdsma, A.: Relative lack of pharmacologic action of 3-methoxy analogue of norepinephrine. *Proc. Soc. Exp. Biol. N. Y. 98*: 74–76, 1958.

F

306. Faivre, G., Sommelet, J., Gilgenkrantz, J. M., Cherrier, F., and Masse, G.: Topographical diagnosis of a pheochromocytoma by determination of catecholamines at various levels of the venacaval system. *Bull. Soc. Med. Hop. (Paris) 113*: 129–137, 1962.

307. Falck, B., Ljungberg, O., and Rosengren, E.: On the occurrence of monoamines and related substances in familial medullary thyroid carcinoma with pheochromocytoma. *Acta Pathol. Microbiol. Scand. 74*: 1–10, 1968.

308. Fanning, G. L., Dykes, M. H. M., and May, A. G.: Anaesthetic management of pheochromocytoma: A case report. *Can. Anaesth. Soc. J. 17*: 261–268, 1970.

309. Farley, S. E., and Smith, C. L.: Unusual location of pheochromocytoma in the urinary bladder. *J. Urol. 81*: 130–132, 1959.

310. Farquhar, J. W.: Phaeochromocytoma in childhood; case report and a brief review of 56 others recorded in the literature. *J. R. Coll. Surg. Edinburg. 3*: 300–310, 1958.

311. Feist, J. H. and Lasser, E. C.: Pheochromocytoma with large cystic calcification and associated sphenoid ridge malformation. *Radiology 76*: 21–26, 1961.

312. Ferris, T. F., Toxemia of Pregnancy. *In:* Beeson, P. B., and McDermott, W., eds., *Cecil-Loeb Textbook of Medicine,* 13th edition. Phila., London, Toronto, W. B. Saunders, 1971, pp. 1199–1200.

313. Finegold, M. J., and Haddad, J. R.: Multiple endocrine tumors. *Arch. Pathol. 76*: 449–455, 1963.

314. Fink, G. D., and Fisher, J. W.: The role of the adrenergic nervous system in erythropoietin production. *Fed. Proc. 33*: 544, 1974 (Abstr. 1879) .

315. Fischer, J. A., Blum, J. W., and Binswanger, U.: Acute parathyroid hormone response to epinephrine in vivo *J. Clin. Invest. 52*: 2434–2440, 1973.

316. Fleisher, D. S., Voci, G., Cresson, S. L., and Karafin, L.: Preoperative localization of pheochromocytoma. *J. Pediat. 64*: 711–715, 1964.

317. Fletcher, J. R.: Medullary (solid) carcinoma of the thyroid gland. *Arch. Surg. 100*: 257–262, 1960.

318. Flink, E. B.: Heavy Metal Poisoning: Lead Poisoning. *In:* Beeson, P. B., and McDermott, W., eds.,

Cecil-Loeb Textbook of Medicine, 13th ed. Philadelphia, London, Toronto, W. B. Saunders, 1971, pp. 63–66.

319. Flint, L. D.: A urologist's experience with 17 cases of pheochromocytoma. *J. Urol. 90:* 491–499, 1963.

320. Flint, L. D., and Bartels, C. C.: Ten years' experience with 15 operated cases of pheochromocytoma. *Surg. Clin. North Am. 42:* 721–732, 1962.

321. Folkow, B.: The haemodynamic consequences of adaptive structural changes of the resistance vessels in hypertension. *Clin. Sci. Mol. Med. 41:* 1–12, 1971.

322. Forde, T. P., Yormak, S. S., and Killip, T. III: Reflex bradycardia and nodal escape rhythm in pheochromocytoma. *Am. Heart J. 76:* 388–392, 1968.

323. Foster, G. V.: Calcitonin (thyrocalcitonin). *N. Engl. J. Med. 279:* 349–360, 1968.

324. Fox, L. P., Grandi, J., Johnson, A. H., Watrous, W. G., and Johnson, M. J.: Pheochromocytoma associated with pregnancy. *Am. J. Obstet. Gynec. 104:* 288–295, 1969.

325. Frankel, F.: Ein Fall von doppelseitigem, völlig latent verlaufenen Nebennierentumor und gleichzeitiger Nephritis mit Veränderungen am Circulationsapparat und Retinitis. *Virchows Arch. Pathol. Anat. Physiol. 103:* 244–263, 1886

326. Fred, H. L., Allred, D. P., Garber, H. E., Retiene, and Lipscomb, H.: Pheochromocytoma masquerading as overwhelming infection. *Am. Heart J. 73:* 149–154, 1967.

327. Freeman, N. E., Freedman, H. and Miller, C. C.: The production of shock by the prolonged continuous injection of adrenalin in unanesthetized dogs. *Am. J. Physiol. 131:* 545–553, 1941.

328. Freiha, F. S., Kavaney, P. B. Cunningham, J. J., Fajardo, L. F., and Castellino, R. A.: Extra-adrenal pheochromocytoma causing renal artery stenosis. *Urology 2:* 303–307, 1973.

329. French, C., and Campagna, F. A.: Pheochromocytoma with shock, marked leukocytosis, and unusual electrocardiograms. Case report and review of the literature. *Ann. Intern. Med. 55:* 127–134, 1961.

330. Friedberg, R.: Pheochromocytoma and adrenocortical function. *Danish Med. Bull. 3:* 213–216, 1956.

331. Friedman, M., Rosenman, R. H., and Carroll, V.: Changes in the serum cholesterol and blood clotting time in men subjected to cyclic variation of occupational stress. *Circulation 17:* 852–861, 1958.

332. Fries, J. G., and Chamberlin, J. A.: Extra-adrenal pheochromocytoma: Literature review and report of a cervical pheochromocytoma. *Surgery 63:* 268–279, 1968.

333. Fritz, I. and Levine, R.: Action of adrenal cortical steroids and norepinephrine on vascular responses of stress in adrenalectomized rats. *Am. J. Physiol. 165:* 456–465, 1951.

334. Frohlich, E. D., Dustan, H. P., and Page I. H.: Hyperdynamic beta-adrenergic circulatory state. *Arch. Intern. Med. 117:* 614–619, 1966.

335. Frohlich, E. D., Tarazi, R. C., and Dustan, H. P.: Hyperdynamic beta-adrenergic circulatory state. *Arch. Intern. Med. 123:* 1–7, 1969.

336. Fry, I. K., Kerr, I. H., Thomas, M. L., and Starer, F.: Value of aortography in diagnosis of pheochromocytoma. *Clin. Radiol. 18:* 276–281, 1967.

337. Furchgott, R. F.: The classification of adrenoceptors (adrenergic receptors). An evaluation from the standpoint of receptor theory. *In:* Blaschko, H., and Muscholl, E., eds., *Catecholamines.* Berlin, Heidelberg, New York, Springer-Verlag, 1972. pp. 283–335.

338. Futterweit, W., Allen, L., and Moser, M.: Pheochromocytoma with radioactive iodine uptake and electrocardiographic abnormalities. *Metabolism 11:* 589–599, 1962.

G

339. Gabriel, R., and Harrison, B. D. W.: Meningioma mimicking features of a phaeochromocytoma. *Br. Med. J. 2:* 312, 1974.

340. Gagel, R. F., Melvin, K. E. W., Tashjian, A. J. Jr., Miller, H. H., Feldman, Z. T., Wolfe, H. J., DeLellis, R. A., Cervi-Skinner, S., and Reichlin, S.: Natural history of the familial medullary thyroid carcinoma-pheochromocytoma syndrome and the identification of preneoplastic states by screening studies: A five year report. *Trans Assoc. Am. Physicians 88:* 177–191, 1975.

341. Ganem, E. J., and Cahill, G. F.: Pheochromocytomas coexisting in adrenal gland and retroperitoneal space, with sustained hypertension. *N. Engl. J. Med. 238:* 692–697, 1948.

342. Geffen, L. B., Rush, R. A., Louis, W. J., and Doyle, A. E.: Plasma catecholamine and dopamine-β-hydroxylase amounts in phaeochromocytoma. *Clin. Sci. 44:* 421–424, 1973.

343. Geffen, L. B., Rush, R. A., Louis, W. J., and Doyle, A. E.: Plasma dopamine-β-hydroxylase and noradrenaline amounts in essential hypertension. *Clin. Sci. 44:* 617–620, 1973.

344. Gelfman, N. A., Landau, S. J., Mulrow, P. J., Friedewald, T. W., and Dalessio, D. J.: Unresectable pheochromocytoma: Response to α-methyldihydroxy-L-phenylalanine. *J. Chronic Dis. 16:* 217–222, 1963.

345. Gélinas, R., Pellerin, J., and D'Iorio, A.: Biochemical observations of a chromaffin tumour. *Rev. Can. Biol. 16:* 445–450, 1957.

346. Gemmell, A. A.: Phaeochromocytoma and the obstetrician. *J. Obstet. Gynaecol. Br. Commonw. 62:* 195–202, 1955.

347. Gendel, B. R., and Ende, M.: Pheochromocytoma: report of an unusual case with gastro-intestinal bleeding. *Gastroenterology 19:* 344–348, 1951.

348. German, W. J., and Flanigan, S.: Pituitary adenomas, a follow-up study of the Cushing series. *Clin. Neurosurg. 10:* 72–81, 1964.

349. Gersack, J. R., and Riba, L. W.: Pheochromocytoma and ureteral obstruction. *J. Am. Med. Assoc. 189:* 60–61, 1964.

350. Gerst, E. C., Steinsland, O. S., and Wolcott, W. W.: Use of constant temperature and sodium borohydride in the trihydroxyindole method for catecholamines. *Clin. Chem. 12:* 659–669, 1966.

351. Gifford, R. W., Jr.: Hypertensive emergencies and their treatment. *Med. Clin. North Am. 45:* 441–452, 1961.

352. Gifford, R. W., Jr., Kvale, W. F., Maher, F. T. Roth, G. M., and Priestley, J. T.: Clinical features, diagnosis and treatment of pheochromocytoma: a review of 76 cases. *Mayo Clin. Proc. 39*: 281–302, 1964.

353. Gifford, R. W. Jr., Roth, G. M., and Kvale, W. F.: Evaluation of new adrenolytic drug (Regitine) as test for pheochromocytoma. *J. Am. Med. Assoc. 149*: 1628–1634, 1952.

354. Gifford, R. W., Jr., and Tweed, D. C.: Spurious elevation of urinary catecholamines during therapy with alpha-methyldopa: A diagnostic pitfall. *J. Am. Med. Assoc. 182*: 493–495, 1962.

355. Gilliland, I. C. and Daniel, O.: Phaeochromocytoma presenting as an abdominal emergency. *Br. Med. J. 2*: 275–277, 1951.

356. Gillman, J., Gilbert, C., and Spence, I.: Phaeochromocytoma in the rat: Pathogenesis and collateral reactions and its relation to comparable tumours in man. *Cancer 6*: 494–511, 1953.

356a. Giroux, L., Delorme, F., and Bettez, P.: Syndrome des névromes muqueux multiples. *Union Med. Can. 104*: 605–610, 1975.

357. Gitlow, S. E.: Catecholamines and the circulatory system: summary of discussion and commentary. *Pharmacol. Rev. 18*: 707–711, 1966.

358. Gitlow, S. E., Mendlowitz, M., and Bertani, L. M.: The biochemical techniques for detecting and establishing the presence of a pheochromocytoma. A review of ten years' experience. *Am. J. Cardiol. 26*: 270–279, 1970.

359. Gitlow, S. E., Mendlowitz, M., Khassis, S., Cohen, G., and Sha, J.: The diagnosis of pheochromocytoma by determination of urinary 3-methoxy-4-hydroxymandelic acid. *J. Clin. Invest. 39*: 221–226, 1960.

360. Gitlow, S. E., Mendlowitz, M., Kruk, E., and Khassis, S.: Diagnosis of pheochromocytoma by assay of catecholamine metabolites. *Circ. Res. 9*: 746–754, 1961.

361. Gitlow, S. E., Mendlowitz, M., Wilk, E. K., Wilk, S., Wolf, R. L., and Bertani, L. M.: Excretion of catecholamine metabolites by normal children. *J. Lab. Clin. Med. 72*: 612–620, 1968.

362. Gitlow, S. E., Mendlowitz, M., and Wolf, R. W.: The diagnosis of pheochromocytoma. *J. Mt. Sinai Hosp. (N. Y.) 28*: 159–179, 1961.

363. Gitlow, S. E., Ornstein, L., Mendlowitz, M., Khassis, S., and Kruk, E.: A simple colorimetric urine test for pheochromocytoma. *Am. J. Med. 28*: 921–926, 1960.

364. Gitlow, S. E., Pertsemlidis, D., and Bertani, L. M.: Management of patients with pheochromocytoma. *Am. Heart J. 82*: 557–567, 1971.

365. Gjessing, L. R.: Studies of functional neural tumors. VI. Biochemical diagnosis. *Scand. J. Clin. Lab. Invest. 16*: 661–669, 1964.

366. Gjøl, N., Dybkaer, R., and Funder, J.: Shock in phaeochromocytoma treated with noradrenaline. *Br. Med. J. 2*: 673–675, 1957.

367. Glenn, F.: Surgical treatment of chromaffin tumors. *Am. Surg. 37*: 6–11, 1971.

368. Glenner, G. G., Crout, J. R., and Roberts, W. C.: A functional carotid-body-like tumor secreting levarterenol. *Arch. Pathol. 73*: 230–240, 1962.

369. Glenner, G. G., Crout, J. R., and Roberts, W. C.: A noradrenaline-secreting carotid-body-like tumor. *Lancet 2*: 439, 1961.

370. Glenner, G. G., and Grimley, P. M.: Tumors of the extraadrenal paraganglion system (including chemoreceptors). *In: Atlas of Tumor Pathology*, 2nd series, fascicle 9. Washington, D.C., Armed Forces Institute of Pathology, 1974, 90 pp.

371. Glushien, A. S., Mansuy, M., and Littman, D. S.: Pheochromocytoma: Its relationship to the neurocutaneous syndromes. *Am. J. Med. 14*: 318–327, 1953.

372. Gold, R. E., Wisinger, B. M., Geraci, A. R., and Heinz, L. M.: Hypertensive crisis as a result of adrenal venography in a patient wtih pheochromocytoma. *Radiology 102*: 579–580, 1972.

373. Goldberg, H. C., and Marsden, C. A.: Catechol-O-methyl transferase: Pharmacological aspects and physiological role. *Pharmacol. Rev. 27*: 135–206, 1975.

374. Goldberg, L. I.: Dopamine—clinical uses of an endogenous catecholamine. *N. Engl. J. Med. 291*: 707–710, 1974.

375. Goldenberg, M.: Adrenal medullary function. *Am. J. Med. 10*: 627–641, 1951.

376. Goldenberg, M., and Aranow, H., Jr.: Diagnosis of pheochromocytoma by the adrenergic blocking action of benzodioxan. *J. Am. Med. Assoc. 143*: 1139–1143, 1950.

377. Goldenberg, M., Aranow, H., Jr., Smith, A. A., and Faber, M.: Pheochromocytoma and essential hypertensive vascular disease. *Arch. Intern. Med. 86*: 823–836, 1950.

378. Goldenberg, M., Pines, K. L., Baldwin, E. DeF., Green, D. G., and Roh, C. E.: The hemodynamic response of man to norepinephrine and epinephrine and its relation to the problem of hypertension. *Am. J. Med. 5*: 792–800, 1948.

379. Goldenberg, M., and Rapport, M. M.: Norepinephrine and epinephrine in human urine (Addison's disease, essential hypertension, pheochromocytoma). *J. Clin. Invest. 30*: 641–642, 1951.

380. Goldenberg, M., Serlin, I., Edwards, T., and Rapport, M. M.: Chemical screening methods for the diagnosis of pheochromocytoma. I. norepinephrine and epinephrine in human urine. *Am. J. Med. 16*: 310–327, 1954.

381. Goldenberg, M., Snyder, C. H., and Aranow, H., Jr.: New test for hypertension due to circulating epinephrine. *J. Am. Med. Assoc. 135*: 971–976, 1947.

382. Goldfien, A.: Pheochromocytoma: Diagnosis and anesthetic and surgical management. *Anesthesiology 24*: 462–471, 1963.

382a. Goldfien, A., Zileli, S., Goodman, D., and Thorn, G. W.: The estimation of epinephrine and norepinephrine in human plasma. *J. Clin. Endocrinol. Metab. 21*: 281–295, 1961.

383. Goldstein, M., Prochoroff, N., and Sirlin, S.: A radioassay for dopamine-β-hydroxylase activity. *Experientia 21*: 592–593, 1965.

384. Goldzieher, J. W., McMahon, H. E., and Goldzieher, M. A.: Coarctation of the abdominal aorta simulating pheochromocytoma. *Arch. Intern. Med. 88*: 835–839, 1951.

385. Goodall, McC., and Stone, C.: Adrenaline and

noradrenaline producing tumors of the adrenal medulla and sympathetic nerves. *Ann. Surg. 151*: 391–398, 1960.

386. Goodman, L. S., and Gilman, A.: *The Pharmalogical Basis of Therapeutics, 5th edition.* Goodman L. S., and Gilman, A., eds., New York, Macmillan, 1975, 1704 pp.

387. Gordon, A. S., and Zanjani. E. D.: The renal erythropoietic factor (erythrogenin) and erythropoietin (ESF). *In:* Stohlman, F., Jr., ed., *Hemopoietic Cellular Proliferation.* New York, Grune and Stratton, 1970, pp. 97–111.

388. Gordon, R. D., Küchel, O., Liddle, G. W., and Island, D. P.: Role of the sympathetic nervous system in regulating renin and aldosterone production in man. *J. Clin. Invest. 46*: 599–605, 1967.

389. Gordon, R. S., Jr., and Cherkes, A.: Unesterified fatty acid in human blood plasma. *J. Clin. Invest. 35*: 206–212, 1956.

390. Gorlin, R. J., and Mirkin, B. L.: Multiple mucosal neuromas, pheochromocytoma, medullary carcinoma of the thyroid and marfanoid body build with muscular wasting. Syndrome of hyperplasia and neoplasia of neural crest derivatives—an unitarian concept. *Z. Kinderheilkd 113*: 313–325, 1972.

390a. Gorlin, R. J., Sedano, H. O., Vickers, R. A., and Červenka, J.: Multiple mucosal neuromas, pheochromocytoma and medullary carcinoma of the thyroid—a syndrome. *Cancer 22*: 293–299, 1968.

391. Gould, J., and Mundal, A. L.: Multifocal ventricular tachycardia induced by Etamon in a case of pheochromocytoma. *Am. Heart J. 42*: 460–466, 1951.

392. Graham, J. B.: Pheochromocytoma and hypertension. An analysis of 207 cases. *Int. Abstr. Surg. 92*: 105–121, 1951.

392a. Gray, T. K., Bieberdorf, F. A., and Fordtran, J. S.: Thyrocalcitonin and the jejunal absorption of calcium, water, and electrolytes in normal subjects. *J. Clin. Invest. 52*: 3084–3088, 1973.

393. Green, D. M.: Pheochromocytoma and chronic hypertension *J. Am. Med. Assoc. 131*: 1260–1265, 1946.

394. Green, D. M., Johnson, A. D., Lobb, A., and Cusick, G.: The effects of adrenalin in normal and hypertensive patients in relation to the mechanism of sustained pressure elevations. *Lab. Clin. Med. 33*: 332–346, 1948.

395. Green, D. M., and Peterson, E. M.: Hypertensive encephalopathy after administration of Benzodioxan. *J. Am. Med. Assoc. 142*: 408–409, 1950.

396. Greenberg, R. E., and Gardner, L. I.: Catecholamine metabolism in a functional neural tumour. *J. Clin. Invest. 39*: 1729–1736, 1960.

397. Greenberg, R., Rosenthal, I., and Falk, G. S.: Electron microscopy of human tumors secreting catecholamines: Correlation with biochemical data. *J. Neuropathol. Exp. Neurol. 28*: 475–500, 1969.

398. Greenblatt, D. J., Ransil, B. J., Harmatz, J. S., Smith, T. W., Duhme, D. W., and Koch-Weser, J.: Variability of 24-hour urinary creatinine excretion by normal subjects. *J. Clin. Pharmacol. 16*: 321–328, 1976.

398a. Greenhouse, A.: Pheochromocytoma and menin-

gioma of the foramen magnum. *Ann. Intern. Med. 55*: 124–127, 1961.

399. Greer, M., Anton, A. H., and Williams, C. M. Echevarria, R. A.: Tumours of neural crest origin. *Arch. Neurol. 13*: 139–148, 1965.

400. Greer, W. E. R., Robertson, C. W., and Smithwick, R. H.: Pheochromocytoma—diagnosis, operative experience and clinical results. *Am. J. Surg. 107*: 192–201, 1964.

401. Griffin, W. O., Dilts, P. V., and Roddick, J. W.: Non-obstetric surgery during pregnancy. *In: Current Problems in Surgery.* Chicago, Year Book Medical Publishers, 1969, pp. 1–56.

402. Griffith, M. I., Felts, J. H., James, F. M., Meyers, R. T., Shealy, G. M., and Woodruff, L. F., Jr.: Successful control of pheochromocytoma in pregnancy. *J. Am. Med. Assoc. 229*: 437–439, 1974.

403. Grimley, P. M., and Glenner, G. G.: Histology and ultrastructure of carotid body paragangliomas. Comparison with the normal gland. *Cancer 20*: 1473–1488, 1967.

404. Grimson, K. S., Longino, F. H., Kernodle, C. E., and O'Rear, H. B.: Treatment of patient with pheochromocytoma: Use of adrenolytic drug before and during operation. *J. Am. Med. Assoc. 140*: 1273–1274, 1949.

405. Guazzi, M., Boccelli, G., and Zanchetti, A.: Carotid body chemoreceptors: Physiological role in buffering fall in blood pressure during sleep. *Science 153*: 206–208, 1966.

406. Gupta, K. K.: Phaeochromocytoma and myocardial infarction. *Lancet 1*: 281–282, 1975.

H

407. Habermann, E. T., Millheiser, P. J., and Castin, D. F.: Pheochromocytoma in the organ of Zuckerkandl presenting with gastro-intestinal symptoms. *J. Clin. Endocrinol. Metab. 24*: 334–338, 1964.

408. Hagen, K. O. von, and Barrows, H. S.: Familial pheochromocytoma with ependymoma of the spinal cord: Case report and review of the literature. *J. Neurosurg. 20*: 600–604, 1963.

409. Haimovici, H.: Evidence for an adrenergic component in the nervous mechanism of sweating in man. *Proc. Soc. Exp. Biol. Med. 68*: 40–41, 1948.

410. Halpern, M., and Currarino, G.: Vascular lesions causing hypertension in neurofibromatosis. *N. Engl. J. Med. 273*: 248–252, 1965.

411. Halvorsen, S.: The central nervous system in regulation of erythropoiesis. *Acta Haematol. 35*: 65–79, 1966.

412. Hamberger, C.-A., Hamberger, C. R., Wersäll, J., and Wågermark, J.: Malignant catecholamine-producing tumour of the carotid body. *Acta Pathol. Microbial. Scand. 69*: 489–492, 1967.

413. Hamberger, C. A., Ritzen, M., and Wersäll, J.: Demonstration of catecholamines and 5-hydroxytryptamine in the human carotid body. *J. Pharmacol. Exp. Ther. 152*: 197–201, 1966.

414. Hamilton, B. P. M., Landsberg, L., Levine, R. J., and Tashjian, A. H., Jr.: Sipple's syndrome: Results of screening a large family. *Clin. Res. 21*: 979, 1973 (Abstr.).

415. Hamilton, J. E.: Pheochromocytoma of the adrenal

with paroxysmal hypertension: a case relieved by surgery. *K. Med. J. 38*: 572–575, 1940.

416. Hamilton, M., Litchfield, J. W., Peart, W. S., and Sowry, G. S. C.: Phaeochromocytoma. *Br. Heart J. 15*: 241–249, 1953.

417. Hamrin, B.: Sustained hypotension and shock due to an adrenaline-secreting phaeochromocytoma. *Lancet 2*: 123–124, 1962.

418. Hansson, L., Hunyor, S. N., Julius, S., and Hoobler, S. W.: Blood pressure crisis following withdrawal of clonidine (Catapres, Catapresan), with special reference to arterial and urinary catecholamine levels, and suggestions for acute management. *Am. Heart J. 85*: 605–610, 1973.

419. Harbitz. F.: Tumors of the sympathetic nervous system and the medulla of the adrenal glands, especially malignant neuroblastoma. *Arch. Intern. Med. 16*: 312–328, 1915.

420. Harkin, J. C., and Reed, R. J.: Tumors of the peripheral nervous system: *In*: *Atlas of Tumor Pathology*, 2nd series, fascicle 3. Washington, D.C., Armed Forces Institute of Pathology, 1969. 174 pp.

421. Harrison, T. S., Bartlett, J. D., Jr., and Seaton, J. F.: Current evaluation and management of pheochromocytoma. *Ann. Surg. 168*: 701–713, 1968.

422. Harrison, T. S., Birbari, A., and Seaton, J. F.: Malignant hypertension in pheochromocytoma: Correlation with plasma renin activity. *Johns Hopkins Med. J. 130*: 329–332, 1972.

423. Harrison, T. S., and Freier, D. T.: Pitfalls in the technique and interpretation of regional venous sampling for localizing pheochromocytoma. *Surg. Clinics N. Am. 54*: 339–347, 1974.

424. Harrison, T. S., Seaton, J. F., Cerny, J. C. Brookstein, J. J., and Bartlett, J. D., Jr.: Localization of pheochromocytoma by caval catheterization. *Arch. Surg. 95*: 339–343, 1967.

425. Hatfield, P. M., James, A. E., and Schulz, M. D.: Chemodectomas of the glomus jugulare. *Cancer 30*: 1164–1168, 1972.

426. Haug, W. A., and Baker, H. W.: Malignant paraganglioma of the organ of Zuckerandl. *Arch. Pathol. 62*: 335–339, 1956.

427. Haverback, B. J., Stubrin, M. I., and Majcher, S. J.: Serotonin and related substances: *In*: Dowling, H. F., ed., *Disease-a-Month*. Chicago, Year Book Medical Publishers, April, 1966. 40 pp.

428. Hazard, J. B., Hawk, W. A., and Crile, G., Jr.: Medullary (solid) carcinoma of the thyroid, a clinicopathologic entity. *J. Clin. Endocrinol. 19*: 152–161, 1959.

429. Heath, D., Edwards, C., and Harris, P.: Post-mortem size and structure of the human carotid body. *Thorax 25*: 129–140, 1970.

430. Hecht, H. H., Crandall, R., and Samuels, A. J.: Adrenergic blockade in man by a new imidazole derivative C-7337. *Fed. Proc. 9*: 283–284, 1950.

431. Hegglin, R., and Holzmann, M.: Elektrokardiographische Befunde beim Paragangliom der Nebenniere. *Deut. Arch. Klin. Med. 180*: 681–691, 1937.

432.. Helly, C.: Zur pathologie der Nebenniere. *Münch. Med. Wochenschr. 60*: 1811–1812, 1913.

433. Helson, L., Fleisher, M., Bethune, V., Murphy, M. L. Schwartz, M. K.: Urinary cystathionine, catecholamine, and metabolites in patients with neuroblastoma. *Clin. Chem. 18*: 613–615, 1972.

434. Hendee, A. E., Martin, R. D., and Waters, W. C.: Hypertension in pregnancy: toxemia or pheochromocytoma? *Am. J. Obstet. Gynecol. 105*: 64–72, 1969.

435. Hennessy, T. G., Stern, W. E., and Herrick, S. E.: Cerebellar hemangioblastoma: erythropoietic activity by radioiron assay. *J. Nucl. Med. 8*: 601–606, 1967.

436. Henry, M. U.: A case of phaeochromocytoma without hypertension. *Br. Med. J. 2*: 344, 1954.

437. Hermann, H., and Mornex, R.: Human Tumours Secreting Catecholamines: Clinical and Physiopathological Study of the Pheochromocytomas. Oxford, New York, Pergamon Press, 1964, 207 pp.

438. Hervonen, A.: Development of catecholamine-storing cells in human fetal paraganglia and adrenal medulla: A histochemical and electron microscopical study. *Acta Physiol. Scand. (Suppl.) 368*: 94, 1971.

439. Heymans, C., and Neil, E.: *Reflexogenic Areas of the Cardiovascular System*. Boston, Little, Brown, 1958.

440. Higgins, P. McR., and Tresidder, G. C.: Phaeochromocytoma of the urinary bladder. *Br. Med. J. 2*: 274–277, 1966.

441. Hill, C. S., Ibanez, M. L., Samaan, N. A., Ahern, M. J., and Clark, R. L.: Medullary (solid) carcinoma of the thyroid gland: an analysis of the M. D. Anderson Hospital experience with patients with the tumor, its special features, and its histogenesis. *Medicine 52*: 141–171, 1973.

442. Hillarp, N.-Å.: Some problems concerning the storage of catechol amines in the adrenal medulla. *In*: Wolstenholme, G. E. W., and O'Connor, M. P., eds., *Ciba Foundation Symposium on Adrenergic Mechanisms*. Boston, Little, Brown, 1960, pp. 481–501.

443. Hillarp, N.-Å.: The construction and functional organization of the autonomic innervation. *Acta Physiol. Scand. 46 (Suppl.)*: 157, 1959.

444. Hillarp, N.-Å., and Hökfelt, B.: Evidence of adrenaline and noradrenaline in separate adrenal medullary cells. *Acta Physiol. Scand. 30*: 55–68, 1953.

445. Hillarp, N.-Å., Hökfelt, B., and Nelson, B.: The cytology of the adrenal medullary cells with special reference to the storage and secretion of the sympathomimetic amines. *Acta Anat. 21*: 155–167, 1954.

446. Hillarp, N.-Å., Lindqvist, M., and Vendsalu, A.: Catecholamines and nucleotides in pheochromocytoma. *Exp. Cell. Res. 22*: 40–44, 1961.

446a. Himms-Hagen, J.: Effects of catecholamines on metabolism. *In*: Blaschko, H., and Muscholl, E., eds., *Catecholamines*. Berlin, Heidelberg, New York, Springer-Verlag, 1972, Chap. 11, pp. 363–462.

446b. Hiner, L. B., Gruskin, A. B., Baluarte, H. J., Cote, M. L., Sapire, D. W., and Levitsky, D.: Plasma renin activity and intrarenal blood flow distribution in a child with a pheochromocytoma. *J. Pediatr. 89*: 950–952, 1976.

447. Hines, E. A., Jr., and Brown, G. E.: Cold pressor test for measuring reactability of the blood pressure. *Am. Heart J. 11*: 1–9, 1936.

448. Hingerty, D., and O'Boyle, A.: *Clinical Chemistry*

of the Adrenal Medulla. Kugelmass, I. N., ed., Springfield, C. C. Thomas, 1972, 124 pp.

449. Hinterberger, H., and Bartholomew, R. J.: Catecholamines and their acidic metabolites in urine and in tumour tissue in neuroblastoma, ganglioneuroma, and pheochromocytoma. *Clin. Chim. Acta 23:* 169–175, 1969.

450. Hirschman, S. Z., Feingold, M., and Boylen, G.: Mercury in house paint as a cause of acrodynia. Effect of therapy with N-acetyl-D-L-penicillamine. *N. Engl. J. Med. 269:* 889–893, 1963.

451. Hoeldtke, R. D., and Martin, W. R.: Urine volume and catecholamine excretion. *J. Lab. Clin. Med. 75:* 166–174, 1970.

452. Hökfelt, B.: Noradrenaline and adrenaline in mammalian tissues; distribution under normal and pathological conditions with special reference to the endocrine system. *Acta Physiol. Scand. (Supp. 92) 25:* 1–134, 1951.

453. Hollenhorst, R. W.: The ocular changes associated with pheochromocytoma. *Am. J. Med. Sci. 216:* 226–233, 1948.

454. Hollinshead, W. H. Anatomy of the endocrine glands. *Surg. Clin. North Am. 32:* 1115–1140, 1952.

454a. Hollister, L. E. and Moore, F.: Factors affecting excretion of catecholamines in man: Urine flow, urine pH, and creatinine clearance. *Res. Commun. Chem. Pathol. Pharmacol. 1:* 193–202, 1970.

455. Holsti, L. R.: Malignant extra-adrenal phaeochromocytoma. *Br. J. Radiol. 37:* 944–947, 1964.

456. Holton, P.: Noradrenaline in tumors of the adrenal medulla. *J. Physiol. 108:* 525–529, 1949.

457. Holtz, P., Credner, K., and Koepp, W.: Die enzymatische Entstehung von Oxytyramin im Organismus und die physiologische Bedeutung der Dopadecarboxylase. *Arch. Exp. Pathol. Pharmak. 200:* 356–388, 1942.

458. Holtz, P., Credner, K., and Kroneberg, G.: Über das sympathicomimetische pressorische Prinzip des Harns ("Urosympathin") *Arch. Exp. Pathol. Pharmakol. 204:* 228–243, 1947.

459. Horn, H. L.: Pheochromocytoma: A case of paroxysmal hypertensive attacks induced by eating and changes in position. *Ann. Intern. Med. 51:* 129–140, 1959.

460. Horwitz, D., and Sjoerdsma, A.: Some interrelationships between elevation of blood pressure and angina pectoris. *In: Hypertension. Vol. 13. Proceedings of the Council for High Blood Pressure Research.* New York, American Heart Association, 1964.

461. Howard, E. B., and Nielsen, S. W.: Pheochromocytomas associated with hypertensive lesions in dogs. *J. Am. Vet. Med. Assoc. 147:* 245–252, 1965.

462. Howard, J. E., and Barker, W. H.: Paroxysmal hypertension and other clinical manifestations associated with benign chromaffin cell tumors (phaeochromocytoma). *Bull. Johns Hopkins Hosp. 61:* 371–410, 1937.

463. Huang, S.-N., and McLeish, W. A.: Pheochromocytoma and medullary carcinoma of thyroid. *Cancer 21:* 302–311, 1968.

464. Hubble, D.: Phaeochromocytoma in children. *Arch. Dis. Child. 26:* 340–350, 1951.

465. Hulst, L. A.: Megacolon van ongewone oorsprong. *Ned. Tijdschr. Geneeskd. 95:* 3368–3375, 1951.

466. Hume, D. M.: Pheochromocytoma in the adult and in the child. *Am. J. Surg. 99:* 458–496, 1960.

467. Hume, D. M., and Porter, R. R.: Acute dissecting aortic aneurysms. *Surgery 53:* 122–154, 1963.

468. Huston, J. R., and Stewart, W. R. C.: Hemorrhagic pheochromocytoma with shock and abdominal pain. *Am. J. Med. 39:* 502–504, 1965.

469. Hutchinson, G. B., Evans, J. A., and Davidson, D. C.: Pitfalls in the diagnosis of pheochromocytoma. *Ann. Intern. Med. 48:* 300–309, 1958.

470. Hyman, A., and Mencher, W. H.: Pheochromocytoma of the adrenal gland. *J. Urol. 49:* 755–771, 1943.

I

471. Ibanez, M. L., Cole, V. W., Russell, W. O., and Clark, R. L.: Solid carcinoma of the thyroid gland. Analysis of 53 cases. *Cancer 20:* 706–723, 1967.

472. Imura, H., Kato, Y., Masaki, I., Masachika, M., and Mikio, Y.: Effect of adrenergic blocking or stimulating agents on plasma GH, IRI and blood FFA levels in man. *J. Clin Invest. 50:* 1069–1079, 1971.

473. Iseri, L. T., Henderson, H. W., and Derr, J. W.: Use of adrenolytic drug, Regitine, in pheochromocytoma. *Am. Heart J. 42:* 129–136, 1951.

474. Ishibashi, M., Takeuchi, A., Yokoyama, S., Yamaji, T., Tsuchimochi, T., Tanaka, T., Kurihara, H., and Ikeda, M.: Pheochromocytoma with renal artery stenosis and high plasma renin activity. *Jpn. Heart J. 16:* 741–748, 1975.

475. Itoh, C., Yoshinaga, K., Sato, T., Ishida, N., and Wada, Y.: Presence of N-methylmetadrenaline in human urine and tumor tissue of phaeochromocytoma. *Nature 193:* 477–478, 1962.

476. Iversen, L. L.: Dopamine receptors in the brain: a dopamine-sensitive adenylate cyclase models synaptic receptors illuminating antipsychotic drug action. *Science 188:* 1084–1089, 1975.

477. Iversen, L. L.: Uptake of circulating catecholamines into tissues. *In:* Blaschko, H., Sayers, G., and Smith, D. A., eds. *Vol. VI. Adrenal Gland. Handbook of Physiology, Sect. 7. Endocrinology.* Washington, D.C. Am. Physiological Society. 1975. pp. 713–722.

477a. Iversen, L. L., Salt, P. J. and Wilson, H. A.: Inhibition of catecholamine uptake in the isolated rat heart by haloalkylamines related to phenoxybenzamine. *Br. J. Pharmacol. 46:* 647–657, 1972.

478. Ivy, H. K., Schirger, A., Fuller, H., Jr., and McConahey, W. M.: Hypertension associated with hyperthyroidism. *In:* Manger, W. M., ed., *Hormones and Hypertension.* Springfield, Ill., C. C. Thomas, 1966, Chap. 9, pp. 238–250.

J

479. Jackson, C. E., Tashjian, A. H., Jr., and Block, M. A.: Detection of medullary thyroid cancer by calcitonin assay in families. *Ann. Intern. Med. 78:* 845–852, 1973.

480. Jacob, H. S.: The polycythemias and their relationship to erythropoietin. *In:* Dowling, H. F., ed., *Disease-a-Month,* Chicago, Year Book Medical Publishers, August, 1974.

481. Jacobson, W. E., Hammarsten, J. F., and Heller, B. I.: The effects of adrenaline upon renal function and electrolyte excretion. *J. Clin. Invest. 30*: 1503–1506, 1951.

482. Jaim-Etcheverry, G., and Zieher, L. M.: Cytochemical localization of monoamine stores in sheep thyroid gland at the electron microscope level. *Experientia 24*: 593–595, 1968.

483. James, R. E., Baker, H. L., Jr., and Scanlon, P. W.: The roentgenologic aspects of metastatic pheochromocytoma. *Am. J. Roentgenol. Radium Ther. Nucl. Med. 115*: 783–793, 1972.

484. Javaheri, P., and Raafat, J.: Malignant phaeochromocytoma of the urinary bladder. *Br. J. Urol. 47*: 401–404, 1975.

485. Jelliffe, R. S.: Phaeochromocytoma presenting as a cardiac and abdominal catastrophe. *Br. Med. J. 2*: 76–77, 1952.

486. Jiang, N-S, Machacek, D., and Wadel, O. P.: Further study on the two-column plasma catecholamine assay. *Mayo Clin. Proc. 51*: 112–116, 1976.

487. Jiang, N-S, Stoffer, S. S., Pikler, G. M., Wadel, O., and Sheps, S. G.: Laboratory and clinical observations with a two-column plasma catecholamine assay. *Mayo Clin. Proc. 48*: 47–49, 1973.

488. Joasoo, A., and Freeman, Z.: Tyramine and glucagon in pheochromocytoma. *Lancet 2*: 726, 1967.

489. Johns, V. J., Jr., and Brunjes, S.: Pheochromocytoma. *Am. J. Cardiol. 9*: 120–125, 1962.

490. Johnson, L. R., Reese, M., and Nelson, D. H.: Interference in Pisano's urinary metanephrine assay after use of x-ray contrast media. *Clin. Chem. 18*: 209–211, 1972.

491. Julian, W. A., Cole, A. T., and Fried, F. A.: Renovascular hypertension: A rare complication of excision of pheochromocytoma. *J. Urol. 111*: 722–723, 1974.

K

492. Kahn, M. T., and Mullon, D. A.: Pheochromocytoma without hypertension—Report of a patient with acromegaly. *J. Am. Med. Assoc. 188*: 74–75, 1964.

493. Kahn, P. C., and Nickrosz, L. V.: Selective angiography of the adrenal glands. *Am. J. Roentgenol. Radium Ther. Nucl. Med. 101*: 739–749, 1967.

494. Kalff, G.: Anaesthesiologische Probleme bei Patienten mit Phäochromocytom. *Anaesthesist 17*: 43–47, 1968.

495. Kaplan, E. L., Peskin, G. W., and Arnaud, C. D.: Nonsteroid, calcitonin-like factor from the adrenal gland. *Surgery 66*: 167–174, 1969.

496. Karsner, H. T.: Tumors of the adrenal. *In: Atlas of Tumor Pathology*. Section VIII, fascicle 29. Washington, D.C., Armed Forces Institute of Pathology, 1950. 68 pp.

497. Käser, H.: Catecholamine-producing neural tumors other than pheochromocytoma. *Pharmacol. Rev. 18*: 660–665, 1966.

498. Katz, R. L., and Wolf, C. E.: Pheochromocytoma. *In: Mark, L. C. and Ngai, S. H. eds., Highlights in Clinical Anesthesiology*. New York, Harper and Row, 1971, Chap. 7, pp. 55–65.

499. Kaude, J. V., and Agee, O. F.: Angiographic diagnosis of pheochromocytoma. *J. Am. Med. Assoc. 207*: 1353, 1969.

500. Kaufman, S., and Friedman, S.: Dopamine-β-hydroxylase *Pharmacol. Rev. 17*: 71–100, 1965.

501. Kaumann, A. J.: Potentiation of the effects of isoprenaline and noradrenaline by hydrocortisone in cat heart muscle. *Naunyn Schmiedeberg's Arch. Pharmacol. 273*: 134–153, 1972.

502. Kawashima, K.: Über einen Fall von maltiplen Hautfibromen met Nebennierengeschwulst. *Virchows. Arch. 203*: 66–74, 1911.

502a. Keim, H. J., Drayer, J. I., Case, D. B., Lopez-Ovejero, J., Wallace, J. M., Weber, M. A., and Laragh, J. H.: A role for renin in rebound hypertension and encephalopathy after infusion of saralasin acetate (sar1-ala8-angiotension II). *N. Engl. J. Med. 295*: 1175–1177, 1976.

503. Keir, F. E.: Removal of pheochromocytoma during pregnancy. *J. Int. Coll. Surg. 24*: 316–321, 1955.

503a. Keiser, H. R., Beaven, M. A., Doppman, J., Wells, S., and Buja, L. M.: Sipple syndrome: medullary thyroid carcinoma, pheochromocytoma and parathyroid disease. *Ann. Intern. Med. 78*: 561–579, 1973.

504. Keith, N. M., Wagener, H. P., and Barker, N. W.: Some different types of essential hypertension: Their course and prognosis. *Am. J. Med. Sci. 197*: 332–343, 1939.

505. Kelleher, J., Walters, G., Robinson, R., and Smith, P.: Chemical tests for phaeochromocytoma. *J. Clin. Pathol. 17*: 399–404, 1964.

506. Kelly, H. M., Piper, M. C., Wilder, R. M., and Walters, W.: Case of paroxysmal hypertension with paraganglioma of the right suprarenal gland. *Mayo Clin. Proc. 11*: 65–70, 1936.

507. Kennedy, J. S., Symington, T., and Woodger, B. A.: Chemical and histochemical observations in benign and malignant pheaochromocytoma. *J. Pathol. Bacteriol. 81*: 409–418, 1961.

508. Kerr, J. H., Corbett, J. L. Prys-Roberts, C., Crampton-Smith, A., and Spalding, J. M. K.: Involvement of the sympathetic nervous system in tetanus. *Lancet 2*: 236–241, 1968.

509. Kerzner, M. S., Reeves, J. A., De Nyse, D., and Claunch, B. C.: Pheochromocytoma with renal artery compression in an identical twin. *Arch Intern. Med. 121*: 91–94, 1968.

510. Keys, A.: The response of the plasma potassium level in man to the administration of epinephrine. *Am. J. Physiol. 121*: 325–330, 1938.

510a. Khairi, M. R. A., Dexter, R. N., Burzynski, N. J., and Johnston, C. C., Jr.: Mucosal neuroma, pheochromocytoma and medullary thyroid carcinoma: Multiple endocrine neoplasia type 3. *Medicine 54*: 89–112, 1975.

511. Killins, J. A., and Eberbach, C. W.: Pheochromocytoma: A cause of two unanticipated surgical deaths. *Wis. Med. J. 56*: 277–280, 1957.

512. Kinkhawala, M. N., and Conradi, H.: Angiography of extra-adrenal pheochromocytomas. *J. Urol. 108*: 666–668, 1972.

513. Kirkendahl, W. M., Liechty, R. D., and Culp, D. A.: Diagnosis and treatment of patients with

pheochromocytoma. *Arch. Intern. Med. 115*: 529–536, 1965.

514. Kirshner, N., Goodall, McC., and Rosen, L.: Metabolism of dl-adrenaline-2-C14 in the human. *Proc. Soc. Exp. Biol. Med. 98*: 627–630, 1958.

515. Kitajima, W., Saruta, T., Kondo, K., Yamada, R., Aoki, S., and Nagakubo, I.: A case of secondary aldosteronism induced by pheochromocytoma. *J. Urol. 114*: 141–143, 1975.

516. Kleinschmidt, A., and Schümann, H. J.: Strukturuntersuchungen über die Adrenalin- und Noradrenalinspeichernden Granula des Nebennierenmarkes. *Neunyn-Schiedeberg's Arch. Pharmakol. Exp. Pathol 241*: 260–272, 1961.

517. Kline, I. K.: Myocardial alterations associated with pheochromocytomas. *Am. J. Pathol. 38*: 539–552, 1961.

517a. Hochberg, F. H., Dasilva, A. B., Galdabini, J., and Richardson, E. P. Jr.: Gastrointestinal involvement in von Recklinghausen's neurofibromatosis. *Neurology 24*: 1144–1151, 1974.

518. Koehler, A. E., Marsh, N., and Hill, E.: Effect of epinephrine injected intravenously at a constant rate in normal and hypertensive cases. *J. Biol. Chem. 119*: 59, 1937.

519. Kohn, A.: Das chromaffine Gewebe. *Z. Anat. Entwicklungsgesch. 12*: 253, 1902.

519a. Kontras, S. B.: Urinary excretion of 3-methoxy-4-hydroxymandelic acid in children with neuroblastoma. *Cancer 15*: 978–986, 1962.

520. Koonce, D. H., Pollock, B. E., and Glassy, F. J.: Bilateral pheochromocytoma associated with neurofibromatosis. Death following aortography. *Am. Heart J. 44*: 901–909, 1952.

521. Kopin, I. J.: Metabolic degradation of catecholamines. The relative importance of different pathways under physiological conditions and after administration of drugs. *In:* Blaschko, H. and Muschool, E., eds., *Catecholamines.* Berlin, Heidelberg, New York, Springer-Verlag, 1972. Chap. 8, pp. 270–282.

522. Koplin, I. J.: Storage and metabolism of catecholamines: The role of monoamine oxidase. *Pharmacol. Rev. 16*: 179–191, 1964.

523. Kopin, I. J., and Axelrod, J.: Presence of 3-methoxy-4-hydroxyphenylglycol and metanephrine in phaeochromocytoma tissue. *Nature 185*: 788, 1960.

524. Kopin, I. J., Axelrod, J., and Gordon, E.: The metabolic fate of H3-epinephrine and C14-metanephrine in the rat. *J. Biol. Chem. 236*: 2109–2113, 1961.

525. Kopriva, C. J., and Eltringham, R.: The use of enflurane during resection of a pheochromocytoma. *Anesthesiology 41*: 399–400, 1974.

526. Kramer, W.: Lesions of the central nervous system in multiple neurofibromatosis. *Psychiatr. Neurol. Neurochirurgia. 74*: 349–368, 1971.

527. Kraupp, O. Stormann, H., Bernheimer, H., and Obenaus, H.: Vorkommen und Diagnostische Bedeutung von Phenolsäuren im Harn beim Phäochromocytom. *Klin. Wochenschr. 37*: 76–80, 1959.

528. Kremer, D. N.: Medullary tumor of the adrenal glands with hypertension and juvenile arterio-sclerosis. *Arch. Intern. Med. 57*: 999–1007, 1936.

529. Kreul, J. F., Dauchot, P. J., and Anton, A. H.: Hemodynamic and catecholamine studies during pheochromocytoma resection under enflurane anesthesia. *Anesthesiology 44*: 265–268, 1976.

530. Kukreja, S. C., Hargis, G. K., Rosenthal, I. M., and Williams, G. A.: Pheochromocytoma causing excessive parathyroid hormone production and hypercalcemia. *Ann. Intern. Med. 79*: 838–840, 1973.

531. Kuni, C. C. Extra-adrenal pheochromocytoma with metastasis in Down's syndrome. *J. Pediatr. 83*: 835–836, 1973.

532. Kurnick, N. B.: Autonomic hyperreflexia and its control in patients with spinal cord lesions. *Ann. Intern. Med. 44*: 678–686, 1956.

533. Kvale, W. F.: Clinical aspects of pheochromocytoma. *Minn. Med. 41*: 291–295, 1958.

534. Kvale, W. F., Roth, G. M., Manger, W. M., and Priestley, J. T.: Pheochromocytoma, *Circulation 14*: 622–630, 1956.

535. Kvale, W. F., Roth, G. M., Manger, W. M., and Priestley, J. T.: Present-day diagnosis and treatment of pheochromocytoma. A review of fifty-one cases. *J. Am. Med. Assoc. 164*: 854–861, 1957.

L

536. L'abbé, M., Tinel, J., and Doumer, E.: Crises solaires et hypertension paroxystique en rapport avec une tumeur surrénale. *Bull. Soc. Méd. Hôp. 46*: 982–990, 1922.

537. LaBrosse, E. H., Axelrod, J., and Kety, S. S.: O-Methylation, the principal route of metabolism of epinephrine in man. *Science 128*: 593–594, 1958.

538. LaBrosse, E. H., Axelrod, J., and Sjoerdsma, A.: Urinary excretion of normetanephrine by man. *Fed. Proc. 17*: 386, 1958.

539. LaBrosse, E. H., and Hertting, G.: Bilary excretion of dl-epinephrine metabolites. *Fed. Proc. 19*: 398–404, 1964.

540. LaBrosse, E. H., Mann, J. D., and Kety, S. S.: The physiological and psychological effects of intravenously administered epinephrine and its metabolism in normal and schizophrenic men—III. *J. Psychiatr. Res. 1*: 68–75, 1961.

541. Lacy, P. E.: The pancreatic beta cell: Structure and function. *N. Engl. J. Med. 276*: 187–195, 1967.

542. Lagos, J. C., and Gomez, M. R.: Tuberous sclerosis: Reappraisal of a clinical entity. *Mayo Clin. Proc. 42*: 26–49, 1967.

543. Laham, A. J., and Schrock, J. B.: Pheochromocytoma with persistant hypertension and thoracolumbar sympathectomy. *Surgery 27*: 935–938, 1950.

544. Lake, C. R., Ziegler, M. G. Coleman, M., and Kopin, I. J.: Plasma norepinephrine and dopamine-beta-hydroxylase in hypertension. *Fed. Proc. 35* (Abstr. 1063): 398, 1976.

545. Langemann, H., Boner, A., and Müller, P. B.: Aminosäurendecarboxylase in Phäochromocytom- und Karzinoidgewebe. *Schweiz. Med. Wochenschr. 92*: 1621–1623, 1962.

545a. Langer, S. Z.: Presynaptic regulation of catecholamine release. *Biochem. Pharmacol. 23*: 1793–1800, 1974.

546. Langford, H. G.: Hemodynamic consequences of renin tachyphylaxis and norepinephrine failure of response. *Am. J. Physiol. 198*: 561–564, 1960.

547. Langman, J.: *Medical Embryology*, 2nd ed. Baltimore, Maryland. Williams and Wilkins, 1969, 386 pp.

548. Lanner, L. O., and Rosencrantz, M.: Arteriographic appearances of phaeochromocytoma. *Acta Radiol., (Diagn.) 10*: 35–48, 1970.

549. Lattes, R.: Nonchromaffin paraganglioma of ganglion nodosum, carotid body, and aortic-arch bodies. *Cancer 3*: 667–694, 1950.

550. Lattes, R., and Waltner, J. G.: Nonchromaffin paraganglioma of the middle ear (carotid body-like tumor; glomus-jugulare tumor). *Cancer 2*: 447–468, 1949.

551. Laumonier, R., Marche, C., and Marche, J.: Etude ultrastructurale d'une phaeochromocytome. *Ann. Anat. Pathol. Anat. Norm. Med. Chir. 13*: 137–146, 1968.

552. Lauper, N. T., Tyce, G. M., Sheps, S. G., and Carney, J. A.: Pheochromocytoma: Fine structural, biochemical and clinical observations. *Am. J. Cardiol. 30*: 197–204, 1972.

553. Lawrence, A. M.: A new provocative test for pheochromocytoma. *Ann. Intern. Med. 63*: 905–906, 1965. (Abstr.)

554. Lawrence, A. M.: Glucagon and pheochromocytoma. *Ann. Intern. Med. 73*: 852–853, 1970.

555. Lawrence, A. M.: Glucagon provocative test for pheochromocytoma. *Ann. Intern. Med. 66*: 1091–1096, 1967.

556. Leather, H. M., Shaw, D. B., Cates, J. E., and Walker, R. M.: Six cases of phaeochromocytoma with unusual clinical manifestations. *Brit. Med. J. 1*: 1373–1378, 1962.

557. LeDouarin, N., and LeLièvre, C.: Démonstration de l'originic neurale des cellules à calcitonine du corps ultimobranchial chez l'embryon de poulet. *C. R. Acad. Sci. Ser. D 770*: 2857–2860, 1970.

558. Leduc, J.: Catecholamine production and release in exposure and acclimation to cold. *Acta Physiol. Scand. 53 (Suppl. 183)*: 1–101, 1961.

559. Leduc, J., and D'Iorio, A.: Biochemical studies of two cases of pheochromocytoma. *Rev. Can. Biol. 19*: 34–52, 1960.

560. Lee, R. E., and Rousseau, P.: Pheocnromocytoma and obesity. *J. Clin. Endocrinol. Metab. 27*: 1050–1052, 1967.

561. Leestma, J. E., and Price, E. B., Jr.: Paraganglioma of the urinary bladder. *Cancer 28*: 1063–1073, 1971.

562. Lefebvre, P. J., Cession-Fossion, A., and Luyck, A. S.: Glucagon test for pheochromocytoma. *Lancet 2*: 1366, 1966.

563. Lefkowitz, R. J.: β-adrenergic receptors; recognition and regulation. *N. Engl. J. Med. 295*: 323–328, 1976.

564. Lehman, D. J., and Rosof, J.: Massive hemorrhage into an adrenal pheochromocytoma. Report of a case with sudden death. *N. Engl. J. Med. 254*: 474–476, 1956.

565. L'Esperance, F. A., Jr.: Hemobarometry. Preliminary report of a new diagnostic technique. *Am. J. Ophthalmol. 75*: 266–278, 1973.

566. Levan, G., Mitelman, F., and Telenius, M.: Chromosomes in Sipple's syndrome. *Lancet 1*: 1510, 1973.

567. Lever, A. F., Mowbray, J. F., and Peart, W. S.: Blood flow and blood pressure after noradrenaline infusions. *Clin. Sci. 21*: 69–74, 1961.

568. Lever, J. D., Lewis, P. R., and Boyd, J. D.: Observations on the fine structure and histochemistry of the carotid body in the cat and rabbit. *J. Anat. 93*: 478–490, 1959.

569. Levey, G. S., Weiss, S. R., and Ruiz, E.: Characterization of the glucagon receptor in a pheochromocytoma. *J. Clin. Endocrinol. Metab. 40*: 720–723, 1975.

570. Levi-Montalcini, R., and Booker, B.: Excessive growth of the sympathetic ganglia evoked by a protein isolated from mouse salivary glands. *Proc. Nat. Acad. Sci. U.S.A. 46*: 373–384, 1960.

571. Levit, S. A., Sheps, S. G., Espinosa, R. E., Remine, W. H., and Harrison, E. G., Jr.: Catecholamine-secreting paraganglioma of glomus-jugulare region resembling pheochromocytoma. *N. Engl. J. Med. 281*: 805–811, 1969.

572. Levitt, M., Spector, S., Sjoerdsma, A., and Udenfriend, S.: Elucidation of the rate-limiting step in norepinephrine biosynthesis in the perfused guinea-pig heart. *J. Pharmacol. Exp. Ther. 148*: 1–8, 1965.

573. Lieberman, L. M., Beierwaltes, W. H., Conn., J. W., Ansari, A. N., and Nishiyama, H.: Diagnosis of adrenal disease by visualization of human adrenal glands with 131I-19-Iodocholesterol. *N. Engl. J. Med. 285*: 1387–1393, 1971.

574. Lima, F. X. P., Barros, N. M., Jr., and Franca, H. H.: Feochromocitoma: Considerções sôbre provas diagnosticas, com apresentação de um caso. *Rev. Paul. Med. 50*: 111–120, 1957.

575. Lindau, A.: Studien über Kleinhirncysten; Bau, Pathogenesis und Beziehungen zur Angiomatosis Retinae. *Acta Pathol. Microbiol. Scand. (Suppl.) 1*: 1–128, 1926.

576. Lindau, A.: Zur Frage der Angiomatosis Retinae und ihrer Hirnkomplikationen. *Acta Ophthalmol. 4*: 193–226, 1927.

577. Linde, P.: Unusual tumor (pheochromocytoma) in infant 5 months old. *Nord. Med. 12*: 897, 1924.

578. Lindsey, C. M., DeHart, H. S., and Glenn, J. F.: Pheochromocytoma of the urinary bladder. *Urol. 7*: 210–211, 1976.

579. Litchfield, J. W., and Peart, W. S.: Pheochromocytoma with normal excretion of adrenalin and noradrenalin. *Lancet 2*: 1283–1284, 1956.

580. Ljungberg, O.: On medullary carcinoma of the thyroid. *Acta Pathol. Microbiol. Scand. (Suppl.) 231*: Section A, 1–57, 1972.

581. Ljungberg, O., Cederquist E., von Studnitz, W.: Medullary thyroid carcinoma and pheochromocytoma: A familial chromaffinomatosis. *Br. Med. J. 1*: 279–281, 1967.

582. Loehning, R. W., and Massa, R. I.: Possible nephrotoxicity from enflurane anesthesia in a patient with severe renal disease. *Anesthesiology 40*: 203–205, 1974.

583. Lopez, J. F.: Pheochromocytoma of the adrenal gland with granulosa cell tumor and neurofibromatosis: Report of a case with fatal outcome following abdominal aortography. *Ann. Intern. Med. 48*: 187–199, 1958.

584. Louis, W. J., and Doyle, A. E.: The use of a double-isotope derivative plasma assay for nor-adrenaline and adrenaline in the diagnosis and localization of pheochromocytoma. *Aust. N. Z. J. Med. 3*: 212–217, 1971.

585. Louis, W. J., Doyle, A. E., and Anavekar, S.: Plasma norepinephrine levels in essential hypertension. *N. Engl. J. Med. 288*: 599–601, 1973.

586. Louis, W. J., Doyle, A. E., Heath, W. C., and Robinson, M. J.: Secretion of dopa in phaeochromocytoma. *Br. Med. J. 4*: 325–327, 1972.

587. Lovenberg, W., Bruckwick, E. A., Alexander, R. W., Horwitz, D., and Keiser, H. R.: Evaluation of Serum Dopamine-β-Hydroxylase Activity as an Index of Sympathetic Nervous Activity in Man. *In*: Usdin, E., ed., *Neuropsychopharmacology of Monoamines and Their Regulatory Enzymes*. New York, Raven Press, 1974. pp. 121–128.

588. Lucia, S. P., Leonard, M. E., and Falconer, E. H.: The effect of the subcutaneous injection of adrenalin on the leukocyte count of splenectomized patients and of patients with certain diseases of the hematopoietic and lymphatic systems. *Am. J. Med. Sci. 194*: 35–43, 1937.

589. Lulu, D. J.: Pheochromocytoma of the organs of Zuckerkandl. *Arch. Surg. 99*: 641–644, 1969.

590. Lund, A.: Adrenaline and noradrenaline in blood and urine in cases of pheochromocytoma. *Scand. J. Clin. Lab. Invest. 4*: 263–265, 1952.

591. Lund, A.: Simultaneous fluorimetric determinations of adrenaline and noradrenaline in blood. *Acta Pharmacol. Toxicol. 6*: 137–146, 1950.

592. Lund, A., and Møller, K. O.: Adrenaline concentration in the blood of patients dying of adrenaline poisoning. *Acta Pharmacol. Toxicol. 14*: 363–366, 1958.

593. Lund, A., and Møller, K. O.: Nor-epinephrine in blood in pheochromocytoma. *Ugeskr. laeg. 133*: 1068, 1951.

594. Lund-Johansen, P.: Shock after administration of phenothiazines in patients with pheochromocytoma. *Acta. Med. Scand. 172*: 525–529, 1962.

595. Lupulescou, A.: Les phéochromocytomes expérimentaux. *Ann. Endocrinol. 22*: 459–468, 1961.

596. Lurvey, A. Yusin, A., and DeQuattro, V.: Pseudo-pheochromocytoma after self-administered isoproterenol. *J. Clin. Endocrinol. Metab. 36*: 766–769, 1973.

596a. Lynch, J. D., Sheps, S. G., Bernatz, P. E., ReMine, W. H., and Harrison, E. G., Jr.: Neurofibromatosis and hypertension due to pheochromocytoma or renal-artery stenosis. *Minn. Med. 55*: 25–31, 1972.

M

597. Mackay, G., and Rosenheim, S. H.: Pathology of tumors of the adrenal medulla. *In: Endocrine and Nonendocrine Hormone-Producing Tumors. M. D. Anderson Hospital & Tumor Institute, Houston, Texas*. Chicago, Year Book Medical Publishers, 1971, pp. 241–255.

598. MacKeith, R.: Adrenal-sympathetic syndrome: chromaffin tissue tumor with paroxysmal hypertension. *Br. Heart J. 6*: 1–12, 1944.

599. MacKenzie, D. W.: Discussion of Hyman, A. and

Mencher, W. H.: Pheochromocytoma of the adrenal gland. *J. Urol. 49*: 772–776, 1943.

600. Maddox, K., and Rothwell, F. L.: Pheochromocytoma of long duration. *M. J. Aust. 2*: 123–125, 1958.

601. Maebashi, M., Miura, Y., Yoshinaga, K., and Sato, K.: Plasma renin activity in pheochromocytoma. *Jpn. Circ. J. 32*: 1427–1432, 1968.

602. Mahaux, J. E., Schaepdryver, A. F., de, Veriniory, A., Enderle, J., Smets, W., Reinhold, H., Rood, M. de, and Meunier, A.: Pheochromocytoma with pseudohyperthyroid symptoms. Localization of the tumor by retropneumoperitoneum and by graded determination of catecholamines in the inferior vena cava. *Ann. Endocrinol. 24*: 93–101, 1963.

603. Mahoney, E. M., Friend, D. G., Dexter, L., and Harrison, J. H.: Localization of (adrenal and extra-adrenal) pheochromocytomas by vena caval blood. *Surg. Forum 14*: 495–496, 1963.

604. Maier, H. C.: Intrathoracic pheochromocytoma with hypertension. *Ann Surg. 130*: 1059–1065, 1949.

605. Maier, H. C., and Humphreys, G. H. II: Intrathoracic pheochromocytoma, including a case of multiple paragangliomas of the functional and nonfunctional type. *J. Thorac. Surg., 36*: 625–641, 1958.

606. Malbin, B.: Excess urinary catecholamines without pheochromocytoma. *Ann. Intern. Med. 51*: 613–617, 1959.

607. Malm, R. J., Manger, W. M., Sullivan, S. F., Papper, E. M., and Nahas, G. G.: The effect of acidosis on sympatho-adrenal stimulation. *J. Am. Med. Assoc. 2*: 121–125, 1966.

608. Maloney, J. M.: Pheochromocytoma in pregnancy. *N. Engl. J. Med. 253*: 242–243, 1955.

609. Malter, I. J., and Koehler, P. R.: Angiographic findings in pheochromocytomas of the organs of Zuckerkandl. *Radiology 97*: 57–58, 1970.

610. Manasse, P.: Über die hyperplastischen Tumoren der Nebennieren. *Virchow. Arch. Pathol. Anat. 133*: 391–404, 1893.

611. Manasse, P.: Zur Histologie und Histogenese der primären Nierengeschwülste. *Virchows. Arch. Pathol. Anat. 145*: 113–157, 1896.

611a. Manger, W. M.: Observations on plasma catecholamines in patients with diastolic hypertension. *Am. J. Cardiol. 9*: 731–742, 1962.

612. Manger, W. M: Pressor amines in pheochromocytoma. *Minn. Med. 41*: 296 and 321, 1958.

613. Manger, W. M., and Bessis, M.: White cell uptake of *l*-dihydroxyphenylalanine (*l*-dopa), catecholamines (CAs) and 5-hydroxytryptamine (5-HT). *The Pharmacologist 11* (Abstr. 188): 263, 1969.

614. Manger, W. M., Bollman, J. L., Maher, F. T., and Berkson, J.: Plasma concentration of epinephrine and norepinephrine in hemorrhagic and anaphylactic shock. *Am. J. Physiol. 190*: 310–316, 1957.

615. Manger, W. M., Davis, S. W., Chu, D. S., Freedman, L. S., Ebstein, R. P., Park, D. H., Levitz, S. M., and Goldstein, M.: Effect of a modified cold pressor test on plasma catecholamines (CA) and dopamine-β-hydroxylase (DBH). *Fed. Proc. 33* (Abstr. 1117): 408, 1974.

616. Manger, W. M., Flock, E. V., Berkson, J., Bollman, J. L., Roth, G. M., Baldes, E. J., and Jacobs, M.: Chemical quantitation of epinephrine and norepi-

nephrine in thirteen patients with pheochromocytoma. *Circulation 10*: 641–652, 1954.

617. Manger, W. M., Frolich, E. D., Gifford, R. W., and Dustan, H. P.: Norepinephrine infusion in normal subjects and patients with essential or renal hypertension: Effect on blood pressure, heart rate, and plasma catecholamine concentrations. *J. Clin. Pharmacol. 16*: 129–141, 1976.

617a. Manger, W. M., Hart, C. J., Hulse, M., and Dufton, S.: Correlation between tumor catecholamines (CA) and blood pressure (BP) in 38 patients with pheochromocytoma. *Fed. Proc. 36 (Abstr. 309)*: 328, 1977.

618. Manger, W. M., Nahas, G. G., Papper, E. M. and Habif, D. V.: Effect of pH control and oxygen administration on the course of prolonged hypovolemic shock. *Ann. Surg. 156*: 503–509, 1962.

619. Manger, W. M., Schwartz, B. E., Baars, C. W., Wakim, K. G., Bollman, J. L., Peterson, M. C., and Berkson, J.: Epinephrine and arterenol (norepinephrine) in mental disease. *Arch. Neurol. Psychiatry. 78*: 396–412, 1957.

620. Manger, W. M., Steinsland, O. S., Nahas, G. G., Wakim, K. G., and Dufton, S.: Comparison of improved fluorometric methods used to quantitate plasma catecholamines. *Clin. Chem. 15*: 1101–1123, 1969.

621. Manger, W. M., von Estorff, I., Davis, S., Chu, D., Wakim, K., and Dufton, S.: Inadequacy of plasma catecholamines as an index of adrenergic activity. *Fed. Proc. 34* (Abstr. 2853) : 723, 1975.

622. Manger, W. M., and Wakim, K. G.: The place of norepinephrine and epinephrine in the etiology of diastolic hypertension. *Z. Klin. Chem. 2* (3) : 65–75, 1964.

623. Manger, W. M., and Wakim, K. G.: The role of norepinephrine and epinephrine in the etiology of diastolic hypertension. *In*: Manger, W. M., ed., *Hormones and Hypertension*. Springfield, Ill., C. C. Thomas, 1966, Chap. 2, pp. 41–86.

624. Manger, W. M., Wakim, K. G., and Bollman, L. J.: Chemical Quantitation of Epinephrine and Norepinephrine in Plasma. Springfield, Ill., C. C. Thomas, 1959, 398 pp.

625. Manger, W. M., Wakim, K. G., and Bollman, J. L.: Effect of increased intracranial pressure on pressor amine concentration in blood. *Fed. Proc. 14*: 98, 1955.

626. Mannhart, M., Ludin, H., Veyrat, R., and Zieger, W. H.: Secondary hyperaldosteronism caused by cervical phaeochromocytoma cured by ablation of the tumor. *Helv. Med. Acta. 35*: 479–483, 1969–70.

627. Manning, P. C. Jr., Molnar, G. D., Black, B. M., Priestley, J. T., and Woolner, L. B.: Pheochromocytoma, hyperparathyroidism and thyroid carcinoma occurring coincidentally. *N. Engl. J. Med. 268*: 68–72, 1963.

628. Marc-Aurele, J., Brouillet, J., Leboeuf, G., Vitye, B., Barbeau, A., and Genest, J.: A peculiar form of clinical shock. *Can. Med. Assoc. J. 78*: 589–591, 1958.

629. Marchetti, G.: Beitrag zur Kenntnis der pathologischen Anatomie der Nebennieren. *Virchows Arch. Pathol. Anat. 177*: 227–248, 1904.

630. Margolis, F. L., Roffi, J., and Jost, A.: Norepineph-

rine methylation in fetal rat adrenals: *Science 154*: 275–276, 1966.

631. Marine, D., and Baumann, E. J.: Hypertrophy of adrenal medulla of white rats in chronic thiouracil poisoning. *Am. J. Physiol. 144*: 69–73, 1945.

631a. Marks, A. D., and Channick, B. J.: Extra-adrenal pheochromocytoma and medullary thyroid carcinoma with pheochromocytoma. *Arch. Intern. Med. 134*: 1106–1109, 1974.

632. Marley, E., and Blackwell, B.: Interactions of monoamine oxidase inhibitors, amines, and foodstuffs. *Adv. Pharmacol. Chemother., 8*: 185–239, 1970.

633. Marshall, D., Saul, G. B., and Sachs, E., Jr.: Tuberous sclerosis: A report of 16 cases in two family trees revealing genetic dominance. *N. Engl. J. Med. 261*: 1102–1105, 1959.

633a. Masheter, H. C.: Pheochromocytoma, astrocytoma and neurofibromatosis in one patient. *Br. Med. J. 2*: 1518, 1963.

634. Mason, G. A., Hart-Mercer, J., Millar, E. J., Strang, L. B., and Wynne, N. A.: Adrenaline-secreting neuroblastoma in an infant. *Lancet 2*: 322–325, 1957.

635. Mathias, C. J., Christensen, N. J., Corbett, J. L. Frankel, H. L., Goodwin, T. J., and Peart, W. S.: Plasma catecholamines, plasma renin activity and plasma aldosterone in tetraplegic man, horizontal and tilted. *Clin. Sci. Mol. Med. 49*: 291–299, 1975.

635a. Mathias, C. J., Christensen, N. J., Corbett, J. L., Frankel, H. L., and Spalding, J. M. K.: Plasma catecholamines during paroxysmal neurogenic hypertension in quadriplegic man. *Circ. Res. 39*: 294–308, 1976.

636. Mayo, C. H.: Paroxysmal hypertension with tumor of retroperitoneal nerve. Report of case. *J. Am. Med. Assoc.. 89*: 1047–1050, 1927.

637. Mazey, R. M., Kotchen, T. A., and Ernst, C. B.: A syndrome resembling pheochromocytoma following a stroke. Report of a case. *J. Am. Med. Assoc. 230*: 575–577, 1074.

637a. Mazze, R. I., Trudell, J. R., and Cousins, M. J.: Methoxyflurane metabolism and renal dysfunction. Clinical correlation in man. *Anesthesiology 35*: 247–252, 1971.

638. McAlister, W. H., and Kochler, P. R.: Hemorrhage into a pheochromocytoma in a patient on anticoagulants. *J. Can. Assoc. Radiol. 18*: 404–406, 1967.

639. McCoy, G. E., and Bridgeman, M. L.: Use of drugs in the diagnosis and treatment of pheochromocytoma. *Pediatrics 6*: 286–298, 1950.

640. McCullagh, E. P., and Engel, W. J.: Pheochromocytoma with hypermetabolism. Report of two cases. *Ann. Surg. 116*: 61–75, 1942.

641. McGavack, T. H., Benjamin, J. W., Speer, F. D., and Klotz, S.: Malignant pheochromocytoma of the adrenal medulla (paraganglioma) : report of case simulating carcinoma of the adrenal cortex with secondary adrenal insufficiency. *J. Clin. Endocrinol. 2*: 332–338, 1942.

642. McGuire, L. B., and Fox, L. M.: Recurrent pheochromocytoma and recognition of site of metastasis by means of venous catheterization. *Ann. Intern. Med. 60*: 125–130, 1964.

643. McLeish, G. R., and Adler, D.: Case of intrathoracic pheochromocytoma and hypertension. *Acta Med. Scand. 306 (suppl)*: 135, 1955.

644. McMillan M.: Identification of hydroxytyramine in a chromaffin tumour. *Lancet 2*: 284, 1956.

645. McNeill, A. D., Groden, B. M., and Neville, A. M.: Intrathoracic phaeochromocytoma. *Br. J. Surg. 57*: 457–462, 1970.

646. Meaney, T. F., and Buonocore, E.: Selective arteriography as a localizing and provocative test in the diagnosis of pheochromocytoma. *Radiology 87*: 309–314, 1966.

647. The Medical Letter. On Drugs and Therapeutics. Should propranolol be stopped before surgery? Vol. 18, No. 10 (Issue 452), May 7, 1976. The Medical Letter, Inc., Mark Abramowicz, Editor, 56 Harrison St., New Rochelle, N.Y. 10801.

648. Melicow, M. M.: Hibernating fat and pheochromocytoma. *Arch. Pathol. 63*: 367–372, 1957.

649. Melicow, M. M., Uson, A. C., and Veenema, R. J.: Malignant non-functioning pheochromocytoma of the organ of Zuckerkandl masquerading as a primary carcinoma of the prostate with metastases. *J. Urol. 110*: 97–103, 1973.

650. Melmon, K. L., Sjoerdsma, A., and Mason, D. T.: Distinctive clinical and therapeutic aspects of the syndrome associated with bronchial carcinoid tumors. *Am. J. Med. 39*: 568–581, 1965.

651. Melville, K. I., Blum, B., Shister, H. E., and Silver, M. D.: Cardiac ischemic changes and arrythmias induced by hypothalamic stimulation. *Am. J. Cardiol. 12*: 781–791, 1963.

652. Melvin, K. E. W., Miller, H. H., and Tashjian, A. H., Jr.: Early diagnosis of medullary carcinoma of the thyroid gland by means of calcitonin assay. *N. Engl. J. Med. 285*: 1115–1120, 1971.

653. Melvin, K. E. W., and Tashjian, A. H., Jr.: The syndrome of excessive thyrocalcitonin produced by medullary carcinoma of the thyroid. *Proc. Nat. Acad. Sci. 59*: 1216–1222, 1968.

654. Mena, E., Bookstein, J. J., Holt, J. F., and Fry, W. J.: Neurofibromatosis and renovascular hypertension in children. *Am. J. Roentgenol. Radium Ther. Nucl. Med. 118*: 39–45, 1973.

655. Mencher, W. H.: Perirenal insufflation. *J. Am. Med. Assoc. 109*: 1338–1341, 1937.

656. Menof, P.: Sudden enlargement of thyroid gland. *Lancet 2*: 996–999, 1954.

657. Meyer, J. S., Hutton, W. E., and Kenny, A. D.: Medullary carcinoma of the thyroid gland. Subcellular distribution of calcitonin and relationship between granules and amyloid. *Cancer 31*: 443–441, 1973.

657a. Meyer, J. S., Stoica, E., Pascu, L., Shimazu, K., and Hartmann, A.: Catecholamine concentrations in CSF and plasma of patients with cerebral infarction and haemorrhage. *Brain 96*: 277–288, 1973.

658. Meyer, P., Alexandre, J.-M., Devaux, C., Leroux-Robert, C., and Milliez, P.: Détermination de l'activité rénine plasmatique chez 261 hypertendus. *Presse Med. 74*: 2025–2030, 1966.

659. Meyers, M. A.: Characteristic radiographic shapes of pheochromocytomas and adrenocortical adenomas. *Radiology 87*: 889–892, 1966.

660. Meyers, M. A.: *Diseases of the Adrenal Glands: Radiologic Diagnosis with Emphasis on the Use of Presacral Retroperitoneal Pneumography.* Springfield, Ill., C. C. Thomas, 1963. 97 pp.

661. Meyers, M. A., and King, M. C.: Unusual radiologic features of pheochromocytoma. *Clinical Radiol. 20*: 52–56, 1969.

662. Mićić, R., Kićić, M., and Adanja, S.: Pheochromocytoma of urinary bladder. *Acta Endocrinol. 39*: 1–12, 1962.

663. Miles, R. M. Pheochromocytoma—interesting experiences with three cases. *Ann. Surg. 149*: 925–934, 1959.

664. Milhaud, G., Tubiana, M., Parmentier, C., and Coutris, G.: Epithélioma de la thyroide sécrétant de la thyrocalcitone. *C. R. Acad. Sci. Ser. (D) 266*: 608–610, 1968.

665. Miller, G. L., and Wynn, J.: Acromegaly, pheochromocytoma, toxic goiter, diabetes mellitus and endometriosus. *Arch. Intern. Med. 127*: 299–303, 1971.

665a. Miller, H. H., Melvin, K. E. W., Gibson, J. M., and Tashjian, A. H., Jr.: Surgical approach to early familial medullary carcinoma of the thyroid gland. *Am. J. Surg. 123*: 438–443, 1972.

666. Miller, J. W.: Ein paragangliom des Brustsympathicus. *Centralbl. Allg. Pathol. Anat. 35*: 85–94, 1924.

667. Miller, S. S., Sizemore, G. W., Sheps, S. G., and Tyce, G. M.: Parathyroid function in patients with pheochromocytoma. *Ann. Intern. Med. 82*: 372–375, 1975.

668. Minno, A. M., Bennett, W. A., and Kvale, W. F.: Pheochromocytoma. A study of 15 cases diagnosed at autopsy. *N. Engl. J. Med. 251*: 959–965, 1954.

669. Misugi, K., Misugi, N., and Newton, W. A.: Fine structural study of neuroblastoma, ganglioneuroblastoma, and pheochromocytoma. *Arch. Pathol. 86*: 160–170, 1968.

670. Mitchell, S. C., Blount, S. G., Jr., Blumenthal, S., Hoffman, J. I. E., Jesse, M. J., Lauer, R. M., and Weidman, W. H.: The pediatrician and hypertension. *Pediatrics 56*: 3–5, 1975.

671. Miyahara, M.: Catecholamines and hemodynamic changes in hypertension. *Jpn. Circ. J. 30*: 157–162, 1966.

672. Moertel, C. G., Beahrs, O. H., Woolner, L. B., and Tyce, G. M.: "Malignant carcinoid syndrome" associated with non-carcinoid tumors. *N. Engl. J. Med. 273*: 244–248, 1965.

673. Moir, W. W., and Crummy, A. B.: Calcified pheochromocytoma of the para-aortic body. *J. Urol. 107*: 15–16, 1972.

674. Montalbano, F. P., Baronofsky, I. D., and Ball, H. H.: Hyperplasia of the adrenal medulla. A clinical entity. *J. Am. Med. Assoc. 182*: 264–267, 1962.

675. Moon, H. D., Koneff, A. A., Li, C. C., and Simpson, M. E.: Pheochromocytomas of adrenals in male rats chronically injected with pituitary growth hormone. *Proc. Soc. Exp. Biol. Med. 93*: 74–77, 1956.

676. Moon, H. D., Simpson, M. E., Li, C. H., and Evans, H. M.: Neoplasms in rats treated with

pituitary growth hormone. II. Adrenal glands. *Cancer Res. 10*: 364–370, 1950.

677. Moon, H. D., Simpson, M. E., Li, C. H., and Evans, H. M.: Neoplasms in rats treated with pituitary growth hormone III. Reproductive organs *Cancer Res. 10*: 549–556, 1950.

678. Moon, H. D., Simpson, M. E., Li, C. H., and Evans, H. M.: Neoplasms in rats treated with pituitary growth hormone V. Absence of neoplasms in hypophysectomized rats. *Cancer Res. 11*: 535–539, 1951.

679. Moon, V. H.: *Shock: Its Dynamics, Occurrence and Management.* Philadelphia: Lea & Febiger, 1942, p. 48.

680. Moorhead, E. L. II, Caldwell, J. R., Kelly, A. R., and Morales, A. R.: The diagnosis of pheochromocytoma. Analysis of 26 cases. *J. Am. Med. Assoc. 196*: 1107–1113, 1966.

681. Moser, M., Sheehan, G., and Schwinger, H.: Pheochromocytoma with calcification simulating cholelithiasis. Report of a EGSC. *Radiology 55*: 855–858, 1950.

682. Moser, M., Watkins, D., Morris, N., Prandoni, A. G., and Mattingly, T. W.: Effect of Dibenzyline on skin temperature, peripheral blood flow, and vasomotor responses in normal patients and patients with increased vaso-constrictor tone. *Circulation 8*: 224–231, 1953.

683. Moskowitz, M. A., and Wurtman, R. J.: Catecholamines and neurologic diseases. (First of two parts.) *N. Engl. J. Med. 292*: 274–280, 1975.

684. Moskowitz, M. A., and Wurtman, R. J.: Catecholamines and neurologic diseases. (Second of two parts.) *N. Engl. J. Med. 292*: 332–338, 1975.

685. Moyer, J. H., and Handley, C. A.: Norepinephrine and epinephrine effect on renal hemodynamics. *Circulation 5*: 91–97, 1952.

685a. Mudge, G. H., Jr., Grossman, W., Mills, R. M., Jr., Lesch, M., and Braunwald, E.: Reflex increase in coronary vascular resistance in patients with ischemic heart disease. *N. Engl. J. Med. 295*: 1333–1336, 1976.

686. Mueller, P. S., and Horwitz, D.: Plasma free fatty acid and blood glucose responses to analogues of norepinephrine in man. *J. Lipid Res. 3*: 251–255, 1962.

687. Mullholland, S. G., Atuk, N. O., and Walzak, M. R.: Familial pheochromocytoma associated with cerebellar hemangioblastoma. A case history and review of the literature. *J. Am. Med. Assoc. 207*: 1709–1711, 1969.

688. Mulrow, P. J., Cohn, G. L. and Yesner, R. R.: Isolation of cortisol from a pheochromocytoma. *Yale J. Biol. Med. 31*: 363–372, 1959.

689. Munk, Z. M., Tolis, G.: Furosemide screening test and pheochromocytoma. *Ann. Intern. Med. 83*: 739–740, 1975.

690. Murphy, M., Prior, F. N., and Joseph, S.: Halothane and blood transfusion for phaeochromocytoma. A case report. *Br. J. Anaesth. 36*: 813–815, 1964.

691. Muscholl, E.: Die Hemmung der Noradrenalin-Aufnahme des Herzens durch Reserpin und die Wirkung von Tyramin. *Naunyn-Schmiedeberg's Arch. Pharmakol. Exp. Pathol. 240*: 234–241, 1960.

N

692. Naftchi, N. E., Lowman, E. W., Sell, G. H., and Rusk, H. A.: Peripheral circulation and catecholamine metabolism in paraplegia and quadriplegia. *Archives Phys. Med. Rehabil. 53*: 357–361, 1972.

693. Naftchi, N. E., Wooten, G. F., Lowman, E. W., and Axelrod, J.: Relationship between serum dopamine-β-hydroxylase activity, catecholamine metabolism, hemodynamic changes during paroxysmal hypertension in quadriplegia. *Circ. Res. 35*: 850–861, 1974.

694. Nagatsu, T., Levitt, M., and Udenfriend, S.: Tyrosine hydroxylase—the initial step in norepinephrine biosynthesis. *J. Biol. Chem. 239*: 2910–2917, 1964.

695. Nagatsu, T., Yamamoto, T., and Nagatsu, I.: Partial separation and properties of tyrosine hydroxylase from the human pheochromocytoma. Effect of Norepinephrine. *Biochim. Biophys. Acta 198*: 210–218, 1970.

696. Nahas, G. G., Manger, W. M., Mittleman, A., and Ultman, J. E.: The use of 2-amine-2-hydroxymethyl-1, 3-propanediol in the correction of addition acidosis and its effect on sympathoadrenal activity. *Ann. N. Y. Acad. Sci. 92*: 596–616, 1961.

697. Nahas, G. G., Zagury, D., Milhaud, A., Manger, W. M., and Pappas, G. D.: Acidemia and catecholamine output of the isolated canine adrenal gland. *Physiol. 213*: 1186–1192, 1967.

698. Nakada, T., Momose, G., and Yoshida, T.: Diagnosis of adrenal hypertension. I. Selective adrenal venography and pharmacological evaluation using catheter technique for detecting pheochromocytoma. *J. Urol. 109*: 757–760, 1968.

699. Nakano, Y., Imura, H., Yawata, M., Shinpo, S., Ikeda, M., Morimoto, M., Manabe, S., Kato, Y., and Fukase, M.: 3rd. International Congress of Endocrinology, Mexico, D.G., 1968. Abstracts of Brief Communications, Gual, C., ed. *Excerpta Medica Foundation*, Amsterdam, New York, 1968, p. 63.

700. Neff, F. C., Tice, G. M., Walker, G. A., and Ockerblad, N.: Adrenal tumor in female infant with hypertrichosis, hypertension, overdevelopment of external genitalia, obesity, but absence of breast enlargement. *J. Clin. Endocrinol. 2*: 125–127, 1942.

701. Neil, D. W., Carre, I. J., McCorry, R. L., and Thompson, R. H.: A possible source of error in diagnosis of pheochromocytoma. *J. Clin. Pathol. 14*: 415–417, 1961.

702. Neill, C. A., and Smith, G.: Bilateral phaechromocytoma in a 6-year-old boy. *Arch. Dis. Child. 27*: 286–290, 1952.

703. Neimann, N., Pierson, M., Lesure, J., Vert, P., and Gilgenkranz, G.: Pheochromocytoma in a 10-year-old girl. Topographic diagnosis by determination of blood catecholamines at different levels. *Arch. Fr. Pediatr. 16*: 1372–1377, 1959.

704. Neville, A. M.: The Adrenal Medulla. *In:* Symington, T., ed., *Functional Pathology of the Human Adrenal Gland*, Baltimore, Williams and Wilkins, 1969. pp. 217–324.

705. Newton, T. H., Smith, G. I., Kolb, F. O., and Smith, D. R.: Successful use of Regitine (phentolamine) in the diagnosis and surgical management of

a case of pheochromocytoma; an apraisal of its clinical usefulness. *N. Engl. J. Med. 252*: 974–979, 1955.

706. Nibbelink, D. W., Peters, B. H., and McCormick, W. F.: On the association of pheochromocytoma and cerebeller hemangioblastoma. *Neurology 19*: 455–460, 1969.

707. Nickerson, M.: The pharmacology of adrenergic blockade. *Pharmacol. Rev. 1*: 27–101, 1949.

708. Nickerson, M., and Collier, B.: Drugs inhibiting adrenergic nerves and structures innervated by them. *In*: Goodman, L. S. and Gilman, A., eds., *The Pharmacological Basis of Therapeutics*, 5th ed. New York, Macmillan, 1975, Chap. 26, pp. 533–564.

709. Niijima, T., Takata, M., Shimizu, K., and Ohashi, T.: Surgical diseases of the adrenal. Clinical observation of 7 cases of pheochromocytoma. *Acta Urol. Japonica 19*: 1021–1029, 1973.

710. Northfield, T. C.: Cardiac complications of phaeochromocytoma. *Br. Heart J. 29*: 588–593, 1967.

711. Nourok, D. S.: Familial pheochromocytoma and thyroid carcinoma. *Ann. Intern. Med. 60 (Suppl. 5)*: 1028–1040, 1964.

712. Nourok, D. S., Gwinup G., and Hamwi, G. J.: Phentolamine-resistant pheochromocytoma treated with sodium nitroprusside. *J. Am. Med. Assoc. 183*: 841–844, 1963.

713. Nyman, D., and Wahlberg, P.: Necrotic phaeochromocytoma with gastric haemorrhage, shock, and uncommonly high catecholamine excretion. *Acta Med. Scand. 187*: 381–383, 1970.

O

714. Oberling, C., and Jung, G.: Paragangliome de la surrénale avec hypertension artérielle; à propos du choc obstétrical. *Bull. Soc. R. Belge Gynecol. Obstet. 16*: 279–283, 1927.

715. Ogata, T., and Ogata, A.: Über die Henle'sche Chromreaktion der sogenannten chromaffinen Zellen und den mikrochemischen Nachweis des Adrenalins. *Beitr. Pathol. Anat. Allg. Pathol. 71*: 376–387, 1923.

716. O'Gorman, L. P.: Improved technique for the estimation of VMA in serum. *Clin. Chim. Acta 23*: 247, 1969.

717. O'Higgins, N. J., Cullen, M. J., and Hefferman, A. G.: A case of acromegaly and phaeochromocytoma. *J. Ir. Med. Assoc. 60*: 213–216, 1967.

718. Öhman, U., Granberg, P.-O., Hjern, B., and Sjöberg, H. E.: Pheochromocytoma, *Acta Chir. Scand. 140*: 660–666, 1974.

719. Oliver, D. O.: The diagnosis and management of phaeochromocytoma. *Hosp. Med. 2*: 1279–1284, 1968.

720. Oliver, M. F., Kurien, V. A., and Greenwood, T. W.: Relation between serum-free-fatty-acids and arrhythmias and death after acute myocardial infarction. *Lancet 1*: 710–714, 1968.

721. Olson, H. H., Paulson, P. S., Beilin, L. B., and Ohtake, C.: Pheochromocytoma: Current concepts of diagnosis and management. A report of combined pheochromocytoma and multiple hepatic hamartomas. *Am. Surg. 37*: 455–466, 1971.

722. Orgain, E. S.: Pheochromocytoma: The value of certain tests used routinely in diagnosis. *Ann. Intern. Med. 43*: 1178–1194, 1955.

723. Ortega, P. Jr.: Malignant paraganglioma arising from the organs of Zuckerkandl. Report of a case with autopsy observations. *Arch. Pathol. 53*: 78–86, 1952.

724. Ortiz, F. T., and Diaz, P. M.: Use of enflurane for pheochromocytoma removal. *Anesthesiology 42*: 495–497, 1975.

725. Otten, U., and Theonen, H.: Circadian rhythm of tyrosine-hydroxylase induction by short-term cold stress: modulatory action of corticoids in newborn and adult ráts. *Proc. Natl. Acad. Sci. U.S.A. 72*: 1415–1419, 1975.

726. Overholt, R. H., Ramsay, B. H., and Meissner, W. A.: Intrathoracic pheochromocytoma; Report of a case. *Dis. Chest. 17*: 55–62, 1950.

P

727. Page, I. H.: Syndrome simulating diencephalic stimulation occurring in patients with essential hypertension. *Am. J. Med. Sci. 190*: 9–14, 1935.

728. Page, L. B., and Copeland, R. B.: Pheochromocytoma. *In*: Dowling, H. F., ed., Chicago. *Disease-a-Month*. Chicago Year Book Medical Publishers, January, 1968.

729. Page, L. B., and Jacoby, G. A.: Catecholamine metabolism and storage granules in pheochromocytoma and neuroblastoma. *Medicine 43*: 379–386, 1964.

730. Page, L. B., Raker, J. W., and Berberich, F. R.: Pheochromocytoma with predominant epinephrine secretion. *Am. J. Med. 47*: 648–652, 1969.

731. Palmer, R. S., and Castleman, B.: Paraganglioma (chromaffinoma, pheochromocytoma) of the adrenal gland simulating malignant hypertension: Report of a case. *N. Engl. J. Med. 219*: 793–796, 1938.

732. Paloyan, E., Paloyan, D., and Harper, P. V.: Glucagon-induced hypocalcemia. *Metabolism 16*: 35–39, 1967.

733. Pampari, D., and Lacerenza, C.: Intrathoracic pheochromocytoma. *J. Thoracic Surg. 36*: 174–181, 1958.

734. Paulshock, B. Z., and Miller, E. R.: Unsuspected pheochromocytoma resulting in postoperative death. *Ann. Intern. Med. 44*: 573–575, 1956.

735. Pearse, A. G. E.: Common cytochemical and ultrastructural characteristics of cells producing polypeptide hormones (the APUD series) and their relevance to thyroid and ultimobranchial C cells and calcitonin. *Proc. Roy. Soc. London, Ser. B 170*: 71–80, 1968.

736. Pearse, A. G. E.: Cytochemical evidence for the neural crest origin of mammalian ultimobranchial C cells. *Histochemie 27*: 96–102, 1971.

737. Pearse, A. G. E.: The genesis of APUD amyloid in endocrine polypeptide tumors: Histochemical distinction from immunoamyloid. *Virchows Arch. B 10*: 93–107, 1972.

737a. Pearson, K. D., Wells, S. A., and Keiser H. R.: Familial medullary carcinoma of the thyroid, adrenal pheochromocytoma and parathyroid hyperplasia. *Radiology 107*: 249–256, 1973.

738. Peart, W. S.: Persistence of hypertension after

removal of phaeochromocytoma where excretion of adrenaline and noradrenaline is normal, *In*: Wolstenholme, G. E. W. and Cameron, M. P., eds., *Ciba Foundation Symposium on Hypertension: Humoral and Neurogenic Factors.* Boston, Little, Brown, 1954. pp. 104–121.

739. Peelen, J. W., and DeGroat, A.: Pheocyromocytoma complicated by pregnancy: Case report. *Am. J. Obstet. Gynec. 69*: 1054–1061, 1955.

740. Pekkarinen, A.: Adrenaline and noradrenaline in blood and urine. *Pharmacol. Rev. 6*: 35–37, 1954.

741. Pekkarinen, A., Scheinin, T. M., and Näntö, V.: Localization of pheochromocytoma by vena caval catheterization and determination of plasma catecholamines. *Ann. Chir. Gynaecol. Fenn. 56*: 419–423, 1967.

742. Pelkonen, R., and Pitkanen, E.: Unusual electrocardiographic changes in pheochromocytoma. *Acta Med. Scand. 173*: 41–44, 1963.

743. Penfield, W.: Diencephalic autonomic epilepsy. *Arch. Neurol. and Psychiatry 22*: 358–374, 1929.

744. Perez, P. E., Harrison, E. G., Jr., and ReMine, W. H.: Vagal-body tumor (chemodectoma of the glomus-intravagale). *N. Engl. J. Med. 263*: 1116–1121, 1960.

745. Perrin, A., Mornex, R., Mansuy, L., Aimard, G., and Tomasi, M.: Phéochromocytome intrarachidien. *Rev. Lyon. Med. 18*: 577–580, 1969.

746. Perrin, A., Normand, J., Mornex, R., and Froment, R.: Phéochromocytome et athérosclérose coronarienne précoce. *Rev. Atheroscler. 2*: 211–221, 1960.

747. Perry, L. B., and Gould, A. B., Jr.: The anesthetic management of pheochromocytoma: Effect of preoperative adrenergic blocking drugs. *Anesth. Analg. (Cleveland) 51*: 36–40, 1972.

748. Pertsemlidis, D., Gitlow, S. E., Siegel, W. C., and Kork, A. E.: Pheochromocytoma: 1. Specificity of laboratory diagnostic tests. 2. Safeguards during operative removal. *Ann. Surg. 169*: 376–385, 1969.

749. Philips, B.: Intrathoracic pheochromocytoma. *Arch. Pathol. 30*: 916–921, 1940.

750. Philips, P. J., Coles, M. E., and Wise, P. H.: Cost of Diagnosis of phaeochromocytoma. *Med. J. Aust. 2*: 406–407, 1975.

751. Pick, L.: Das Ganglioma embryonale sympathicum (Sympathoma embryonale), eine typische bösartige geschwuestform des sympathischen nervensystems. *Berl. Klin. Wochenschr. 49*: 16–22, 1912.

752. Pickering, G. W.: *High Blood Pressure*, 2nd ed. New York, Grune and Stratton, 1968, 717 pp.

753. Pickering, R. S., Hartman, G. W., Weeks. R. E., Sheps, S. G., and Hattery, R. R.: Excretory urographic localization of adrenal cortical tumors and pheochromocytomas. *Radiology 114*: 345–349, 1975.

754. Pickles, B. G.: Pheochromocytoma complicating pregnancy. Maternal and/or fetal death following natural delivery. *J. Obstet. Gynaecol. Br. Emp. 65*: 1010, 1958.

755. Pincoffs, M. C.: A case of paroxysmal hypertension associated with suprarenal tumor. *Trans. Assoc. Am. Physicians 44*: 295–299, 1929.

756. Pinet, A., Mornex, R., Perrin, J., Tran Minh, V., and Veyret, Ch.: Une cause rare de sciatalgies:

phéochromocytome de la concavité sacrée érodant le sacrum et l' os iliaque. *J. Radiol. Electrol. 53*: 851–855, 1972.

757. Pisano, J. J.: A simple analysis for normetanephrine and metanephrine in urine. *Clin. Chim. Acta 5*: 406–414, 1960.

758. Pisano, J. J., Crout, J. R., and Abraham, D.: Determination of 3-methoxy-4-hydroxymandelic acid in urine. *Clin. Chem. Acta 7*: 285–291, 1962.

759. Pochedly, C.: *Neuroblastoma.* Acton, Mass., Publishing Sciences Group, 1976. 314 pp.

760. Poliquin, P. A., and Dupuis, P.: Adrenal pheochromocytoma without hypertension. *J. Am. Med. Assoc. 142*: 1021, 1950 (Abstr.).

761. Pollack, R. S.: Carotid body tumors—Idiosyncracies. *Oncology 27*: 81–91, 1973.

762. Polmieri, G., Ikkos, D., and Luft, R.: Malignant pheochromocytoma. *Acta Endocrinol. (Copenhagen) 36*: 549–560, 1961.

763. Poloyan, E., Scann, A., Straus, F. H., Pickleman, J. R., and Poloyan, D.: Familial pheochromocytoma, medullary thyroid carcinoma and parathyroid adenomas. *J. Am. Med. Assoc. 214*: 1443–1447, 1970.

764. Porte, D., Jr., Graber, A. L., Kuzuya, T., and Williams, R. H.: The effect of epinephrine on immunoreactive insulin levels in man. *J. Clin. Invest. 45*: 228–236, 1966.

765. Portnoy, B., Engleman, K., and Wyatt, R.: Plasma catecholamines in hypertensive and psychiatric disorders. *Clin. Res. 17*: 258, 1969.

766. Postlethwait, R. W.: Gastrointestinal carcinoid tumors: A review. *Postgrad. Med. 40*: 445, 1966.

767. Potter, E. L., and Parrish, J. M.: Neuroblastoma, ganglioneuroma, and fibroneuroma in a stillborn fetus. *Am. J. Pathol. 18*: 141–151, 1942.

768. Potter, L. T., and Axelrod, J.: Properties of norepinephrine storage particles of the rat heart. *J. Pharmacol. Exp. Ther. 442*: 299–305, 1963.

769. Poutasse, E. F., and Gifford, R. W., Jr.: Pheochromocytoma: diagnosis and treatment. *Prog. Cardiovasc. Dis. 8*: 235–252, 1965.

770. Prichard, B. N. C., and Ross, E. J.: Use of propranolol in conjunction with alpha receptor blocking drugs in pheochromocytoma *Am. J. Cardiol. 18*: 394–398, 1966.

771. Prout, B. J., and Wardell, W. M.: Sweating and peripheral blood flow in patients with pheochromocytoma. *Clin. Sci. 36*: 109–117, 1969.

772. Pryse-Davies, J., Dawson, I. M. P., and Westbury, G.: Some morphologic, histochemical and chemical observations on chemodectomas in the normal carotid body, including a study of the chromaffin reaction and possible ganglion cell elements. *Cancer 17*: 185–202, 1964.

773. Prys-Roberts, C., Corbett, J. L., Kerr, J. H., Crampton-Smith, A., and Spalding, J. M. K.: Treatment of sympathetic overactivity in tetanus. *Lancet 1*: 542–546, 1969.

774. Pullman, T. N., and McClure, W. W.: The effect of L-nor-adrenaline on electrolyte excretion in normal man. *J. Lab. Clin. Med. 39*: 711–719, 1952.

775. Pyörälä, K., Pitkänen, E., and Toivonen, S.: Alphamethyl-p-tyrosine in the symptomatic treatment of

patients with malignant pheochromocytoma. *Ann. Med. Intern. Fenn. 57*: 65–73, 1968.

R

776. Raab, W.: *Hormonal and Neurogenic Cardiovascular Disorders: Endocrine and Neuro-endocrine Factors in Pathogenesis and Treatment.* Baltimore, Williams and Wilkins, 1953, pp. 320–326.

777. Rabin C. B.: Chromaffin cell tumor of the suprarenal medulla (Pheochromocytoma). *Arch Pathol. 7*: 228–243, 1929.

778. Radtke, W. E., Kazmier, F. J., Rutherford, B. D., and Sheps, S. G.: Cardiovascular complications of pheochromocytoma crisis. *Am. J. Cardiol. 35*: 701–705, 1975.

779. Ramey, E. R., Goldstein, M. S., and Levine, R.: Action of nor-epinephrine and adrenal cortical steroids on blood pressure and work performance of adrenalectomized dogs. *Am. J. Physiol. 165*: 450–455, 1951.

780. Ramsay, L. D., and Langlands, J. H. M.: Phaeochromocytoma with hypotension and polycythaemia. *Lancet 2*: 126–128, 1962.

781. Ranges, H. A., and Bradley, S. E.: Systemic and renal circulatory changes following the administration of adrenin, ephedrine, and paradrinol to normal man. *J. Clin. Invest. 22*: 687–693, 1943.

782. Ratzenhofer, M., Auböck, L., and Müller, O.: Zur Kenntnis vom Feinbau und Sekretionsmechanismus der Phäochromocytome. *Beitr. Pathol. 137*: 36–64, 1968.

783. Reese, H. H. F.: Skin lesions and central nervous system diseases. *Postgrad. Med. J. 10*: 230–236, 1951.

784. Remine, W. H., Chong, G. C., van Heerden, J. A., Sheps, S. G., and Harrison, E. G., Jr.: Current management of pheochromocytoma. *Ann. Surg. 179*: 740–748, 1974.

785. Renzini, V., Brunori, C. A., and Valori, C.: A sensitive and specific fluorimetric method for the determination or noradrenaline and adrenaline in human plasma. *Clin. Chim. Acta 30*: 587–594, 1970.

786. Reynolds, J. L., and Gilchrist, T. F.: Congenital heart disease and pheochromocytoma. *Am. J. Dis. Child. 112*: 251–255, 1966.

787. Richards, A. N., and Plant, O. H.: Urine formation in the perfused kidney: The influence of adrenalin on the volume of the perfused kidney. *Am. J. Physiol. 59*: 184–190, 1922.

788. Richards, V., and Hatch, F. N.: Surgical experiences with pheochromocytoma. *Ann. Surg. 134*: 40–54, 1951.

789. Richardson, J. A., and Woods, E. F.: The effects of increased intracranial pressure on plasma catechol amine levels. Blood pressure and ventricular contractility. *J. Pharmacol. Exp. Ther. 119*: 179, 1957.

790. Richardson, K. C.: The fine structure of autonomic nerve endings in smooth muscle of the rat vas deferens. *J. Anat. 95*: 427–442, 1962.

791. Richmond, J., Frazer, S. C., and Millar, D. R.: Paroxysmal hypotension due to an adrenaline-secreting phaeochromocytoma. *Lancet 2*: 904–906, 1961.

792. Riddell, D. H., Schull, L., Frist, T. F., and Baker, T. D.: Experience with pheochromocytoma in 21 patients. Use of dichloroisoproterenol hydrochloride for cardic arrhythmia. *Ann. Surg. 157*: 980–988, 1963.

793. Riemer, R.: Sobre um caso de syndrome de Addison produzida por "paraganglioma da capsula suprarenal." *Folha Med. 8*: 33, 1927.

794. Riley, C. M.: Familial dysautonomia. *In*: Levine, S. Z., ed., *Advances in Pediatrics, Vol. 9.* Chicago, Year Book Medical Publishers, 1957, pp. 157–190.

795. Ritzel, G., Berger, H., and Roulet, D. L.: Increased catecholamine excretion in case of acrodynia (Pink disease). *Ann. Paediat. (Basel) 198*: 81–88, 1962.

796. Rizack, M. A.: An epinephrine-sensitive lipolytic activity in adipose tissue. *J. Biol. Chem. 236*: 657–662, 1961.

797. Roach, P. J.: Gastrointestinal bleeding in pheochromocytoma and following the administration of norepinephrine (Arterenol). *Arch. Intern. Med. 104*: 175–179, 1959.

798. Robertshaw, D.: Catecholamines and control of sweat glands. *In*: Blaschko, H., Sayers, G., and Smith, D. A., eds. *Vol. VI. Adrenal Gland. Handbook of Physiology, Sect. 7. Endocrinology.* Washington, D.C. Am. Physiological Society. 1975. pp. 591–603.

799. Robertson, A. I. G.: Anaesthetic management of phaeochromocytoma. *Proc. R. Soc. Med. 55*: 432–436, 1962.

799a. Robertson, D. M., Sizemore, G. W., and Gordon, H.: Thickened corneal nerves as a manifestation of multiple endocrine neoplasia. *Trans. Am. Acad. Ophthalmol. Otolaryngol. 79*: 772–787, 1975.

800. Rodin, F. H.: Hypertensive retinopathy associated with adrenal medullary tumor (pheochromocytoma). A new clinical entity. *Arch. Ophthalmol. 34*: 402–407, 1945.

801. Rogoff, J. M., Quashnock, J. M., Nixon, E. N., and Rosenberg, A. W.: Adrenal function and blood electrolytes. *Proc. Soc. Exp. Biol. Med. 73*: 163–169, 1950.

802. Roland, C. B.: Pheochromocytoma in pregnancy: report of a fatal reaction to phentolamine (Regitine) methane-sulfonate. *J. Am. Med. Assoc. 171*: 1806–1809, 1959.

803. Rollason, W N.: Halothane and phaeochromocytoma. A case report. *Br. J. Anaesth. 36*: 251–255, 1964.

804. Rosati, L. A., and Augur, N. A., Jr.: Ischemic enterocolitis in pheochromocytoma. *Gastroenterology 60*: 581–585, 1971.

805. Rose, A. G.: Catecholamine-induced myocardial damage associated with phaeochromocytomas and tetanus. *S. Afr. Med. J. 48*: 1285–1289, 1974.

806. Rosenberg, E. B.: The carcinoid syndrome and hypertension. *Arch. Intern. Med. 121*: 95–96, 1968.

807. Rosenberg, J. C., and Varco, R. L.: Physiologic and pharmocologic considerations in the management of phaeochromocytoma. *Surg. Clin. North Am. 47*: 1453–1460, 1967.

808. Rosenstein, B. J., and Engelman, K.: Diarrhea in a child with a catecholamine-secreting ganglio-

neuroma. Case report and review of the literature. *J. Pediatr. 63*: 217–266, 1963.

809. Rosenthal, I. M., Greenberg, R., Goldstein, R., Kathan, R., and Cadkin, L.: Catecholamine metabolism in a pheochromocytoma. Correlation with electron micrographs. *Am. J. Dis. Child. 112*: 389–395, 1966.

810. Rosenthal, I. M., Kathan, R. Falk, G. W., and Wong, R.: Catecholamine metabolism of ganglioneuroma; correlation with electromicrographs. *Pediatr. Res. 3*: 413–424, 1969.

811. Ross, E. J.: Clinical aspects of phaeochromocytoma. *Proc. R. Soc. Med. 65*: 16–17, 1972.

812. Ross, E. J.: The management of cases of pheochromocytoma. Clinical Staff Conference, University College Hospital, London. *Proc. R. Soc. Med. 55*: 427–436, 1962.

813. Ross, E. J., Prichard, B. N. C., Kaufman, L., Robertson, A. I. G., and Harries, B. J.: Preoperative and operative management of patients with pheochromocytoma. *Br. Med. J. 1*: 191–198, 1967.

814. Ross, L. L.: Electron microscopic observations of the carotid body of the cat. *J. Biophys. Biochem. Cytol. 6*: 253–262, 1959.

815. Ross, R. D.: False positive reaction to the Regitine test for pheochromocytoma: Report of a case. *Ann. Intern. Med. 41*: 1061–1066, 1954.

816. Rosse, W. F., and Waldmann, T. A.: A comparison of some physical and chemical properties of erythropoiesis-stimulating factors from different sources. *Blood 24*: 739–749, 1964.

817. Rossi, P., Young, I. S., and Panke, E. F.: Techniques, usefulness, and hazards of arteriography in pheochromocytoma. A review of 99 cases. *J. Am. Med. Assoc. 205*: 547–553, 1968.

818. Roth, G. M.: Laboratory diagnosis of pheochromocytoma. *Minn. Med. 41*: 297–300, 1958.

819. Roth, G. M., Dockerty, M. B., and Hightower, N. C., Jr.: Pheochromocytoma from the laboratory standpoint. *Surg. Clin. North Am. 32*: 1065–1077, 1952.

820. Roth, G. M., Flock, E. V., Kvale, W. F., Waugh, J. M., and Ogg, J.: Pharmacologic and chemical tests as an aid in the diagnosis of pheochromocytoma. *Circulation 21*: 769–778, 1960.

821. Roth, G. M., Hightower, N. C., Jr., Barker, N. W., and Priestley, J. T.: Familial pheochromocytoma: Report on three siblings with bilateral tumors. *Arch. Surg. 67*: 100–109, 1953.

822. Roth, G. M., and Kvale, W. F.: Tentative test for pheochromocytoma. *Am. J. Med. Sci. 210*: 653–660, 1945.

823. Roth, G. M., Kvale, W. F., Manger, W. M., and Priestley, J. T.: Pheochromocytoma. *Circulation 14*: 622–630, 1956.

824. Roth, G. M., Manger, W. M., Flock, E. V., and Kvale, W. F.: Difficulties and precautions concerned with the tests used as an aid in diagnosis of pheochromocytoma. *Acta Cardiol. 12*: 130, 1957 (Abstr.).

825. Roth, R. H., Stjärne, L., Levine, R. L., and Giarman, N. J.: Abnormal regulation of catecholamine synthesis in pheochromocytoma. *J. Lab. Clin. Med. 72*: 397–403, 1968.

826. Roux: Thesis, Lausanne, 1926. Cited by Barbeau, A., Marc-Aurèle, J., Brouillet, J., Vityé, B., Leboeuf, G., Cartier, P., Mignault, G., and Genest, J. Le phéochromocytome bilatéral: Presentation d'un cas et revue de la littérature. *Union Med. Can. 87*: 165–178, 1958.

827. Roux-Berger, J. L., Naulleau, J., and Contiadès, X. J.: Cortico-surrénalome malin. Aortographie. Exérèse. Guérison opératoire. *Bull. Mem. Soc. Chir. (Paris) 60*: 791–802, 1934.

828. Rowntree, L. G., and Ball, R. G.: Diseases of the suprarenal glands. *Endocrinol. 17*: 263–294, 1933.

829. Russell, D. S., and Rubenstein, L. J.: *Pathology of Tumuors of the Nervous System*, 3rd edition. Lumsden, C. E., ed., Baltimore, Williams and Wilkins, 1971, 344 pp.

830. Ruthven, C. R. J., and Sandler, M.: Estimation of homovanillic acid in urine. *Anal. Biochem. 8*: 282–292, 1964.

S

831. Saavedra, J. M., Grobecker, H., and Axelrod, J.: Adrenaline-forming enzyme in brain stem: elevation in genetic and experimental hypertension. *Science 191*, 483–484, 1976.

832. Sack, H., and Koll, J. F.: Das Phäochromocytom. *Ergeb. Inn. Med. Kinderheilk. 19*: 446–555, 1963.

833. Sack, H., and Koll, J.: *Der Symptomatische Hochdruck*. Stuttgart, Ferdinand Enke Verlag, 1959, pp. 19 and 45.

834. Sagher, F., and Even-Paz, Z.: *Mastocytosis and the Mast Cell*. Chicago, Year Book Medical Publishers, 1967, 427 pp.

835. Saint-Pierre, A., Lejosne, Ch., and Perrin, A.: Aspects electrocardiographiques des pheochromocytomes. *Coeur Med. Interne 13*: 59–73, 1974.

836. Saint-Pierre, A., Perrin, A., Mornex, R., and Pouzeratte, J.-P.: Les troubles du rythme cardiaque dus aux phéochromocytomes (et forme rythmique pure). *Coeur et Med. Interne 9*: 3–11, 1970.

837. Salo, M., and Laaksonen, V.: The maintenance of the circulation during anaesthesia in patients with phaeochromocytoma. *Ann. Chir. Gynaecol. Fenn. 61*: 142–151, 1072.

838. Salo, M., and Vapaavuori, M.: Anaesthesiological aspects of the operative treatment of phaechromocytoma. *Ann. Chir. Gynaecol. Fenn. 61*: 129–132, 1972.

839. Saltz, N. J., Luttwak, E. M., Schwartz, A., and Goldberg, G. M.: Danger of aortography in the localization of pheochromocytoma. *Ann. Surg. 144*: 118–123, 1956.

840. Samaan, H. A.: Risk of operation in a patient with unsuspected phaeochromocytoma. *Br. J. Surg. 57*: 462–465, 1970.

841. Samols, E., Marri, G., and Marks, V.: Interrelationship of glucagon, insulin and glucose. The insulinogenic effect of glucagon. *Diabetes 15*: 855–866, 1966.

842. Samuels, A. J.: Primary and secondary leucocyte changes following the intramuscular injection of epinephrine hydrochloride. *J. Clin. Invest. 30*: 941–947, 1951.

843. Sandberg A. A., Nelson, D. H., Palmer, J. G., Samuels, L. T., and Tyler, F. H.: The effects of epinephrine on the metabolism of 17-hydroxycorticosteroids in the human. *J. Clin. Endocrinol. 13*: 629–647, 1953.

844. Sandler, M. Karim, S. M. M., and Williams, E. D.: Prostaglandins in amine-peptide-secreting tumours. *Lancet 2*: 1053–1054, 1968.

845. Sandler, M., and Ruthven, C. R. J.: Estimation of catecholamine metabolites in urine. *Assoc. of Clin. Pathologists Broadsheet 82*: 1–7, 1974.

846. Sandler, M., and Ruthven, C. R. J.: The measurement of 4-hydroxy-3-methoxymandelic acid and homovanillic acid. *Pharmacol. Rev. 18*: 343–351, 1966.

847. Sands, M. J., McDonough, M. T., Cohen, A. M., Rutenberg, H. L., and Eisner, J. W.: Fatal malignant degeneration in multiple neurofibromatosis. *J. Am. Med. Assoc. 233*: 1381–1382, 1975.

848. Santos, D. E., de la Paz, A., Ninos, N. P., Tobin, J. R., and Gunnar, R. M.: Phentolamine (Regitine) test in cerebrovascular accidents. *Arch. Intern. Med. 117*: 752–756, 1966.

849. Sapira, J. P., Altman, M., Vandyk, K. D., and Shapiro, A. P.: Bilateral adrenal pheochromocytoma and medullary thyroid carcinoma. *N. Engl. J. Med. 273*: 140–143, 1965.

850. Sarosi, G., and Doe, R. P.: Familial occurrence of parathyroid adenomas, pheochromocytoma, and medullary carcinoma of the thyroid with amyloid stroma (Sipple's syndrome). *Ann. Intern. Med. 68*: 1305–1309, 1968.

851. Sato, T., Ishida, N., Itoh, C., Wada, Y., and Yoshinaga, K.: Studies on the metabolism of catecholamines in pheochromocytoma. *Tohoku J. Exp. Med. 76*: 313–318, 1962.

852. Sato, T., Kobayashi, K., Miura, Y., Sakuma, H., Yoshinaga, K., and Nakamura, K.: High epinephrine content in the adrenal tumors from Sipple's syndrome. *Tohoku J. Exp. Med. 115*: 15–19, 1975.

853. Sato, T., Ono, I., Miura, Y., and Yoshinaga, K.: Increased catecholamine excretion during normotensive phase in paroxysmal type of pheochromocytoma. *Jpn. Heart J. 12*: 214–220, 1971.

854. Sato, T., Saito, H., Yoshinaga, K., Shibota, Y., and Sasano, N.: Concurrence of carotid body tumor and pheochromocytoma. *Cancer 34*: 1787–1795, 1974.

855. Sato, T. L., and Sjoerdsma, A.: Urinary homovanillic acid in pheochromocytoma. *Br. Med. J. II*: 1472–1473, 1965.

856. Sayer, W. J., Moser, M., and Mattingly, T. W.: Pheochromocytoma and the abnormal electrocardiogram. *Am. Heart J. 48*: 42–53, 1954.

857. Schaepdryver, A. F., de: Cited by Maynert, E. W., in summary of discussion and commentary of Sect. IV, Properties of adrenergic tissues. Second symposium on catecholamines. *Pharmacol. Rev. 18*: 457–458, 1966.

858. Schaepdryver, A. F., de: Fluorimetric estimation of adrenaline and noradrenaline in urine and blood and diagnosis of chromaffin cell tumors. *Arch. Int. Pharmacodyn. 121*: 489–505, 1959.

859. Schaepdryver, A. F., de, and Leroy, J. G.: Urine volume and catecholamine excretion in man. *Acta Cardiol. 16*: 631–638, 1961.

860. Schafer, E. L.: Hypertonie bei hormonalen Erkrankungen und ihre Therapie. *Med. Welt 39*: 1824, (1959).

861. Schega, W.: Chirurgie des Nebennierenmarks, *Chirurg. 40*: 304–308, 1969.

862. Schenkein, I., Bueker, E. D., Helson, L., Axelrod, F., and Dancis, J. Increased nerve-growth stimulation in disseminated neurofibromatosis. *N. Engl. J. Med. 290*: 613–614, 1974.

863. Schenker, J. G., and Chowers, I.: Pheochromocytoma and pregnancy. *Obstet. and Gynecol. Surg. 26*: 739–747, 1971.

864. Schimke, R. N., and Hartmann, W. H.: Familial anyloid-producing medullary thyroid carcinoma and pheochromocytoma. A distinct genetic entity. *Ann. Intern. Med. 63*: 1027–1039, 1965.

865. Schimke, R. N., Hartmann, W. H., Prout, T. E., and Rimoin, D. L.: Syndrome of bilateral pheochromocytoma, medullary thyroid carcinoma and multiple neuromas. A possible regulatory defect in the differentiation of chromaffin tissue. *N. Engl. J. Med. 279*: 1–7, 1968.

866. Schlegel, G. G., von: Neurofibromatose Recklinghausen und Phäochromocytom. *Schweiz. Med. Wochenschr. 90*: 31–39, 1960.

867. Schmid, R.: Porphyria. *In*: Beeson, P. B., and McDermott, W., eds., *Cecil-Loeb Textbook of Medicine*, 13th edition. Philadelphia, London, Toronto, W. B. Saunders, 1971, pp. 1704–1706.

868. Schnelle, N., Carney, F. M. T., Didier, E. P., and Faulconer, A., Jr.: Anesthesia for surgical treatment of pheochromocytoma. *Surg. Clin. North Am. 45*: 991–1001, 1965.

869. Schnelle, N., Ferris, D. O., and Schirger, A.: The use of blood volume determination in patients undergoing surgery for pheochromocytoma. *Anesth. Analg. (Cleveland) 43*: 641–645, 1964.

870. Schoket E., and Teloh, H. A.: Case report: Aganglionic magacolon, pheochromocytoma, megaloureter and neurofibroma: concurrence of several neural abnormalities. *Am. J. Dis. Child. 94*: 185–191, 1957.

871. Scholes, G. B., Eley, K. G., and Bennett, A.: Effect of prostaglandins on intestinal motility. *Gut 9*: 726, 1968.

872. Schümann, H. J.: Hormon-und ATP-Gehalt des menschlichen Nebennierenmarks und des Phäochromocytomgewebes. *Klin. Wochenschr. 38*: 11–13, 1960.

873. Schümann, H. J.: The distribution of adrenaline and noradrenaline in chromaffin granules from the chicken. *J. Physiol. 137*: 318–326, 1957.

874. Schurch, W., Messerli, F. H., and Genest, J.: Arterial hypertension and neurofibromatosis. Renal artery stenosis and coarctation of abdominal aorta. *Can. Med. Assoc. J. 113*: 879–885, 1975.

875. Schwartz, D. T.: Relation of intestinal carcinoid to renal hypertension. *Angiology 21*: 568–574, 1970.

875a. Scott, H. W., Jr., Oates, J. A., Nies, A. S., Burko, H., Page, D. L., and Rhamy, R. K.: Pheochromocytoma: Present diagnosis and management. *Ann. Surg. 183*: 587–593 1976.

876. Scott, H. W., Jr., Riddell, D. H., and Brockman, S. K.: Surgical management of pheochromocytoma. *Surg. Gynecol. Obstet. 120:* 707–724, 1965.

877. Scott, W. W., and Eversole, S. L.: Pheochromocytoma of the urinary bladder. *J. Urol. 83:* 656–664, 1960.

877a. Seegal, B. C., Hsu, K. C., Lattimer, J. K., Habif, D. V., and Tannenbaum, M.: Immunoglobulins, complement and foreign antigens in human tumor cells. *Intern. Arch. Allergy,* in press.

878. Sellwood, R. A., Wapnick, S., Breckenridge, A. Williams, E. D., and Welbourn, R. B.: Recurrent phaeochromocytoma. *Br. J. Surg. 57:* 309–312, 1970.

879. Shand, D. G.: Propranolol. *In:* Dowling, H. F., ed. *Disease-a-Month.* Chicago, Year Book Medical Publishers, Oct., 1974.

880. Shapiro, A. P., Baker, H. M., Hoffman, M. S., and Ferris, E. B.: Pharmacologic and physiologic studies of a case of pheochromocytoma. *Am. J. Med. 10:* 115–130, 1951.

881. Shaw, K. N. F., and Trevarthen, J.: Exogenous sources of urinary phenol and indole acids. *Nature 182:* 797–798, 1958.

882. Shepherd, D. M., and West, G. B.: Hydroxytyramine and the adrenal medulla. *J. Physiol. 120:* 15–19, 1953.

883. Sheps, S. G.: Tests for pheochromocytoma. *N. Engl. J. Med. 279:* 45–46, 1968.

884. Sheps, S. G., Kottke, B. A., Tyce, G. M., and Flock, E. V.: Effect of methyldopa on the metabolism of catecholamines and tryptophan in metastatic pheochromocytoma: Report of two cases. *Am. J. Cardiol. 14:* 641–649, 1964.

885. Sheps, S. G., Kottke, B. A., Tyce, G. M., and Flock, E. V.: Effect of methyldopa on the metabolism of catecholamines and tryptophan in two cases of metastatic pheochromocytoma. *Circulation 28:* 804, 1963 (abstr.).

886. Sheps, S. G., and Maher, F. T.: Comparison of the histamine and tyramine hydrochloride tests in the diagnosis of pheochromocytoma. *J. Am. Med. Assoc. 195:* 265–267, 1966.

887. Sheps, S. G., and Maher, F. T.: Histamine and glucagon tests in diagnosis of pheochromocytoma. *J. Am. Med. Assoc. 205:* 895–899, 1968.

888. Sheps, S. G., Tyce, G. M., Flock, E. V., and Maher, F. T.: Current experience in the diagnosis of pheochromocytoma. *Circulation 34:* 473–483, 1966.

889. Sherwin R. P.: Histopathology of pheochromocytoma. *Cancer 12:* 861–877, 1959.

890. Sherwin, R. P.: The adrenal medulla, paraganglia and related tissues. *In:* Bloodworth, J. M. B., Jr., ed., *Endocrine Pathology.* Baltimore, Williams and Wilkins 1968, pp. 256–315.

891. Shimbo, S., and Nakano, Y.: A case of malignant pheochromocytoma producing parathyroid hormone-like substance. *Calcif. Tissue Res. 15:* 155–156, 1974.

892. Shipley, A. M.: Paroxysmal hypertension associated with tumor of the suprarenal. *Ann. Surg. 90:* 742–749, 1929.

893. Shishito, S., and Watanabe, H.: Blood pressure control after the removal of pheochromocytoma. *Urol. Int. 22:* 301–311, 1967.

894. Shrago, G. G., McKinnon, C. M., and Clark, R.: Adrenal tumors simulating intrarenal lesions. *Am. J. Roentgenol. Radium Ther. Nucl. Med. 121:* 518–522, 1974.

895. Silbergeld, E. K., and Chisolm, J. J.: Lead poisoning: Altered urinary catecholamine metabolites as indicators of intoxication in mice and children. *Science 192:* 153–155, 1976.

896. Silverman, L., Dahlin, D. C. Tyce, G. M. and Stickler, G. B.: Ganglioneuroblastoma. Studies of pathologic changes and content of catecholamine. *Am. J. Clin. Pathol. 42:* 145–151, 1964.

897. Sipple, J. H.: The association of pheochromocytoma with carcinoma of the thyroid gland. *Am. J. Med. 31:* 163–166, 1961.

898. Siqueira-Filho, A. G., Sheps, S. G., Maher, F. T., Jiang, N.-S., and Elveback, L. R.: Glucagon-blood catecholamine test: Used in isolated and familial pheochromocytoma. *Arch. Intern. Med. 135:* 1227–1231, 1975.

899. Sivapragasam, S., Nickerson, G., and Morgan, O.: Systemic hypertension in the Guillain-Barré syndrome. *IRCS J. Med. Sci. 4:* 342, 1976.

900. Sivula, A.: Recurrence of benign phaeochromocytoma by intraoperative implantation. *Acta Chir. Scand. 140:* 334–339, 1974.

901. Sizemore, G. W., Beahrs, O. H., Capen, C. C., *et al.*: Multiple endocrine neoplasia, Type 2b: A familial syndrome of mucosal neuromas and connective tissue abnormalities with C-cell hyperplasia or medullary carcinoma of the thyroid gland, pheochromocytoma, and normal parathyroid glands. In press.

902. Sizemore, G. W., and Go, V. L. W.: Stimulation tests for diagnosis of medullary thyroid carcinoma. *Mayo Clin. Proc. 50:* 53–56, 1975.

903. Sizemore, G. W., Go, V. L. W., Kaplan, E. L., Sanzenbacher, L. J., Holtermuller, K. H., and Arnaud, C. D.: Relations of calcitonin and gastrin in the Zollinger–Ellison syndrome and medullary carcinoma of the thyroid. *N. Engl. J. Med. 288:* 641–644, 1973.

903a. Sizemore, G. W., and Heath, H., III.: Pentagastrin injection is superior to calcium infusion for the diagnosis of familial medullary thyroid carcinoma. *Clin. Res. 24:* Abstr. 584A, 1976.

904. Sizemore, G. W., and Winternitz, W. W.: Autonomic hyper-reflexia-supression with alpha-adrenergic blocking agents. *N. Engl. J. Med. 282:* 795, 1970.

905. Sjoerdsma, A.: Catecholamine metabolism in patients with pheochromocytoma. *Pharmacol. Rev. 11:* 374–378, 1959.

906. Sjoerdsma, A.: Newer biochemical approaches to treatment of hypertension. *Ann. N.Y. Acad. Sci. 88:* 933–938, 1960.

907. Sjoerdsma, A.: Sympatho-adrenal system: Pheochromocytoma. *In:* Beeson, P. B., and McDermott, W., eds., *Cecil-Loeb Textbook of Medicine,* 13th edition. Philadelphia, London, Toronto, W. B. Saunders, 1971, pp. 1832–1836.

908. Sjoerdsma, A., Engelman, K., Spector, S., and Udenfriend, S.: Inhibition of catecholamine synthe-

sis in man with alpha-methyl tyrosine, an inhibitor of tyrosine hydroxylase. *Lancet 2*: 1092–1094, 1965.

909. Sjoerdsma, A., Engelman, K., Waldmann, T. A., Cooperman, L. H., and Hammond, W. G.: Pheochromocytoma: Current concepts of diagnosis and treatment. *Ann. Intern. Med. 65*: 1302–1325, 1966.

910. Sjoerdsma, A. Leeper, L. C., Terry, L. L., and Udenfriend, S.: Studies on the biogenesis and metabolism of norepinephrine in patients with pheochromocytoma. *J. Clin. Invest. 38*: 31–38, 1959.

911. Sjöstrand, T.: After-potentials in the electrocardiogram. *Acta Physiol. Scand. 24*: 247–260, 1951.

912. Skopin, I. V., Tatarinova, T. E., Freidman, S. L., and Bender, K. I.: Simulated arterial hypertension produced with large doses of ephedrine and theophedrine. *Terk. Arkh. 32*: 64–65, 1960.

913. Slavotinek, A., de la Lande, I. S., and Head, R.: Medullary thyroid carcinomas with bilateral phaeochromocytomas. *Aust. Ann. Med. 17*: 320–326, 1968.

913a. Sleisenger, M. H.: Diseases of the gallbladder and bile ducts. *In*: Beeson, P. B. and McDermott, W., eds. *Cecil and Loeb Textbook of Medicine*, 13th edit. Philadelphia, London, Toronto. W. B. Saunders, 1971, p. 1406.

913b. Sletten, K., Westermark, P., and Natvig, J. B.: Characterization of amyloid fibril proteins from medullary carcinoma of the thyroid. *J. Exp. Med. 143*: 993–998, 1976.

914. Smith, A. A., and Dancis, J.: Exaggerated response to infused norepinephrine in familial dysautonomia. *N. Engl. J. Med. 270*: 704–707, 1964.

914a. Smith, A. A., and Dancis, J.: Response to intradermal histamine in familial dysautonomia—a diagnostic test. *J Pediatr. 63*: 889–894, 1963.

915. Smith, A. D., Gitlow, S., Gall, E., Wortis, S. B., and Mendlowitz, M.: Effect of disulfiram and ethanol on the metabolism of dl-beta-H³-norepinephrine. *Clin. Res. 8*: 367, 1960.

916. Smith, A. D., and Winkler, H.: Fundamental mechanisms in the release of catecholamines. *In*: Blaschko, H., and Muscholl. E., eds. *Catecholamines*. Berlin, Heidelberg, New York, Springer-Verlag, 1972, Chap. 13, pp. 538–605.

917. Smith, A. M.: Phaeochromocytoma and pregnancy. *J. Obstet. Gynaecol. 80*: 848–851, 1973.

917a. Smith, C. J., Hatch, F. E., Johnson, J. G., and Kelly, B. J.: Renal artery dysplasia as a cause of hypertension in neurofibromatosis. *Arch. Intern. Med. (Chicago) 125*: 1022, 1970

918. Smithwick, R. H.: Surgical measures in hypertension. *In*: DeBakey, M., and Spurling, R. G., eds., *American Lectures in Surgery*. Springfield, Ill., C. C. Thomas, 1950, 95 pp.

919. Smithwick, R. H.: The Surgical physiology of hypertension. *Surg. Clin. N. Am. 29*: 1699–1730, 1949.

920. Smithwick, R. H., Greer, W. E. R., Robertson, C. W., and Wilkins, R. W.: Pheochromocytoma; a discussion of symptoms, signs and procedures of diagnostic value. *N. Engl. J. Med. 242*: 252–257, 1950.

921. Smits, M.: *Een Studie over familiair voorkomen van phaeochromocytoma*. Thesis, Utrecht, 1959, 51 pp.

921a. Smits, M., and Huizinga, J.: Familial occurrence of phaeochromocytoma. *Acta Genet. Stat. Med. 11*: 137–153, 1961.

922. Snyder, S. H., Axelrod, J., and Zweig, M.: A sensitive and specific fluorescence assay for tissue serotonin. *Biochem. Pharmacol. 14*: 831–835, 1965.

923. Sobonya, R. E., Weaver, J. P., and Anton, A. H.: Extra-adrenal epinephrine-producing pheochromocytoma with fatal shock. *Res. Commun. Chem. Pathol. Pharmacol. 5*: 241–251, 1973.

924. Sode, J., Getzen, L. C., and Osborne, D. P.: Cardiac arrhythmias and cardiomyopathy associated with pheochromocytomas. *Am. J. Surg. 114*: 927–931, 1967.

925. Söderström, N., Telenius-Berg, M., and Akerman, M.: Diagnosis of medullary carcinoma of the thyroid by fine needle aspiration biopsy. *Acta Med. Scand. 197*: 71–76, 1975.

926. Sourkes, T. L., Denton, R. L., Murphy, G. F., Chavez, B., and Saint Cyr, S.: The excretion of dihydroxyphenylalanine, dopamine and dihydroxyphenylacetic acid in neuroblastoma. *Pediatrics 31*: 660–668, 1963.

927. Spalding, J. M. K.: A case of pheochromocytoma. *Br. Med. J. I*: 564–565, 1947.

928. Spatt, S. D., and Grayzel, D. M.: Pheochromocytoma of the adrenal medulla. *Am. J. Med. Sci. 216*: 39–50, 1948.

929. Spector, S., Sjoerdsma, A., and Udenfriend, S.: Blockade of endogenous norepinephrine synthesis by alpha-methyl-tyrosine, an inhibitor of tyrosine hydroxylase. *J. Pharmacol. Exp. Ther. 147*: 86–95, 1965.

930. Spergel, G., Bleicher, S. J., and Ertel, N. H.: Carbohydrate and fat metabolism in patients with pheochromocytoma. *N. Engl. J. Med. 278*: 803–809, 1968.

931. Spergel, G., Levy, L. J., Chowdhury, F. R., Rodman, H. M., Ertel, N. H., and Bleicher, S. J.: A modified phentolamine test for diagnosis of pheochromocytoma. *J. Am. Med. Assoc. 211*: 266–269, 1970.

932. Staats, E. F., Brown, R. L., and Smith, R. R.: Carotid body tumors, benign and malignant. *Laryngoscope 76*: 907–916, 1966.

933. Stackpole, R. H., Melicow, M. M., and Uson, A. C.: Pheochromocytoma in children. *J. Pediatr. 63*: 315–330, 1963.

934. Stallings, J. H., Jr.: Pheochromocytoma: Report of a cure in a 12 year old girl. *Clin. Proc. Child. Hosp. 11*: 158–163, 1955.

935. Starr, I., Jr.: The production of albuminuria by renal vasoconstriction in animals and in man. *J. Exp. Med. 43*: 31–51, 1926.

936. Staszewska-Barczak, J., and Vane, J. R.: The release of catechol amines from the adrenal medulla by histamine. *Br. J. Pharmacol. Chemother. 25*: 728–742, 1965.

937. Stefanini, P., Baglioni, A., Fiorani, P.: Le pheochromocytome. *Lyon Chir. 65*: 195, 1969.

938. Steiner, A. L., Goodman, A. D., and Powers, S. R.: Study of a kindred with pheochromocytoma, medullary thyroid carcinoma, hyperparathyroidism and

Cushing's disease: Multiple endocrine neoplasia, type 2. *Medicine 47*: 371–409, 1968.

938a. Stevens, B. F. and Waite, W. W.: Pheochromocytoma. Case report with autopsy findings. *Tex. Med. 35*: 469–471, 1939.

938b. Stjärne, L., and Brundin, J.: Dual adrenoceptor-mediated control of noradrenaline secretion from human vasoconstrictor nerves: Facilitation by β-receptors and inhibition by α-receptors. *Acta Physiol. Scand. 94*: 139–141, 1975.

939. Stjärne, L., Euler, U.S. von, and Lishajko, F.: Catecholamines and nucleotides in phaeochromocytoma. *Biochem. Pharmacol. 13*: 809–818, 1964.

940. Stolz, F.: Ueber Adrenalin und Alkylaminoacetobrenzatechin. *Ber. Dtsch. Chem. Ges. 37*: 4149–4154, 1904.

940a. Stone, R. A., Lilley, J. J., and Golden, J.: Plasma dopamine-beta-hydroxylase activity in phaeochromocytoma. *Clin. Endocrin. 5*: 181–185, 1976.

941. Stott, A. W., Robinson, R., and Smith, P.: Total metadrenaline excretion in patients treated with α-methyldopa. *Lancet 1*: 266–267, 1963.

942. Strickler, C. W., Jr.: Pheochromocytoma: Operative failure. *South. Surgeon 11*: 193–199, 1942.

943. Strieder, N., Ziegler, E., Winkler, H., and Smith, A. D.: Some properties of soluble proteins from chromaffin granules of different species. *Biochem. Pharmacol. 17*: 1553–1556, 1968.

944. Strömbeck, J. P., and Hedberg, T. P.: Tumor of the suprarenal medulla associated with paroxysmal hypertension. Report of case preoperatively diagnosed and cured by extirpation after capsular incision. *Acta Chir. Scand. 82*: 177–189, 1939.

945. Strömblad, B. C. R., and Nickerson, M.: Accumulation of epinephrine and norepinephrine by some rat tissues. *J. Pharmacol. Exp. Ther. 113*: 154–159, 1961.

946. Studnitz, W. von: Effect of Marsilid on excretion of 3-methoxy-4-hydroxymandelic acid in man. *Scand. J. Clin. Lab. Invest. 11*: 244–225, 1959.

947. Studnitz, W. von: Glukagontest Und Phäochromozytomdiagnostik. *Schweiz. Med. Wachenschr. 100*: 1023–1026, 1970.

948. Studnitz, W., von: Methodische und Klinische untersuchungen über dit Ausscheidung der 3-methoxy-4-hydroxymandelsaure un urin. *Scand. J. Clin. Lab. Invest. 12 (Suppl. 48)*: 30–33, 1960.

949. Studnitz, W. von: On the excretion of 3-methoxy-4-hydroxymandelic acid in patients with serotonin producing tumours. *Scand. J. Clin. Lab. Invest. 11*: 309–310, 1959.

950. Studnitz, W. von, Käser, H., Sjoerdsma, A.: Spectrum of catechol amine biochemistry in patients with neuroblastoma. *N. Engl. J. Med. 269*: 232–235, 1963.

951. Sturman, M. F., Moses, D. C., Beierwaltes, W. H., Harrison, T. S., Ice, R. D., and Dorr, R. P.: Radiocholesterol adrenal images for the localization of pheochromocytoma. *Surg. Gynecol. Obstet. 138*: 177–180, 1974.

952. Stutz, I. L., Rosenburg, S. A., Cohen, H. M., Chamovitz, R., and Bogarad, I.: Pheochromocytoma and pregnancy. *Ann. Intern. Med. 47*: 801–812, 1957.

953. Suba, A. R.: Bilateral pheochromocytoma with megacolon. Case report. *Mo. Med. J. 68*: 256–258, 1971.

954. Sullivan, J. M., and Solomon, H. S.: The diagnosis of pheochromocytoma. Overnight excretion of catecholamine metabolites. *J. Am. Med. Assoc. 231*: 618–619, 1975.

955. Sunderman, C. R., Sunderman, F. W., Jr., and Ballinger, W. F.: Measurements of serum vanilmandelic acid in a patient with pheochromocytoma. *Am. J. Clin. Pathol. 43*: 122–129, 1965.

956. Sunderman, F. W.: Measurements of vanilmandelic acid for the diagnosis of pheochromocytoma and neuroblastoma. *Am. J. Clin. Pathol. 42*: 481–497, 1964.

957. Suzuuki, S.: Ueber zwei Tumoren aus Nebennierenmarkgewebe. *Berlin Klin. Wochenschr. 47*: 1623–1625, 1910.

958. Swinton, N. W., Jr., Clerkin, E. P., and Flint, L. D.: Hypercalcemia and familial pheochromocytoma. Correction after adrenalectomy. *Ann. Intern. Med. 76*: 455–457, 1972.

959. Symington, T., and Goodall, A. L.: Studies in phaeochromocytoma: I. Pathological aspects. *Glasgow Med. J. 34*: 75–96, 1953.

960. Szanto, P. B.: Non-chromaffin paraganglioma. *Int. Surg. 57*: 236–240, 1972.

961. Szent-Györgyi, A.: Observations on the function of peroxidase systems and the chemistry of the adrenal cortex. *Biochem. J. 22*: 1387–1409, 1928.

962. Szijj, I., Csapó, Z., Lászlo, F. A., Kovács, K.: Medullary cancer of the thyroid gland associated with hypercorticism. *Cancer 24*: 167–173, 1969.

T

963. Takahashi, K., Kawanishi, H., Kashiwai, K., Matsuda, M., Sakaguchi, T., Nagtomo, T., and Fuju, K.: Paraganglioma (pheochromocytoma) of the urinary bladder. *Acta Urol. Japonica 21*: 723–729, 1975.

964. Tan, T.-L., and Young, B. W.: Pheochromocytoma of the bladder: case report. *J. Urol. 87*: 63–67, 1962.

965. Tannenbaum, M.: Ultrastructural pathology of adrenal medullary tumors. *In:* Sommers, S. C., ed., *Pathology Annual.* New York, Appleton-Century-Croft, 1970, pp. 145–171.

966. Tarazi, R. C., Dustan, H. P., Frohlich, E. D., Gifford, R. W., Jr., and Hoffman, G. C.: Plasma volume and chronic hypertension. Relationship to arterial pressure levels in different hypertensive diseases. *Arch. Intern. Med. 125*: 835–842, 1970.

967. Tarazi, R. C., Frohlich, E. D., and Dustan, H. P.: Plasma volume changes with long-term beta-adrenergic blockade. *Am. Heart J. 82*: 770–776, 1971.

968. Tashjian, A. H., Jr., Howland, B. G., Melvin, K. E. W., and Hill, C. S., Jr.: Immunoassay of human calcitonin: Clinical measurement, relation to serum calcium and studies in patients with medullary carcinoma. *N. Engl. J. Med. 283*: 890–895, 1970.

969. Tashjian, A. H., Jr., and Melvin, K. E. W.: Medullary carcinoma of the thyroid gland: Studies of

thyrocalcitonin in plasma and tumor extracts. *N. Engl. J. Med. 279*: 279–283, 1968.

970. Tassman, I. S.: *The Eye Manifestations of Internal Diseases.* St. Louis, C. V. Mosby Co., 1942, pp. 55, and 451.

971. Taubman, I., Pearson, O. H., and Anton, A. H.: An asymptomatic-catecholamine-secreting pheochromocytoma. *Am. J. Med. 57*: 953–956, 1974.

972. Tcherdakoff, Ph., Simoni, G., and Milliez, P.: Caractères évolutifs du phéochromocytome. Etude de 42 cas personnels. *Nouv. Presse Méd. 3*: 861–864, 1974.

973. Tenzer, C.: Quelques aspects electrocardiographiques d'un phéochromocytome. *Acta Cardiol. 9*: 532–541, 1954.

974. Terry, R. B., Tobin, J. R., and O'Connor, R. B.: Intravenous phentolamine for pheochromocytoma and "adrenaline shock." *Br. Med. J. 2*: 771–772, 1958.

975. Tevetoğlu, F., and Lee, C. H.: Adrenal pheochromocytoma simulating diabetes insipidus. Report of a case and review of the other pediatric cases. *Am. J. Dis. Child. 91*: 365–379, 1956.

976. Thomas, J. E., Rooke, E. D., and Kvale, W. F.: The neurologist's experience with pheochromocytoma. A review of 100 cases. *J. Am. Med. Assoc. 197*: 754–753, 1966.

977. Thompson, C. E., and Witham, A. C.: Paroxysmal hypertension in spinal-cord injuries. *N. Engl. J. Med. 239*: 291–294, 1948.

978. Tisherman, S. E., Gregg, F. J., and Danowski, T. S.: Familial pheochromocytoma. *J. Am. Med. Assoc. 182*: 152–156, 1962.

979. Triplett, J. C., and Atuk, N. O.: Dissecting aortic aneurysm associated with pheochromocytoma. *South. Med. J. 68*: 748–753, 1975.

980. Twedt, D. C., Tilley, L. P., Ryan, W. W., Liu, S. K., Wilkins, R. J., and Johnson, G. F.: Pheochromocytoma in the canine (Grand Rounds conference). *J. Am. Anim. Hosp. Assoc. 11*: 491–496, 1975.

981. Tyce, G. M., Sheps, S. G., and Flock, E. V.: Determination of urinary metabolites of catecholamines after the administration of methyldopa. *Proc. Staff. Meet. Mayo Clin. 38*: 571–576, 1963.

U

982. Udenfriend, S.: *Fluorescence Assay in Biology and Medicine, Vol. 1.* New York, Academic Press, 1962, p. 141.

983. Underdahl, L. O., Woolner, L. B., and Black, B. M.: Multiple endocrine adenomas—report of eight cases where the parathyroids, pituitary and pancreatic islets were involved. *J. Clin. Endocrinol. Metab. 13*: 20–47, 1953.

V

984. Vallance, W. B.: Sudden death from an asymptomatic pheochromocytoma. *Br. Med. J. I*: 686–687, 1957.

985. Valorie, C. Thomas, M., and Shillingford, J.: Free noradrenaline and adrenaline excretion in relation to clinical syndromes following myocardial infarction. *Am. J. Cardiol. 20*: 605–617, 1967.

986. Vane, J. R.: The Second Gaddum Memorial Lecture. The release and fate of vasoactive hormones in the circulation. *Br. J. Pharmacol. 35*: 209–242, 1969.

987. Van Epps, E. F., Hyndman, O. R., and Greene, J. A.: Clinical manifestations of paroxysmal hypertension associated with pheochromocytoma of adrenal. Report of a proved and of a doubtful case. *Arch. Intern. Med. 65*: 1123–1129, 1940.

987a. Van Hagen, K. V., and Barrows, H. S.: Familial pheochromocytoma with ependymoma in the spinal canal. *J. Neurosurg. 20*: 600–604, 1963.

988. Van Vliet, P. D., Burchell, H. B., and Titus, J. L.: Focal myocarditis associated with pheochromocytoma. *N. Engl. J. Med. 274*: 1102–1108, 1966.

989. Van Way, C. W., III, Michelakis, A. M., Alper, B. J., Hutcheson, J. K., Rhamy, R. K., and Scott, H. W., Jr.: Renal vein renin studies in a patient with renal hilar pheochromocytoma and renal artery stenosis. *Ann. Surg. 172*: 212–217, 1970.

990. Van Way, C. W., III, Scott, H. W., Jr., Page, D. L., and Rhamy, R. K.: Pheochromocytoma. *In*: Ravitch, M. M., ed., *Current Problems in Surgery*. Chicago, Year Book Medical Publishers, 1974, pp. 1–59.

991. Vaquez, H., and Donzelot, E.: Les crises d'hypertension artérielle paroxystique. *Presse Méd. 34*: 1329–1331, 1926.

991a. Vega, C. E., de la Slater, S., Ziegler, M. G., Lake, C. R., and Murphy, D. L.: Reduction in plasma norepinephrine during fenfluramine treatment. *Clin. Pharmacol. Ther. 21*: 216–221, 1977.

992. Vendsalu, A.: Studies on adrenaline and noradrenaline in human plasma. *Acta Physiol. Scand. 49 (Suppl. 173)*: 1–123, 1960.

992a. Vetter, H., Fischer, N., Bayer, J. M., Schnitz, Th.E., Werning, C., and Vetter, W.: Aldosteron, Cortisol und Plasma-Renin-Aktivität beim Phäochromocytom. *Klin. Wochenshr. 52*: 719–721, 1974.

993. Viljoen, J. F.: Technique for weaning patient from propranolol therapy before elective surgery. *J. Am. Med. Assoc. 234*: 1272, 1975.

994. Viveros, O. H., Arqueros, L., and Kirshner, N.: Release of catecholamines and dopamine-β-oxidase from the adrenal medulla. *Life Sci. 7*: 609–618, 1968.

995. Vogt, M.: Medullary cortical relationships in the adrenals. *In*: Wolstenholme, G. E. W., and Cameron, M. P., eds., *Ciba Foundation Colloquia on Endocrinology. Vol. 8 The Human Adrenal Cortex*. Boston, Little, Brown, 1955, pp. 241–253.

996. Volhard, F.: Die doppelseitigen hämatogenen Nierenerkrankungen. *Handbuch. d. inn. Med. v. Bergmann-Stähelin.* Vol. VI. Berlin. J. Springer. 1931. Cited in reference 776, this volume.

997. Voorhess, M. L.: Functioning neural tumors. *Pediatr. Clin. North Am. 13*: 3–18, 1966.

998. Voorhess, M. L.: The catecholamines in tumour and urine from patients with neuroblastoma, ganglioneuroblastoma and pheochromocytoma. *J. Pediatr. Surg. 3*: 147–148, 1968.

999. Voorhess, M. L., Stuart, M. J., Stockman, J. A., and Oski, F. A.: Iron deficiency anemia and in-

creased urinary norepinephrine excretion. *J. Pediatr. 86:* 542–547, 1975.

1000. Voûte, P. A., Jr., Wadman, S. K., and van Putten, W. J.: Congenital neuroblastoma. Symptoms in the mother during pregnancy. *Clin. Pediatr. J. 9:* 206–207, 1970.

W

1001. Waaler, E.: A chromaffine tumuor simulating Graves' disease. *Acta Med. Scand. 123:* 1–11, 1945.

1002. Waldmann, T. A., and Bradley, J. E.: Polycythemia secondary to a pheochromocytoma with production of an erythropoiesis-stimulating factor by the tumor. *Proc. Soc. Exp. Biol. Med. 108:* 425–427, 1961.

1003. Waldmann, T. A., Levin, E. H., and Baldwin, M.: The association of polycythemia with a cerebellar hemangioblastoma. *Am. J. Med. 31:* 318–324, 1961.

1004. Waldmann, T. A., Rosse, W. F., and Swarm, R. L.: The erythropoiesis-stimulating factors produced by tumors. *Ann. N.Y. Acad. Sci. 149:* 509–515, 1968.

1005. Walker, C. H.: Migraine and its relationship to hypertension. *Br. Med. J. 2:* 1430–1433, 1959.

1006. Warren, S., Grozdev, L., Gates, O., and Chute, R. N.: Radiation–induced adrenal medullary tumors in the rat. *Arch. Path. 82:* 115–118, 1966.

1007. Washington, E. L., Callahan, W. P., Jr., and Edwards, E. W.: Pheochromocytoma of the adrenal medulla. Its role in the pathogenesis of malignant hypertension. *J. Clin. Endocrinol. 6:* 688–698, 1946.

1008. Watanabe, H., and Morita, M.: Eccrine sweat gland sensitivity to catecholamines in patients with pheochromocytoma and primary aldosteronism. *Tohoku J. Exp. Med. 115:* 377–384, 1975.

1009. Watkins, D. B.: Pheochromocytoma: A review of the literature. *J. Chronic Dis. 6:* 510–527, 1957.

1010. Watson, R. L., and Hansen, H. R.: Pheochromocytoma—cardiac stability during methoxyflurane anesthesia for surgical removal. *Anesth. Analg. (Cleveland) 46:* 324–329, 1967.

1011. Weaver, J. C., Kawata, N., and Hinman, F., Jr.: Renal cyst simulating pheochromocytoma. *Postgrad. Med. 11:* 294–298, 1952.

1012. Weichert, R. F., III: The neural ectodermal origin of the peptide-secreting endocrine glands: A unifying concept for the etiology of multiple endocrine adenomatosis and the inappropriate secretion of peptide hormones by nonendocrine tumors. *Am. J. Med. 49:* 232–241, 1970.

1013. Weil-Malherbe, H.: Factors affecting the excretion of catecholamines and recent methods for their determination. *In:* Mattar, E., de Brong Mattar, G., and James, V. H. T., eds., *Recent Advances in Endocrinology, Proceedings of the Seventh Pan-American Congress of Endocrinology. Sao Paulo, 1970,* Amsterdam, Excerpta Medica, 1971, pp. 35–42.

1014. Weil-Malherbe, H.: Phaeochromocytoma catechols in urine and tumour tissue. *Lancet 2:* 282–284, 1956.

1015. Weil-Malherbe, H.: II. The fluorimetric estimation of catecholamines. *In:* Quastel, J. H., ed.,

Methods in Medical Research. Chicago, Year Book, 1961, Vol. 9, pp. 130–146.

1016. Weil-Malherbe, H.: The simultaneous estimation of catecholamines and their metabolites. *Z. Klin. Chem. 2:* 161–167, 1964.

1017. Weil-Malherbe, H., Axelrod, J., and Tomchick, R.: Blood-brain barrier for adrenaline. *Science 129:* 1226–1227, 1959.

1018. Weil-Malherbe, H., and Bone, A. D.: Adrenergic amines of human blood. *Lancet 1:* 974–977, 1953.

1019. Weil-Malherbe, H., and Bone, A. D.: Chemical estimation of adrenaline-like substances in blood. *Biochem J. 51:* 311–318, 1952.

1020. Weinshilboum, R. M., Thoa, N. B., Johnson, D. G., Kopin, I. J., and Axelrod, J.: Proportional release of norepinephrine and dopamine-β-hydroxylase from sympathetic nerves. *Science 174:* 1349–1351, 1971.

1021. Weise, V. K., McDonald, R. K., and Labrosse, E. H.: Determination of urinary 3-methoxy-4-hydroxymandelic acid in man. *Clin. Chim. Acta. 6:* 79–86, 1961.

1022. Weiss, S. R.: Testing in pheochromocytoma and another endocrine tumor. *Ann. Intern. Med. 81:* 116–117, 1974.

1023. Wellhöner, H. H., Erdmann, G., and Wiegand, H.: Neural transport of tetanus toxin. *Science 192:* 158, 1976.

1024. Wells, A. H., and Boman, P. G.: The Clinical and pathologic identity of pheochromocytoma. *J. Am. Med. Assoc. 109:* 1176–1180, 1937.

1025. Wells, S. A., Jr., Ontjes, D. A., Cooper, C. W., Hennessey, J. F., Ellis, G. J., McPherson, H. T., and Sabiston, D. C., Jr.: The early diagnosis of medullary carcinoma of the thyroid gland in patients with multiple endocrine neoplasia, type II. *Ann. Surg. 182:* 362–370, 1975.

1026. Wermer, P.: Genetic aspects of adenomatosis of the endocrine glands. *Am. J. Med. 16:* 363–371, 1964.

1026a. Wermer, P.: The diagnosis of polyadenomatosis of endocrine glands. *Radiologic Clinics N. Am. 5:* 349–354, 1967.

1027. Werning, C. Ziegler, W. H., Baumann, K., Enders, P., Gysling, E., Weidmann, P., and Siegendthaler, W.: Die Plasma-Renin-Aktivität beim Phäochromozytom. *Dtsch. Med. Wochenschr. 95:* 117–125, 1970.

1028. Wertlake, P. T., Wilcox, A. A., Haley, M. I., and Petersen, J. E.: Relationship of mental and emotional stress to serum cholesterol levels. *Proc. Soc. Exp. Biol. Med. 97:* 163–165, 1958.

1029. West, G. B., Shepherd, D. M., and Hunter, R. B.: Adrenaline and noradrenaline concentration in adrenal glands at different ages and in some diseases. *Lancet 261:* 966, 1951.

1030. West, G. B., Shepherd, D. M., Hunter, R. B., and MacGregor, A. R.: The function of the organs of Zuckerkandl. *Clin. Sci. 12:* 317–325, 1953.

1031. West, J. L.: Bovine pheochromocytoma: case report and review of literature. *Am. J. Vet. Res. 36:* 1371–1373, 1975.

1032. Weston, J. A.: The migration and differentiation of neural crest cells. *Advances Morphog. 8:* 41–114, 1970.

1033. Whitby, L. G., Axelrod, J., and Weil-Malherbe, H.: The fate of H³-norepinephrine in animals. *J. Pharmacol. Exp. Ther.* 132: 193–201, 1961.

1034. White, L. W., Levy, R. P., and Anton, A. H.: Comparison of biochemical and pharmacological testing for pheochromocytoma. *Res. Commun. Chem. Pathol. Pharmacol.* 5: 252–262, 1973.

1035. Wilber, J. F., Turtle, J. R., and Crane, N. A.: Inhibition of insulin secretion by pheochromocytoma. *Lancet* 2: 733, 1966.

1036. Wilk, E. K., Gitlow, S. E., and Bertani, L. M.: A modification of the Taniguchi method for the determination of normetanephrine and metanephrine. *Clin. Chim. Acta* 20: 147–148, 1968.

1037. Wilk, S., Gitlow, S. E., Clarke, D. D., and Paley, D. H.: Determination of urinary 3-methoxy-4-hydroxyphenylethylene glycol by gas-liquid chromatography and electron capture detection. *Clin. Chim. Acta.* 16: 403–408, 1967.

1038. Wilk, S., Gitlow, S. E., Mendlowitz, M., Franklin, M. J., Carr, H. E., and Clarke, D. D.: A quantitative assay for vanillylmandelic acid (VMA) by gas-liquid chromatography. *Anal. Biochem.* 13: 544–551, 1965.

1039. Wilkerson, J. A., Van de Water, J. M., and Goepfert, H.: Role of embryonic induction in benign transformation of neuroblastomas. *Cancer* 20: 1335–1342, 1967.

1040. Wilkie, B. N., and Krook, L.: Ultimobranchial tumor of the thyroid and pheochromocytoma in the bull. *Pathol. Vet.* 7: 126–134, 1970.

1041. Wilkins, R. W., Greer, W. E. R., Culbertson, J. W., Halperin, M. H., Litter, J., Burnett, C. H., and Smithwick, R. H.: Extensive laboratory studies of a patient with pheochromocytoma before and after successful operation. *Arch. Intern. Med. 86*: 51–78, 1950.

1042. Williams, C. M., and Greer, M.: Homovanillic acid and vanilmandelic acid in diagnosis of neuroblastoma. *J. Am. Med. Assoc. 183*: 836–840, 1963.

1043. Williams, E. D.: A review of 17 cases of carcinoma of the thyroid and phaeochromocytoma. *J. Clin. Pathol. 18*: 288–292, 1965.

1044. Williams, E. D., Brown, C. L., and Doniach, I.: Pathological and clinical findings in a series of 67 cases of medullary carcinoma of the thyroid. *J. Clin. Pathol. 19*: 103–113, 1966.

1045. Williams, E. D., Karim, S. M. M., and Sandler, M.: Prostaglandin secretion by medullary carcinoma of the thyroid. A possible cause of the associated diarrhea. *Lancet 1*: 22–23, 1968.

1046. Williams, E. D., and Pollock, D. J.: Multiple mucosal neuromata with endocrine tumours: A syndrome allied to von Recklinghausen's disease. *J. Pathol. 91*: 71–80, 1966.

1047. Willis, R. A.: *Pathology of Tumours.* London, Butterworth, 1953, p. 607.

1048. Willis, R. A.: *Pathology of Tumours,* 4th ed. London, Butterworth, 1967, pp. 886–887.

1049. Wilson, R. J., Craig, G. M., and Mills, I. H.: Metabolic studies in a patient with a phaeochromocytoma associated with hypokalaemia and hyperaldosteronism. *J. Endocrinol. 56*: 69–78, 1973.

1050. Wingo, C. F., Williams, J. P., and Wade, F. A.: Pheochromocytoma: Two case reports with unusual reactions and a general review. *Ann. Intern. Med. 42*: 856–872, 1955.

1051. Winkler, H.: Isolierung und Charakterisierung von Chromaffinen Noradrenalin-Granula aus Schweine-Nebennierenmark. *Naunyn-Schmiedeberg's Arch. Pharmacol.* 263: 340–357, 1969.

1052. Winkler, H., and Smith, A. D.:' Catecholamines in phaeochromocytoma: Normal storage but abnormal release? *Lancet 1*: 793–795, 1968.

1053. Winkler, H., and Smith, A. D.: Pheochromocytomas and other catecholamine-producing tumors. *In*: Blaschko, H., and Muscholl, E., eds., *Catecholamines.* Berlin, Heidelberg, New York, Springer-Verlag, 1972, Chap. 20, pp. 900–933.

1054. Winkler, H., Zeigler, E., and Strieder, N.: Gewinnung und Eigenschaften der Katecholamin-speichernden Granula eines Phäochromocytoms. *Klin. Wochenschr.* 45: 1238–1241, 1967.

1055. Wintrobe, M. M.: *Clinical Hematology,* 5th ed. Philadelphia, Lea and Febiger, 1961, p. 245.

1055a. Wiswell, J. G., Hurwitz, G. E., Coronko, V., Bing, O. H. L., and Child, D. L.: Urinary catecholamines and their metabolites in hyperthyroidism and hypothyroidism. *J. Clin. Endocrin. Met.* 23: 1102–1106, 1963.

1055b. Witham, A. C. and Fleming, J. W.: The effect of epinephrine on the pulmonary circulation in man. *J. Clin. Invest. 30*: 707–717, 1951.

1056. Wolf, P. L., Dickenman, R. C., and Langston, J. D.: Fibrosarcoma of the pulmonary artery, masquerading as a pheochromocytoma. *Am. J. Clin. Pathol. 34*: 146–154, 1960.

1057. Wolf, R. L., Mendlowitz, M., Roboz, J., and Gitlow, S. E.: New rapid test for pheochromocytoma: Urinary assay of normetanephrine, metanephrine, and 3-methoxy-4-hydroxyphenylglycol. *J. Am. Med. Assoc. 188*: 859–861, 1964.

1058. Wolfe, H. J., Melvin, K. E., Cervi-Skinner, S. J., et al.: C-Cell hyperplasia preceding medullary thyroid carcinoma. *N. Engl. J. Med. 289*: 437–441, 1973.

1059. Wurtman, R. J.: *Catecholamines.* Boston, Little, Brown, 1966, 111 pp.

1060. Wurtman, R. J.: Control of epinephrine synthesis in the adrenal medulla by the adrenal cortex: Hormonal specificity and dose-response characteristics. *Endocrinology 79*: 608–614, 1966.

1061. Wurtman, R. J., and Axelrod, J.: Control of enzymatic synthesis of adrenaline in the adrenal medulla by adrenal cortical steroids. *J. Biol. Chem. 241*: 2301–2305, 1966.

1062. Wurtman, R. J., Kopin, I. J., and Axelrod, J.: Thyroid function and the cardiac disposition of catecholamines. *Endocrinology, 73*: 63–74, 1963.

1063. Wurtman, R. J., Pohorecky, L. A., and Baliga, B. S.: Adrenocortical control of the biosynthesis of epinephrine and proteins in the adrenal medulla. *Pharmacol. Rev.* 24: 411–426, 1972.

1064. Wurtman, R. J., Axelrod, J., Vesell, E. S., and Ross, G. T.: Species differences in inducibility of phenylethanolamine-N-methyl transferase. *Endocrinology 82*: 584–590, 1968.

Y

1065. Yankopoulos, N. A., Montero, A. C., Curd, W. G., Jr., Kahil, M. E., and Condon, R. E.: Observations on myocardial function during chronic catecholamine oversecretion. *Chest 66*: 585–587, 1974.

1066. Yanowitz, F., Preston, J. B., and Abildskov, J. A.: Functional distribution of right and left stellate innervation to the ventricles. *Circ. Res. 18*: 416–428, 1966.

1067. Yokoyama, M., and Takayasu, H.: An electron microscopic study of the human adrenal medulla and pheochromocytoma. *Urol. Int. 24*: 79–95, 1969.

1068. Yoshinaga, K., Sato, T., and Ishida, N.: Studies on the role of noradrenaline in the pathogenesis of hypertension. *Tohoku J. Exp. Med. 72*: 301–308, 1960.

Z

1069. Zauder, H. L., ed.: *Clinical Anesthesia. Pharmacology of Adjuvant Drugs.* Vol. 10, No. 1. Philadelphia, F. A. Davis, 1973. 349 pp.

1070. Zelch, J. V., Meaney, T. F., and Belhobek, G. H.: Radiologic approach to the patient with suspected pheochromocytoma. *Radiology 111*: 279–284, 1974.

1071. Ziegler, W. H., Langemann, H., and Müller, P. B.: Vergleichende Untersuchungen an Tumorgeweben von Phäochromocytom und Karzinoid. *Schweiz. Med. Wochenschr. 97*: 1731–1734, 1967.

1072. Zileli, M. S., Hamlin, J. T., III, Reutter, F. W., and Friend, D. G.: Evaluation of catechol amine levels in renal insufficiency. *J. Clin. Invest. 37*: 409–413, 1958.

1073. Zimmerman, I. J., Biron, R. E., and McMahon, H. E.: Pheochromocytomas of the urinary bladder. *N. Engl. J. Med. 249*: 25–26, 1953.

1074. Zuspan, F. P.: Adrenal gland and sympathetic nervous system response in eclampsia. *Am. J. Obstet Gynecol. 114*: 304–313, 1972.

Index